Dr Wayne Jonas

How Healing Works

get well and stay well using your body's power to heal itself

SCRIBE

Melbourne • London

Scribe Publications
18–20 Edward St, Brunswick, Victoria 3056, Australia
2 John Street, Clerkenwell, London, WC1N 2ES, United Kingdom

This edition published by arrangement with Lorena Jones Books, an imprint of the
Crown Publishing Group, a division of Penguin Random House LLC, New York.

Published by Scribe 2018

Over the past three decades, the author has seen hundreds of patients. Throughout
this book, he has drawn on the stories they have generously shared to illustrate the
vast range of treatment experiences. Many of the case histories you will read are
composites. When the author has based examples on particular patients, he has
changed their names and distinguishing features in order to protect their identity.
Any resulting resemblance to persons alive or dead is entirely unintentional and
coincidental.

In addition, the information and advice presented in this book are not meant to
substitute for the advice of your family physician or other trained health-care
professionals. You are advised to consult with health-care professionals with regard
to all matters pertaining to you and your family's health and well-being.

As of press time, the URLs displayed in this book link or refer to existing websites
on the internet. The publisher is not responsible for and should not be deemed to
endorse or recommend any website other than our own or any content available on
the internet (including without limitation, any website, blog post, or information
page) that is not created by the publisher.

Illustrations by Six Half Dozen Design Studio

Printed and bound in the UK by CPI Group (UK) Ltd, Croydon CR0 4YY

Scribe Publications is committed to the sustainable use of natural resources and the
use of paper products made responsibly from those resources.

9781911344636 (UK edition)
9781925322538 (Australian edition)
9781925548709 (e-book)

CiP records for this title are available from the British Library. and the National
Library of Australia.

scribepublications.co.uk
scribepublications.com.au

Contents

INTRODUCTION

The Need for a New Understanding of Healing   vii

SECTION 1: RETHINKING HEALING

Chapter 1 *The Paradox of Healing*   1

Chapter 2 *How We Heal*   16

Chapter 3 *How Science Misses Healing*   40

Chapter 4 *A Science for Healing*   65

SECTION 2: THE DIMENSIONS OF HEALING

Chapter 5 *Coming Home*   92

Chapter 6 *Acting Right*   113

Chapter 7 *Loving Deeply*   143

Chapter 8 *Finding Meaning*   172

SECTION 3: YOUR HEALING JOURNEY

Chapter 9 *Integrative Health*   206

Chapter 10 *Creating Healing*   240

APPENDICES

The HOPE Consultation   260

Constructing Your Healing Journey   268

Additional Reading on Integrative Health   297

Notes   298

Acknowledgments   316

Index   318

Introduction

The Need for a New Understanding
of Healing

Most of the treatments we think produce healing do not work when exposed to rigorous scientific scrutiny. Yet people often get better. Why? How?

This book argues that the vast majority of healing comes from a few basic principles that can be used effectively by any system—ancient or modern, conventional or alternative, proven or unproven—and by both doctors and patients in their daily lives. The secret: to elicit a meaningful response in the person who requires healing.

My approach is based on almost forty years of seeing patients as a mainstream family doctor, as a trained scientist, and as an explorer of many medical systems. I discovered how healing happens through my work with patients, as director of the Office of Alternative Medicine at the National Institutes of Health (NIH), and as a research scientist at the World Health Organization (WHO), Walter Reed Army Institute of Research, and Samueli Institute.

In this book, I'm going to give you a simple, systematic approach to real healing. Drawing on the most rigorous scientific evidence available as well as wisdom from ancient healing traditions, I will show you that:

- Only 20% of healing comes from the "treatment agent" that the doctor applies to you—whether that is surgery, drugs, acupuncture needles, herbs and supplements, diet, or anything else external to you.
- A full 80% of healing comes from constructing a meaningful treatment response, unique to you, which is internal and highly personal, using simple principles and components.
- You can activate your own inherent healing processes and get your physician and others on board to help accelerate your healing journey, making any approach more effective, safer, and less expensive. And these processes can prevent the majority of chronic diseases in the future.

I am not arguing, as some others do, that you can simply think yourself into healing. And I am well aware that understanding what stimulates healing or prevents disease will not fix a broken bone, cure cancer, or stop a heart attack. However, the top ten reasons for seeing a doctor, according to a study by the Mayo Clinic, include pain (especially back pain), fatigue, cognitive dysfunction, hypertension, diabetes, obesity, chronic heart or lung problems, or brain diseases such as Alzheimer's, Parkinson's, or depression. Almost all of these conditions accelerate and increase as we age, so even if you feel healthy now, chances are if you live long enough, you will get more than one of these conditions, unless you seek out ways to prevent them.

If you understand how healing really works for the most common chronic conditions, you can take greater control of your own recovery, increase the likelihood that any specific treatment will be effective, prevent many of the diseases of aging, and radically reduce your dependence on the medical industry. *How Healing Works* provides a way for merging curing and healing—producing true integrative health. Now I invite you to travel with me to see how I discovered this.

SECTION I

Rethinking Healing

Chapter 1

The Paradox of Healing

What we think heals often doesn't, but
almost anything can heal.

Most of what we think produces health actually does not. But there is an inherent healing capacity within us all that, when properly released, can produce remarkable recovery, health, and happiness. The healing process is understood and applied in many wisdom traditions and by wise physicians today, but has been obscured by modern medicine's obsession with small parts, and the technologies, techniques, and chemicals that manipulate them. While many of these technologies are extremely valuable, this hyperfocus and the economic rewards driving them has largely squeezed out the essence of what medicine is all about—how to guide a person to healing, wholeness, and well-being.

Let's take a closer look at how we heal.

HIEN

We were miles into the jungle, and my best buddy, Hien, was injured. I was scared. How would we get him out? Although we spoke hardly a word of each other's language—his, Vietnamese, and mine, English—our communication was clear. How would he get back? Would he die out here? There was a war going on, wasn't there? Hien's ankle was markedly swollen. Large amounts of blood collected under the skin. He could barely stand, much less walk on it. Maybe I could run out of the jungle, find my dad, and see if he could call in one of those American military helicopters. I tried to say that to Hien's father, who was the scout master, but he looked unconcerned. We would camp there that night, he said in Vietnamese, and continue hiking in the morning. Then he turned to me and said in broken English, "Hien be okay, Wen. No worry." But I didn't see how he would be okay.

Hien and I were both nine years old, and I was his only American friend, which was not surprising, given that I was the only nine-year-old American boy in Nha Trang, Vietnam, in early 1964. My father was a chaplain in the military, assigned to serve the spiritual needs of American service men and women in Vietnam. At the time, America was not engaged in active combat, and military advisors could bring families there. My father had asked us to come. So, with four kids, ages two to twelve, in tow, my mother packed us up and we moved to Nha Trang, a lovely coastal village in the center of the country. We lived near the beach, in a four-bedroom French "villa," on a fenced-off half-acre lot complete with biting red ants, large gecko lizards often found in the house, and pigs running through the yard. The weather was hot. My mother was occupied with volunteer activities and taking care of my two younger siblings; my older brother was off at boarding school. I was largely free to roam the town. "Just be back before dark," my mom would instruct. Trust and faith seemed to be part of both my parents' natures. A bicycle allowed me to get around the town at will to explore. My father spent most of the week ministering to soldiers in far-off posts and would return on weekends to execute his church duties, visit people in the hospital, and hold services on the base.

I met Hien at the Vietnamese school run by French missionaries that we attended every morning. We became friends while playing marbles. He was a great long-range shooter, and I was good close-up, so when we played team marbles on the playground, we were tough to beat. We won a lot of trading cards—the marble game betting currency of the schoolchildren. After Vietnamese school, I rode my bike across town to do Calvert tutoring lessons in order to keep up with American schools back home. One day while en route, I saw Hien going into a building with his great-grandmother. She was clearly ill, being carried in by her family. Curious, I rode my bike around the back and climbed up a short stone wall to see what was inside. It was a Vietnamese hospital, staffed with traditional practitioners and lots of sick patients, many of them lying outside in the yard.

This traditional Vietnamese hospital was fascinating. It was not at all like the American military hospital a few miles away, with its clean sheets, IVs, and electronic monitors. In the American hospital, nurses and doctors in white uniforms attended to patients, clergy visited on Saturdays, and a few volunteers—like my mother—would open mail and give back massages. Otherwise, the patients were left alone. In the Vietnamese hospital, however, most patients were cared for by their families. Families brought food, cleaned them, and administered herbal medicines, applied hot and cold packs, and gave other types of treatments. There were always people around the patients. The traditional doctors used mostly acupuncture and herbs—and cupping and *moxa*, a curious treatment in which an herb was burned while resting on an acupuncture point, and then was knocked off before actually burning the patient. The contrast in resources to the American hospital—but more important, to their approaches—was startling. I spent hours looking over the wall, watching people come and go, wondering what medical conditions they had and what the doctors and families were doing.

One day I saw Hien and his family with his great-grandmother. Like many other patients who were outside because there weren't enough beds inside the Vietnamese hospital, Hien's grandmother was lying on a mat on the hard ground—weak, frail, and near death's door. My friend was dutifully taking care of her, bringing her soup and feeding it to her one spoonful at a time, and cleaning her up when she had accidents. Despite her weakness, she would lift her head periodically and smile, and they would converse in Vietnamese. The doctors would come out, put needles in different parts of her body, do curious twisting motions with her legs and arms, and occasionally place a poultice of herbal concoctions on her abdomen or forehead. The family was constantly there, with Hien's mother coming for long periods to take care of her. Hien's great-grandmother seemed quite happy and comfortable. One day I rode my bike down and climbed up to look over the wall, and they were gone. I learned later that she had died peacefully, her family around her.

Hien and I joined a Boy Scouts troop, and that's how we ended up together on that backpacking trip when he sprained his ankle. Again, it looked pretty bad to me, very swollen and with blood under the skin just below the leg bone. He couldn't walk on it, and I figured we would have to carry him out the next day. I had brought along a small first aid kit I'd gotten from the American hospital; the treatments for a sprained ankle consisted of tape, Ace bandages, and some aspirin. But that evening, Hien's father pulled out a powder of green herbs and mixed it with water into a paste. He applied the paste to Hien's ankle and put two acupuncture needles in his leg above the sprain. He removed the needles after one hour and left the poultice on overnight. The next day, Hien's ankle was almost normal again, and we resumed the hike. He seemed to have no pain.

How had this happened? At age nine, I had not yet thought of becoming a doctor, but I wondered how these two different approaches to healing—the low-tech acupuncture/herbal/family care approach from traditional Vietnamese practices on the one hand, and the high-tech surgery/drugs/professionals approach of the Americans—could both work. I had seen American medicine work, but now I had seen a completely different system bring comfort to a terminally ill great-grandmother as she died, and also rapidly resolve an ankle sprain without aspirin, ice, or an Ace bandage. How could healing be happening with two such completely different approaches? Later in life, I had pretty much forgotten Hien and his great-grandmother. During medical school, I was taught that those acupuncture needles and herbs were ineffective and unscientific. Modern approaches were considered better—more effective, safer, and faster. I learned to rely on "gold standard" science, especially evidence from randomized, double-blind, placebo-controlled trials. I threw myself fully into modern medicine and science, determined to use the most rigorous evidence to separate what worked from what didn't.

Then Norma came along.

NORMA

"You are such a sweet boy," Norma would say at the start of every visit. "You are the best doctor ever." I blushed. She knew how to handle me. Norma was seventy-nine, with multiple chronic health problems. She loved having a family doctor—a "one-stop shop," she said—to know her and take care of most of her ills. The one problem that affected her most was her osteoarthritis, the joint disease that now impacts one in every five American adults and more than half of those her age. She didn't complain about the pain. What bothered her most was her decreasing ability to volunteer at the hospital. This was one of the greatest sources of joy and meaning in her life. I would see her frequently in the hospital halls, pushing around the free-book cart for patients and guests. She got to know the regular visitors who were the most chronically ill and brought them specific books she thought they would like. The arthritis mostly affected her hands and knees, which made it difficult to handle the books and hand them out.

Norma came to see me often and loved to have me "practice" on her, but all I had to offer her were painkillers and recommendations for heat and stretching. Those didn't help much, and her disease progressed. Her volunteer visits declined and she became sad. Then I read about something that might help—niacinamide, a form of vitamin B_3. I had found an old book about it in my medical school's discard pile. It was written by a doctor named William Kaufman and published in 1949. Dr. Kaufman had given niacinamide in high doses to thousands of patients with arthritis over long periods of time. What was unusual for a doctor in private practice was that he had carefully measured and documented the pain, strength, and range of motion in every patient who took it. He reported that the patients' pain diminished and their strength, range of motion, and moods improved considerably and steadily when taking niacinamide. It seemed perfect for Norma. The one problem was that niacinamide had never been tested scientifically—in a randomized, double-blind, placebo-controlled trial. It did not have the kind of evidence I needed to prescribe or recommend it. So I decided to do such a study myself with Norma and arthritis patients like her.

When I opened enrollment for the study, Norma joined immediately and was an enthusiastic participant. She did all the baseline measurements and agreed to be randomly assigned to get either niacinamide or an identical-looking placebo pill. Neither she nor I would know which one she was getting until after the study was completed. She started her treatment, which involved taking two pills, three times a day. Within a week and then continuing for the three months of the study, she and her arthritis got steadily better in all ways. She began telling everyone that they should sign up for the study; she became my best unofficial recruiter. Soon she stopped using her cane, resumed her daily volunteer book rounds at the hospital, and reported better mood and sleep. Others observed that her normally stiff muscles moved more easily. Her daughter came in at one visit to personally thank me for helping her mother. Norma was smiling more, she said. She was happy. And I was happy. I had found a cure for arthritis! I would be famous! Or so I thought.

When the study was over, I broke the blinding code to find out what she was taking—niacinamide or the placebo pill. Norma had been taking the placebo pill. I was stunned! I thought something was wrong with the label made by the pharmacologist. I checked and double-checked the shipping labels, randomization codes, and the pharmacist's process for dispensing the pills. Nothing was wrong. Norma had gotten remarkably better, perhaps 80% overall, as she took a completely inert pill.

Niacinamide did work—a little. When we statistically analyzed the differences in response between those on the niacinamide and those on the placebo, the niacinamide did work better than the placebo, but by only a small amount. On average, those on the vitamin improved by 29%, compared to a 10% worsening in those on the placebo. While this was statistically significant in favor of the vitamin, the overall difference was small—and the placebo had fewer side effects. High-dose niacinamide can cause liver problems in some people. I was disappointed. I had not found a cure for arthritis after all. But I continued to wonder why Norma had gotten so much better. Something had triggered her healing. Was she just an unusual patient—an aberration? Did I just pick the wrong patients to include in the study? Did I do the study wrong? Pick the wrong treatment?

It was not an aberration. When examined through rigorous science, using randomization, double-blinding, and placebo controls with adequate numbers of patients, most treatments for the most common chronic conditions either do not work or work only 20% to 30% of the time. Most of the drugs prescribed for pain, mental health, ulcers, hypertension, diabetes, Parkinson's disease, and many other conditions show little benefit, with improvement in a minority of those studied. Even surgery, the king of modern medicine, works very little for chronic diseases (especially pain) when studied in a rigorous manner. For example, in a pooled analysis of over eighteen thousand patients, drawn from studies where half the patients got sham (fake) acupuncture (needles are put in the wrong points or not inserted into the skin at all) and the other half got real acupuncture, the groups getting the fake acupuncture had a healing rate of over 80% of that experienced by the those getting real acupuncture. While this rate of improvement from a fake treatment may seem stunning to many readers, it is actually a rather routine finding and also occurs with modern, scientifically developed treatments. For example, studies in which sham (fake) surgery (an imitation of surgery without the actual tissue manipulation) is "performed" on half of a patient test group with chronic pain, it produces 87% as much improvement as seen in those who receive the real surgery. In some studies, the fake surgery worked better than the real surgery and produced fewer side effects. In fact, this type of improvement with fake treatments is found in many areas of modern medicine. The majority of improvement for many treatments occurs with the fake or placebo treatment, whether the placebo is mimicking a drug, herb, needle, or knife. Can treatments still heal even when science has proven them wrong? Impossible, I thought. It took another patient to teach me that this was not impossible at all.

SERGEANT MARTIN

Sergeant Martin crawled from the tangled web of steel that had been his truck, bleeding from every orifice. Although dazed, he got to his buddy, who was lying unconscious and exposed in the middle of the road, and pulled him to safety. Sergeant Martin had suffered an insidious and incapacitating brain injury. Unfortunately, he is one of many: nearly three hundred thousand American service members are living with traumatic brain injury (TBI) suffered while fighting in Afghanistan or Iraq. Rather than penetrate the brain like a bullet, an improvised explosive device (IED) usually produces a close-range shock wave that impacts the brain as a whole. Damage and bleeding in the brain is often global, with small areas of injury spread throughout. Often the extent of the injury is not fully evident for months and gets worse until it stabilizes. The victim is left with multiple functional problems, from memory loss to language problems, mood swings, sleep disturbances, and chronic pain, especially headaches.

Sergeant Martin had all these problems. He would duck at the sound of a door slamming. He avoided social gatherings, worried that something bad might happen. He had almost daily headaches and was constantly on painkillers. He would wake at night in a panic, sure that someone was breaking into the "green zone." He was emotionally labile—sometimes acting like a loving kid, other times screaming at his wife to lock the doors. One morning his wife found a loaded handgun under his pillow. She told him to get rid of it. He said he needed it to sleep at night. They argued. Finally, he agreed to make sure it was not loaded. She threw the ammunition away but worried how this might end. He told her and everybody else that he was not suicidal. He said he had seen what happened to people who said they were; they were locked up in a mental ward.

There is no cure for this type of brain injury. I juggled drugs for Sergeant Martin's headaches, anxiety, sleep disturbances, and other symptoms. I sent him to physical therapy, group therapy, individual psychological counseling, and music therapy. Of those, the only one he really liked was music therapy. He especially loved to listen to

Beethoven's Ninth Symphony.

I asked him to rest and work with several specialists in brain injury and PTSD. Over time he improved—but only incrementally and marginally. Soon he settled into chronic dysfunction and left the service with a permanent disability. From then on, all I could do for him was palliation, tweaking his medicines to minimize the side effects and providing him with slightly more relief. It was a discouraging practice. When I told him I had nothing new left to offer him, he dismissed me as his doctor. "I won't accept that," he said on his last visit with me. "You are keeping me stuck in Beethoven's first movement. I know there is more." He paused. "Friend," he said (he had never called me that before), "when I was in Iraq and we hit that roadside bomb, I don't recall pulling my buddy to safety from the road. Others told me I did that. The only thing I remember after the bomb is waking up in the hospital in a daze. I am still in that daze; and I need to wake up again." He made no more appointments. Just like on the battlefield, Sergeant Martin was not going to give up. He was determined to win this battle, too. I only hoped he would eventually win the war going on inside himself.

Doctors don't like to give patients what they call "false hope." The idea is that, when there are no effective treatments for a condition, it is better for patients to learn to cope with reality than seek ineffective and possibly harmful treatments that are unlikely to work. Science helps us determine what works and what does not—and so, we believe, distinguishes true hope from false hope. Sometimes patients interpret this to mean *no* hope and either fall into despair or, like Sergeant Martin, reject the suggestion that they must live with their condition.

Before Sergeant Martin, I thought I knew how to determine true from false hope for my patients using science. Sergeant Martin, however, taught me that it was more complicated than I thought. Distinguishing true from false hope was not just a matter of science—it had to be done jointly by physician and patient together. Neither one alone had a lock on how to handle hope.

Here is what happened: Several months later, I saw Sergeant Martin in the hallway of the hospital, and I hardly recognized him. He had improved remarkably. He said he had fewer headaches, better sleep, and less pain. He spoke more clearly. He was off most of the drugs I had prescribed. He was going back to school, had a part-time job, and was getting along with his family. What had he done, I asked?

"Hyperbaric oxygen," he answered.

"Really?" I asked in disbelief.

"Yep," he continued. "Got forty treatments, and it cured me." He was not cured, but he was clearly much better than I had ever seen him. *It couldn't be from that treatment*, I thought to myself. I had studied hyperbaric oxygen (HBO) therapy and rejected it, as had most scientists, because the research evidence showed that it did not work.

But Sergeant Martin did not care what I said about the science. He had done the impossible when he rescued his buddy after the bomb went off. He would face the impossible now and try to rescue himself. My opinion did not stop him. He had heard from his buddies that HBO might help brain injury, so he had done forty HBO treatments.

I asked him to come in and tell me more about what he had done. He explained that it was his father who found the HBO center and agreed to pay for the treatment sessions, which were not covered by insurance. These sessions involved going into a special HBO center and entering a large chamber where ten patients were treated at once. At the HBO center, Sergeant Martin met a physician, an HBO specialist, who described the treatment and the expected effects and evaluated patients for their baseline symptoms and function. Sergeant Martin went every day (except weekends) and would sit in the chamber with a group of other patients for an hour while breathing 100% oxygen through a mask. He often saw the same patients there each day, several of whom also had a brain injury. The air pressure in the chamber was turned up, which he could feel in his ears, sort of like when you dive down below the surface in a swimming pool.

The technicians explained to him what HBO would do. The theory was that pressurized oxygen diffused into the brain and stimulated healing in damaged areas that had only been "stunned" by the bomb blast and were dormant. The extra oxygen was said to "wake up" the stunned brain and speed it on the road to healing. I didn't buy that explanation, but Sergeant Martin did. And there he stood before me—largely healed.

He had reached the final movement of his symphony. He had sung his "Ode to Joy."

He was not the only one. The advocates of HBO presented case after case of apparently miraculous healing. They convinced the United States Congress to authorize federal funding and test whether it truly worked, using rigorous scientific methods. The study conducted by the U.S. military cost more than $30 million. It compared three groups: real HBO; "fake" HBO subjects, who were told they got high oxygen but really got room air; and the usual treatment without either real or fake HBO. The study found that HBO did not work any better than a fake version of the treatment using room air instead of 100% oxygen. That didn't satisfy the advocates of HBO, who said they knew it worked. They claimed they saw improvements in patients with brain injury every day. They also alleged that the study had been done poorly by skeptics who biased the results. At that point, the military asked an independent organization—Samueli Institute, which I directed at the time—to analyze all the studies on HBO (within and outside the military) and, with the help of a panel of experts, including both advocates and skeptics of HBO, to make a final determination on its effectiveness.

The data was clear. The review confirmed that HBO did not work any better than a fake version, which involved sitting in a slightly pressurized chamber breathing room air for forty sessions. But the study revealed something few others had noticed: patients with brain injuries who received either real HBO or the fake HBO treatment did much better than those who got standard treatment alone—the kind of treatment I had provided Sergeant Martin. And the benefit was not small. Those who sat in the chamber for the full forty sessions had more than twice the improvement of those who received only drugs and other therapies. Adding oxygen did not increase that improvement, but going through the treatment helped. There was something about the ritual and delivery of the treatment that produced a dramatic healing effect. Perhaps it was the patients' and physicians' beliefs, perhaps it was the social engagement during the treatment, or perhaps it was some other factor. But it was not the oxygen. The military rejected the treatment after the HBO theory was disproved. But Sergeant Martin was right—he had hope, and he was better. I was happy for him, but confused. Was this another glimpse of a sleeping giant in modern medical research— the placebo effect—that I was to come to know well later in my career? What was I supposed to recommend to the next patient with a brain injury who came into my office? How could I trust my own judgment in medical practice to use the best treatment? And not to give false hope?

CHARLEY

As it turns out, many other physicians were also beginning to doubt their own experience—and with good reason. From the 1960s to the 1990s, a series of scholars using rigorous scientific methods showed repeatedly that many widely used treatments—even those considered "standard of care"—were not only ineffective but actually harmful. Medical opinion should be distrusted, they said, and in its place, a careful and structured process for summarizing clinical research, called "systematic reviews," should be used. This was the approach Samueli Institute used to examine the effect of HBO on brain injury. While I believed in good evidence, the importance of this did not hit me until I inadvertently contributed to the death of a patient by using the standard of care. It still feels like a punch in the gut—and it's no consolation knowing that medical errors are the third leading cause of death in the United States.

Charley was a sixty-six-year-old former Marine whom I hospitalized with a suspected heart attack in 1985. It was a routine admission and management. He had chest pain and nausea that sounded like a possible heart attack; his EKG showed signs of possible heart ischemia (low oxygen) and irregular heartbeats. In 1985, it was routine to hospitalize someone with these symptoms and treat them with bed rest, morphine to ease the pain, nitrates to expand their coronary vessels, beta blockers to slow their heart rate and lower their blood pressure, and antiarrhythmic drugs to prevent the heartbeat from becoming irregular. Most patients improved and were discharged a few days later. Some went on to have further complications.

Charley looked stable when I checked up on him before I went home that evening; he seemed perfectly comfortable. Blood tests indicated he had had a mild heart attack and would likely recover quickly. "See you in the morning," I said.

But that night, I was catching up on my medical journal reading and came across a study that showed I might be harming Charley with the antiarrhythmic drugs. The study randomized patients like Charley to receive either antiarrhythmic drugs or a placebo. Those who received this routine care and got the drugs actually died at a higher rate than those who did not. I put the article aside and decided I would bring it up in morning report. Had anyone else seen this article, I wondered? Should we stop giving these drugs?

I didn't get the chance to discuss it with my colleagues. At about 4 a.m. I got an urgent call from the hospital, telling me that Charley had died. His heart had gone into a fatal rhythm that could not be reversed. I rushed to the hospital to find his wife in his room weeping. What had happened? she asked. I didn't know what to say. Did his heart attack spread and cause the fatal arrhythmia? An autopsy later showed no evidence of that. Had I killed him by giving him the antiarrhythmic drug, as the new study implied? That was the most likely explanation.

The routine use of antiarrhythmics was stopped after the study I had read was confirmed. All in all, it was estimated that at the peak of antiarrhythmic drug use for suspected heart attacks, the medical profession was killing up to fifty thousand people a year. Expert clinical experience was harming patients. Only a placebo-controlled study revealed that.

For thousands of years, medical treatments have been selected and passed down using clinical experience as the best approach to truth. But could accumulated medical wisdom, both from ancient practices like acupuncture and modern drugs like the one given to Charley, be wrong? If so, how could we explain healing?

PARADOX

Since 1991, I have had the good fortune to have jobs that allow me to explore these questions. First, as the director of the Medical Research Fellowship at Walter Reed Army Institute of Research, it was my job to teach the research fellows how to think critically about medical science and apply rigorous methods in their research. Each year we had five or six fellows who were taught in-depth research methods and learned critical evaluation skills. Each fellow did research on a cutting-edge medical topic and carried the study through from start to finish. I adopted evidence-based teaching methods that emerged from Oxford and McMaster universities to teach physicians how to counter the errors of clinical experience. The NIH later adopted some of those teaching methods in their courses on clinical research. Did these same principles apply to ancient healing methods and alternative healing approaches used by most people in the world? I had the opportunity to examine that when I took over as the director of the Office of Alternative Medicine at the NIH and a WHO Traditional Medicine Center of Excellence in 1996 and 1998, respectively. Later, when I was CEO of Samueli Institute, a nonprofit organization dedicated to exploring the science of healing, my team had the chance to do scientific deep dives into ancient and modern healing practices.

This series of jobs allowed me to work with physicians, healers, patients, and researchers around the world to examine three main questions: First, to what extent do the health care practices from diverse traditions actually work when rigorously studied using gold-standard science? Second, what degree of improvement is found from these health care practices when used in regular clinical practice? And, third, are there any common characteristics that cut across all these traditions, ancient or modern, that can explain how their healing happens?

I call what has emerged from this exploration the "paradox of healing." When rigorously studied, ancient traditional practices such as acupuncture and herbal remedies, as well as more recent complementary and alternative treatments such as homeopathy, dietary supplements, and manual therapies, show disappointing results and only small effects.

Likewise, data on most of our modern conventional treatments show the same thing. Most drugs for pain, mental health, ulcers, hypertension, and diabetes, for example, show little benefit—often only 20% to 30%. Furthermore, the more carefully the studies are done, the smaller the effects. Even more startling, only about one-third of well-done studies— executed in the laboratory or in the clinic—can be independently replicated. Thus our confidence that even a 20% improvement can be repeatedly obtained is low. Even surgery (when not simply changing anatomy, like fixing a leg or removing a tumor) works minimally. And when these treatments do work, it is often not for the reasons scientists think they do.

Yet the paradox is that all these approaches can work, if applied properly. When we looked at the rate of improvement in patients who received very different types of treatments from around the world, we found that 70% to 80% of people will get better. Later in this book, I will describe Parkinson's patients who get better with treatments as different as ancient Ayurvedic medicine and electrical stimulation of the brain, soldiers with PTSD who get better with yoga or psychotherapy, patients with pain who get better with acupuncture or opioids, and patients whose health improves when under the care of a homeopath or surgeon, even when rigorous studies show little if any effect from these treatments. We need to understand *why* they get better.

Chapter 2

How We Heal

Placebo research reveals what most medical science conceals

There is a sleeping giant in modern medical research that has yet to awaken and reveal itself fully. When it does, it will lay waste to what we think we know about healing. It plays no favorites and so is equally devastating to ancient healing claims, complementary medicine, and mainstream health care. It is called the "placebo response." Failure to understand the importance of the placebo response led me (and all of biomedicine) down the path that contributed to the deaths of patients like Charley. Likewise, failure to use the placebo response causes us to throw out powerful treatments like the ritual used by Sergeant Martin, which could markedly help other soldiers with brain injury. This giant can subvert the good intentions behind how we deliver healing with patients every day. By failing to acknowledge the negative aspects of placebo—called the "*nocebo* response"—we often inadvertently harm with our treatments. Knowing how the placebo response works opens a door to healing that few in medicine enter. But you don't have to wait. In this chapter, I will summarize what we know about the placebo response (and its underlying causes) and how you and your doctor can use it for healing. You will get an inside view of what is coming before our understanding of placebo in medicine has fully awakened.

NORMA

How was I going to tell Norma, my patient with debilitating arthritis, that she had been taking the placebo? She had gotten remarkably better in almost all ways. She remarked to me many times during the study on how well the vitamin was working. She had less pain, was more active, and had returned to her volunteer job at the hospital. She was happier. Others noticed and commented on her improved mood and ability to move. Now I had to tell her. I worried about what would happen when I did. Would she be devastated? Embarrassed? Angry? I worried she would regress to her former state of pain and limited mobility. But I was required both ethically and legally to inform her about what she had been taking.

Norma was a tall, thin woman with long gray hair who still had the sparkle of a young woman in her eye. She reminded me of a reed, easily blown about by the wind. Her psychological nature fit her physical stature to a T. She was gentle and empathetic. She was always willing to follow my suggestions. She was one of my most compliant patients. My fear that she would regress in her healing was based on two long-held assumptions in medicine: first, that her improvement had all been based on her own "belief" that she was getting active treatment; second, that she was a good "placebo responder," usually thought of as someone who is "suggestible" and easily influenced by the opinions of others—especially authorities, like me, her doctor. The premise that some people are suggestible in this way has a long history in medical science. After Anton Mesmer, a German physician in the seventeenth century, claimed he could heal using "animal magnetism," in 1797, his claim was tested by a team that included Benjamin Franklin. They used one of the first double-blind testing methods, in which patients did not know if they were getting the real treatment or a fake version and physicians did not know which patients received the real treatment. One method was placing a blanket or curtain between the therapist and the patient. Patients were told that they were being treated at times when they were not. Other patients were blindfolded so they could not see the therapist or what he was doing. Franklin reported that patients would respond to the suggestion of treatment and this response occurred even when no treatment was given.

This idea that belief and suggestibility were key factors in many patients' healing eventually led to the use of blinded tests of other therapies to see if their efficacy was real. Double-blind methods were first applied to "alternative" treatments like homeopathy by a skeptical medical profession. Eventually these blinding approaches were used for conventional treatments, too, especially new drugs. Soon the double-blind method became accepted as the gold standard for determining whether a treatment worked. All treatment effects had to be separated from the effects of belief to be considered effective.

Both Norma and I had believed she was on the real treatment. Would I harm her if I undermined that belief by telling her she was on the placebo? I thought I would, which would violate my oath to "do no harm," as a physician. But I had to tell the truth.

I waited several weeks to inform her, hoping she would enjoy her good results for a little longer. Fortunately, during that time a way out of this dilemma emerged. The statistician who analyzed the study came back with the overall results. The vitamin had proved to be effective. When comparing the overall improvement in the group taking the niacinamide compared with those taking the placebo pill, the niacinamide group improved about 8% more than the placebo group. This was considered a significant effect; that is, it had a p-value of less than 0.05 in the statistical tests. A p-value of less than 0.05 means that if we did one hundred more studies like the one Norma was in, there would be a 95% chance we would still get at least an 8% or more improvement in the niacinamide group compared with the placebo group. It does not mean the effect of the vitamin was large (it wasn't), only that the small effect we saw was probably real. Probably, but not for certain. To know for sure, most scientists would suggest that the study be repeated a few more times to see if the effect persists. But, at least for this study, the probability was considered high enough by scientific convention for me to tell Norma I had found a viable treatment for her. So several weeks later, when I sat down with Norma to let her know that she was taking the placebo, I could immediately tell her that the study had found the vitamin to be effective and that, if she wanted, we could switch her to the real treatment. In other words, I tried to gloss over the fact that she had gotten better because of her belief, focusing on the prospect of even greater improvement. Fortunately, she was happy with that and continued to do well on the niacinamide. I was off the hook. I chalked up the experience to Norma's suggestibility and assumed that she was an exception rather than the rule. That is, until I met Bill.

BILL

Bill arrived in my office to seek help for his chronic back pain. He came in only at the urging of his wife, as he was skeptical that any doctor could fix him. He had been to many doctors. Finally, he agreed to come in after the pain was so bad that he had to cancel a car trip to see his grandchildren. He told me that his Korean-born wife urged him to see an acupuncturist because acupuncture is used to treat back pain in Korea. So, reluctantly, he came to see me, not because I was an acupuncturist but because he wanted to know if acupuncture could help him or if, as he said, it is "all just placebo."

Bill is the opposite of suggestible. In fact, he doesn't believe that any doctors or treatment can help at all. I could tell by his opinions, his body, and his body language that it is hard to influence him. He has husky round shoulders and a thick belly. He lumbers more than walks into the room and has a limp favoring his right side, which is where he feels most of his back pain.

He sat down slowly in a chair facing me and crossed his arms in front of him. He had that kind of look that says, *Go ahead and try to help—I have already been through it all.*

Nevertheless, he'd come in to see me. He said he did so mainly to "get his wife off of his back" and because I am a physician who practices in the military. He had been in the military and figured I won't make money off any treatment I recommend, so I'm less likely to push something on him. I had about twenty minutes to answer his questions and see if I could help him.

I started by saying there is no easy answer, which he already knew. But then it hit me that I was saying that because he was completely different from Norma, and I, too, didn't actually expect him to get better. I looked over the list of treatments he had tried. These included analgesics; nonsteroidal anti-inflammatory drugs (NSAIDS), such as aspirin or ibuprofen; muscle relaxants; antidepressants; chiropractic manipulation; and injections. At one point he was told to go to bed and rest. Later, he was told to get up and be more active. He was given exercises and physical therapy. He went to a chiropractor. Fortunately, he had not been given traction (which *is* harmful for patients with back pain), but a couple of decades earlier he would have been given that as well. What really put him off about doctors was that he had been told to see a psychiatrist because it was "all in his head." The psychiatrist treated him for depression (which he was sure he did not have) and then finally told Bill not to come back until he really wanted to get well. "The gall of that guy," he told me. "Like I *want* to have this!"

Patients with chronic musculoskeletal pain like Bill are very common; in fact, musculoskeletal conditions are the number-one cause of suffering and the number-one chronic condition that spurs people to visit a doctor, making up over 8% of all visits per year. Back pain is the most common of those musculoskeletal conditions, affecting over 70% of all adults sometime during their life, and is the leading cause of limited activity in the world. It costs the United States over $100 billion per year. There is no measure of how much meaningful life is lost, typified by Bill's inability to see his grandchildren. It is common for patients like Bill with chronic back pain to have undergone multiple treatments. It is common for physicians to prescribe a variety of treatments. Bill came to me because his wife made him ask me about acupuncture, but he didn't believe in it.

"Doc," he asked, "should I try acupuncture? Is it effective or a waste of time? I have to pay for it, because this is not going to be reimbursed by my insurance; should I spend the time, the effort, and the expense? Do I have to believe in it?"

It was a reasonable question, for which I owed him a reasonable answer. I was not sure I had one.

Acupuncture can stimulate natural painkillers in the brain, called endogenous opioids—even in animals. This makes us think the effects are real and not due to the placebo effect. Comparisons of acupuncture treatment for back pain with other treatments, such as drugs, physical therapy, and education, show that it works well. But so does sham acupuncture. This makes the effects seem largely due to the placebo effect. So even though the treatment seemed to be mostly placebo, similar to the vitamin I had tested on Norma, the downside—other than the cost and time spent on treatment—was small. So I suggested to Bill that he try it, but with a limited number of treatments, and then determine if it was working for him. I tried to keep a neutral and objective tone, trying not imply that there was not much hope for it to work. More like a personal experiment. Bill seemed to like that tone and was glad I was not an advocate for the treatment, like his wife, and that I could be objective.

I sent him to an acupuncturist I knew and trusted. After eight sessions, his pain was not much better, and he and I decided it was not worth continuing. While we gave up on the acupuncture, I didn't want to give up on Bill. I asked him if he would like to explore other treatments, and he said he would, but there were not many he hadn't already tried.

His X-rays showed a narrowing of the disk space in his lower spine from arthritis, so I suggested he see a surgeon. Bill was his usual skeptical self. He didn't want to be cut on, and he had friends who had undergone surgery with little benefit. Some were even worse. But Bill had already done almost every treatment available, including intensive physical therapy. So, reluctantly, and with little belief that it would help, he had the surgical procedure. The procedure involved injection of a cementlike substance into his collapsing disk. He thought this seemed less invasive than opening his back up and fusing the disk with rods. The effects were dramatically positive. Three weeks after the procedure, his pain was the lowest it had been in years. He and his wife promptly got in the car and drove ten hours to see their grandchildren. They were very happy. Because Bill was not a suggestible person and did not believe in this treatment, I decided that this confirmed my opinion that "real" treatments were those that worked in those who did not believe. For the suggestible, placebo treatments might be more appropriate.

THE PLACEBO EFFECT

I was wrong. In 1995, I brought together a small group of investigators at the NIH who were studying why placebo seemed to work in some people and not in others. We were interested in understanding why an inert or inactive substance, such as a sugar or salt solution or distilled water with no known pharmacological value, could be effective and how often this happened. This question was popularized in a 1955 article on placebo by Henry Beecher, MD, in the *Journal of the American Medical Association*. Beecher reported that about one-third of all effects seen in medicine were due to the placebo response. This became medical gospel for decades, even though several studies after that reported an approximate 70% response rate to treatments that were later shown to be inert. At the meeting in 1995, Professor Dan Moerman, an anthropologist from the University of Michigan, showed findings that floored the audience. He had collected data from around the world that completely undermined the placebo gospel of Henry Beecher, the belief of most of the medical profession, and my belief that Norma and Bill had each improved for different reasons—one because of suggestibility and belief and the other because of the treatment.

Professor Moerman revealed that the healing effect from fake treatments could vary from 0% to 100%—*even for the same disease and same treatment—depending on the context and cultural meaning* in which they were delivered. One review, for example, studied 117 placebo-controlled trials of a drug treatment for stomach ulcers done across multiple countries. These studies showed objectively that the same inert treatment (a sugar pill) had a wide range of effects from country to country. The healing rate in Germany, for example, was very high, but in the Netherlands and Denmark it was low. In Brazil, hardly any patients with ulcers healed when given placebo. The dramatically varying results were influenced by country, context, delivery, and the patient's interpretation of that delivery. In other words, the cultural context influenced the meaning, which in turn influenced the biology, the pathology, and the outcome. The effects were very specific. For example, in Germany, the placebo healing rates of patients with high blood pressure were low, not high as for ulcers. In fact, the meaning and context surrounding how a treatment was delivered had a much greater impact on healing than the treatment modalities themselves. Inert treatments for pain like Bill's, for example, worked better if you gave them by needle rather than pill; gave them in the hospital rather than at home, applied them more often rather than less frequently, charged more for them rather than less, and delivered them with a positive and confident message rather than a neutral or skeptical message. Acupuncture was found to be more effective the closer the study was conducted to China, where acupuncture was developed and is widespread. I suspect surgery works better in the West, though no one has studied that. It seemed that the magnitude of a person's healing depended less on the suggestibility and belief of the individual patient than on the collective belief of the culture and the ritual created to deliver that belief.

Professor Ted J. Kaptchuk, director of the Center for Placebo Studies at Harvard Medical School, is one of the world's most respected researchers on the placebo response. In a recent analysis, he sheds light on the variability of these effects by comparing three types of healing encounters: Navajo ceremonial chants, acupuncture treatment in the Western world, and the biomedical provision of health care. He describes each encounter as being surrounded by beliefs, narratives, "multi-sensory dramas," and culturally defined influences, all of which can be described as rituals in the treatment of illness. Depending on the setting and the practitioner, such rituals may take the form of communal chanting and practices led by a medicine man; the insertion of needles that takes place in an office redolent with representations of Asian culture; or authoritative white-coated clinicians presiding over complex biomedical testing and treatment technology. Looking at this research, I began to wonder: did my patient Bill get better from surgery not because it was "real," but because surgery was more culturally meaningful to him than the other treatments he had undergone? I was skeptical of this explanation. Bill had been through many treatments and should have benefited even if they were from placebo effects. But two studies conducted after I had seen Bill seemed to contradict this assumption. In those studies, patients were randomly assigned to get either the cement or balloon injections into collapsing disks (like Bill had received) or a fake procedure that mimicked the real injections but did not manipulate the spinal disk in any way. In both studies, patients who underwent the fake procedure did just as well as those who got the real procedure.

I still found this hard to believe. Bill was resistant to treatments and was not in any way suggestible. Could it be that, at least for pain, the meaning and context of a treatment produced much of the healing, even in patients who were not suggestible? Even when "hard" procedures were used, such as surgery, that manipulated tissues and corrected anatomy? To test this assumption, my team and I did a meta-analysis of all surgery studies of chronic pain, whether in the back, knees, abdomen, or heart. We selected studies that compared real surgery to sham surgery, in which patients and doctors went through the ritual of surgery but no real correction of anatomy was done. We were able to determine the quality of the studies and then combine results into a single estimate of the contribution to healing pain from "true" surgery. The final analysis showed equally good improvement of any pain condition when the ritual of surgery was applied to the patient but no actual surgery was done. These sham surgery studies showed that, at least for pain treatments, healing occurs from something else. Could it be that the millions of surgeries done every year to treat pain produce healing because they are powerful types of ritual placebos? Could it be that the healing that occurred in Norma and Bill were not so different after all? As different as they were, could it be that they both had tapped into their own inherent healing capacity in different ways, and that healing was connected to their beliefs and behavior and to those around them more than the specific treatment they received?

Professor Kaptchuk has done two studies exploring to what extent the effect of treatment depends on collective belief verses individual belief. In one study, all patients with a painful abdominal condition (irritable bowel syndrome, or IBS) were given a fake treatment—sham acupuncture. However, the social ritual was varied between groups to enhance the dose of collective belief. In one group, the practitioner came in and said very little and delivered the treatment. In a second group, the practitioner explained how the treatment works and set the expectation that the treatment will work. In the third group, a prominent physician from a prominent medical school delivered the treatment with a full explanation and a story about the good results others had obtained with the treatment. All the patients held about the same amount of individual belief in acupuncture at the beginning of the study. But the greater the social meaning produced by the ritual, the better the effect. In the third group, the benefit the patients experience is greater than that achieved by the best drugs approved for treatment of IBS.

In a second study by Kaptchuk, patients were actually told ahead of time that the treatment was fake. One group was given placebo pills with this description: "Placebo pills made of an inert substance, like sugar pills, that have been shown in clinical studies to produce significant improvement in IBS symptoms through mind-body, self-healing processes." This statement created an expectation that even these placebos have an effect. A second group of IBS patients was given no treatment but with the same quality of interaction with providers. The group given the placebo (and who knew it was placebo) had significantly better pain reduction and improved quality of life.

No matter what form the ritual takes, says Kaptchuk, these can have powerful influences on the healing process. "We cannot explain the effects of rituals using placebo treatments simply by belief and expectation," Kaptchuk explains. "While belief may contribute some to the outcome in these studies, the effects produced by healing rituals are much larger than can be explained by what the patient believes about the treatment. The main reasons these effects occur is still a mystery." Research suggests that healing rituals are associated with modulations of symptoms through neurobiological mechanisms, just like we see from drugs. They can not only affect pain, but change the immune system, alter organ function, shift brain processing, and even influence specific cell receptors and genes. One study, done by renowned placebo researcher Professor Fabrizio Benedetti of the University of Turin, Italy, demonstrated that if you link a placebo treatment ritual to a painkiller, you can continue to get pain relief with the placebo after withdrawing the painkiller. And even more remarkably, the placebo will work using the same cellular mechanism of the painkiller to which it was linked. The body not only can learn to heal, it can be taught which specific mechanism in the body to use to produce the effect. Placebo effects, writes Kaptchuk, are often described as "non-specific." He suggests instead that they should be considered—and further researched—as the "specific" effects of healing rituals.

THE 80% EFFECT

The giant is stirring. Sugar pills and fake needles or sham surgeries do not heal. Healing comes from the meaning and context in which these various treatment agents get deployed. Modern medicine uses placebo in research not to optimize healing but to separate the effects of belief and meaning from those of the drug or technique itself. According to current convention in science, it is the drug or technique that is the "real" effect. Yet by turning the microscope around and looking at what causes healing when no real treatment is used, science has begun to uncover the underlying mechanisms of how we heal that span all modalities—ancient and modern, alternative or mainstream. Since that NIH meeting in 1995, research on the placebo response has exploded and is dissecting the underlying processes and magnitude of our capacity to heal. This research is now being collated and accelerated by the Society for Interdisciplinary Placebo Science (SIPS). Started in 2015, SIPS has become a forum for looking at how healing works by investigating the underlying mechanisms of the placebo response.

And that healing capacity is large, providing close to 80% of the effects we see in medicine. Since the 1950s, when Henry Beecher first put forth his idea that placebo heals, major placebo responses have been reported in over forty conditions with more being added each year. And the magnitude of those effects is often 60%, 70%, and even 80% for many common conditions. These effects can be produced by any agent—including needles, pills, radiation, chants and prayers, touch, surgery, and talk—provided those treatments are delivered in a way that fits the patient and their expectations and is done using a ritual their culture finds meaningful. For many of these conditions, the effect of the social ritual and the meaning it creates for a patient produces a larger rate of healing than the treatment itself. In many cases, the color of pills, their shape, and the way they are delivered determines their effectiveness as much as—or more than—the medicine they contain. In fact, if you optimized all the factors that produce healing in the "placebo" group of a study, it is possible to push the improvements patients get up to a level that often dwarfs the benefit from the "real" treatment.

From the perspective of science and good evidence, a proven treatment needs to show that it works better than the placebo arms of a study and—preferably—for the reasons the scientists think it works. This is called the "specific effect" and is what good science gives us. From a patient's perspective, however, optimized effects are preferred—whether they are called placebo, "non-specific," or ritual-based. Of course, ideally these treatment rituals are not unsafe, too expensive, or too difficult to do. The effect is like the treatment you see on the right side of the illustration. But when the placebo and ritual effects are enhanced, it becomes very difficult to prove the agent used in these rituals adds much to the effect. So in the context of an optimized treatment, the supposed "real" treatment cannot be proven.

The work of Kaptchuk, Moerman, Benedetti, and others explained why my proven treatments were not working as well as the ones my patients had found. My proven treatments were not optimized or meaningful for them. My evidence-based medicine was coming into conflict with person-centered care.

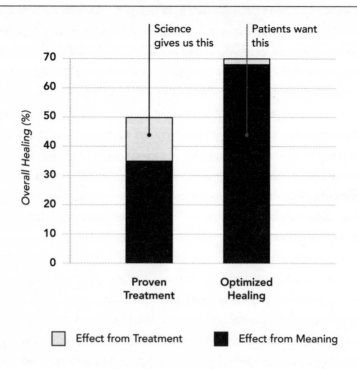

TREATMENT VERSUS MEANING

THE COMMON THREAD

I now began to understand how Norma, Bill, Sergeant Martin, and many other patients I had treated got better, sometimes because of me, often despite me. When Sergeant Martin described the details of his hyperbaric oxygen (HBO) treatment for brain injury, he was describing how, after going against my recommendations, he had entered a ritual that induced underlying mechanisms of healing. How did he do that? First, he expected it to work. It was not just a matter of his own expectation, however; his father, who encouraged and paid for the treatment, was enthusiastic. Second, the nurses, technicians, doctors, and other patients created a milieu that infused that belief with social meaning. The group that underwent treatment each week shared their stories, experiences, and lives, building cultural meaning into the ritual. They became friends and mutual supporters in healing. Finally, the experience of healing—in his case, breathing what he understood to be lifesaving oxygen—was repeated, reinforced, and conditioned in his experience and his physiology. The treatment agent—oxygen—had no therapeutic value in itself for a damaged brain, but it gave him a feeling that something was happening and a sense of well-being, reinforced each week. In the same way pain drugs were "educated" to work in the study by Professor Fabrizio (page 25), Sergeant Martin's brain was taught how to heal each week through social and classical conditioning. Researchers at SIPS have now shown that three main mechanisms—belief and expectation, meaningful social learning, and reinforcement or conditioning—are the underlying mechanisms of the placebo response, and the likely explanation for the majority of human healing in any system or from any treatment.

MAKING MEANING

In an article that Professor Moerman and I wrote several years ago, we suggested that the so-called placebo response can occur and result in healing, whether a proven or unproven substance is used. Every physician and every medical practitioner wants to try to enhance the therapeutic effects of their treatments. I certainly wanted to. I had been sobered by the death of Charley. And I was sobered further when I saw patients get better, often despite my recommendations. However, my greatest worry was whether the approach to science I was using prevented me from optimizing healing. Whether a treatment is labeled as placebo or not is more of an academic and economic question than the primary concern of the clinician and patient. The question for a patient was not whether a treatment was better than placebo, but the likelihood that a patient would get better after the treatment. I realized that in order to maximize the effect of any treatment I offered, I needed to maximize the response from the context and meaning of the treatment for the patient and culture. Research on placebo was making that process visible in a way I had never seen before. Moerman and I suggested that physicians replace the term "placebo effect" with the words "meaning, context, and learning response" or simply the "meaning response." We redefined placebo effect as the physiological, psychological, and clinical effects of meaning when a placebo (or inert treatment) is used. That response is really about healing, and the use of placebos or inert substances in research were of value only to help us understand *how* to heal, not what to heal with. I was beginning to suspect that what health care was mostly about was learning how to heal through meaning. Could it be that many of the thousands of treatments being pushed by practitioners all over the world were just the tools to induce healing by manipulating belief, social meaning, and conditioning through ritual? Was the process of healing being obscured by our constant search for "good evidence" in medicine in which the only "real" treatments are those that can be separated from meaning and context? Was the majority of healing due to the agency of the patient rather that the agent used? The giant was stirring.

BILL FINDS HIS WAY

About eleven months after his surgery, Bill came lumbering back into my office again. He was limping, favoring the right, as before. His wife was not with him this time, but the look of "I have done this before" was. He sat down carefully; I could tell he was in pain. He told me what had happened. After the surgery, he'd felt great. Within three weeks, he had the least amount of pain he'd had in over a decade. So naturally, he became more active, which, he said, "was the whole point." He and his wife drove several times to see the grandchildren. He could play with them, even sitting on the floor for short periods, something he could not do before. About six months after the surgery, he noticed a slight twinge in his back while he was mowing the lawn. At first it seemed minor. Still, he rested for a bit and did some of the physical therapy stretches he knew. Then, at nine months to the day after his surgery, he was reaching over to pick up a toy from the ground and felt a "pop" in the right side of his back. He couldn't stand up straight. The pain was excruciating. He went back to the surgeon. X-rays and CT scans showed "nothing different," and the surgeon did not recommend another surgery. "Give it some time," he was told. But the pain was back, and continued to worsen. Now it was just as bad as before the surgery. He was back on medications and doing physical therapy—and not driving to see the grandchildren anymore. It had been two more months since he felt his back "pop."

"So why have you come back to see me?" I asked. Bill paused and took a deep breath sort of like he was letting go of something he had held on to for a long time. He leaned forward and put his hands on his knees. "When I was in here last time, asking about acupuncture and asking you did you think it would help my pain, you asked me some questions that I thought were strange. Questions like, did I have any stress and how did I manage it, how did I sleep, and what my diet was like, and did I have any friends. Things like that."

"Yes," I said, "I recall."

Bill took another breath. "Why did you ask those questions? What did that have to do with my pain?"

"Well," I said, "I have learned that a path toward healing often involves things not related to the main conditions people come in to see me for—the pain, for example. I was trying to see how open you were to exploring other aspects of your life that might help you feel well, or if you were just seeking another treatment for your back pain. At the time, it seemed you were just seeking another treatment."

Bill leaned back again but did not cross his arms this time. "I was," he said. "My wife wanted me to try acupuncture, and I came to see if there was any science behind it. You said there was a little bit, so we tried it."

"Yes," I replied. "We tried it, and it didn't work, so we went on to see the surgeon, and it helped." I was not sure where he was going with the discussion, but then he came out with it.

"Dr. Jonas," he said, leaning forward again, "how much science is there to support surgery?"

Now I was a bit worried. Was he angry? Was he looking for ammunition against the surgeon? Or me?

"Well," I said, "about 75% of people get better after surgery and, as it turns out, so do many of those who get fake surgery. So it seems that the ritual of going through surgery has a lot to do with people getting better. They seem to do other things—like being more mentally positive and physically active. That is likely a large part of the healing."

Bill took this in. "Just like acupuncture?" he asked.

I thought for a moment. "Yes," I said, "just like with acupuncture."

After Bill's pain had returned, he had begun to look back at all the treatments he had done, almost a dozen of them. He had noticed that most of them helped for a while but then the pain would return. Some, like surgery, were dramatic but not long lasting; others, like acupuncture were gradual or did not work at all. What Bill wanted to know was if his continued search for "cures" for this pain was the right approach. He had been thinking about the questions I had asked—about stress, sleep, diet, friends, and life balance—and the role it might play in his healing. "The most important thing in life for me is to be available to my kids and grandkids, to be active with them, and to be able to do things with my wife—like traveling once in a while. But I spend so much time dealing with the back pain or going to get treatments for it, I have not been able to do that. When you asked those questions about my life, it started me thinking that I needed to focus more on those rather than all the pain treatments. I want you to help me do that."

Remarkably, Bill, the "fix me" guy, was starting to realize from his personal experience what I was also coming to from my professional and research experience. That healing and curing, though connected, were not the same. Curing involved what he had been going through—getting a diagnosis and trying out various treatments based on the scientific evidence. That evidence was gathered from research and reviews of research comparing one treatment to another treatment, or to no treatment or to a placebo or sham treatment, to see if it was "real." These studies examined whether the collective response of a group to a treatment was better than the collective response in another group that was given placebo, no treatment, or another treatment. If the treatment group had acceptable side effects and costs, the treatment was said to have "worked" and was recommended to patients. These studies averaged out the effects in groups. But no individual is average.

Healing, on the other hand, was a more subtle and individual process. It involved finding out what gave a person a sense of well-being. Doing what was most meaningful to them. It involved more than seeking a treatment for a specific symptom or condition; it involved finding and engaging in activities that brought joy and satisfaction. It had more to do with caring for one's deeper self than with getting health care for the body. It involved paying attention to the "meaning and context" of a behavior—the very factors that the research of professors Moerman, Kaptchuk, and Benedetti, and I had found produced the placebo response. It was this meaning and context that my questions to Bill where meant to get at.

"I would be happy to help you do that, Bill," I replied, "if you will help me understand what processes are most helpful for you in getting well. Can we make it a partnership of learning together—finding out how healing happens in your case?"

Bill agreed. So we started to build a healing ritual unique to him.

THE HEALING JOURNEY

Bill became one of the first of many patients to work with me to traverse a healing rather than a cure-focused journey and to learn a process that would help others unlock their inherent healing capacity: the capacity that placebo research indicated contributed up to 80% of the benefit from many treatments and in many conditions. We started by looking at the scientific evidence for the treatments Bill had done over the past fifteen years and for any treatment or self-care method he might be interested in using. We were especially interested in these questions:

- What was the overall improvement from doing the ritual of the treatment, as measured in the placebo group of a study?
- Was the treatment better than no treatment at all?
- Was it better than other treatments for the same condition?
- What were the side effects and harms?
- How complicated was it and what did it cost?

EFFECTIVENESS OF BILL'S LOWER BACK PAIN TREATMENTS

TREATMENT	BETTER THAN PLACEBO?	BETTER THAN NO TREATMENT?	EQUAL OR BETTER THAN A PROVEN TREATMENT?
Acupuncture	YES	UNKNOWN	UNKNOWN
* Advice to stay active	UNKNOWN	UNKNOWN	UNKNOWN
* Analgesies	UNKNOWN	POSSIBLY	YES
* Antidepressants	POSSIBLY	UNKNOWN	UNKNOWN
* Bed rest	UNKNOWN	NO	NO
Biofeedback	POSSIBLY	UNKNOWN	POSSIBLY
* Exercises	UNKNOWN	UNKNOWN	POSSIBLY
Injections (facet joint and trigger point)	POSSIBLY	UNKNOWN	UNKNOWN
* Manipulation	POSSIBLY	UNKNOWN	POSSIBLY
* Muscle relaxants	UNKNOWN	UNKNOWN	NO
* Nonsteroidal anti-inflammatory drugs	YES	YES	YES
* Physical therapies	UNKNOWN	UNKNOWN	UNKNOWN
Traction	NO	NO	UNKNOWN

KEY

○ UNKNOWN
◔ POSSIBLY
◑ NO
● YES

* Already used by the patient prior to the first visit

We placed all this information in a chart. What immediately emerged is that very few treatments—conventional or alternative—had good evidence that they worked in the long run. Most had never been compared to a placebo ritual, and when they had been, almost all of them added only a small amount to the overall outcome—often less than 20%. Some worked slightly better than others, but most treatments had not been compared to each other directly, so it was rare that we could determine whether one treatment was better than another. Almost all of them were better than doing nothing. It appeared that you needed to do *something* to get the most benefit out of the healing ritual, but the specifics of that something was less important than we thought.

While the overall response rate between treatments varied little, the adverse side effects, on the other hand, varied considerably. Major interventions, such as surgery and medication, produced unwanted side effects in more patients than benefited from them. Often 50% to 60%

of patients would experience a side effect. Gentler treatments, such as yoga or music, had fewer and less severe side effects—but they were not without problems. Often the research did not even bother to measure side effects, which created a gap in information about them.

When we stepped back and looked at our handiwork, we both immediately saw a pattern emerge. Most treatments did not work better than the ritual and so were not thought to be "real" and were not offered or encouraged by doctors, including me. But looked at another way, almost all the treatment rituals actually helped people get better—often producing improvements in 60%, 70%, or even 80% of patients in the group—just as seen in the placebo literature. Bill commented, "So instead of not having any treatments that work, it looks like I have a wealth of options. I just need to decide which ones I like, can do, and [can] afford." His insight was profound. Bill had gone from a cycle of "Fix me or let me try another treatment I don't like" to a smorgasbord of options. He now had to decide only which ones were the most meaningful to him—that is, the ones he could and wanted to do to achieve his goal of playing with the grandkids. Freed from a mind-set that was looking to the next magic cure for his pain, he could go about building a pathway to well-being based on what was meaningful for him.

To help find and select the most meaningful treatments, Bill started by keeping a journal in which he wrote down observations about what made him feel well and what did not. The "strange" questions I had asked him on his first visit to me became the basis for these observations. They did not have to be linked to his pain. It could be anything he observed that helped him feel better about himself—helped him feel happy and well. After two months of keeping this journal, Bill came back with several insights.

First, his back felt the worst when he did not get enough sleep. He was in a habit of overeating into the evening, usually accompanied by several drinks and reading the stock market on his cell phone before going to bed. He snored a lot and woke up frequently. His doctor had put him on a night breathing treatment called CPAP but he did not like the apparatus. He never took naps. His doctor had also told him he was overweight and needed to lose fifty pounds or he would become diabetic like his father had been. He was already prediabetic. The dietitian he went to gave him a calorie-restricted diet and told him to stop drinking.

Second, he found that he was constantly on the go all day. About what, he wasn't sure, but things just seemed to always be required of him—mostly by his wife, who wanted him to help keep the house repaired and to run errands. While he and his wife had always had a good relationship, after the journaling, he realized that he really didn't talk with her—or anyone else for that matter—about his experiences or worries. For example, when his father had died a few years before, he had done all that was needed for the funeral and burial. His father was an alcoholic, and they had not had been close. He had not engaged much with Bill and his brother, except to yell at them and occasionally hit them. Bill never talked about his relationship with his father with anyone, including his wife, and did not discuss his feelings about his father's death with anyone.

OPENING UP

As we continued to explore questions on healing and Bill continued his journaling, he noted that he did a number of things that made him feel better. A hot shower followed by putting pressure on his back lessened the pain. Stretching had always helped, but he found it difficult to make himself do it because it was painful. Before the pain, he had enjoyed hunting and spending long hours in the woods. Being outdoors in his backyard, watching the birds, now soothed him. In one journal entry Bill wrote the following: "Good night's sleep last night, woke up rested and serene. Katie [his four-year-old grandchild, who was visiting] came in to play; sat for an hour on the floor with a tea set and dolls. No pain. She is such a joy." This triggered a memory for Bill from his childhood. He was about five years old and came running home from school excited about a clay ashtray he had made for this father. His father had come home early with a headache and had been drinking for several hours. On reaching the house, Bill burst into the living room and ran up to his father to show him the ashtray. Startled from his stupor, his father grabbed the ashtray and hurled it across the room, smashing it against the wall. Bill ran to his room and shut the door. He remembers crying for hours. From that day forward, he would tiptoe around his father, uncertain as to how he would react to any situation. He never cried again.

"I don't know why I remembered that episode," Bill said, "There were many others. Maybe being with Katie reminded me of my childhood. I made sure I was not that way with my kids, but I never recall him just sitting on the ground playing tea." He took a deep breath. "I don't know why I told you that story. I have never told anyone that story."

Little did Bill know that opening up to difficult traumas and telling them to someone or writing them down is one of the most effective self-healing behaviors. Extensive research has shown that as little as a single episode of deep self-engagement, usually around a trauma or hurt, can have prolonged healing effects. Research by social psychologist Professor James Pennebaker and others has documented psychological, physiological, and immunological changes from such episodes in well-conducted randomized controlled trials—the gold standard of science. Others have shown that these meaningful engagements can improve pain relief in arthritis, lung function in asthmatics, and immune function in the elderly. They also reduce the need for medical care and lower costs. By giving himself space to observe and map his own healing path, Bill had discovered this for himself.

BILL'S BODY STARTS TO RESPOND

Bill's healing had begun, not from psychotherapy (he would never submit to that) but by observing what he valued most in life, what made things worse, and what made things better. By finding meaning and linking it to the behavior and treatments he wanted, he was building his own self-care rituals. We mapped out a plan. He decided to tackle sleep first. When rested, he felt better all around. He agreed to limit his drinks to two a night; before bed, he would take a hot shower and listen to an audio recording of nature sounds to help him relax. He stopped all electronic reading from bed and darkened his room with blackout curtains, covering up any electronic clocks. We put him on a small amount of the herb valerian (proven in randomized placebo-controlled studies to help people go to sleep) and low-dose, slow-release melatonin (not yet proven in randomized controlled studies), just for a month to assist in conditioning a deep relaxation and help him get into that habit at night. He also took his pain medications as needed. For one month, we did nothing specifically for Bill's pain or back. For the first time in years, it was not the focus of his visits to my clinic or of his daily routine. Yet he reported feeling better. He still had pain, but it did not bother him as much. He was moving more. He was taking less medication.

We then began to work on Bill's body. Pressure helped, so he thought he would like a selective use of massage. It just so happens my group had done a good meta-analysis of massage that showed effectiveness for chronic musculoskeletal pain like Bill's—especially compared to doing nothing, but even a little bit better when compared to sham massage, which involved very light touch. He also found stretching useful but had tried physical therapy and did not want that again. Also, he said he didn't want to keep coming into the hospital or clinic to receive treatment "with all those sick people." Bill was starting to no longer identify as a patient. We chose yoga instead.

There happens to be good research evidence that yoga is effective for easing back pain. The year before, my organization had conducted a comprehensive systematic review of nondrug approaches to pain. Yoga had emerged as one of the best. Recently, the American College of Physicians, the top group of internal medicine doctors in the United States, added yoga and massage to their guidelines for managing back pain. But someone like Bill, with long-term chronic pain, needs to do yoga carefully. Bill could easily set off spasms and fall into a downward spiral if his stretching was not done right. He had injured himself with stretching before. We decided to combine a periodic massage with gentle restorative yoga done slowly and under professional guidance. Soon, he learned how to control the stretches himself and was doing them three times a week—twice a week at home. After about four weeks, he found that when he did the massage/yoga combination, he didn't need his nighttime pain medication, and the yoga alone allowed him to cut his daily medication in half.

Eventually, Bill began to ask about the role of food for his weight and prediabetes. He wanted to explore how he could connect better with this wife and friends. By the time he was ready to explore those issues, however, his back pain was 80% better. Perhaps more important, he knew how to take charge of his own healing. He now knew how to use various agents to enhance his own healing agency.

THE PAIN POINT

Worldwide, chronic pain affects over one in five adults. Primary care settings in Asia, Africa, Europe, and the Americas report persistent pain in 10% to 25% of adults. Worldwide costs from all this pain total in the hundreds of billions per year. But the true costs of pain cannot be measured in money. Chronic pain, like most chronic illnesses, is a multifactorial, multidimensional condition that affects not just the body, but also the mind, the spirit, and the social environment.

Sometimes, a specific cause can be found and fixed. For acute disease, trauma, most infections, and an a few chronic diseases, a specific cure is possible. But for chronic pain and many chronic illnesses, there are no single cures. Bill spent fifteen years looking for a pain cure. What he needed was healing. He needed to become aware of those factors in this life that helped him feel better in general and get well. And he needed assistance in incorporating those into his life. He needed someone to help coach him in the process of self-care.

Most treatment approaches for chronic pain cannot be proven using the gold standard of research—the double-blind, randomized, placebo-controlled trial. Even when studied using this method, the contribution of proven therapies adds only a small amount (on average about 20%) to improvement compared to improvement that comes from meaning and context. The meaning factors produce the other 80% of improvement. Was the impact of the meaning response true for other chronic conditions? Was science missing the cause of improvement in areas other than pain?

Chapter 3

How Science Misses Healing

The science of the small and particular.

Is preventing two deaths from heart disease worth the cost to the ninety-eight people who will not get any benefit and the twenty people who will suffer major complications from a treatment? This is an ongoing debate in medicine about a real drug. To put the question bluntly: is preventing death in a few worth producing suffering in many? These are not easy questions to answer and are at their core not scientific questions. They are questions about values. Yet the way we do science obscures this discussion of values. Rarely are the details of the full risks and benefits of a treatment discussed with patients. Doctors and regulators just accept these questions as academic debates. And then plow through with their recommendations. Yet the uncertainty in bioscience is huge. If a patient is at high risk for heart disease, their likelihood of benefit outweighing harm goes up. If they are at low risk—like most of us—their likelihood of being more harmed than helped goes up. And we can't tell ahead of time which category a person falls into. This dilemma confronts us not because the science is bad; rather, it's because of the

40

way we do science—seeking specific effects for particular biological targets that contribute to a disease and then using this information to treat complex, whole people who respond only partially in ways we want, and frequently in ways we don't want. The problem, I discovered, is in the science of the small and particular. The very type of science that benefits us so well for acute disease now harms us when treating chronic disease. This is the consequence of a reductionist science that started with the invention of the microscope and continues with even smaller units of analysis, like single molecules in our genes. For all the power of this type of science, we have not appreciated the limitations and harm it also produces. In this chapter, I will explain how patients who found holistic paths to healing eviscerated my arrogance about the certainty of reductionist science and opened up my mind to discover how healing works.

AADI

Aadi had been tremor-free for more than a year—again. This was the third time he had been "cured." A prominent businessman from Bangalore, India, Aadi had built a highly successful export business that made him quite wealthy. But at age fifty he developed Parkinson's disease. Parkinson's is a chronic and progressive disease in which vital nerve cells in the brain malfunction and die. Over time, the Parkinson's sufferer is unable to control body movements. Aadi's disease progressed rapidly, striking fear in him as he experienced the increasingly severe tremors and rigidity. Darkness descended over his life. He could imagine, he told me when I interviewed him later, all he had built—his business, his family of five girls and one boy, his prominent home and community life—all crumbling before him. He had to "fix it," he said. So he channeled all the drive he had used to build his business into finding a cure. He made trips to the top Parkinson's specialty centers in New Delhi, Bangalore, London, and finally the United States. They confirmed the diagnosis, and he ended up on two drugs designed to boost the chemical dopamine in his brain, along with an antidepressant that he didn't like because he said it made it harder to think. These were all the therapies that have been proven to help in Parkinson's. But Aadi experienced only moderate benefit from the treatment, reducing but not stopping the tremors and doing little for his advancing rigidity and sunken mood. Since he had the means, he looked even wider for possible cures, but all he found were some experimental treatments, such as implanting dopamine-producing cells or electrical devices into his brain. He was desperate enough to consider these therapies.

His wife intervened at this point. Seeing how the disease was ruining her husband and destroying their family, she was desperate, too, but she took a different approach to finding a solution. "You are Indian," she would scold him. "You should go see an Ayurvedic doctor. It is the oldest medical system in the world—developed right here in this country. Why do you fly all over the world seeking a cure when the answer might be right under your nose?"

As a man stern in both business and family life, Aadi resisted. "I don't want that quackery," he said. He tried to ignore her. But he continued to deteriorate. So Aadi's wife visited a local Ayurvedic hospital to inquire if they could treat Parkinson's. They said they could help.

Ayurveda, a word that means "life-knowledge" in Sanskrit, is an ancient traditional Indian medical system—as Aadi's wife had said, one of the oldest medical systems in the world—and is still being practiced widely in India today. It is a prescientific system. Although its origins are likely more than five thousand years old, there has been very little research to verify its claims of healing. Like most traditional health care practices, it is widely used throughout India but less so by the educated and well-off like Aadi. It has been practiced on billions of people for thousands of years but has not been subjected to modern scientific evaluation. Aadi was skeptical when his wife suggested he try it, especially when the first step involved reading his astrological chart to help discern the "spiritual" forces contributing to his Parkinson's. Aadi did not believe in any of that stuff, but his wife continued to insist that he go to an Ayurvedic hospital outside Bangalore and at least try it for a month. After all, she pointed out, he had exhausted all other options and had only gotten worse. Reluctantly, he agreed. That was six years ago.

When I met Aadi, he was about to be discharged from the Ayurvedic hospital for the third time. The hospital is a large complex with rooms and buildings over a number of acres in rural India, about five hours from Bangalore. In addition to simple rooms for patients to stay in overnight, it has temples, massage rooms, group yoga rooms, a large herbal garden and manufacturing facility, and a bath house where hydrotherapy and oil treatments were administered. In the last six years, Aadi had come to the hospital three times, staying four to six weeks each time. The first time he went begrudgingly. The second time, skeptically. This time, enthusiastically. Each time he had walked out largely symptom-free; his tremors were 90% improved, his rigidity gone, his energy improved, and his mood lifted. After each visit he could again focus on his business and family. This time, he had spent five weeks at the Ayurvedic hospital engaging in daily intensive treatments that touched all aspects of his mind, body, and spirit.

Aadi told me that each time he visited the hospital, the treatments largely eliminated his symptoms. The first time, the improvement lasted almost two years. Gradually he had gotten busy and not returned to the doctor. He began to drop off the program of meditation, special diets, herbs, and oil massages that had been prescribed for him to follow. Slowly his symptoms returned. This time, he volunteered to come back for a "booster" treatment. Although he admitted that he was not cured—the tremor was not completely gone—nevertheless he was now fully functional and ready to return home. And he was off all other medications. "Magic," he said, with a smile and a shrug. He still didn't believe in magic, but he knew this worked.

Aadi let me examine him. A full neurological exam showed only a minor tremor that came out with certain tests, and minor dysfunction in his reflexes. Everything else was normal. Had I seen him in my office, I would not have diagnosed him with Parkinson's. Aadi said he went back to the Ayurvedic hospital every twelve to eighteen months for a month of intensive treatment. "What kind of treatment do they provide?" I asked. "Well," said Aadi, "you must ask Dr. Manu about that; he is the head doctor here. I do a lot of things, but most of it seems to be directed toward getting my head back on straight; helping me see what is important in life. In the business of my normal life when I forget who I really am, that is when I get sick. I come here to find out why I was born. They also do a lot of 'cleansing' of my body—with cathartics, oil massages, herbs, and things. I have stopped asking the details. I just know it works. Dr. Manu can explain it better, I am sure," he shrugged. "Go talk to him."

MANU

Dr. Manu Padimadi—or Dr. Manu, as they called him at the Ayurvedic hospital—is a tall, confident man. When he speaks to you, he looks at you intensely, as if he is peering into your soul. It is a bit unsettling. He had managed the hospital for seven years, after fourteen years of study. His father and grandfather had run the hospital before him. His English was an impeccable high British, which, I learned later, he perfected while studying chemistry and molecular biology at Oxford. I didn't know that the first time we met. I was at his hospital in southern India as part of my job as director of a WHO Collaborating Center for Traditional Medicine, seeking to further the scientific understanding of traditional healing systems like Ayurveda. Dr. Manu had set up a process for collecting data on Ayurvedic treatments and was eager to advance research on it. He explained the basic philosophy and approach of ayurveda to me. The primary goal of Ayurveda, he said, was to help the mind experience "universal consciousness." Once that was experienced, he explained, healing arises "because you have found your true self." Aadi, he said, had lost the purpose of his life, pursuing business at the expense of his family, his community, and even his own personal health and growth. Ayurveda began with a spiritual exploration for why he had fallen away from his divine purpose and then designed practices to help bring both his mind and body into better alignment with that purpose. It did this by evaluating the balance of a person's *doshas*. Doshas, Manu explained, are a combination of constitutional characteristics that define each individual. Made up of characteristics of body type and a person's mental and emotional nature, they serve as guides for "personalizing" each patient's path to wellness. In Ayurveda, he explained, there is no distinction between mind and body. Physiology and spiritual elements are all interacting parts of a whole person. In addition, the person needs to be "nudged" toward healing by using small stresses, such as cathartics and herbs. Slightly toxic substances were given infrequently. Fasting and exercise—especially yoga—were also part of the healing regime.

The goal of these treatments, Manu went on, was to "wake up" a person's inherent healing processes—to create mental and physical disturbances that, when applied in the context of life's purpose and direction, helped the person reorder himself or herself, become more whole, and heal. When people had the right elements around them to nourish their bodies, minds, and spirits, and those elements were stimulated to heal in this manner, he explained, patients recover and find new levels of balance and health. "Once wholeness is achieved, it can only be maintained if they continue to connect their actions—including their treatments—to the core meaning in their life," Manu said. "This is what increases the probability that they remain well." Profound stuff, I thought, but what did it mean in daily life?

Each morning, Aadi would get up early and go through a series of rituals and prayers to help him center and become more mindful. He was on a special diet, designed to help balance his dosha energy, and took various herbs and exercises designed to relax and cleanse the body and mind. Breathing and meditation, yoga and fasting were all part of the program. After a month of such a routine, his body would have come back into "balance" and heal itself. Aadi had experienced this now three times. And his Parkinson's had all but resolved each time.

While Dr. Manu's explanation of creating the right meaning and context made sense from my experiences with Norma, Bill, Sergeant Martin, and other patients, the description of doshas, the use of cathartics and small doses of toxins, and especially the role of astrology in guiding treatments seemed like superstition and nonsense. I told Dr. Manu that. Had any of these treatments been rigorously studied or proven in randomized, controlled trials? Had ayurvedic physicians shown that any of them actually caused the healing and recovery they claimed? Was there proof that doshas existed? Could they be measured and manipulated? We knew that Parkinson's disease was caused by low dopamine production in a specific part of the brain—the *substantia nigra*. Had any of the treatments been shown to increase dopamine in that part of the brain, I asked?

No, Manu admitted, they had not measured the production of dopamine in the brain produced by Ayurvedic treatments. He was open to that. In fact, he said, if there was a noninvasive way to track the biochemical markers of disease improvement for the conditions they treated, he imagined this would markedly help them improve and personalize this ancient system more—and make it more scientific. But, he warned, simply focusing on what produced a rise of dopamine in one area of the brain over a short period of time would be misguided. What was needed to properly study Ayurveda, he explained, was a research approach to monitoring the response of the whole person. More objective ways of tracking that response would be welcome as long as they were not used in ways that interfered with the ability of the whole person to respond as a complex, adaptive system. "Looking at only one small part of a person's disease and treating only that is harmful. First, do no harm," he said with a flash of irony, repeating part of the Hippocratic oath that all Western doctors repeat when they get their degrees.

I was skeptical and a bit annoyed to receive a lecture on the science and ethics of Western medicine from a non-Western doctor in the middle of rural India. Surely, I thought, some of what Aadi was being subjected to was harmful. I had seen studies of toxic heavy metals in Ayurvedic herbs and couldn't imagine how inducing diarrhea and vomiting with cathartics could be good for you. I pointed this out to him.

"Look," said Manu with a slight sigh, "forget the doshas and the astrology and the cathartics for a minute." He went to a whiteboard on the wall of his office and began drawing. "Every major healing system, including modern Western medicine, acknowledges that a person is more than just their body and biochemistry; that to truly treat the whole person, we must acknowledge that they are physical, social, mental, and spiritual." He drew a series of concentric circles on the whiteboard. "Well-being and healing arise when a person is both treated and experiences themselves as a whole person. Our job as physicians is to assist them to understand and make those connections—to find out what is deeply meaningful for them—and then nudge their body and mind with treatments to help them respond in a way that restores balance and wholeness."

MANU'S DRAWING OF THE AYURVEDIC MODEL OF A PERSON

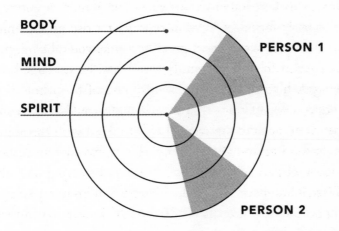

Manu drew a line from the outside circle—the one representing the body—down through the other layers of a person to the spiritual level and then back again. "When this connection is made, wholeness and healing happen. After all, the word *heal* comes from the Old English word *haelan*, from which we also get the words *whole* and *holy*."

I was again struck by the irony that an Indian doctor in an ancient healing center in rural India was giving me an English lesson.

"When Aadi leaves the hospital tomorrow," he continued, "he will leave experiencing that sense of wholeness, balance, and well-being. He will be 90% better in the symptoms of his Parkinson's disease also. Even if I could show you that one of the herbs he takes increases dopamine in the substantia nigra of his brain by 100%, I would still need to deliver that therapy within the context of his whole life to make it work well.

His challenge, when he leaves, will be to try and maintain meaning, wholeness, balance, and even holiness in his daily life and reinforce it with behaviors such as periodic fasting and yoga to keep those healing processes active."

XIAO AND MR. COUSINS

I had to admit that some of what Manu said made sense. We are not just bags of chemicals; at any rate, we cannot treat ourselves that way without causing harm. But Manu was proposing a universal process for healing, not requiring knowledge of the specific effect of a treatment on a biological mechanism or outcome. Whatever the explanation for Aadi's remarkable improvement, one thing was clear: he had tapped into it repeatedly, and he was much better than before he engaged in this ancient healing system. Although I was glad to see Aadi's improvement from an otherwise incurable disease, I was distressed at Manu's explanation of how it happened.

Clearly, Dr. Manu was well educated in Western science and medicine as well as ancient Ayurvedic practices. He was one of those rare individuals fully trained in two entirely different systems.

While Manu's explanation made intuitive sense, what bothered me was that I could find practically no evidence to support that his treatments improved Parkinson's disease. And that I could not accept. One of the hallmarks of good scientific evidence in medicine is being able to isolate and prove that a specific treatment produces a specific effect through a specific mechanism. If you looked at all the interventions and treatments Aadi underwent, there were no clinical studies or even basic science studies indicating that those treatments influenced the core biological problem in Parkinson's—the level of dopamine in the substantia nigra part of the brain. Instead, the treatments appeared to be for general wellness enhancement or to stress his system and induce a reactive response not specific to Parkinson's. A review of his interventions revealed that only one had been shown to produce dopamine in the brain. This was a dietary intervention using lentils as part of his meals. A small clinical study found that this food improved dopamine production, but not to a sufficient extent to explain Aadi's remarkable improvement. In addition, dopamine production can be produced by many things, including placebo interventions, as long as the patient expects them to work. There was no reason to think that the herb was any more effective than any other treatments Aadi had done, provided he believed—and the culture believed—that they were going to help him. From what I could tell, Aadi had gotten better because he had some basic health and wellness support (nutrition, exercise, rest), a physiological stress or two to get his system changing (fasting, cathartics, toxins), and manipulation of his belief by a bunch of placebos.

This pattern was not isolated to Ayurvedic. But how common was it? To find out, I set up a program to travel around the world and explore a variety of healing systems. As director of both a WHO Center for Traditional Medicine and the NIH Office of Alternative Medicine, I was specifically interested in examining these systems for their impact on patient outcomes and the scientific foundation they might have. The pattern I saw at the Ayurvedic clinic with Aadi turned out to be quite common within other systems, each of which had its own unique framework, set of interventions, explanations, and rituals. Yet all seemed to follow a basic pattern.

An example was a visit to the Great Wall Hospital outside of Beijing, China, which specializes in treating a disease called ankylosing spondylitis (AK). AK is a progressive autoimmune disease that causes erosion, fibrosis, sclerosis, and freezing of the joints, especially of the spine. It is a genetic disease that affects males more than females, reducing strong, energetic boys and men to invalids in a matter of a few years. In AK, there is a general weakening of the person with an increase in inflammation and pain and a decrease in motion and function. There are no effective treatments. Readers may recall seeing a story by the writer Norman Cousins, who claimed to have cured himself of ankylosing spondylitis with high doses of vitamin C and laughter therapy, neither of which had been proven to reverse the disease. At the Great Wall Hospital, they provided several treatments, but the primary one was a flat-needled microsurgery technique that broke up the fibrosis around the spine. The technique looked very painful, as long, flat acupuncture needles were placed along the spine and wiggled until they broke up the connective tissue. This "microsurgery" was repeated weekly, providing a rather strong nudge—more like a jolt—to the body from which it had to recover and repair itself. These microsurgeries were delivered, however, within a context very similar to what I had seen at Aadi's Ayurvedic Clinic. Families were present everywhere, providing food and care for the patients, supporting and encouraging them as they underwent the therapy. Physical manipulation called *tui na*—a type of body massage (very different from the massages Aadi had undergone)—was also provided. Daily exercise in the form of tai chi was prescribed, along with long periods of rest and sleep between treatments. The herbal medicines given were mixtures said to encourage a proper "balance of chi" or "life energy" and to calm the immune system after the needle treatments. All this was guided by determining how each patient's life energy was impacted by the environment, the seasons, his family, and the stars. Each of these factors was said to guide the chi and to reorder, balance, and heal the patient.

I remember following a young man of twenty-four named Xiao who had progressive and advancing AK. As an only boy in China's one-child policy system, he was prized and doted on by his entire extended family. Quite a gifted athlete, he had joined the track and field team at school and at one point was even being considered for the Olympic team in pole vaulting. But at eighteen-years-old he noticed an increasing pain in his pelvis and back. When heat and physical therapy did not help, his parents took him to the Beijing hospital. X-rays of the spine revealed the characteristic cloudiness of AK between spinal disks and the pelvis. A blood test confirmed that he had HLA-27, a gene associated with 25% of those with the disease—and usually the more severe type. By age twenty-four, Xiao had progressed further, now with more stiffness (called a bamboo spine in medical circles), fatigue, inflammation in the eye (also a rare symptom of AK), and some early cardiac symptoms. When we first met, Xiao joked, "I used to bend the pole in track and field—now I am the pole."

Xiao's mother saw my uncertainty in how to react to this statement.

Was he being sarcastic? She put me at ease. "Typical Xiao," she said with a smile, "always joking. Even with advancing disease, he has kept his humor."

"I was lucky to be born into this family," he would say. "I may not be able to vault my body any more to new heights, but I can still vault my spirit."

When Xiao first arrived at the Great Wall Hospital, his family said he was in a wheelchair and unable to walk. He could not turn from right to left or bend forward more than twenty degrees. He was totally dependent on their care. When I examined him, six weeks after he came to the Great Wall Hospital, he was up on his own feet and walking with a cane. He could now turn almost forty-five degrees from side to side. He said he was much better: happier, with more energy, and significantly less pain. He would be there about two more months undergoing other traditional Chinese medicine treatments. Dr. Yu Chen, the hospital director, told me that they got about 60% excellent improvement in patients with ankylosing spondylitis after one to three months of treatment. When I followed Xiao around, the parallels to other medical approaches that produced healing were uncanny: teams of caregivers, including doctors and family members, and specialists in spiritual therapy (Chinese medicine has no psychotherapy as we know it in the West, but uses astrology as in India). Special diets high in spices were prescribed, and combinations of Chinese herbs, some of which contained toxic materials (as do some Ayurvedic treatments), were given. And there was a lot of exercise in the form of tai chi, exposure to the natural environment, and rest and sleep. Xiao and his family were overjoyed at the improvement he had sustained. Dr. Chen said that about half the patients maintain these good effects for several years, but others regress. He had no data to back up any of his claims and had done no clinical trials to demonstrate that this overall procedure worked. A few of the spices and herbal products had been studied in the laboratory for their immune modulation ability, but none of them had been studied in clinical trials with AK patients.

After seeing Xiao I reflected on what Norman Cousins wrote about his own treatment of ankylosing spondylitis. Unable to find an integrative center in the United States, he essentially created his own treatment plan—visiting specialists at UCLA and "alternative" practitioners separately, and then putting together a general health enhancement program involving high-dose vitamin C and laughter over a period of several months. The laughter involved watching old comedy movies such as those of Charlie Chaplin, followed by significant rest and sleep. Strangely, it seemed that both Xiao and Norman Cousins came to laughter as a treatment for their disease. They had other things in common. Cousins was also surrounded by family and friends and mentioned the importance of immersing himself in a natural environment that induced calm—a relaxation response—during what was otherwise a very stressful time. Xiao would take daily walks and do his tai chi in the woods—often with one of his aunts or hospital friends.

Like the Great Wall Hospital's healing environment, the one Norman Cousins produced for himself also had no research to back it up. Subsequent studies of high-dose vitamin C demonstrated very small to negligible effects on the disease. Cousins didn't know it at the time, but when given at the doses he was taking, vitamin C is a toxin—an oxidant rather than an antioxidant—and so produced repeated stress on his body. As for laughter and the immune system, only a small amount of research had been done. Yet Cousins reported that with these treatments, he improved almost to the point of a complete cure.

HOW COMMON?

I wondered: how common is this pattern—support, stimulus, and belief—in healing? To find out, my team and I conducted a series of field investigations on a variety of practices in several countries. Our goal was to analyze what the practices did and what kind of results they were getting. We visited and performed in-depth evaluations of more than thirty centers around the world. And we saw this same pattern in all of them. Under the right conditions, results like that those experienced by Norma, Bill, Sergeant Martin, Aadi, Xiao, and Mr. Cousins were common. These centers and clinics often produced marked clinical effects. And like the others, they lacked scientific proof. We saw that healing was, in fact, possible and could be induced for many chronic diseases. But when we sought to isolate any one treatment component from the rest and measure its contribution on one outcome—as is required by good science to prove them—the effects diminished, disappeared, or at most contributed only 20% to 30% to a patient's improvement. The process and ritual of treatment produced the rest. Was this a common pattern when science was applied to healing no matter the treatment—be it herbs, diet, or drugs?

The more I deeply dove into the science, the weaker what I thought I knew from medical training became. I'd seen Norma, Bill, Sergeant Martin, and other patients flounder under my care, while I was using the best evidence—and then get markedly better after using nonscientific methods, despite my skepticism. Seeing patients like Aadi and Xiao, whose diseases are presumed to be incurable, resolve their symptoms using ancient systems of healing, based on no real science, caused my world to fray around the edges.

There was no good evidence that prayer or astrology, massage, cathartics, or herbs cured Parkinson's disease. Similarly, there was no scientific basis for the belief that needles and tai chi could cure ankylosing spondylitis, or that vitamins cured arthritis, or surgery reversed back pain, or oxygen treated brain injury. How widespread were these phenomena? How often did healing occur? How often did science miss it? And why? Was this simply from lack of research on healing treatments, or was there something in the way we tried to prove healing that interfered with our seeing it? It seemed that the secret to 80% of healing was right under my nose. But how could we test it if we could not even see it? Then I remembered Sarah.

SARAH

Sarah and her baby were not supposed to be in Germany. Her husband, an Army truck mechanic working for an engineering battalion, was on a one-year tour without family. But she came anyway. As a twenty-one-year-old, newly married and a new mother, she did not want to be away from him. So she moved to the town of Dexheim, Germany. I was the physician responsible for the military unit in Dexheim—a small American outpost. Sarah and her husband were both from Kansas, and now Sarah was depressed. This was not surprising, given her environment. She lived off post in a rundown apartment. She hadn't graduated from high school and didn't speak any German. She had a new baby. And she was far away from home. When her husband would come home from days in the field, he would often find the house in a mess and his wife sleeping or crying in her bed with the baby. They came to me for help.

I diagnosed Sarah with postpartum depression, began some counseling, and started her on an antidepressant medication, a type of medication called a selective serotonin reuptake inhibitor, or SSRI. About a month later, she came back in and said she had stopped the medication. Since starting it, she had lost all interest in sex or intimacy, which before the baby had been a major part of life for her and her husband. She was sure it was the medication, since the drop-off in interest had occurred right after she started taking it.

"Doctor," she said, "while my moods are somewhat better, it is making our marriage worse. My husband is understanding, but don't you have anything better?"

I doubted that her decrease in desire for intimacy was due to the medication. More likely, it was a continuing symptom of her postpartum depression. But to counter her opinion would be counterproductive. I asked them to come in together the following week so we could talk about it and I could do a bit more counseling.

Later that week, I was at a medical meeting and consulted one of my colleagues about what to do. The small clinic I ran was in a remote section of Germany, and German doctors did our emergency transport service when we had car accidents or drug overdoses on the post—something that happened about once a month. I spoke German from living in Germany as a child and knew many of the local doctors. On this occasion, I asked one of my closest German colleagues about Sarah's case. "Oh yes," he said, "I've seen many women like this—far from home and homesick. Young and without a social support network, they now have the full responsibilities of a baby and the demands of a husband."

This doctor suggested two things. "First, give her the homeopathic remedy *Gelsemium* and then add the herb *Hypericum*," he said. "Its common name is St. John's wort. It works just as well as the antidepressants, but doesn't have the side effects that you describe. Make sure you explain what it is for and what it should do."

I had never heard of these treatments. I went back to my office and looked for any research on them. *Gelsemium* was a homeopathic remedy that not been studied but, from what I could tell from its very low dose, had to be a placebo. The homeopathic books said it was good for homesickness and described cases similar to Sarah's—but with no testing or proof. St. John's wort, on the other hand, had been studied several times for depression and was slightly better than placebo in randomized controlled trials. It had a good safety profile.

It seemed that there was little downside to these treatments, so I made note of these two additional tools for when I met with Sarah and her husband.

Because her husband had described how their home was quite cluttered and dirty because of her depression, I suggested that we have someone come in and provide household help. I also asked if they would be willing to have someone come watch the baby a couple times a week so Sarah could go to events on the post; she agreed. I then told them about the two remedies that my German colleague had recommended.

I read to her the indications from the book about *Gelsemium* (good for homesickness) and translated the description of St. John's wort from a German flyer. It was "an ancient herb with a beautiful yellow flower— like a ray of sunshine in a plant." Not only did studies show that it lifted mood, but it would be less likely to produce a decline in sexual interest. After hearing that these didn't have the side effects Sarah thought were produced by the antidepressant, they both said, "Absolutely, Doc, we want to try that."

The two medications were not in the military pharmacy, so I told them to go to their local German apothecary to pick them up. I asked them to come back in three weeks.

When she returned, Sarah reported feeling much better. Her husband was out on another a field exercise, but she had not been crying as much and had gone to several of the women's support sessions on base. "I met another woman from Kansas," she said. "She grew up a couple hours from where I did. We meet for coffee now between the women's meetings. And get this," she said, with more animation than I had ever heard from her before. "She is three months pregnant!"

Sarah made a plan to clean up the house with a friend while her husband was gone. I asked her to continue the medicines and come back again in another three weeks, this time with her husband. Three weeks later—now six weeks after the change in environment and treatment— they came in, both smiling.

"Doc," said her husband, "that St. Germ's wort really works! She is feeling much better. Thank you so much."

I never found out how their love life was going, but I assumed a bit better. I followed them for another six months before they returned to the United States, and Sarah continued to do well and the baby began to thrive. I found out on one of the last visits before they left to go home that she had stopped taking both *Gelsemium* and St. John's wort but had continued to function and cope.

Certainly, something had helped Sarah. Perhaps it was the change in the physical environment in her house after someone came in to clean it. Perhaps it was the friend she had made. Perhaps it was because their sex life had improved. Perhaps it was the homeopathic *Gelsemium* (most likely a placebo) or the herb St. John's wort (a mild antidepressant). I wondered, though: was it really the St. John's wort? Her improvement was quite dramatic.

When I looked at the research literature, the evidence indicated that the herb did help with mild to moderate depression, but the effect was small—not much larger than what you'd see with placebo. Was it the herb, the friend, the clean house, or the presumed intimacy that healed her? Why had it worked when the drug did not?

ST. JOHN'S WORT

A few years later, I had the great fortune to test this question directly by helping to design and fund a large clinical study of the same herb and drug for depression that I had given Sarah. It was an unusual type of study, more rigorous than most drug tests. Normally, new drugs are tested in two-armed studies in which patients are randomly assigned to the active treatment (drug or herb, for example) or an identical-looking placebo. These types of clinical studies are expensive, so before a drug gets to such a test, a series of laboratory studies are usually done to show the drug is absorbed into the brain and affects the chemicals thought to be involved in depression. If these first studies are not done, a clinical study comparing a drug to placebo is usually not done. The scientific community was skeptical about St. John's wort's effectiveness because these types of preliminary studies either had not been done or did not show direct effects in the brain. While antidepressants could be explained because of the known effect they had on certain chemicals in the brain—SSRIs, for example, impacted a neurotransmitter called serotonin—there was no specific chemical in a sufficient amount in St. John's wort to affect any known brain chemical related to depression. The herb contained small amounts of several chemicals, and one in particular, called hypericin, seemed to impact the brain in a variety of ways, but the amounts of hypericin in the herb—including the amount I gave to Sarah—were too low to reasonably explain these effects. Most scientists in the United States thought the studies done in Germany, which were funded by the herbal companies who made them, were probably biased, and that the data showing benefit was wrong. Even though I offered to fund the study from my budget at the NIH, the other NIH institutes were hesitant to undertake the test.

Finally, Dr. Bob Temple, one of the most respected researchers at the FDA, had a solution. We should do a three-armed study in which patients were randomly assigned to the herb, a placebo, or a proven FDA-approved antidepressant drug: sertraline (brand name Zoloft), one of the SSRIs with a known mechanism of action and clinical effects, which I had prescribed for Sarah. With this design, the director of the

National Institute of Mental Health at NIH agreed to conduct the study. He had always wanted to have his institute run an independent drug study on depression (most were done by pharmaceutical companies), and a direct comparison with the herb and placebo had never been done. We found one of the most respected mental health researchers in the country to do it—Dr. Jonathan Davidson from Duke University. I had known Dr. Davidson for years. A wonderful psychiatrist, originally from England, he was not only a great researcher but also a compassionate and careful physician, the type of psychiatrist who listens carefully to you and spends the time needed to understand you. Like Dr. Manu, he possessed an unusual presence—a healing presence—and his British accent lent an air of sophistication and authority to any encounter.

Dr. Davidson carefully constructed a study designed to separate the placebo and his own healing effects from those of the herb and drug. However, when we approached the companies to supply the herbs and drug—standard procedure even for government-run studies—the drug company balked. They did not want to participate in the study. They made more than a billion dollars a year on the sale of sertraline. When I offered to make public their noncooperation, they relented and agreed to supply the drug. However, before the NIH study began they launched their own, two-armed study, comparing the herb to placebo—exactly the type of study not recommended by the FDA, because it did not have a positive (proven drug) control group. In that study, they selected patients who had worse depression than we planned to test—worse than Sarah had and worse than the subjects of the German studies. Those patients were less likely to respond to the herb. By spending a great deal of money, they sped the trial to completion in an attempt to beat the NIH and show that St. John's wort did not work. And they did, publishing a negative study—St. John's wort and placebo had equivalent effects—a full year before the NIH study was done. The conclusions of this study—that St. John's wort did not work—spread widely. Sales of the herb dropped.

Unlike the public, my colleagues held out for the results of the more rigorous, three-armed study by Dr. Davidson. His study picked the right types of patients; gave them the right doses; did proper blinding with placebo, so no one knew who was getting the herb, drug, or placebo; and included a large enough number of patients to rule out chance. What would it show? Would the herb beat the drug? Likely not, I thought. Would it beat placebo? It should. Would it have fewer side effects than the drug? If Sarah's experience was any indication, it would.

When the data was analyzed and they had broken the blinding code to see the effect in each group, I waited with anticipation. It had been nearly ten years since I had treated Sarah with both the drug and the herb, and it took three years to complete the study. My bet was that the drug and herb would work better than placebo but the herb would not work as well as the drug—but with fewer side effects.

Turns out I was wrong. All three groups—whether they were taking the herb, drug, or placebo—got better at the same rate. There was no difference in the rate or degree of improvement in depression. The herb and placebo had fewer side effects than the drug, however, confirming what I had seen with Sarah.

I was flummoxed. When the study was published in the prestigious *Journal of the American Medical Association* (*JAMA*), the news headlines around the world reported that a major NIH study had shown that St. John's wort did not work. Sales of the herb dropped further. What few people picked up on, however, was that *the proven drug had also not worked any better than placebo*. This was the most important finding of the study, and it was totally missed. The healing effect of the ritual—of just getting treated and seen in the placebo group—was as powerful as both the drug and the herb.

Knowing Dr. Davidson and his bedside manner, I was not surprised that many of the patients got better, including the ones on placebo. I had seen it in my own studies and with patients such as Norma. But the scientists and the public were so focused on whether the herb or drug added more than placebo—by even a small amount—that the actual reasons for healing were completely overlooked. Something about the way we were going about our science—always attempting to reduce it to the smallest, most specific focus—was causing us to miss out on healing.

THE DECLINE EFFECT

The publicity around the *JAMA*-reported study implied that drug treatment was more effective than St. John's wort, and it heightened the likelihood that the drug and not the herb would be prescribed by other physicians. I interpreted it quite differently—as did many of my FDA colleagues. To me, it was further evidence that something other than the agent produced healing. Previous research had demonstrated that between 70% and 80% of the improvement seen in clinical studies with both St. John's wort and antidepressants was also seen in those taking placebo. The single study by Dr. Davidson had simply confirmed this. And this, as it turns out, is more often the rule than the exception. The more rigorously one looks at almost any treatment, the smaller and smaller the effect size becomes compared to placebo; as the science gets better, the difference between placebo and the real treatment diminishes.

This is known as the "decline effect." We see it over and over again in clinical research. The more rigorous and larger a study, the smaller the actual contribution of the active treatment. Early studies, especially smaller pilot studies, frequently show large effects, which encourage physicians and patients to use the treatment. Usually those smaller studies are not enough for FDA approval or to be accepted by the mainstream community as standard of care; therefore, additional and larger studies follow. As those larger and more rigorous studies are done, the effects diminish. When you combine the results of those studies in a method called meta-analysis, frequently the effects became so small as to become irrelevant for use in practice.

What's more, the effects of even proven treatments frequently cannot be replicated by others when taken out of the hands of the original investigators. This "replicability problem" has been extensively reported by Dr. John Ioannidis, chair of the Department of Medicine at Stanford University, and others. In a startling analysis of clinical research published in the *Journal of the American Medical Association* in 2012, Ioannidis showed that only about one-third of proven results can be replicated. These were not just pilot studies, whose test treatments often show a decline effect in subsequent studies; these were failures at replications of established and proven therapies—like the antidepressant I had prescribed to Sarah. Soon, others began to look at research outside of clinical medicine and found that replicability was a general problem in science. Even laboratory and basic research—where we control many more factors than in clinical research—can be replicated only about 30% to 40% of the time. While the decline effect shows that initial findings often shrink or even disappear in the end, the replicability problem shows that even what are thought to be proven effects are usually not replicable. If someone else tries to repeat a study, often the effects of the active agent disappear. What is left are other nonspecific or unknown factors variously attributed to the "placebo effect." As I explain later, I prefer to call these effects—the component that hold the majority of healing—"the meaning effect."

THE DECLINE EFFECT

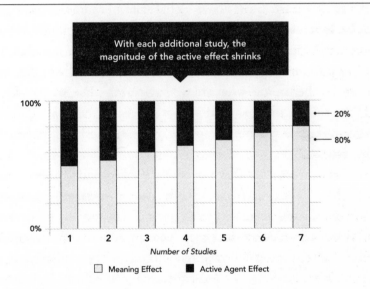

What helped Sarah and her husband was not the fact that the St. John's wort worked for her depression; rather, it was the way I delivered it and the ritual and social events that followed—an ordered house, making a friend, and intimacy—that nudged her out of depression and produced the healing. I couldn't say whether she got a lift in mood from the *Gelsemium*, the St. John's wort, or the sertraline, but I could say that the way she engaged in the treatment allowed her to get out of bed and become her own healing agent. As I had seen with other patients, the treatment context and the meaning response were more important than whether the specific treatment had been proven in rigorous research for her condition.

CERTAINTY FALLS APART

Depression is one of the most common and burdensome conditions in the world. It causes a lot of suffering. And it frequently accompanies other chronic diseases. Sarah had depression after her baby was born. Bill had depression because of his back pain. Sergeant Martin was depressed after his brain injury. Depression frequently accompanies Parkinson's disease. SSRIs have global sales of more than $11 billion a year. St. John's wort, even with all the negative publicity from the NIH studies, still tops $50 million a year in sales. But if more than 80% of improvement in depression from any treatment is from the way it is delivered—the ritual—what are we paying for when we pay for a drug or herb or other treatment? If we are not using the treatment in a way to maximize the meaning response, *we may be* mostly paying for *the side effects.*

Proven treatments that target specific molecular pathways and so create their intended effects, usually also have effects on unintended targets, producing unwanted side effects. Thus, the very treatments that work—those producing the benefit seen in 20% to 30% in randomized studies—also produce unwanted effects. Those unwanted effects frequently impact 50% to 70% of those who take them, including when the treatment did not work. In short: in complex systems like the human body, "specific" treatments have a higher probability of causing harm than good. Judging whether the harms are worth the benefits is the challenge in all of medicine.

STATIN SIDE EFFECTS

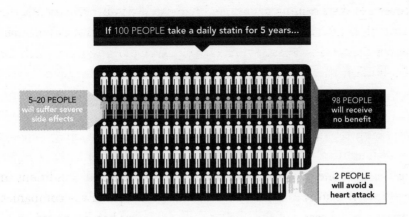

If 100 PEOPLE take a daily statin for 5 years...

5–20 PEOPLE will suffer severe side effects

98 PEOPLE will receive no benefit

2 PEOPLE will avoid a heart attack

The figure illustrates this for one of the most common and beneficial treatments we have for preventing the number-one killer in developed countries: heart disease. That treatment is statin drugs for reducing cholesterol. For every one hundred people who take a statin, two will have their potential death from a heart attack prevented, and ninety-eight will derive no benefit. Most of those same one hundred people will experience some type of side effect, and between five and twenty of those will experience a serious side effect, like major muscle pain or the development of type 2 diabetes.

Not only was my confidence in what I had been taught under threat, but the very scientific basis on which it rested was starting to look shaky. In his 2015 book, *The Laws of Medicine*, Pulitzer Prize–winning author Siddhartha Mukherjee says the laws of medicine "are really the laws of uncertainty, imprecision, and incompleteness. They apply equally to all disciplines of knowledge where these forces come into play. They are the laws of imperfection." He goes on to describe how attempts to apply rigorous science often fall short of giving us a good basis for decisions in health care. Even rigorously done experiments give us only probabilities or shifts in likelihood of benefit. And despite applying strict rules of research and critical thinking to science, decisions are still full of bias—statistical, clinical, linguistic, perceptual, regulatory, and financial bias—which can undermine our efforts at objectivity and certainty. What is more, only about one-third of what is published and "proven" using rigorous, experimental research can be replicated, leaving a two-thirds uncertainty for the gold standard—the best of the best of evidence.

Finally, the negative effects of those treatments for the whole person—with all of his or her complex reactions—are frequent, varied, and often poorly recognized. Layer upon layer of uncertainty began to pile on top of what I had based my whole medical career on, what I had taught to students, what I had used to treat patients. If only a small proportion of healing was from the treatments I dished out, and if most patients were getting side effects from those treatments, then was I throwing out most of the healing—and perhaps producing harm—by always looking for the small and particular effects? To make matters worse, this type of science is also being reinforced with money—lots of money—from companies seeking to get their products approved even when they might be doing more harm than good. Drugs get FDA-approved when they show their benefits go beyond placebo, even by a small amount. This requires very large and expensive studies. Proof now has to be purchased. A "real" treatment must separate itself from the daily processes of healing. It was patients like Aadi and Sergeant Martin who went beyond these rules of evidence and pointed me to the underlying rules of healing, prompting me to think there has to be a better way to heal.

Chapter 4

A Science for Healing

The science of the large and the whole.

Before science, we had only superstition or intuition to guide us to truth. Both were flawed when it came to healing. With science, we have approaches for testing our ideas in small ways and making incremental advancements in our understanding. Occasionally, these incremental advances result in a major impact—such as with the discovery of penicillin or vaccines. Before science, an epidemic was considered an act of God. After science, it became a containment challenge. We could now do more than pray. While science is a major improvement over superstition, it does not solve the uncertainty in healing. We sometimes lose sight of this. We think that by precisely defining and classifying disease, by rigorously measuring and instituting robust controls, we can determine the best treatments that will give us the most consistent results. And for many conditions this type of science does just that. When biomedical science works, it can work dramatically—especially when what ails us has a simple or a single cause—an infectious agent, a trauma, or a sudden anatomical manifestation of a chronic process, like during a heart attack. This is when the application of science in health care shines. We find miracle cures and produce magic bullets.

We save millions through the application of these discoveries in public health, and we keep individuals alive when they would have died on the battlefield or on the highway or at the end of their life.

We love those discoveries, and we get lured into using this type of science for everything, looking for the cure in an attempt to eliminate the disease we have named. We train our scientists and practitioners to look for those cures. We structure our health care system to look for those cures and treat all diseases and illnesses as if we have found the cures. We pay for these treatments, even when the benefit of the treatment is small, the risks large, and the harms poorly understood. We love this type of science—the science of the small and particular. We love it so much that we use it when we should not. Left to our own intuitive devices, we will pick an attempt to cure over healing or prevention almost all the time. Like the fox who sees a rabbit only when it moves and not the hundred others hiding in the grass, we too tend not to see what happens in our life until something changes. Most of life remains hidden in the background, unless we initially bring those elements into our vision.

Thus the science that successfully stops infections, treats trauma, and saves our lives from acute diseases doesn't work very well for chronic diseases. Not only does it not work well, but it can also mislead us and harm us—by giving us partial treatments for diseases and producing side effects that need to be managed. And by causing us to ignore simpler approaches that produce larger and more whole-person effects. This is why when we do apply a new discovery to chronic illness, we usually get only modest effects—on average about 20% to 30%. Yet there are health care systems and patients who get much better results than that. They have tapped into the other 70% to 80% of what is possible. There is nothing wrong with incremental science, but there is something wrong with the way we apply that science to healing.

WHOLE SYSTEMS SCIENCE

Imagine for a moment that all the chemical, energetic, psychological, and social exchanges of a person could be visualized as a web-like ball composed of millions of interactions occurring every second. When in optimal health, the ball is perfectly round and the interactions are occurring rapidly through a network of nodes or intersections in this web of interconnected links or pathways.

The primary goal of these interactions is to maintain the web-ball's shape—the smooth flow of interactions—even in the face of traumas from the outside and breakdowns in pathways on the inside. When the ball is resilient, whenever a stress or trauma is put on it, the ball rebounds to its established shape and function and so maintains its health and wholeness. This epitomizes resilience. The network of the web also has multiple redundant pathways internally with which to maintain the chemical, energetic, psychological, and social flows when any of the individual links slow or break. Strong pathways can compensate for the weakest links.

Each node and link in the web involves hundreds of thousands of interdependent interactions that create complex chemical and energetic exchanges—billions and billions of simultaneous interactions—all designed to keep us surviving, functioning, and flourishing within a narrow range. If flow and shape are maintained, we experience health. If they break down or are disturbed, we experience disease or illness. We experience these interactions in our life as physical sensations and responses, symptoms and dysfunctions, emotions and feelings, thoughts and perceptions, social interactions with others—and sometimes as connections to unknowable forces beyond ourselves, which give rise to spiritual feelings and insights.

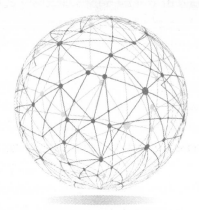

Whole Systems Science looks at the web of connections within our bodies.

When we are healthy and resilient, this web of interactions exists in dynamic balance and vibrancy. Think of a young child reaching out and playing with his environment; a growing preteen curious and learning about himself and the world; an athlete or an artist at the top of her game and in the zone. We have all seen it. We have all felt it. We have all been there. When we are a person experiencing love, appreciation, peace, joy, and awe and are fully connected in body, mind, social interactions, and spiritual purpose, we then have a taste of full health and well-being. We are in the state that our body and mind is constantly trying to maintain. That is health.

We are not just a sack of chemicals, however. If we open the ball and look inside, we see at least four dimensions that make up a whole person. Manu drew a version of a whole person with three dimensions on his whiteboard when he was explaining to me how Ayurveda approached Aadi and his Parkinson's treatment to me. Modern science has discovered similar (and additional) dimensions that we use for healing. If we were to cut into this web-ball-person, we would see that their network consists of a physical domain on the outside (I call that the body), a set of behaviors under that, a network of social and emotional interactions and then an "inner domain"—involving our thoughts, expectations, intentions, and personal experiences—what we call the mind or spirit.

If we deal with only one aspect of a person—say, the body or the mind parts—we get only partial results, and we produce reverberations (often unwanted) throughout the rest of the person. To fully heal and be well, we need to enhance connections across all four dimensions of a human—body, behavior, social, and spiritual. Healing works by making those connections stronger and inducing us to become more whole and responsive in the world.

THE WHOLE PERSON FROM THE PERSPECTIVE OF SYSTEMS SCIENCE

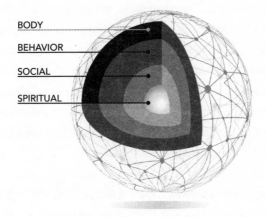

BODY
BEHAVIOR
SOCIAL
SPIRITUAL

Every person has an inherent, automatic set of processes that continually seeks to maintain balance and vibrancy across all these dimensions and maintain the integrity of the entire network. The goal of a whole systems approach is to keep this in balance when we are well (in medical terms this is called prevention); to return balance when we are thrown off (this is called recovery); and to grow, interact, and flourish even if we have a chronic disease. This latter state is often referred to as well-being and can happen even when we have an incurable disease or are at the end of life. We have all experienced this sense of wholeness, vibrancy, and balance, even if only for a moment. This is health and well-being. Healing is the process that constantly strives to keep us in this state if we are healthy, and seeks to restore us to it when we are hit by trauma, stress, or illness. In medicine this view is called the "biopsychosocial" or "whole person" model of health care, and the science used to study it is called "whole systems science." Whole systems science is the science of the large and the whole. It is the foundation for the future of health care. But you can use it now.

So what happens when things are not working properly and we cannot return to homeostasis? Chronic illness happens when something goes wrong with a person, such that their web of health and healing is distorted.

From the whole systems science perspective, disease is a distortion in the shape or in the web of pathways. When an outside disturbance like a stress or trauma occurs, symptoms are produced as the person attempts to rebound, repair itself, and restore order and harmony again. If the disturbance is from a single cause or event, such as an acute trauma or infection, removing that cause will allow the person to come back to harmony rapidly. As we saw in the last chapter, if the causes are multiple, as is usual in chronic illness, attempts to control or remove the main distortions may partially control the disease but usually produce only a small or modest response.

DISEASE DISTORTS THE WEB OF HEALTH, BREAKS DOWN CONNECTIONS & INFLAMES NODES

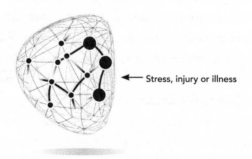

Stress, injury or illness

DISEASE-FOCUSED APPROACH

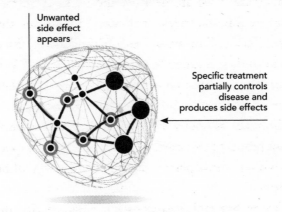

Unwanted
side effect
appears

Specific treatment
partially controls
disease and
produces side effects

A specific treatment is used to control the main disease manifestation. It may do that, but it also produces unwanted side effects in other areas of the body and mind. This is what happens when we apply only specific treatments—treatments derived from the science of the small and particular. It is also why so many of us end up on multiple drugs— each one designed to produce a specific effect. This is how we usually apply science when seeking cures.

THE MEANING RESPONSE

Whole systems science and the biopsychosocial model offer a different approach to healing. It's an approach that taps into this inherent capacity of a whole system to return to balance and maintain its integrity—and to produce the other 70% to 80% of healing. This approach stimulates and supports the person as a whole—connecting all four dimensions and nudging them to recover, rebalance, and restore the harmony that existed prior to the illness.

HEALING-FOCUSED APPROACH

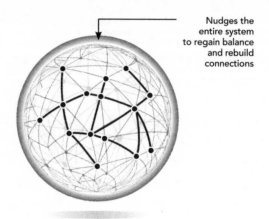

Nudges the entire system to regain balance and rebuild connections

I call how this type of healing happens the "meaning response." Why? The definition of "meaning" is "the intended significance of something: the gist, drift, trend, or purpose." But this word is a bit too cerebral for what actually happens during healing. The word "response" means a reaction to a stimulus, whether that stimulus is a physical environment, a change in behavior, a social interaction, a medical or spiritual ritual, or a word. By combining the word "meaning" with the word "response," we get closer to the dynamic nature of what my patients experienced and what well-delivered health care systems can produce. When the meaning response occurs, the whole person—not just one specific part of the person—is stimulated and supported to return to balance, health and well-being.

This is what my patients had discovered and taught me—though it went against my established knowledge and opinions at the time. Healing works through the meaning response by improving the connections across all the dimensions of a person—by stimulating their response in a meaningful way.

Given our complex, redundant web of pathways, each person's journey to induce their meaning response can follow a different path and may use different tools and modalities. Some enter their healing journey using pills and potions, like Norma did. Some may completely change the setting in which they live, like Aadi. Some may find their journey starts with a change in attitude, like Bill. Whatever human activity is used as the entry point—through the body/external, behavior/lifestyle, social/emotional, or spiritual/mental—the pathway and processes for releasing our inherent healing capacity are similar for everyone. First, a deeply meaningful experience is found—often by engaging in a ritual of care. This helps us find the unique, best, and most enduring path for each of us. Second, all the core dimensions of a person are acknowledged—body/external, behavior/lifestyle, social/emotional, and spiritual/mental. This supports complex healing processes to the full extent and helps us use as many redundant pathways as possible. Finally, we engage in some stimulus for healing—usually a stress or challenge—followed by removal of the stimulus, then rest, so that we can rebound and recover. Periodic repetition of this stimulus keeps our body and mind resilient and responsive and on a continuous healing path.

To help organize this when I work with patients, and to help you organize this in your own life, I define four dimensions of healing for a person—body/external, behavior/lifestyle, social/emotional, and spiritual/mental—within which there are many available approaches, tools, and agents. I then use three processes to activate those dimensions for healing: meaning, support, and stimulus. When a person is well and wants to keep well, or when a person is ill and wants to recover their health, or when a person is dying and wants to find well-being, their healing journey involves exploring these four dimensions and engaging in these three processes. When that happens, healing emerges spontaneously and order is restored—like a healthy child recovering from a cold or an athlete rebounding from an injury or an elder dying in peace.

Healing approaches using whole systems science are just beginning to be developed in health care. As with any emerging discipline, it currently goes by many names, including the biopsychosocial model, complexity science, systems biology, systems medicine, personalized medicine, and most recently precision medicine and precision health. The NIH has recently embraced whole systems science with its Precision Medicine Initiative (PMI). PMI performs ongoing data collection on more than a million people in most of the dimensions of human functioning—from genetics to epigenetics—including behavior, medical treatment, and social interactions. Once collected, this database will become a rich source of information for better application of whole systems science and the meaning response in health care.

In the meantime, there are already examples of the power of whole systems science being applied in health care. These also go by various names, such as person-centered care, systems wellness, scientific wellness, precision wellness, functional medicine, and integrative health care. (In the second section of this book, I describe some of these systems and how you can find and use them.)

The late Professor David D. Price, a prominent research psychologist at the NIH, and world-renowned Italian neuroscientist Professor Fabrizio Benedetti analyzed all the research on how meaning and context impact chronic diseases: diseases with pain, like Norma and Bill's; Parkinson's disease, like Aadi's; or depression, like Sarah's. They and others have shown that our brains can produce large amounts of painkillers, anti-Parkinson's neurotransmitters, anti-depression chemicals, and immune modulators—an internal pharmacy used by the meaning response to heal. These chemicals are induced in the brain through rituals and behaviors that not only influence our beliefs and expectations but also stimulate and condition our bodies to respond to those rituals and behaviors in physical ways. Often these rituals involve the use of therapeutic agents such as pills or potions, drugs or herbs, needles or knives; or sophisticated technologies such as implanted electrodes or cell transplants; or softer methods such as massages or physical therapy. From the whole systems perspective, when we set out to heal chronic diseases, the specific agent used is less important than how the treatment is administered; that is, how the ritual of healing is constructed and the meaning response is induced. Armed with an understanding from whole systems science and the power of the meaning response, I could now understand how the remarkable recoveries I had seen provided me and others with the tools and processes for making the same thing happen in others' lives. The mystery of healing—why it happens or does not—was revealed.

BACK TO NORMA

When Norma had gotten better so dramatically from her arthritis and depression as she started taking the pills in the clinical study, I first thought she was on the active treatment, meaning I had discovered a cure for arthritis. When I found out she was on the placebo pill, I then assumed that she had gotten better because I was a good healer and she was suggestible. Her recovery and well-being must have been because I was a good communicator, I thought: I had induced in her a belief that she could get well, reinforced that belief with the treatment, and persuaded her that she could get better. Surely I was a master of biopsychosocial healing.

One of the most influential books in medicine during the last fifty years is a book called *Persuasion and Healing*, by psychiatrist Jerome Frank. I had read the book in medical school, and it influenced me greatly. Dr. Frank demonstrated that any type of psychotherapy has some basic features that account for its effectiveness: an emotionally charged relationship (I was Norma's favorite doctor), a healing setting (the clinic and hospital I saw her in), and a rationale or myth explaining the symptoms and process for resolving them (my hypothesis was that the vitamin could cure arthritis).

Most doctors like to think when a patient gets better, it is because of their treatment and care. This is what keeps us going. It is self-satisfying to think that. But I soon found that the main explanation for Norma's improvement was not the vitamin I had given her nor my miraculous persuasion powers. Norma's recovery was a lot more mundane and less magical than that. When I revealed to Norma that she had been on the placebo, she was with her daughter. Her daughter told me that getting back to her volunteer job in the hospital was one of the most important things her mom wanted in her current stage of life. Before the study, she did not feel like going to the hospital and sat at home, remaining sedentary for long periods. This made her feel worse. Soon after starting the placebo, Norma began to tell herself she felt better and forced herself to start back at her volunteer job. Even before the treatment was supposed to kick in, her activity level increased. After she started taking the pills she began to go into the hospital regularly—at first once a week, then three times a week, then every day.

Now, we know that one of the most effective ways to prevent deterioration and even improve arthritis is to keep active. Exercise reduces pain, improves mood, and slows or reverses the decline from almost any illness—including arthritis and depression. It is one of those general healing nudges. Norma had an important purpose (her job at the hospital), and joining the study had linked that purpose to a behavior that stressed her body with exercise in a way that improved her pain and function and allowed her to nourish her soul with social contact. Her remarkable recovery had little to do with the vitamin or my powers of persuasion. It occurred because she used a compelling life purpose—meaning—to take her outside her physical comfort zone and stimulate her natural recovery capacity through exercise.

I also discovered that something else had helped induce an improvement. She was taking a pill four times a day.

Medical treatments in many systems involve taking pills and potions, whether they are drugs, herbs, vitamins, or over-the-counter liquids or tinctures. Taking a substance, especially if it is accompanied with a sense of feeling better, induces a "conditioned response" in which the act of doing something—especially something requiring a physical act or a substance with a unique smell or flavor—trains the body to respond in a way that reinforces the improvement. Like Pavlov's dogs, which were conditioned to salivate upon the ringing of a bell, we learn to heal upon the swallowing of a pill—including a placebo pill. Our conditioned stimulus (the event that triggers the response) can be almost anything: a pill or a shot, a taste or smell, a needle, a knife or a touch; even an energy stimulus like a light, a sound, or heat or cold. The conditioned stimulus is how our belief and meaning—the reason we seek healing—gets linked to a physical response in our body in a repeated and continuous way. Dr. Kaufman, who wrote the book on the use of niacinamide—the vitamin I was testing for arthritis—told me that it was very important that patients take frequent doses—a minimum of four times a day rather than using a more slowly absorbed version fewer times a day. His rationale was that the fluctuation of the vitamin in the blood was needed to reduce inflammation in the joints. This, as later studies showed, was not true. Still, he had tried time-released versions of the vitamin that were taken less often, and they didn't work as well, he said. But what he had likely stumbled upon was a universal principle of healing—frequent dosing improves healing through conditioning. In fact, for some conditions, if an effective treatment has the number of pills reduced from four pills a day to two pills a day, a physician has to treat as many as twelve additional patients with the less frequent dosing in order for one patient to benefit. Statisticians call this the "number needed to treat" (NNT). This happens in other diseases also. The effect is seen not just in "soft" outcomes like pain or depression; it even results in different death rates. Several studies have shown that patients with heart disease who take all their medication have a lower death rate than those who do not take all their medications—even when that "medication" is a placebo. Like Norma, they do better if they do it more often. Norma not only took four pills a day during the study, but she was also one of my most eager and compliant patients. At least, I thought, I could take some solace that by interacting with me she had pushed through her pain and gotten on a healing path. What actually happened is that Norma had activated her healing in each dimension of her being. She began to move more (body), she started taking more pills that both she and I believed in (behavior), she engaged with others in her volunteer work (social), and she re-established her purpose in life, which was to help others (spirit). Her healing was not from the agent she took; it was from her own agency she found.

Sergeant Martin found healing through a different path, but by using the same process of finding meaning, whole person support, and using a stimulus to heal.

NORMA'S PATH TO HEALING

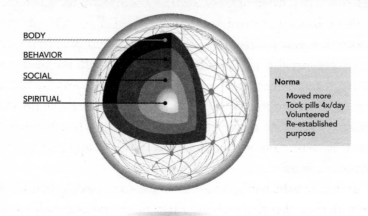

BODY
BEHAVIOR
SOCIAL
SPIRITUAL

Norma
Moved more
Took pills 4x/day
Volunteered
Re-established
purpose

BACK TO SERGEANT MARTIN

Sergeant Martin hated me. It had not always been that way. For over a year, he and I had worked together seeking the best treatment for his traumatic brain injury and PTSD by juggling various medications, counselors, and social workers. We even tried meditation and "exposure therapy"—the proven standard of care for PTSD in which a patient is gradually exposed to the very things that induce fear and nightmares in them until they learn not to react. He stopped after two sessions. "It was terrible," he confessed to me. "Why would I want to relive that memory again?" I was sorry to see him stop, because the science said that it worked. That is when I referred him to music therapy, and he learned about Beethoven's Ninth Symphony. The music therapist said there was something about that symphony that changed him. Perhaps he identified with the struggle the deaf Beethoven had in writing and performing it. Sergeant Martin listened to it repeatedly.

Soon after that, he and his father came in and insisted I refer him to hyperbaric oxygen treatments. It was my turn to draw the line. The science was clear—hyperbaric oxygen did not work. I wasn't going to recommend a "quack" therapy. Both Sergeant Martin and his father left my office angry. I think their last word to me was an expletive. I was pretty sure my powers of persuasion and empathy were not working with them. It was not my finest hour as a healer.

Almost a year later, when I bumped into Sergeant Martin in the hospital hallway, he was markedly better and off medications, but hesitant to talk with me. But I was truly curious as to how he had gotten so much better, and that convinced him to talk. I wondered: had Sergeant Martin also created the fundamentals of healing—meaning, support, and stimulus—with an ineffective therapy and against my recommendations?

"To tell you the truth, Doc," he finally confessed, "when I left your office with my father that day, I was at my wits' end and ready to give up. I mean, I was ready to give up on everything, including my life. I wanted to commit suicide. But my dad convinced me to go to the hyperbaric clinic and said he would pay for it. I felt bad about how he cursed at you, but what could I do? You had your shot with me for over a year."

I knew he was right. We had tried everything I knew to help him.

"When I got to the hyperbaric clinic," Sergeant Martin continued, "I felt I had come home. There were guys there just like me claiming that they were getting better with the oxygen treatment and putting their lives back together. It was the first time I felt hopeful—that I might be able to heal, to have a seminormal life."

What I immediately thought but did not dare voice to Sergeant Martin was that he had found something he believed in and a group to reinforce that belief. I listened instead. Sergeant Martin went on, "After my first oxygen session, I felt better. There was this rush in my ears and fresh air flowing into my lungs. When I left, my mind was clearer; I had more energy. I even mustered a small smile. And the improvements just kept on coming. Soon, I found that I was the one giving hope to other battle buddies coming in. Guys with brain injury and PTSD who came in hopeless. I told them to hang in there. Instead of me always telling my story, I found that I was listening to others tell theirs, and I could really listen now. I could help them."

Sergeant Martin went on to explain how the hyperbaric oxygen worked—an explanation that has been disproven. He explained to me that there were areas of his brain from the injury that could not effectively use oxygen, and when it was forced into his system under pressure, those brain areas "woke up" and began to function again. I say this has been disproven because good studies have shown that breathing even room air—without high oxygen—and at a low pressure also can also improve function. No more oxygen than usual was getting to the brain in those cases, but people got better anyway. In fact, other studies showed that small doses of ischemia—*low* oxygen—can also induce healing responses in the brain. It was the small physiological stress that stimulated healing. Professor Benedetti, whose research on placebo, pain, and performance I described previously, has demonstrated that many of the physiological and functional effects of 100% oxygen can be produced by room air in people working at high altitude when they collectively believe they are getting 100% oxygen and that they will benefit from it.

While Sergeant Martin believed in his own explanation—that more oxygen was penetrating his brain—what he was actually experiencing was a mild stressful stimulus to his body in a positive environment that, as happened to Norma, that conditioned him to improve. But unlike Norma, whose stimulus involved working through the pain of exercise because of an inert pill, Sergeant Martin got an abnormal physiological jolt of a mild toxin—high oxygen—that his body responded to by rallying a repair reaction. Getting high oxygen may seem counterintuitive. After all, isn't oxygen good for you? Sergeant Martin believed (and his practitioners said) that his brain was getting the oxygen it needed. However, the normal concentration of oxygen in the air and the amount the body is used to is about 20%. Oxygen at 100% delivered under high pressure (as Sergeant Martin received) is actually slightly toxic to the body. This induces the body to protect itself by increasing antioxidant production and other repair processes and accelerates healing. The same healing reaction can be induced with no increase in oxygen or even with low oxygen—or other stressors.

I will describe the ritual he did in more detail in a later chapter, but at this point I had learned that Sergeant Martin found, like Norma, a meaningful way to heal himself by helping other service members with brain injury and PTSD. While his condition and treatments were completely different from Norma's, the healing processes he used were the same. He had lined up a meaningful therapy he believed in, done it in a supportive environment, and used high oxygen as a physical stimulus to condition a recovery response that working with me had not.

BACK TO BILL

This world we live in is a relentless place. Often it seems that traumas and stresses come at us continuously, wearing us down, only to hit us with even more difficult ones. Sometimes, they seem to come all at once—a death of a loved one, loss of a job, a car accident, a serious disease. Other times, it is more like water torture—drip, drip, dripping small and continuous stresses that will not let up and have no end in sight. Regardless of which way life brings us traumas, no amount of treatment or therapy will wipe away suffering unless we also build our resilience and recovery capacity. There is no magic cure for suffering, but there is an ability to recover and be happy—if we are willing to walk the labyrinth of healing and use the tools at our disposal to help. Whole systems science and the meaning response teach us that we have a smorgasbord of healing options—proven and unproven—if we adhere to a few basic principles.

Bill showed me, more than any other patient, how to walk that labyrinth. Unlike Norma, Bill was not a believer in any treatment. Nor was I his favorite physician. Unlike Sergeant Martin, he was not antagonistic toward me. Nor was he looking for any particular type of therapy—alternative or conventional. Of course, he wanted the scientifically best treatments for his back pain, if possible, but even more than that, he just wanted to get better. He had tried so many milder treatments that he wanted something "stronger," as he put it. One might think that having a family member with strong beliefs—like his wife, with her belief in acupuncture, might strengthen one's personal beliefs and help with healing. But this is not always the case. Family members, like physicians, are often trying to "fix" a person with chronic illness—getting them to see the doctor, try new treatments, and change behaviors. This pressure can sometimes backfire, however, making the person resistant to those suggestions, or worse, when the treatments fail, reinforcing their despair that recovery from their illness is hopeless. Over the years, Bill had been to the best pain centers in the world—Walter Reed, Johns Hopkins, and veterans' hospitals. He had told his back pain history hundreds of times, and each time someone had tried to help him with one or more treatments. Gradually, as Bill told me when he came in for his pre-op evaluation, he needed something stronger because over the years, he had "become" his back pain. It dominated his life. Others helped reinforce that with all their treatments. He had finally stopped seeing doctors until his wife recommended acupuncture. But, like the other treatments, it had only a mild effect. Surgery was his best hope. He wanted to "cut out the pain," he said.

And it worked for a while. Bill got rapid relief from the surgery. It lasted nine months. Then it came back.

Why did it work? Why did it come back? Bill believed in surgery. So did his doctors. Modern cultures generally believe in surgery. It helped him to do what was most important and meaningful to him—to be with his grandkids. But back surgery of the type Bill had is actually not effective when tested in rigorous research—sham surgery works just as well. Still, surgery can be an excellent stimulus for self-healing. Like other treatments, it can work well when the components of healing—meaning, support, and stimulus—are aligned. However, unlike the four pills a day and regular exercise Norma did or the repeated oxygen and social reinforcement of Sergeant Martin, Bill could not repeat the stimulus. Surgery is usually done only once or twice.

It was after his relapse that Bill came back to see me, this time not to find another "fix," but to do the hard work of navigating the labyrinth of healing processes until he found the combination that helped him sustain self-healing. The journey was not quick, and, for Bill, it involved facing some deep traumas from his childhood that he unveiled during one of our visits after he started to keep a journal. As the meaning of who he was and why he was here began to help him connect his body to the emotional parts of himself, a deeper healing began. Once

Bill understood the connection between his childhood traumas and his bodily reactions he found it easier to do the things he needed to do to keep his back pain at bay—such as managing his sleep and alcohol use, doing regular exercise, stretching, and having periodic massage. Gradually he broke free of his addiction to cures and learned how to support and challenge himself to continually heal. True to his word, he documented his path, and spoke with me throughout the process so I could better understand how he found healing. One day during our discussions of his process, he came out with it bluntly. "Once I stopped seeking a single fix," he told me, "I realized that all these good-intentioned people and wonderful treatments were actually making me worse. When I decided to find out what I needed for a better life in general, that is the moment I began to really heal from my pain." Bill had become his own healing agent.

BACK TO AADI

Armed with the growing tools of whole systems science, I went back to India to explore if it could help me understand what was happening to Aadi and his Parkinson's disease. Did they align with the components of healing and the concepts of whole systems science I was discovering? I took a deep dive into the ancient medicine of Ayurveda with this new lens.

Like Bill, Aadi was not a religious or even very introspective man. His approach to everything was businesslike. He wanted to know what needed to be done and how to do it. Like Bill, problems were to be fixed when they arose so he could move on to the next one. The bottom line of life was the measurable advance in prosperity for him and his family. When Parkinson's disease struck, he approached it in a similar way. Here was something to be fixed too, and the doctors were ready to help him to do just that.

But when visits and treatments from the top doctors in the world did not allow him to get back to work, he grew despondent. That is when his wife visited the Ayurveda hospital and asked for an astrology reading for him. She felt that they needed to seek a deeper understanding for his illness and why the treatments were not working. Aadi thought it was ridiculous. He had no time for "pseudoscience," like astrology or prayer to the Hindu gods, in whom he had no belief. Like Bill, he agreed to go to the clinic to get his wife off his back. Anyway, he thought, it might give him some rest. That, he admitted, he needed.

Like me, Aadi was a bit startled to meet Dr. Manu for the first time, with his impeccable Oxford English and his knowledge of Western science. Dr. Manu said that there was no requirement for Aadi to believe in any of the treatments. "Ayurveda has been honed over thousands of years to produce a fundamental change in your mind and body," he said. "All that is required is that you go through the treatments for at least thirty days. Parkinson's is a serious and difficult problem, so each treatment is essential in restoring balance and recovery." Aadi agreed. He also liked the idea of having my team explore the possible biology of what he was doing.

But the evidence using the science of the small and particular was bleak. First, there was no evidence that the treatments and lifestyle changes Aadi undertook could help Parkinson's specifically. Although he did get some sleep, the process was not a picnic. Each morning he got up early and went to a prayer ceremony in which a Hindu priest went through a long series of chants and rituals. While Aadi did not believe in any of the gods to which they prayed, the rhythmic tone and repetitive motions produced a calming effect to start the day. Since no alcohol was allowed, he soon found his mind much clearer than at home. By the second week, he looked forward to this start of the day. In two weeks, the mental worries around his work and family began to fade. His sleep improved; he began spontaneously waking up early with a clear mind and more energy. Dr. Manu said that Ayurveda had a name for this mental state—*sattvic mind*. This mental state, he said, is one of the core goals of all Ayurvedic treatment and a foundation for healing. In the West, the closest term we have for this state is the *relaxation response*, coined by Dr. Herbert Benson at Harvard Medical School in the 1970s. Dr. Benson was one of the first scientists to study monks in India who meditated for many hours a day. In the 1960s, he measured the profound changes in their brains and bodies that resulted. Since then, he and others have shown mind-body practices that induce what he calls the relaxation response improves physiology, biochemistry, and genetics for a number of conditions. Eight weeks of mindfulness practice (a method to induce the relaxation response), for example, has been shown to grow areas of the brain that often shrink in Parkinson's disease.

Beyond that, however, the morning ceremony and other sattvic mind practices allowed Aadi to explore more deeply why he was so driven to succeed in business. He was the second of five children; his father had always praised his older brother for excelling in school and entrepreneurship, and he'd given him money to develop a small business. Aadi, who was four years younger, could never meet his father's expectations. So he had tried harder. Although he'd become a highly successful businessman, his father had died before seeing his success. Still, the pattern was set from a young age—keep your head down, work hard, compete, and grow wealth. Aadi realized by the end of his thirty days at the Ayurvedic hospital that he had internalized that drive, which often made him callous to others and even caused him to ignore the pain of many whom he loved—and any pain he felt himself. He began to think more about his family and what his life and legacy were about.

Had this been all the mental work Aadi did, it would have been little more than a type of psychotherapy. However, other practices were used to reinforce this relaxation and induce a physical response to the soul he was discovering. The goal was to deepen the meaning he found and embed it into his bodily response. The chief method for this was yoga and diet. One hour of yoga each day not only reinforced the relaxation response and improved circulation to all areas of Aadi's body but also strengthened his muscles and reduced his tremor and unsteadiness. It was not easy; in fact, it was at first downright stressful.

"I didn't like yoga," Aadi admitted. "I was never one to exercise, and this was hard. My muscles were sore the day after the sessions for the first fifteen days." What yoga was doing for Aadi was like what Norma's activity did for her—it introduced a mild traumatic stimulus that produced healing. Over thirty days, Aadi's mobility, strength, balance, and flexibility improved, and parts of the activity—primarily the ending—started to grow on him.

"I loved the ending of the yoga sessions," he said. "It is a posture called 'the corpse' in which you just lie still on your back with arms facing up. It was then that a flood of love would come to me. I would imagine my wife and children and all the affection I had for them and them for me. It was wonderful. I saw and felt what was really important to me."

Finally, his sattvic mind was linked to his body through an oil massage once a week. But the oil massage of Ayurveda is not like the spa treatments given in the West. Two masseurs, one on each side of the body, would rub his body with warm sesame oil in a coordinated and rhythmic pattern, infusing his body with oil and heating it. This was followed by running a small stream of warm oil over his forehead (a procedure called *shirodhara*) with the goal of inducing a sense of relaxation and mental clarity. I asked Manu about this seemingly strange practice.

"Both yoga and shirodhara are done for the same purpose," he said. "To cleanse the body and mind and to help link the understanding Aadi is getting from prayer and meditation to his body, so that both his spiritual and physical life are balanced and function as one."

I did not buy that explanation. When we looked at these and other practices Aadi received, we found the primary molecular changes they produced had nothing to do with cleansing. Instead, they all seemed geared toward inducing nonspecific changes in Aadi's psychological and physical healing responses through repeated mild stress and trauma, followed by deep relaxation during which repair occurred. This happened also with the diet and herbal treatments he underwent. The prayer was followed by a light breakfast, the yoga, a midday meal, and sometimes cathartics and enemas all geared toward "cleansing" as Manu explained. But the food served during his stay was very different than his normal fare. It was all vegetarian and high in curcumin, garlic, and other Indian spices. Fasting was also introduced. Once a week, he fasted for a full twenty-four hours, taking in only vegetable broth and water. Basically, Aadi was undergoing a controlled form of starvation. I was shocked. How could mild starvation help heal Parkinson's?

THE STIMULUS TO HEAL

While periodic starvation may sound harsh and not healing, studies show the exact opposite—when carefully done. Extensive research on large populations, as well as in controlled studies with animals and humans, shows that periodic low-calorie intake, whether through eating foods with lower caloric density (vegetables and fruits), fasting, or simply removing protein from the diet for short periods of time, rapidly stimulates a number of healing responses. Would short episodes of fasting and low protein intake, like those Aadi had been experiencing, increase biochemical mechanisms that preserve and repair damage produced by eating?

To find out, I asked Dr. Mark Mattson, a senior scientist at the National Institute of Aging, part of the NIH. He has been studying effects of diet and fasting on healing and aging for over thirty years. Dr. Mattson is one of the most cited scientists in the world. I asked him, "Could periodic fasting and low-calorie or low-protein intake, like Aadi went through, produce benefit?"

Dr. Mattson had a long and detailed answer, but the short version was a definite yes. Eating both nourishes and causes damage in the body. It supports and feeds the body with nutrients, and it stimulates oxidative and inflammatory processes that, over a lifetime, accelerate aging and damage organs. Refraining from food, or certain types of food, both helps heal some diseases and reduces the risk of chronic disease. Managing the dance between eating and not eating is key to healing and longevity. Periodic fasting (not prolonged starvation), according to Dr. Mattson and other brain researchers, enhances a whole soup of gene and biochemical factors associated with better health, lower disease, and longer life. It also improves mental function and lowers the risk for several diseases of aging, including diabetes, heart disease, brain decline, and cancer. Like exercise, Aadi's lower protein and calorie intake was a periodic stimulus to healing, which conditioned him into a regular pattern.

"The problem," Aadi readily admitted, "is that it was hard to keep up these behaviors once I left the hospital. Outside I relied more on supplements and herbs." But, he concluded, "they were not as powerful as what I got at the hospital. That is why I come back every year or so for a booster." Then he asked me, "So what did you find out about these treatments? Is there any science to them, or are they all just magic?"

They were not magic, but they were also not proven with the science of the small and particular. Were the potions and pills he was given specific treatments for Parkinson's disease? Not likely, I said, given what I had seen about both drug and herbal research for Parkinson's. But from a whole systems science perspective, the rationale of these treatments made a lot of sense. Most of the herbs Aadi was given had anti-inflammatory effects, as did the spices in his food. One, a powder from a tropical legume, *Mucuna pruriens*, had been studied for its effect on the level of L-dopamine in the brain, but the amount was too little to produce the magnitude of improvement he had experienced.

As I pieced together the various approaches Aadi underwent during his stay at the Ayurveda hospital, it became clear that the most likely explanation for his recovery involved the same factors that had healed Norma, Sergeant Martin, and Bill—just differently organized and in a different context. These had helped Aadi find meaning in his life, even though he did not believe in astrology or Hindu gods. The space and time to reflect, think, and talk; his improved sleep; and no alcohol all helped him gain insight and grow new brain cells. This helped him discover meaning and guide him toward recovery. He exercised more, and his nutrition improved with the plant-based diet and spices. More omega-3 and omega-6 fatty acids from the oil massage reduced the inflammation in his brain and nourished his neurons. The herbs and supplements increased his dopamine level—although mostly through the placebo effect from simply taking them. Finally, numerous methods for regularly stimulating a healing response with low-dose stressors were administered. Yoga, fasting, cathartics, massage, heat, and enemas were given rhythmically to keep up a steady response. From a whole systems perspective, these small challenges induce stress proteins and genes that our bodies use to repair and defend itself. These were the nudges to his whole system that induced healing.

The problem with the traditional systems is that the practitioners do not know if what they are doing is, in fact, properly dosed or delivered. While I discovered several healing approaches with factors that could enhance healing, the effects of these treatments were not measured or tracked, except for the patients' subjective reports. No modern science had been applied to them. Of course, that does not mean this science can't be done. Recently, a growing number of studies has looked at the intersection of whole systems science and traditional medical systems. An example of this growing intersection is a course taught at Harvard and the Massachusetts Institute of Technology by Dr. V. A. Shiva Ayyadurai, CEO of a systems science company called CytoSolve. The course examines the relationship of whole systems science and Ayurveda. Clinical verification of these concepts is also beginning. A 2016 study by researchers at the University of California, San Diego, examined more than fifty metabolic pathways altered by a six-day course of treatment using ayurveda approaches like those Aadi had received.

THE PRINCIPLES OF HEALING

In condition after condition, system after system, and person after person, I found three common factors that induced healing: (1) the rituals that helped a person have a meaningful experience, (2) the support of the whole person, and (3) the regular stimulation of a biological response. The specific treatments and agents used varied by person, culture, theory, and place, but the processes were the same. Whole systems science showed us that a person is an ecosystem—*more like a garden to be cultivated than a car to be fixed.* In systems science, the safest and greatest effects occur when the whole person is nudged toward a meaning response, using the universal need to maintain dynamic stability as the healing force. By taking advantage of this force, health and resilience emerge. Instead of manipulating our network nodes and attempting to produce specific effects (and side effects), we strengthen our network links and stimulate our own healing capacity in nonspecific ways to achieve a deeper and more lasting healing.

Healing emerges when we support and strengthen the connections within us—body, behavior, social, and spirit—making us more whole. Using the science of the large and the whole, we now understand that both healing and wholeness involve the same processes and that inducing a meaning response enables both.

Whole systems science, the biopsychosocial model, and the meaning response also allow us to personalize healing in precise ways using almost any agent or behavior. This understanding opens new worlds of opportunity. Treatments usually dismissed—because they do not fit the science of the small and particular—now become available for effective use in a new way. We know that both before and after a diagnosis, and between states of health and disease, there are health-promoting conditions and actions that can prevent, slow, or reverse chronic disease, strengthen overall health, improve function and quality of life, and enhance overall resilience and well-being. We can reduce suffering, regardless of a person's illness or stage of life, provided our behaviors are meaningful, they support and nourish us, and we challenge ourselves to respond.

This is how healing works.

SECTION 2

The Dimensions of Healing

Chapter 5

Coming Home

The place where you live can heal.

Our external physical environment affects our mind and body in ways that heal or hurt us. And that happens mostly outside our awareness. Sometimes, if we simply immerse ourselves in a healing environment, our body responds and we get better. Sometimes the environment is what is making us sick. Cultures around the world have systems to design a space and environment to impact the mind, body, spirit, and well-being. The Japanese tea garden is a well-known example of this. Other approaches include sacred geometry, healing design, feng shui, anthroposophical systems, and Ayurvedic systems. Until recently, modern health care has largely ignored the effect of space on health and well-being. Yet everyone can describe a place they have been where they feel whole and well. And some of us have spent time in "sick buildings."

The key to using the external environment to stay or get well is connecting the physical aspects of your life—the aspects you can see, smell, hear, and touch—with the inner aspects of you—the ones that give your life deep meaning and value. This involves paying attention to how your body and mind already respond to the space you are in, and then organizing the elements of your own healing environment to maintain and restore health. Create your own stage, so to speak, for the drama of healing to happen.

As I sat down to write this part of the book, my wife, Susan, and I were given the challenge of navigating this healing path again. She has given me permission to tell our story.

SUSAN

Our three-month-old grandchild discovered Susan's breast cancer. Well, the baby did not actually discover it, but it was because of him that Susan, who was helping take care of him, found the cancer. Cradled in her arms, the baby's head pressed against the area in her left breast where the cancer was, triggering her to notice the growth. For years, we had been looking forward to having a grandchild, and we were overjoyed when he came. However, his mother had complications after the birth and required some extra care, so my wife enthusiastically volunteered to help care for the baby as our daughter-in-law recovered. Susan loved the job, exhausting as it was, and would hold and carry the baby during the day and even part of the night.

"I think he must have bruised my breast," she told me one evening. "I have a small sore spot where his head presses. But it is not going away."

We both immediately suspected something more ominous. You see, Susan had had breast cancer before—twenty-five years before, and in the same location. She also had a personal and family history full of cancer. Her father had died at fifty-seven of lung cancer. Her paternal aunt and cousin had died at a young age from breast cancer.

This was also her fifth time with some type of cancer—breast, melanoma, basal cell, and squamous cell. Susan's first breast cancer had appeared when she was thirty-five. We had three young children. We cried for days that first time. Her father had suffered a lot as his lung cancer progressed, and we were only a few years out from that experience and his passing.

We had built a treatment and healing ritual that helped her to recover and be cancer-free for twenty-five years. Now, when the MRI and biopsy confirmed another cancer—a different type of breast cancer this time, likely induced by her treatments for the first one—we had a good idea of what we were up against.

The treatments—three types of chemotherapy, a bilateral mastectomy followed by antiestrogen drugs—were going to require that Susan tap deeply into her own capacity to heal, not so much from the disease as from the therapies. As is too often the case in health care today, healing is needed as much to recover from the treatments as to deal with the disease. We are in an age of heroic medicine where there is a thin line between the benefits and harms caused by treatment. This is especially true for cancer treatments. Dealing with the disease *and* the therapy requires resilience and the ability to recover. We needed to tap deeply into her healing capacity.

BABIES AND GRANDBABIES

You would think that the first thing someone would think about after being diagnosed with cancer is survival. And for most this is true. Almost all of medicine and biomedical science is thrown at that issue. Finding a cure for cancer is a constant mantra in medicine; it is what drives some of our most extreme treatments. Alleviating suffering tends to take a backseat. You can see it in the response people have when they hear the diagnosis, and you can hear it in the words our culture uses to fight it—the war on cancer, cut it out, burn it out, poison it, eliminate it, get rid of it, cancer is the enemy, victory over cancer. Oncologists focus on cure data, mostly by doing large studies to calculate the five- and ten-year survival rates under various treatments. You get cured only when the disease is gone—and gone for a long time. When a patient learns she has cancer, she seeks out anything that looks like a magic bullet—something proven to eliminate the disease. Many treatments have permanent effects that people must cope with for the rest of their lives. We usually accept those treatments even if the benefits are small and the side effects large (even when eliminating the tumor is not the most important thing for us). For Susan, the first thing on her mind was not a cure—it was the grandbaby.

It was not that Susan did not want to live long enough to enjoy the child and the family and have more life for other things. It was just that she realized life was more than a quantity; it was also a quality. Because she'd experienced cancer and its treatments before, she knew first-hand the lifelong impact of chemotherapy, radiation, and surgery. And her reasons for long-term survival are different now because all our children are grown and doing well. And she knows from experience the rather modest improvement that treatments make to survival rates. Twenty-five years ago, they did not know if chemotherapy for her type and stage of breast cancer was of any benefit. Now they can tell more precisely what it would add to her chances of living over the years. Whatever the reason for her perspective, the quality of the *now* became as important as the probability of a *later* for her.

None of the physicians asked what her main goals from treatment were. They assumed she would follow their recommendations to increase survival, even by a small margin, at almost any cost. They did not ask what was most important for Susan at this stage in her life. They did not ask if she wanted to weigh the harms of treatment against the potential gains. They did not know about the grandchild. Yet it was our grandchild who dominated many of Susan's decisions for what treatments she would undergo and when, and how she would organize her healing rituals. Without a word, our grandchild not only helped find the cancer but also was influencing its management. The dominating question for her became, how could she undergo the intensive treatments needed and also spend time caring for her grandchild? The path to this was not obvious.

TO CURE OR TO HEAL?

Susan and I have always been very different in our responses to her cancers. I, like most physicians, am a doer—always looking for something to add or manipulate in a person with the idea it will cure them. Susan is more of a be-er—weighing the value of these recommendations with her own values and desires. When faced with a challenge, my instinct is to do it all and look everywhere. If there's a hint of evidence for benefit, I like to try it out, provided the risks are not too great. My wife, on the other hand, is a minimalist; her attitude is "Tell me what I absolutely have to do and I'll do it grudgingly, folding up inside my shell and sleeping until it's over." Healing requires both responses, but not too much of either one. Most important, the response must be created by and meaningful for the person in need of the healing. The methods, whether trying out multiple treatments or holing up in bed, are all simply techniques for navigating the maze of responses when our health and life are threatened.

During her first breast cancer twenty-five years ago, the first thing she did instinctively was to reach out to friends and family and find support for her children as she underwent treatment. Fortunately, our children attended a school that was extremely nurturing to everyone in the family and took special attention to care for them during the process. Second, Susan had an older friend who became a surrogate grandmother and "adopted" us. A joyful and caring woman, she not only helped Susan through chemotherapy, surgery, and radiation, she nurtured the children as well. This support network (and Susan's age) allowed her to undergo intensive chemotherapy and recover rather rapidly, but not without some long-term residual problems including increased weight, early onset of menopause, some cognitive impact (called "chemo brain" in the medical literature), lymphedema, and mild damage to her nerves—peripheral neuropathy, which causes numbness and tingling in the fingers and toes.

Meanwhile, I was out looking for cures. At that time, I fully drank the biomedical Kool-Aid. I was convinced that science- and evidence-based treatments were out there for cancer. I read about and collected articles and books about cancer treatments. I talked to my colleagues to get their thoughts and recommendations. I urged Susan to do many of these treatments. Often, they were not available locally. She complied for a while as we traveled around and tried many of them—me looking for a magic bullet; she rather reluctantly. Most of those treatments turned out to be useless, and some even diminished the quality of her life—and mine. At the time, I did not understand about the decline effect whereby treatments initially look beneficial but further research demonstrates their limited impact. I was only beginning to understand the role of the meaning response in healing.

When Susan was diagnosed with breast cancer the second time, the first thing I explored was the possible benefit of her getting other types of therapies besides the conventional chemo and surgery. I considered supplements to prevent neuropathy and chemo brain, immune therapies to prevent recurrence, and lifestyle changes—exercise and diet— for overall health and recovery. But the evidence for most of these approaches was modest or nonexistent. In addition, the local oncologists had no expertise in these approaches; you had to travel to find them. Susan had promised and wanted to help our son and daughter-in-law take care of the baby. So running off to another part of the world to try other treatments and tests was simply out of the question. Even seeking out those treatments would remove from her one of the most meaningful activities she had in her life.

"We need to find something else," she told me, "close to home and just as good." We then found out that advances in breast cancer management would make that challenging in a different way.

In the last twenty-five years, there have been major advances in the management of breast cancer. These new approaches are guided by genetic testing. The nice thing about genetic tests is they can help tell what the survival benefit from chemotherapy will be for many patients—so they provide that therapy for only those it will help and avoid harming all the others. Susan had those tests and hoped she would not need chemotherapy. Unfortunately, her tests demonstrated that Susan was highly susceptible to a recurrence of the tumor. New chemotherapies like paclitaxel that hadn't existed twenty-five years before might be helpful to reduce that risk. The additional benefits of chemotherapy were modest, improving her ten-year survival chances by 7%—from 88% to 95%. Also, new and sophisticated imaging tests showed that she had atypical cells in her other breast that might become cancer in several years. *Might* was the operative word in this case. We had no idea whether that would happen. Between 30% and 50% of breast cancers detected by these new imaging methods will likely not advance to become problematic. We just don't know which patients those will be, so we treat them all as if they are at high risk. Genetic testing is helping us find out which patients may benefit from treatment and which patients the treatment may harm, but there is uncertainty for many. Still, none of this was known twenty-five years ago. For Susan, however, it soon became clear what she wanted to do. Chemotherapy would reduce her chances of recurrence by 7%. The genetic tests, the abnormal findings in her other breast, and her own personal and family history of previous cancers moved her to decide that the best approach for improving long-term survival involved several rather harsh treatments. She was at high risk for recurrence, so she decided to "hit it with all barrels"—twenty weeks of three types of chemotherapy followed by a double mastectomy followed by ten years of an antiestrogen drug. She would need to tap into her 80% healing capacity just to withstand the cure. The healing would be hard.

So would taking care of the baby. How was she going to undergo all these treatments, attempt the supplements and lifestyle changes I suggested, and be with the baby? These three seemingly incompatible forces converged on her. Navigating between her most meaningful activity—being with our grandchild—and the steamroller of medical treatments that might compromise both her short- and long-term function would be daunting. How could she find the right path toward healing?

Susan was now faced with a dilemma that many of those with chronic illness often confront: the clash of two systems with very different goals. Our cure-focused medical systems are by far the dominant force, populated with well-trained experts and bolstered by the best (but always uncertain) evidence that modern medical research money can buy. Rarely does this system spend the time or money to investigate or provide care for what the whole person needs for healing—their social and emotional situation; the strength of their physical, nutritional, and mental fitness; the lifestyle and behavioral resources available to help them heal; and the value and goals they have for a meaningful life. We have no integrative health system for the delivery of both curing and healing in cancer, for bringing together evidence-based medicine and person-centered care.

Susan and I discussed this dilemma as we sat in the preoperative suite waiting to have a vascular port inserted into her chest through which she would receive her weekly chemotherapy. She lay in bed dressed only in an operating gown, with the nurses, technicians, and physicians moving in and out. They checked the marks where they would open her neck to bury the tube running into the veins. The port would be used every week to draw blood and check her white blood cell count and to deliver the three chemotherapies. How, we wondered, could she be empowered to find a meaningful path forward under these circumstances? It was not obvious. Instead of deciding what to do, she paused in the now, meditated, and listened to her innermost self. She wanted to understand how her current disease and treatment might link to her soul. As they rolled her into the operating room, she heard a song over the intercom. It happened to be a song she had listened to the summer before while walking the Camino de Santiago (The Way to St. James) in France and Spain with our daughter. The song was "All of Me" by John Legend. Suddenly, the memory of that wonderful, spiritual walk came back to her and she felt deeply loved, not just by those around her, but by her own God—even in the midst of this difficult life challenge. She relaxed and released her worries about how to solve the dilemma she now faced. As she drifted off under anesthesia, she had a flash of insight. To embed meaning into her healing and integrate it with her cancer treatment, she would need a healing space in our home. We needed to redo our bedroom.

HEALING SPACES

It may seem strange that what emerges out of a sudden, almost spiritual insight as you are rolled into an operating room is that your bedroom needs to be changed. But this type of sudden and certain insight, which my wife had come to trust, turns out to be one of the best ways to discern a meaningful healing journey. I often work with patients to find ways to increase these insights—using practices like journaling, mindfulness, or dialogue—to help align evidence with intuition and curing with healing. While joy and intuition are important parts of a person—connecting to the emotional and spiritual dimensions—a full healing response must also connect to the external dimension of a person, the physical spaces that impact the body. The physical space is often a good place to start a healing journey. Physical spaces are easy to see and change. Almost everyone knows the calming effect of a beautiful vista, a sunny day, or the sound of flowing water. We have good scientific evidence that physical spaces influences healing for many chronic conditions. And there is a growing understanding of the mechanisms in our brain that do that.

Neuroscientist and immunologist Dr. Esther Sternberg spent thirty years at the NIH investigating the links between stress, stress management, our external environment, and our mental and physical health. She discovered that the physical environment directly impacts our ability to heal, independently of what goes on in that space. While Dr. Price and Professors Kaptchuk and Benedetti have been showing us how the rituals of health care affect our brain's ability to deal with pain, depression, Parkinson's, immune diseases, and other disorders, Dr. Sternberg is showing us how the space itself does the same thing. In her book, *Healing Spaces: The Science of Space and Well-Being*, she summarizes much of that research, demonstrating how the physical environment can trigger our "brain's internal pharmacies," making us sick or healing our ills. She and others have demonstrated that the brain is built to respond to the place we are in—directly, continuously, and unconsciously. The brain structure at the center of our response to space is the hippocampus—a part of the brain that is key to building memories. It also determines whether the physical location we are in is safe, telling us if we need to act to get safe or can relax where we are. It integrates signals from our sensory input—what we see, hear, and smell—to create a sense of place. It also sits near and continually communicates with another brain structure, the amygdala, which controls emotional arousal and response—often called the fight, flight, or freeze response. Thus the hippocampus creates a sensory impression of where we are and connects it to any emotionally laden memory that determines if we should respond or relax. Think of it as the GPS of the brain, which locates us not only in physical space but also in emotional space and puts the two together. This continual arousal or relaxation response produced by where we are signals other organs—including the heart, gut, and immune system—to be on alert or to engage in rest and repair. This happens mostly outside our conscious awareness. The hippocampus reacts to where we are and influences our mind-body response by comparing our space to memories that induce either fear or safety. Through this mechanism our physical space continuously puts our body on alert or into recovery mode, emitting a steady stream of chemicals that can hurt or heal. The place we are in is a powerful pathway to inner healing.

Until the science of this process was understood, the influence of the hospital environment on our internal healing capacity was largely ignored. Hospitals were built for physicians to deliver treatments. The hospital I did my training in was a typical example. Six floors of stacked rooms—usually two to four patients to a room—adjacent to a noisy road with no parking. Doctors had their own entrance in the back, and the emergency room entrance dominated the front of the building. Sirens blasted on and off day and night. Two wings of this concrete block formed the center of the hospital; it was built with little attention to light, noise, color, air flow, or nature. When the hospital needed to expand, other wings were added—usually through long corridors extending from the main lobby. After a few of these were added on, the place became a confusing web of hallways, often without clear markings for directing patients where to go. The larger the hospital became, the more confusing it became—and it had the ambiance of a warehouse rather than a healing environment. This was the typical hospital during most of the twentieth century. Then in 1984, environmental psychologist Roger Ulrich did a pioneering study called "The View from a Window." In that experiment, patients recovering from surgery were randomly assigned to either a room with a window view of a brick wall or a room with a window view of a grove of trees. To everyone's surprise, patients who had a tree view did better in all ways. They had less pain and used less pain medications, needed less nursing care, made fewer complaints about their care, and recovered more rapidly—leaving the hospital a whole day earlier than those looking at the brick wall.

Ulrich launched a research field exploring the effect of space on healing outcomes. So far this growing field has shown that:

- Single-bed rooms in hospitals can reduce infections; reduce falls; improve patient sleep; improve patient, family, and staff communication; and improve satisfaction with care.
- Natural light can reduce medical errors and length of stay; improve sleep, depression, and pain; help premature babies gain weight faster; and improve patient and family satisfaction.
- Exposure to nature can reduce pain, the stress of hospitalization, and the length of the patient's stay, and improve satisfaction.

Other space and environmental characteristics also impact health, including noise, ventilation, artwork, furniture arrangement, and the availability of family and private spaces. Recent research shows that the health care environment can save money, reduce employee turnover, and attract patients—all good for the bottom line. This research is now known as evidence-based design and optimal healing environments (OHE)—an area in which I have focused much of my own work (more on this shortly).

Most changes to create an OHE have been done in acute care. But when used for chronic illness, as done in many cultures over centuries, the impact of an OHE can bring about significant and sustained healing. Clara, a patient of a colleague of mine, used the external dimension to heal herself, when even the best of medicine could not.

CLARA

Clara had been a vibrant and loved teacher at a school for foster children in Baltimore. With three grown children of her own, and a supportive husband, she had retired from teaching to devote her time to community work in the city. All was going well in her life when she was struck by a mysterious illness. It started with fatigue and gradually progressed to muscle weakness and then muscle wasting. She lost an alarming amount of weight and became depressed. Her work in the community was important, but the disease progressed and forced her to give up the work and spend more and more time in bed. Even going to the kitchen to fix breakfast exhausted her. "What is happening to me?" she lamented.

With the help of her husband she began to look for a cure. She had access to and saw specialists throughout the country—at Johns Hopkins, Columbia, Harvard, Wisconsin, Stanford, and UCLA. Multiple hypotheses were entertained. She received multiple diagnoses and tried multiple treatments, some with reasonable evidence, some experimental. What was it? Chronic fatigue syndrome or myalgic encephalomyelitis? Autoimmune myositis? A prion disease? Multiple chemical sensitivity syndrome? Mitochondrial deficiency? Major depression? Psychosomatic disorder? Clara needed a name for her illness, but no one could give her one.

Her hair began to fall out. Soon she needed to hire someone to help her with basic activities of daily living—dressing, cleaning the house, and getting around. She then went to nutritional and alternative medicine doctors. They suggested other causes. Food allergy? Nutritional deficiency? Adrenal fatigue? Yeast overgrowth? Dysbiosis? Chi imbalance? Dosha imbalance? Soul loss? She got a lot of names— but no relief.

It was all the more puzzling because Clara seemed to already have all the elements of health and healing in her life—a supportive family and friends, a good diet, a nice home, and access to the best medical care, both conventional and complementary. Still, she could barely function. One day a friend was visiting and the conversation went from updates on events in the community to Clara's future. Instead of considering what else she could do, her friend asked Clara if there was a place she loved the most and felt happy and well. Clara immediately knew. "Well, yes," she said. "It is in the mountains. My husband and I have a small cabin up in New England. I love being there. It is deep in the woods on a small lake. The animals visit. The light and sounds change by the moment. The silence is wonderful. I can see the mountains from our back porch. The place restores my soul every time I go. But I have not been able to go for a long time because of my illness." There was a pause in the conversation as her friend just waited for her to continue.

In that moment, Clara knew what she was going to do. She had to go to the mountains. It would be difficult, as she could barely take care of herself. But her caregiver would go with her, and between her caregiver, her family, and her friends, she just might be able to stay for a while.

"But what about your doctors and therapy visits?" her friend asked. "What will happen to you if you give those up?"

Clara thought a moment. "I don't know." She took a deep breath. "All the diagnoses and treatments I have done so far have not helped. I think I need to take things into my own hands now." So, with assistance from friends and family, she traveled to her mountain cabin, determined to stay until she either recovered or died.

Her recovery began almost immediately. At first, all she wanted to do was sleep, day and night. "It was," she said later, "as if I was dead most of the time. Except that when I woke up, it was to the peace and silence, the clean water and the cold fresh air. It made me sleep deeper than I had in months. And when I was awake—oh, the beauty. I felt as if I was living in a Mary Oliver poem. I could open my windows and see the glowing green mountains, hear the nearby brook, feel the soft light of the moon at night. Everything changed by the minute. Animals, small and large, crossed my view. Rain and sun moved over me—alternating fire and water. The wind rippled through the trees. They seemed to be in constant prayer." Friends and an assistant helped her eat, bathe, dress, and go outside. For two weeks, other than beholding beauty, her physical condition did not change. And then it did.

It was not a sudden, miraculous improvement. It was slow and incremental, like the waxing and waning of the moon. A little different each day. A bit more energy. A bit less pain. After two more weeks, she was able to go out on the back porch herself. In four weeks, she could walk for thirty yards to the stream behind her house. In six weeks, she ventured into the local town—with help. In eight weeks, she went there on her own. Also on her own, she gradually reduced her medications. Her pain pills, her antidepressants, her steroids. She hoped she would not relapse when she did this—and she did not. After three months in the mountains, Clara woke up one morning, got out of bed, and fixed a cup of coffee before she realized that she had not yet thought of her illness. That is when she knew she was solidly on the path to recovery.

Other things in her life also came together during those three months: the realization that she truly loved her family and wanted to spend more time with them; a clear view of the toll that her sacrifice for others—first teaching and then community service—had taken on her; a deep appreciation for being able to physically move and exercise, which was something she had never liked before. She had a deeper love for her body, as flawed and dysfunctional as it often was. When she returned home, she found that taking care of herself emotionally, physically, and spiritually was no longer an annoying chore, but a privilege—no, a necessity—for her life.

Several years later, Clara confessed to me, "I don't know why I got sick. I had no more understanding of my illness than the doctors had. But I do know that I recovered by doing what I loved most. And in the process, I became more myself—more whole—than I had ever been before." It was a profound and meaningful change in place and space that started Clara on the path to that wholeness—and to healing.

OPTIMAL HEALING ENVIRONMENTS

"Since the beginning of humankind," writes architect Marc Schweitzer, who analyzed data on the effects of environmental design on health, "it is likely that people have been seeking safe shelter in which to heal."

Making simple changes in space can improve healing, function, and well-being inside and outside health care—in homes, worksites, and schools. Patients assigned to a room with a view recovered a full day faster after an operation, and two and a half days faster if hospitalized for mental health problems. Premature babies exposed to full-spectrum light that cycles like daylight gain weight faster than those exposed to continuous light—even though they have literally never seen the light of day. Students in classrooms with windows that open progressed 7% to 8% faster on standardized tests in one year than students in rooms with windows that could not be opened. Children allowed outside to play during school hours have fewer behavioral problems and do better in school, including on tests. Richard Louv, in his book *Last Child in the Woods*, summarizes the remarkable impact that exposure to nature (or lack of such exposure) has on children's health, functioning, and happiness. (The book is a must-read for parents and teachers.)

An increasing number of hospitals around the country are now becoming the OHEs I introduced earlier. Samueli Institute, the organization I directed for fifteen years, created a model to measure whether a health care setting was impacting healing, not just curing. We showed that specific architectural elements—including lighting and interior design—can reduce stress and anxiety, increase patient satisfaction, improve morale and performance of health care workers, and promote the health and healing of patients. OHEs don't just enhance well-being and improve clinical outcomes—they also save money.

Our definition of an OHE is a system and place designed to stimulate and support the inherent healing and wellness capacities of its inhabitants. In short, an OHE delivers healing-oriented practices and environments (HOPE) in a way that integrates them with medical disease treatments. I will show you how I use HOPE later, but for now, simply know that an OHE is a holistic organizing framework applicable to all health care organizations and health care systems. Consistent with its preventive and palliative role, it is also applicable in schools, worksites, and community locations. It is a way of connecting many models of care that share similar goals and philosophies—models such as relationship-centered care, patient-centered care, family-centered care, holistic care, integrative medicine, and the medical home, as well as worksite wellness and optimal learning environments. I briefly describe the OHE in the following section. More detail can be found on my website, DrWayneJonas.com.

THE FOUR DOMAINS OF AN OPTIMAL HEALING ENVIRONMENT

Note that these domains of an OHE parallel the dimensions of a whole person that Dr. Manu drew on his whiteboard in India (see page 46) and also those that whole systems science identified as elemental for how people remain healthy and recover when ill—body, behavior, social, and spiritual. There are four OHE domains as well—internal, interpersonal, behavioral, and external.

Internal Domain

HEALING INTENTION: This is a conscious determination to improve the health of another person or oneself. It incorporates the expectation of an improvement in well-being, the hope that a desired health goal can be achieved, the understanding of the personal meaning that is attached to illness and suffering, and the belief that healing and well-being will occur.

PERSONAL WHOLENESS: This is the experience of well-being that occurs when the body, mind, and spirit are congruent and harmonious. Personal wholeness can be developed and fostered with mind-body practices that reinforce wellness and recovery.

Interpersonal Domain

HEALING RELATIONSHIPS: These are the social and professional interactions that foster a sense of belonging, well-being, and coherence. Nurturing healing relationships is one of the most powerful ways to stimulate, support, and maintain wellness and recovery.

HEALING ORGANIZATIONS: An organization's structure and culture is important for implementing and maintaining an optimal healing environment. The vision and mission of an organization contributes to the development of a healing culture. A successful OHE organization also has a strategic plan for meeting goals, as well as leadership support, stable funding, and a flexible, resilient evaluative culture.

Behavioral Domain

HEALTHY LIFESTYLES: Healthy behaviors can enhance well-being and can prevent, treat, or even cure many diseases. Making appropriate dietary choices, engaging in physical exercise and relaxation activities, and managing addiction are important to lifelong health and wellness.

COLLABORATIVE MEDICINE: This is team-based care that is both person focused and family centered. It also includes thoughtfully blending the best of complementary therapies with conventional medicine.

External Domain

HEALING SPACES: These are built environments designed to optimize and improve the quality of care, outcomes, and experiences of patients and staff. Design components that foster wellness and recovery include evidence-based architectural design, color choices, and access to nature, music, art, and light.

When working with hospitals to use the OHE model, I often find it easiest to start with the external domain and then link it to the other domains. Many hospitals are now putting healing design into action. Next time you seek out a hospital or clinic or ask your insurance plan about coverage, ask if they provide or are becoming an OHE.

HOW TO BRING HEALING HOME

When I assist patients in discovering their own healing capacities, I always ask questions about where they live, work, learn, and play. Exploring these elements with patients helps them find and create the proper physical healing space—the space that their body dimension occupies.

While each of the elements in this bodily external dimension has evidence for its value, the purpose of exploring these is to find just a few—or even one—that is the most meaningful for them. We are seeking how to connect the external space they are in to the patient's inner space of mental, emotional, and spiritual response. Susan would change her bedroom to simplify and sooth her sleep and ease care for her grandchild. Clara changed her location to soak herself in nature. Both used the external environment as an entry point to induce a meaning response for them and pave their path to healing.

ELEMENTS OF THE BODY AND EXTERNAL DIMENSION

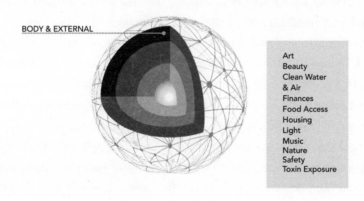

Many healing traditions pay attention to space. In my research group's global studies, we found traditions such as feng shui were used at the Great Wall Hospital for Xiao, and *sthapatya ved*, the ancient healing architecture of India, used at the ayurvedic hospital where Aadi was treated. In some Native American belief systems, "sacred geometry" assigns specific healing properties and meanings to each of the compass directions. Greek temples surrounded patients with nature, music, and art to restore harmony and promote healing. Florence Nightingale attributed differences in the survival rates of patients to differences in crowding, light, and ventilation. And unbeknownst to

Clara, she was engaging in an ancient Japanese practice called *shinrin-yoku,* or "forest bathing." Research has shown that immersing oneself in nature influences the body through more ways than simply the beauty and calm, as important as those are. Trees also emit chemicals called phytoncides that stimulate the immune system, something Clara likely needed. Being in nature also lowers cortisol and reduces heart rate and blood pressure. It increases our brains' natural painkillers. Phytoncides allowed Clara to rest more deeply and experience less pain.

Most people are so familiar with the places they live that they no longer take note of the details of the space or its impact on their lives. However, when I ask them to tell me the ideal environment that evokes a positive memory of joy, awe, or beauty—their ideal place—they can almost always tell me. Is there a window from which to gaze out at nature? What are the colors of the walls and furniture that they love the most? Is there clutter to step over or move aside to get past? What attracts them to a place? Are there elements of a place that allow them to look beyond a chaotic, disorganized space to an image that brings peace and a smile? Most people know their own healing space when they see or imagine it. It is easy to tell when someone realizes his or her healing space—the face lightens, the breath deepens, the muscles release. The signs of a healing response become evident in the person's posture and demeanor. My neuroscience mind sees my patient's hippocampus integrating sensory cues of the place the patient is in with the emotional cues that produce relaxing and joyful memories. The patient reacts as if she were settling into her mother's arms, like she has found a home. I then know she has connected her external environment to the inner dimensions of her life—social, emotional, mental, and spiritual—in a meaningful way. If she can make that a permanent space in her life, she more easily taps into the 80% of healing capacity that routine health care leaves largely untouched.

THE BEDROOM

When Susan came out of the operating room after her port placement, she knew how to solve her dilemma. She'd had an insight that she could use our bedroom as a healing sanctuary to recover from the chemotherapy and surgery and also to have a place where our grandson could be with her and play—with help, of course—during the most difficult times. She had never felt our bedroom had been a comfortable place to sleep—it was too cluttered inside and too open to the outside elements through a large French door and palladium window on one wall. And the colors were not right—too dark in some places and too bright in others. It did not feel like a calming, safe place to rest and bring a baby into. So of all the elements in her external dimension, it was the bedroom that Susan found most meaningful for her as she faced cancer and its treatment again.

The bedroom Susan created for herself was a simple, soothing place with natural light bathing the room in a soft, heavenly glow. A new and more comfortable bed was placed against our too exposing (for her) French doors. This allowed the light to penetrate the room indirectly from the top of the room. White opaque curtains were hung from ceiling to floor. The walls were painted a light blue-gray and kept bare except for a solitary painting placed on one wall—an abstract that almost blended into the wall. It looked like angels off in the distance emitting light—harmonizing with the feel of the room. It was painted by a good friend of hers, which further personalized its meaning. A small mobile of folded paper cranes (a Japanese symbol of healing she had come to love) hung from the ceiling. This too was personal—handmade by friends from the school her children had attended and where she had been chairman of the board after her first cancer.

The closet was expanded to eliminate clutter in the bedroom. Every piece of clothing, every shoe, every dress and sock now had a place. If it didn't have a place, she gave it away. A soft gray-and-white stool stood in the middle of the closet.

When the transformation was complete, I thought the room looked as if it was already part of heaven—glowing, ethereal, simple, uncluttered, peaceful—a picture of the world to come. "Just in case I don't end up in heaven if I die," she humored me one day, "I want to feel a little bit of it on earth now."

In the corner, Susan set up a small play area for the baby and some chairs where others could sit when her grandchild was in the room. As she began to take on the weekly onslaught of chemotherapy and then after that the surgery and other medications, she spent a lot of time in that room often feeling deathly ill, but now continuously healing by sleeping, reading, listening to music, visualizing herself in a better place, and being with the baby in a way that was safe for both of them. "Just being there felt close to God," she said, "and those I most loved, whether I was awake or asleep." She had created her own healing space.

More difficult, however, for Susan (and for most people) was the next dimension of healing—changing behavior and lifestyle.

Chapter 6

Acting Right

How behavior heals.

Seventy percent of chronic disease can be prevented or treated with a healthy lifestyle—by not smoking, consuming minimal alcohol, maintaining an improved diet, exercising, and minimizing stress. But which diet works best? A low-fat diet or low carbohydrates? Paleolithic or Mediterranean? Ornish or Atkins? With some alcohol or none? We were told for many years that we should not eat eggs or butter, but now they are okay. Coffee was bad; now it is good. Low fat was good, now it has caused the obesity epidemic. Exercise is good, but increases injuries. Stress is bad, but some stress builds resilience. It can all get rather confusing. Although there is general agreement on some harmful behaviors—smoking is definitely not good for your health, for example—science seems to flip-flop on the specifics of what is good for us. More important, even when we know what healthy behavior is, most people cannot embed those behaviors into their lives. Less than 5% of people engage in these top-five healthy behaviors. It may be good for you, but if you can't or won't do it, it won't do you any good.

What is the secret to the tapping into the 80% of our healing capacity through lifestyle? A patient named Maria taught me even as she learned it herself. The secret to healthy behavior is not willpower; it is something else.

MARIA

"I think we need to start you on insulin," I said to Maria about seven seconds into our visit. "The medicines we are using now are not controlling your diabetes."

I was not prepared for her reaction. "No," she said flatly, "I can't do that."

There was a fire in her voice I had never heard before. Maria had always been a pleasant and cooperative patient, accepting and using all of my recommendations.

"My father started insulin and then soon lost his legs! He went downhill from there and died. I can't do it! I won't do it. I am sorry, doctor." She burst into tears.

"But Maria"—I tried logic, even though it was clear that was not her operating mode at that moment—"it was the diabetes that caused your father's legs to be amputated, not the insulin."

She was not persuaded. "I am sorry, doctor. You are a good doctor. Can't you find me another way besides insulin? I will do anything. What about a special diet? I can go off sugar," she implored. "I can lose weight."

I was skeptical. Maria was from a large Mexican family—the first child of eight. Her mother and grandmother had been her role models for domestic care and order. Maria had married an American and moved away from Mexico, but she'd brought a lot of it with her. She had six children and had created a home of her own, of which she was proud. To say that food was a major part of her home was an understatement. She loved cooking. And her family loved her cooking. She prepared it with love and from scratch, every day, three times a day, seven days a week. Often the family would invite friends to the feasts and enjoy her marvelous meals. She did it because she grew up that way, she knew how, and it made her and others happy. Maria loved food and cooking.

Unfortunately, the food did not love her back—it had given her diabetes.

Maria had been overweight most of her life; she had had diabetes for seven years and was gradually getting worse. I had referred her to the dietitian—twice—with little effect. Would she really be able to stick to a diet? The Diabetes Prevention Study, just completed, demonstrated that lifestyle modification could prevent the progression of prediabetes to diabetes better than medication. But Maria had full-blown diabetes already, and in my opinion she needed insulin. I had her on the maximum doses of an antidiabetic drug called metformin. At the time, none of the newer antidiabetic medications, such as SGLT2 and DPP-4 inhibitors were available. Insulin was the recommended next step.

"Well," I said, unable to conceal my hesitancy, "there are some major dietary and lifestyle changes that might control your diabetes. But you don't have lot of time to show improvement. We could give it a month—two at the most."

Maria looked eager to hear more. So, with little hope and even less thought, I wrote down the names of two books that had reported rapid improvement in diabetes patients who use them. Both involved very low fat, no sugar, and an organic vegan diet. No meat, no processed or packaged foods, no added anything.

"See what you think of these," I said, "and come see me in about two weeks and we will see if these make sense for you."

Despite my lack of enthusiasm, Maria was overjoyed. "Thank you, doctor. I will cure my diabetes. You will see." She left with vigor in her step. *False hope*, I thought.

She didn't return for six weeks. I had just asked my nurse to give her a call and ask her to come back in when I saw her name on my schedule.

She looked much different. "I did it!" were the first words out of her mouth. "I cured my diabetes with your diet."

Maria had lost fifteen pounds, and a check of her short-term blood sugar was normal. I was still skeptical, but pleased. "That is great, Maria," I said. "Let's check your long-term sugar."

That too showed improvement. It was still abnormal, but better. I was impressed and a bit more hopeful.

"How are you feeling?" I asked.

"Just fine, doctor. Can I avoid insulin now?"

I agreed to have her continue and check back with me monthly. Each month we checked her weight and the long-term blood sugar marker called HbA1c. Over the next five months, her weight largely stayed the same, but her blood sugar remained stable and continued to improve. But something else was happening to her that I couldn't quite put my finger on. Her moods had changed. Instead of the cheerful, agreeable Maria I had known, she seemed sad. I wondered if something stressful was going on at home. Had someone died? Were she and her husband not getting along? It took a few more visits for her to finally tell me.

"Doctor," she said flatly, tears now running down her cheeks, "I didn't want to admit this, but I cannot do the diet anymore. At first it was okay—new and different. But over the last several months I have become very sad. My family hates the food I prepare now, so I cook two meals, one for me and one for them. But, frankly, I hate the food, too. We no longer have friends over for dinner. When my family visits from Mexico, they want someone else to cook. I have lost energy for the kitchen. I cannot care for them like this. I can't care for myself like this. I have failed. Put me on insulin. I will lose my legs and life rather than my family."

Now I had tears running down my cheeks. Maria sounded despondent. She had been so afraid of insulin and so determined to cure herself with the new diet that she had gutted her primary identity as a cook and homemaker. She was afraid to talk with me about it because she thought I would confirm that she had failed and put her on insulin—a death sentence in her mind. In the process, she had also likely reduced her fat intake so drastically that it was affecting her neurotransmitters and contributing to her mood problems. But the main problem was that she had tried to make a lifestyle change that she was not ready for, a change that removed joy from her family and her life. Like many who try to make a radical behavior change without linking it to the central purpose and meaning in their life, it could not be sustained.

"Maria," I said gently, "you have not failed. You have succeeded.

Your blood sugars are much better, and you don't need insulin. But for this to last, you will need to find a way to balance this diet change with your love for food and meals that you and your family have always had. Let's work together to figure out a way to do that." She agreed.

We also agreed to take up the conversation in full at another visit. But I actually hadn't the foggiest idea of how to help Maria. In the meantime, she would make herself and her family a wonderful Mexican meal to celebrate her success—and not worry about what was in it.

The next time I saw her, the old sparkle had returned in her eyes. Her blood sugar had also risen a bit. We would work out a plan with her that was better than the last one, I promised. I suspected it would require we bring in not just another dietician, but a chef to help her take her favorite recipes and make them healthier, and a health coach to help her move her goals forward in a more incremental and meaningful manner. I knew that part of Maria's improvement had to do with the lower sugar content in her diet. But part of the improvement was also the partial starvation she induced in herself by such a radical shift in protein and calories. Like Aadi, she had induced her body to begin healing through a physical stress response. But the process could not be maintained if it removed something so important in her life.

LIFESTYLE MEDICINE

Every year, nearly a million people in the United States die prematurely because of unhealthy behaviors. And chronic lifestyle-related diseases are rapidly becoming the major causes of death worldwide—and soon will surpass infectious disease and malnutrition. Behavior is the primary contributor to the six leading causes of death—heart disease, cancer, stroke, respiratory diseases, accidents, and diabetes. These collectively account for almost 75% of all deaths. And they are all largely preventable. Lifestyle also contributes to diseases of the brain, such as depression and Alzheimer's. Even more disturbing is a new trend: the recent increase in adult-onset (type 2) diabetes in children and teens, which is caused by obesity, lack of exercise, and environmental toxicity. The behaviors that can prevent these premature deaths and diseases are fairly simple—no tobacco and minimal alcohol and drug use; maintenance of proper weight; consumption of nutritious, unprocessed food; clean air and water; physical activity; social support; and good stress management. Most people know this. Shelves of popular books are written about this. Multiple national scientific bodies make recommendations on this. Governments try to regulate behavior for this. Yet despite these efforts, less than 5% of people engage in all of these basic behaviors. And, in an ironic alignment of numbers, less than 5% of medical funding is spent on primary prevention—supporting efforts to help people make these behavior changes. We get what we pay for. Willpower is not the solution to this dilemma. Maria had great willpower yet ran into common social and personal obstacles to using behavior as a path to healing. When left to our own devices, often we can't do what's necessary—or we do it wrong.

Behavioral change is difficult for us, not because we are "weak," but because we are unaware of how our environments and experiences— the health care system, our culture, our past personal history, and the media—are influencing us. When we have this awareness, we can create personal environments where healing behavior easily occurs. We do not have to struggle. We can create a new reality, as one of my other patients showed me.

JEFF

Jeff's dad had died short of age sixty-five of a massive heart attack. Jeff, also a smoker, worried this would happen to him, and he hated the coughing and the smell and the cost of his smoking, but he just could not stop. He had tried nicotine patches, smoking cessation classes, vaping, hypnosis, and acupuncture, but nothing worked for more than a few weeks. He was chemically and psychologically addicted. Then he asked me for help. We did a healing-oriented evaluation (a HOPE assessment, which I will describe later), during which I asked him questions about the dimensions of healing in his life—his external environment, his behavior, his relationships, and his inner life. Surprisingly, what emerged from our discussion was the idea of running. He enjoyed running for short distances; it made him feel better, and he loved both being outdoors and the rhythmic, almost meditative movement; he even liked the soreness he felt after a workout. He had played basketball in high school but hadn't been to the gym since he graduated. Despite liking running, he had never run more than one mile at a time. "I don't think I could do more than that," he noted. "Especially since I started smoking."

If Maria had been a ten on the "I can do it" scale, Jeff fell closer to a one or a two.

I heard about a program that offered marathon training for people who had never run before. I suggested that he stop worrying about trying to quit smoking and sign up for this program instead.

"I can't do a marathon, doctor," he scoffed. "I can barely run a mile." But he agreed to check out the program anyway. Neither of us expected what followed.

At the first meeting of the group, the leader asked people to take off their watches and pedometers and just follow him on a short, easy run. They could stop any time during the run and walk instead, if they wanted. They set off at a moderate pace and ran a flat or downhill route.

Jeff had no problem with the run. In fact, he loved it, especially running with others, which he had not done before. When they stopped, he was shocked to learn that he had just run four miles, something he thought he was incapable of doing. He had broken through a mental barrier.

Over the next few weeks, he started making friends with his fellow runners, enjoying both the social contact, being outdoors, and the discipline of the training. He also noticed that he was smoking less and less, even though he had not made any conscious decision to quit. He was simply not craving cigarettes so much anymore. He was craving running instead.

There are biological explanations for Jeff's response. When you smoke, your body is stimulated to produce neurotransmitters such as dopamine, serotonin, and norepinephrine. These transmit messages to receptors in your brain that make you feel good—just as a nicotine high does. This is the reward that smokers are addicted to. When the nicotine is removed, they feel bad. But other behaviors, such as vigorous exercise, switch on some of the same brain receptors stimulated by nicotine. Many runners, myself included, experience this feeling as a runner's high. By stimulating his brain's reward system with running, Jeff was simply substituting running for cigarettes to satisfy his brain's craving and to get the reward. By the time he ran his first half marathon a year later, he had not smoked a cigarette in three months. Rather than futile battles to overcome a negative addiction—smoking—Jeff had a new ritual that became a positive addiction—a healthy one. This method of change can work for many behaviors and negative addictions, including overeating, alcohol, and drugs, by developing a healthy behavior in a manner that feels equally rewarding. A year later, he was still running—and not smoking.

Jeff did that successfully. Maria did not. She and I still needed to figure out how changes in her food behavior could become more rewarding. We had to connect her behavior change more deeply to what she valued in life.

THE PLACEBO LIFESTYLE

Even healthy behaviors can produce both benefits and harms, depending on how we view them and use them. Maria's healthy diet improved her diabetes but harmed her mental well-being and family life. Current biomedical science attempts to tease out what produces the benefit of specific behavior changes by using the science of the small and particular. This type of science approaches behavior, such as eating, as it does drugs, herbs, and other treatments. We examine the content of certain diets and try and separate out the effects of their content—low or high fat, low or high carbohydrate, low or high protein, and so on. We dissect different types of exercise, such as running, walking, swimming, weight lifting, yoga, tai chi, or gardening. When we investigate methods for stress management, we scrutinize various approaches, such as meditation, visualization, music, mindfulness, biofeedback, and intentional breathing. This is all well and good, except that the more rigorously we do these studies—with better controls, larger sample sizes, more accurate measurement methods—the smaller the effect from the specific behavior is—just like with drugs and herbs.

However, there is a different path to such knowledge, especially when we want to put that knowledge into action in a whole person. Whole systems science helps us understand how to use behavior to maximally stimulate our internal healing capacity and minimize the harms. We saw in chapter 4 (see page 87) how the work of Dr. Mark Mattson of the NIH and others showed that fasting and episodic calorie reduction produced a general reparative and healing response—leading to improved function and longer life. Aadi, Xiao, and Maria were all using dietary manipulations similar to fasting to stimulate healing. Other behaviors can be used in a similar fashion. Exercise, for example, stresses the body—especially the heart, lungs, and muscles. It produces inflammation and generates oxidative damage. In addition, it causes small micro traumas in our muscles, which our body repairs during rest. Provided it is not overdone (yes, you can get too much exercise), these stresses and physical microtraumas become small stimulants to healing that induce our whole system to repair itself and keep us in good health. This is largely how exercise maintains health and increases healing. This is the same mechanism that stimulated Norma to function better with less pain from her arthritis, helped Aadi to improve his brain function, and allowed Bill to finally ease his back pain. Dr. Jordan D. Metzl, author of *The Exercise Cure*, has summarized much of the research on physical movement and health and provides a step-by-step approach to improving the time you spend moving, even if you have never purposely exercised. Research shows that even small and incremental steps toward greater movement are beneficial for most people. Only at the extreme athlete level do negative effects begin to appear. The type of exercise matters very little.

This happens with mental exercise also. Differences in the effects of various stress management approaches are minor compared to the general goal of inducing a relaxation response. For more than fifty years, Harvard's Professor Herbert Benson, author of *The Relaxation*

Response, demonstrated that almost any type of relaxation inducer—prayer, meditation, rhythmic breathing, visualization, or biofeedback—can rapidly reverse the more than five hundred genes that are turned on by stress. In addition, those who regularly practice a relaxation method have better long-term health, recover faster from health challenges, and use fewer medical services.

Was the specific content of the food Maria switched to in order to lose weight and control her diabetes the most important part of her improvement? While the emerging evidence currently points to a Mediterranean-type diet as good for overall health, it appears that simply changing our eating patterns to almost any whole-food approach provides the most benefit. In a large network meta-analysis published in 2014 in the journal *JAMA Internal Medicine*, researchers compared all the major diets being used for weight loss—Ornish, Atkins, paleo, Mediterranean, Weight Watchers, high carbohydrate, high fat, and others. While the high-fat diets worked better for weight loss in the short term, in the long run (after a year) all diets were equally effective. How much of the benefit that we get from healthy behaviors comes from the specific behavior we adopt? Is much of it actually—like the benefit from taking a drug, herb, or other treatment—more like a placebo effect, derived from the context and meaning of a behavior?

As you can imagine, it is a bit challenging to create a placebo behavior. Bill and Aadi knew they were doing yoga, and Maria knew she had changed her diet—those are hard to fake. However, researchers have developed ways to improve the rigor of studies on behavior by producing "placebo lifestyle" approaches and modifying the expectation of benefit from a behavior. These studies have found that much of the improvement from behavior change is produced by what people *think* about the behavior they adopt. Professor Alia Crum of Stanford University has been studying this idea of mind-set as a determining factor.

One ingenious study was set up to evaluate the role of mind-set on the benefits of exercise for health. Everyone believes that exercise is good for health—and it is. But is the benefit from the exercise itself or from the belief and meaning we give to it? That was Professor Crum's question, and she devised this study. Hotel workers who clean rooms all day get a lot of exercise—making beds, cleaning bathrooms, as well as vacuuming and hauling stuff—a workout every day. It should be good for them. The researchers divided a group of these hotel workers into two groups. One group was instructed about the health benefits of activity from the work they did. They were given specific information on how their work activity helped their health. The other half was not instructed in any health benefits associated with their work activity. After one month, the researchers asked the groups about their perceived workload and the management about their actual workload. The researchers also did health measures such as weight, blood pressure, and body mass index. On average both groups did about the same amount of daily work activity—each worker cleaning fifteen rooms. However, the group who knew details about the health benefits from their activities and thought they were getting good exercise showed significantly more health improvement than the group who did not have that knowledge. This included improvements in objective measures, such as decreases in weight, blood pressure, body fat, waist-to-hip ratio, and body mass index. It seems that, as with drug effects, what we know and believe about exercise contributes significantly to its health benefits, well beyond the actual exercise itself! A significant part of the "exercise cure," then, is the meaning response.

Does this happen with food, too? We know that how a drug or herb treatment is labeled has a major influence on its psychological and physiological effect. Pairing a smell or taste with substances that produce biological effects enhances those effects through a process called "conditioning"—remember the impact of Norma taking her placebo pills four times a day compared to two times a day? The very act of doing something with the intention of benefit produced an effect. We know that the social environment and learning from others further enhances this process—remember Sergeant Martin and his hyperbaric oxygen group all getting the oxygen together and reinforcing its positive effects with each other? Eating combines all these factors. Think about how you have eaten all your life. Every meal is infused with your belief in its relative health value (or lack thereof); you get daily conditioning of that belief from its smell and taste; and, most of the time you get social reinforcement of that belief from what and how you prepare and eat together with family and friends. Are the health benefits of eating, something you do several times a day, also influenced by the meaning response? Professor Crum also investigated this question by examining the impact of food labeling on our hormone responses. In an experiment called "Mind over Milkshakes," she examined whether the nutritional label and information about food produced biological effects. One milkshake was called Sensishake; the label said it had no fat, no sugar, and only 140 calories, and was "guilt-free." It seemed very sensible from a health point of view. A second shake was called Indulgence; the label said it contained 640 calories of combined fat and sugar— and delivered the "decadence you deserve." In truth, both shakes had 300 calories and the same nutritional content. Before and after people drank one shake or the other, they had their level of a hormone called ghrelin measured. The ghrelin level rises when you are hungry and drops when you are satiated and don't feel like eating any more. It also slows metabolism, so more calories are stored as fat rather than burned. The study found that ghrelin levels dropped three times more when people drank the "indulgent" shake compared to the "sensible" shake. When people thought they had eaten a heavy, calorie-laden food, their bodies responded as if they had. As in drug studies, most of the effect was due to the belief combined with the ritual around the food—not what was in the food itself. Almost all nutritional science tells us what is healthy or not—based on examining the content of what we eat rather that the process of eating itself. This dilemma contributes to the confusing claims.

Does this mean the content of our diet does not matter? Of course not. Lots of research shows it does. However, how much it matters and the health response generated by food content are markedly influenced by the meaning we attach—individually and culturally—to what we eat. Professor José Ordovás, a senior scientist and director of the Nutrition and Genomic Laboratory at Tufts University in Boston, has studied the effects of the Mediterranean diet on genetic factors related to health. He studies what cultures are eating and measures how those food patterns trigger gene changes related to health and disease. While your doctor may measure your cholesterol and blood sugar and recommend diet changes based on these, Professor Ordovás studies how those factors are influenced by the food-gene interactions that are precursors for them and explain much of what your doctor measures—using the very tools of whole systems science. During his Mediterranean diet research, he noticed there are practically no situations in which the food—healthy or otherwise—is ingested in isolation. Most of the people in countries where the Mediterranean diet is consumed prepare and partake of that food in family and community groups—usually in an atmosphere of friendship, fellowship, and love—like Maria did with her family and friends. When Ordovás measured the gene expression (in the urine) attributed to the Mediterranean diet during the meal preparation, he found that many of the gene expression changes attributed to the health benefits of the food were turned on before a single bite was taken. Eating does not just involve taking in a bunch of chemicals—it is a meaningful social and personal behavior solidified around the "agent" of food. The meaning infused into that behavior influences our bodies—from genes to hormones to cholesterol to our weight. So to help Maria, we had to link her healthier behavior around food to its association with her family and the joy it produced in her life. We needed to use food to induce a meaning response.

HEALTHY BEHAVIOR

While there is scientific evidence for the value of each of the elements I explore with patients to help them find and create healthy behavior, I discuss them with patients not in order to tell them what to do, but for them to find just a few—even one or two—that are the most meaningful for them. Jeff used exercise to stop smoking because he loved to run and be outdoors. He used this love to create a positive addiction to replace smoking. Maria used food to facilitate the cure of her diabetes, but in a way that did not bring her joy. Jeff linked his behavior to meaning, which allowed it to penetrate deeper into this life. Maria simply tried to comply with a dietary change that helped her body but created side effects. Both used the behavioral dimension as an entry point on their path to health and healing. Both did the behavior; however, only Jeff induced a meaning response. Maria did not, even though she seemed to have more willpower.

In most major health systems around the world—both ancient and modern—lifestyle is a cornerstone of disease treatment as well as disease prevention. In ancient China, for example, the head of each family paid the doctor only if everyone in the family remained healthy. When someone became ill, the doctor received no money until the patient recovered. (Think how that would go over in today's managed care!) The system used lifestyle (diet, exercise, exposure to nature, and energy "chi" balance) for both prevention and treatment. It applied the same practices and principles at different intensities depending on whether they were meant to maintain health or restore it.

ELEMENTS OF THE BEHAVIOUR AND LIFESTYLE DIMENSION

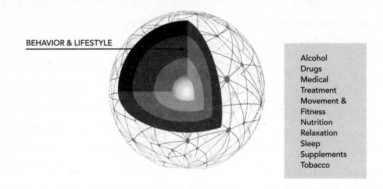

BEHAVIOR & LIFESTYLE

Alcohol
Drugs
Medical
Treatment
Movement &
Fitness
Nutrition
Relaxation
Sleep
Supplements
Tobacco

In the equally ancient Ayurvedic system of India, we saw how Aadi's Parkinson's disease was treated with a personalized regimen of diet, yoga, prayer, meditation, and oil-based massage customized to his body type and emotional makeup. These same approaches were used outside the hospital to prevent the disease's return. Both these medical systems are at least five thousand years old. In another part of the world, in the fourth century BCE, Hippocrates, the pathfinder and inspiration for modern Western medicine, declared that food is the best medicine. The ancient Greek health center of Epidaurus provided gardening for teaching nutrition, sport and exercise to regain physical fitness, theater to work out social and mental health issues, and hot and cold baths to cleanse and stimulate the body to promote healing. Prevention and treatment used the same tools and processes. It was one system. But modern biomedicine has split these goals—prevention and treatment—and developed very different ways to accomplish them.

MINDING THE GAP

In health care today, we have two very different health systems and a gap between them. One system focuses on acute problems such as injury, heart attack, stroke, and infection; the other emphasizes prevention and health promotion through activities like vaccinations, sanitation, and lifestyle changes—like smoking cessation, improved nutrition, exercise, and stress management. The two systems operate in virtual isolation from each other, as if they were in separate buildings—and in most communities, they usually are. What happens, for example, when you have a heart attack? You are rushed by ambulance to a hospital, where elaborate and expensive medical resources are mobilized to help you: a fully equipped emergency room, surgeons, anesthesiologists, nurses, imaging technicians with their machines, and an operating room filled with a dazzling array of medical technology, just to begin. Then, when you have been stabilized with angioplasty, a stent to open up a clogged blood vessel, or surgical removal of a blood clot, you are moved to a hospital room, where nurses, orderlies, technicians and health aides, support staff, and the billing office tend to your needs. All this happens under the supervision of an attending physician, and if you are in a teaching hospital, residents, interns, and medical students join in as well.

After treatment, you need a calm, peaceful environment in which your body can recover from the medical assault. Instead, machines, staff conversations, and loud announcements over the paging system surround you. You are awaked in the middle of the night, stuck with needles to draw blood, and have devices attached to measure your vital signs. If you're in the intensive care unit, these machines are a constant presence, with blinking and beeping readouts on display—blood pressure cuff, finger clip to monitor oxygen levels, electrodes, and maybe a catheter. You are given meals high in sodium, animal fat, and refined carbohydrates like white bread or white rice. And when you are out of acute danger, depleted by the ordeal, you are sent home, usually as soon as possible, with minimal home care planning and often without anyone talking to you about the lifestyle that caused your heart attack in the first place. Once you have been labeled with a disease and have crossed the diagnostic threshold to enter the world of acute care, an entire industry awaits you. Everything in this "building" of the medical system is based on the acute care model of health: namely, that there is a single cause for disease. If an artery is blocked, open it up. If cholesterol or blood pressure is too high, lower it with medication. If you have mild to moderate depression, prescribe mood-elevating drugs. The detailed manipulation of the body by this system is impressive—and expensive.

By contrast, the other "building" in the modern health care focuses on prevention of disease. Here, health care practitioners and public health specialists try to educate you about ways to modify your lifestyle through diet, exercise, stress management, and smoking cessation to address the underlying causes of disease and prevent problems from developing. They supplement your milk and bread with vitamins; your water with chlorine and fluoride; and, repeatedly urge you to eat better, stop smoking, exercise, and, oh, see your doctor for checkups. With a few exceptions, there is still a huge gap between the systems that prevent disease and the systems that treat disease, because they operate from completely different health models.

So, the first step in creating a personal environment that promotes healing behavior is awareness of this gap and exploring ways to fill it in your life. If you find yourself crossing the diagnostic threshold into the acute care system, you can ask your doctor to help you bridge the gap between prevention and treatment by giving you information on and assistance in finding a health behavior change meaningful for you.

Armed with this information, you can then find lifestyle changes that will prevent future problems. At the end of this book, I give you specific tools to help you in that conversation with your doctor.

You must be persistent in finding this help within the medical system, however. Although primary care, like family practice, is supposed to help fill the gap, payment for primary care is still based mostly on the episodic visit in an acute care system, with minimal coverage for prevention, lifestyle, and healing. So even those tasked with bridging the gap usually cannot. Remember, only 5% of the measured expenditures in our health care systems target lifestyle treatments, health promotion, and prevention. And 95% is spent on treatment of acute disease with nonlifestyle approaches, so don't expect the medical industry to do this very well for you. When it comes to bridging this gap between prevention and healing, the situation is changing, but it is nonmedical organizations such as companies and even the military that are leading the way. An example of that is Total Force Fitness in the U.S. military.

TOTAL FORCE FITNESS

One of my assignments in the U.S. Army was to develop ways to close the gap between prevention and health promotion and treatment. The military realized that very often behavior could both prevent and treat disease, and they wanted to help close this gap for service members and their families. In 1991, the Army Surgeon General launched a massive health promotion and prevention program on all Army posts. I was its medical advisor. Every soldier was to get a Health Risk Appraisal Assessment (HRAA). The HRAA screened all soldiers for their lifestyle habits and risk factors, such as smoking, high-fat diet, alcohol use, exercise, and stress. It measured physical health factors such as cholesterol, blood pressure, blood sugar, weight, and percent of body fat. It explored each person's stress management and mental health issues. The HRAA eventually replaced the annual physical, which had been around for over a century and was shown to be largely useless.

Armed with this new information, each post commander was

instructed to work with the hospital commander to take care of any problems that were found. And a lot of problems were found. Although generally healthier than the average population, soldiers were found with previously undetected high blood pressure, cholesterol elevation, smoking and excess alcohol use, weight problems, and depression. What were commanders to do? Most sent these soldiers to the medical treatment clinics, where they received "quick fix" solutions from the acute care system: medications and instructions to change their habits. These clinics and hospitals were all set up on the acute care model of health care that I described earlier. Their environments were neither preventive nor particularly healing. In general, clinic doctors, when confronted with a patient with high cholesterol or high blood pressure, would prescribe medications, rather than taking the time to look at the underlying lifestyle causes of the disorder or manage the more complicated process of behavior change. To be fair, even if they took the time to do this, the acute care system was not organized, nor did it have people with the right knowledge and skills, to deliver effective health promotion. So physicians' hands were largely tied. When commanders realized that a medical solution was not the answer; they created health promotion programs in military units and the community. There was a great need to set up bridges between these two worlds, which was my job. So various "bridging" programs were set up throughout the military and eventually reached the top leadership in all four branches of the military.

In 2007, working with Admiral Mike Mullen, then Chairman of the Joint Chiefs of Staff, my team helped develop an approach called Total Force Fitness. This whole systems science model sought to link healthy behavior not only to health care but also to service members' deeper psychological and spiritual needs. It was a whole person approach designed to address the body and mind and also the person's social and spiritual dimensions. (The whole person healing–oriented approach of Total Force Fitness was subsequently implemented military-wide in a variety of programs and is now being expanded to whole communities such as the Healthy Base Initiative, Operation Live Well, and a seven-state Building Healthy Military Communities program.) Samueli

Institute worked closely with the military to explore ways of bridging specific health behaviors and meaningful daily life. This was done on the military bases, but also in civilian communities, where most service members and their families come from, live, and return to every day. We also assisted programs to address the specific dimensions of healing behavior such as stress management and healthy eating programs. These included programs such as Healthy Kitchens, Healthy Lives, which taught healthy shopping and cooking skills; the Metabolically Optimized Brain, which connected community food access to resilience and enhanced mental health; and the Family Empowerment program, which set standards for implementing science-based, mind-body stress management programs in schools and worksites, teaching people how to improve the relaxation response and build mental fitness. It was from these programs that I learned the key to unleashing the healing power of behavior and lifestyle: connecting behavior change to a personally meaningful life. I didn't see this clearly, however, until another patient, Ensign Rogers, gave it to me straight from his hospital bed. He also gave Maria and me the answer we were looking for.

ENSIGN ROGERS

Ensign Rogers had just had a major heart attack. A retired cook and food service supplier with thirty-four years in the Navy, he had become overweight and developed high blood pressure. After he retired, he developed diabetes. Now he was in the hospital, recovering from the heart attack. I visited him there and we discussed what had happened.

Ensign Rogers' heart attack was, as he put it, "the big one." His recovery was prolonged. It gave him time to think about his life. Rogers, as they called him when he was on active duty, had provided food for sailors throughout his career, first on ships, starting as a server on the line. Then he became a cook and gradually rose in the ranks to become the main supply person for delivering food to ships—from small patrol boats with fewer than twenty passengers to large aircraft carriers with more than six thousand personnel on board. His duties had gone from peeling potatoes, to overseeing food delivery during training, to supplying food to boats during wartime. Later he was responsible for food for entire Navy communities, including families on bases. He knew a thing or two about food. After he retired from the Navy, he became a consultant for food services for the military. Now he advised all four services on how to provide more fresh fruits and vegetables at low cost. "Health food," he said, with some irony, "from scratch. Just like in the old days."

"You know, Doc," he mused, his heart monitor beeping in the background, "unlike medical care, which you only get when you need it, food has to be there all the time—three times a day and 24/7 for all sailors." He had never failed in that job. When he first started, they used to peel the potatoes and cut the vegetables themselves. He learned how to cook then, "from scratch" as he put it. He wasn't a bad cook; not a gourmet chef, but he could put a meal together—usually several hundred at a time, anyway, most from fresh ingredients.

He remembered exactly when cooking from scratch started to change. At first, it was expensive to get the packaged and processed food. But people wanted it. It was quick and easy and scientifically based. "Who wanted to peel all those potatoes every day, anyway?" he reminisced. If you added up the number of people it took to prepare food from scratch, the packaged food became cheaper and easier just to buy—preprocessed food in bulk. "We called it 'industrial food' because it came from the food industry, not our kitchens." he said. Food budgets got thinner and the war mission started to accelerate. "The sailors didn't have as much time to sit around and talk or eat. They needed food quickly and lots of it. They needed high-calorie food, and that's when the cans and packages came in," he reflected.

Instead of ordering pounds of potatoes and carrots, beans, and steak that he had to cut up himself, he received complete meals in packages. Packages of tasty high-fat, high-salt, high-calorie foods—just what the young sailors wanted. "The main drivers of this were the food companies that were selling packaged food at very low prices. And the military could negotiate even lower costs, so things got shifted into those packages," he recalled. Efficiency increased by not having to make food from scratch; now it mostly required only opening and heating. Industrial food had arrived.

Meanwhile, what was labeled "industrial food" inside the military was called "fast food" outside the military. American families were getting conditioned to fast food—a trend that spread and is still spreading around the world. In 1970, only 27.9% of daily meals were eaten outside the home. By 2012, it was over 43%. Ads for high-sugar, high-fat foods began to flood television, further reinforcing fast food as both fun and cool for the modern life. Women, increasingly working outside the home, wanted more rapid ways to feed hungry children. After a full day at work, a drive-through food run became just the ticket.

"The new sailors wanted this food, which they were getting used to as children before they came to the military," Ensign Rogers recalled. "It wasn't too long before the sailors started asking for that kind of food. So, while the industry pushed it as more convenient and cheaper, soon it was the sailors themselves who were the pushers. If we didn't supply it, they would go off base to get it. If they didn't eat in the dining halls, then our budgets were cut further. We couldn't have gone back to fresh foods if we wanted to." He paused for a long time. "I guess now the military leaders want fresh food back again." An even longer pause followed. Finally, he said with a sigh, "I wish them luck."

As the United States entered WWII in 1941, they found so many young men underweight that the military feared they would not be strong enough to endure a grueling war. So the government started feeding programs in schools, including free school lunches, to try and bulk up young men before they entered the military. That, and the need for large amounts of nonperishable, shippable food during the war, had spurred the development of industrial food. What was originally supposed to be a special type of feeding needed for large numbers preparing for battle, soon became the basis for feeding the entire population all the time.

After the war, the military type of fast food was converted into the fast-food industry the succeeding generations now wanted. During this same period, the rate of obesity began rising. Soon being overweight, rather than underweight, became one of the top reasons potential military recruits were turned down. By 2008, over 27% of all recruits and 40% of women wanting to come into the military were too fat to fight. That meant that they were disqualified for entry because they didn't meet the minimum standards for height/weight or fitness that the military considered essential to even start training.

"That is why they hired me as a consultant now, I guess," Rogers said, "to help them reverse this trend. I had seen it happen."

As Ensign Rogers looked up from his hospital bed, we discussed the health consequences of those shifts. He realized that in his career he'd done more than simply find cheaper food to fill the bellies of sailors in less expensive and more rapid ways. He had unwittingly become the architect of his own illness and converted many others into candidates for the costly, high-tech medical care he now received. He was grateful for the procedures, medications, hospital care, and stents that saved his life. He was grateful for the medications that controlled his diabetes and hypertension. He had developed hypertension in his mid-forties and had been put on several medications. He had already been on cholesterol medications. The diabetes medications came a bit later. Toward the end of his career, he didn't meet even the Navy's maximum weight standards, which are generous, and he was afraid he was going to get kicked out early. He starved himself before the biannual weigh-ins. After he retired, his weight ballooned, and that's when the diabetes and hypertension got worse and hard to control. During his thirty years in the Navy, the obesity rates had increased to almost 25% of all service members. He realized now that when he got together with his buddies in the NCO Club, he wasn't the only one with high blood pressure, diabetes, and heart problems. They were all talking about their doctor visits, and almost all were on cholesterol, hypertension, or diabetes medications. He just took it as a normal part of good medical care. After all, they had good medical care even after retirement.

But now, as an advisor to the military, when he recommended that a few million dollars be spent to try to prevent these diseases from happening to others, he heard that either the money was not available or they had to show that buying fresh food would reduce costs. In addition, most of the nutritionists worked at the hospital and didn't have time to help redesign the purchasing and preparation of healthier food. However, he did see a nutritionist when he went in for his diabetes checks, and a great new cooking class had been added to the cardiac rehab program for those with a history of a heart attack. The nutritionists were hired by one part of our health care system—the acute treatment part—but they did not have time to bridge the gap to the other part of our systems—the health promotion and prevention part. The payment system also did not bridge the gap. Military leaders were including only costs for the supply, preparation, and delivery of the food—24/7, three meals a day, without fail. Food was fuel for these young service personnel; they had a mission to accomplish, and that mission came first. They didn't count the cost from the medical consequences that would pop up years later. Nor did they count the personal costs Ensign Rogers now faced.

Like many military members, however, Ensign Rogers had always dedicated his life to service. So even as he talked from his hospital bed, he began to wonder if he could help the admirals and other ensigns with their situation. How could he help them see the long view—a view that had taken him nearly forty years to see himself?

After his discharge from the hospital, he started to attend cardiac rehab. While most of that focused on exercise, he also took a new twelve-week "healthy eating" class for heart patients that the base Community Wellness Center offered—an offshoot of the Total Force Fitness program. In that class, nutritionists and chefs joined forces to teach heart patients how to cook—from scratch, he noticed—in ways that were both healthy and delicious. In addition, the group culture of the class helped people help each other make the behavior changes permanent. If you had a challenge—be it with blanching vegetables or balancing your budget or getting your family on board—usually someone had a similar problem and could help you solve it.

"But," Ensign Rogers told me in a follow-up visit about six months after his heart attack, "for most of these heart patients, the horse had already left the barn. That was not the time to start to prevent their disease. They already had it. I needed it thirty years ago. It can't be just for people who have already had a heart attack."

I agreed.

One year later, Ensign Rogers partnered with a chef and started such a course for everyone at the base Wellness Center. He volunteered his time. "Eat for Life," he called it. Anyone with a risk factor for heart disease—overweight, diabetes, high blood pressure, high cholesterol, smoking, or a family history of early heart problems—could come. Family members could come, too. Meeting once a week for twelve weeks, participants learned how to select, buy, and prepare healthy food; how to make it taste great; and how to involve family and friends in the process.

Brilliant, I thought to myself. It was exactly what I was looking for to help Maria—to see if she could put meaning back into her medium of healthy food. I introduced her to the program as soon as I heard about it. She loved the idea and signed up for the next class.

After taking the class, Ensign Rogers and Maria decided to develop a version focused on Hispanic food—something Maria knew well and Ensign Rogers wanted to learn. With some help from a master chef, and a bit of guidance from a nutritionist, they began a community cooking class for prevention of the country's leading disease killers. Maria found an outlet for her passion, Ensign Rogers for his experience—and both found a new purpose in life. The "side effects" were many. Their diabetes remained under control, their energy improved, and their life expectancy lengthened. And they were helping others do the same. They had tapped into their own healing agency using the "agents" of food and behavior change.

MAKING BEHAVIOR MEANINGFUL

People are creatures of habit. Whole systems science shows that self-regulating systems—like people—constantly work to return to the same form and behavior after they have been stressed or traumatized. That automatic rebound response—the same response that fuels healing and recovery—also makes behavioral changes uncomfortable and hard to implement for many people. Behavioral change can be much more difficult for some than for others. Difficulties implementing long-term behavioral change often occur because of experiences and patterns set in childhood. Maria found a process to merge her healthy eating needs with the contribution she made to family and friends through cooking—something she had learned to do and was rewarded for as a child. Once she linked that meaningful activity to healthy food, the change came naturally and easily.

My wife, Susan, found changing her behavior much more challenging, even when she had reason to do so. Healthy behavior not only prevents disease and reverses many chronic conditions, but it can also blunt the side effects of curative treatments like chemotherapy and surgery. Cancer patients who exercise, eat healthy food, and engage in stress management, tolerate and complete therapy better, recover faster, and suffer fewer consequences of treatment long term. Susan had firsthand experience with the long-term consequences of cancer and its treatment. After her first cancer, she suffered the long-term effects of chemotherapy, including weight gain, nerve damage, and fatigue. Had she been able to engage in extensive behavior change—intensive exercise, careful dietary control, and major stress management—some of the consequences from her disease and treatment could have been mitigated. But Susan was not able to engage in that kind of intensive behavior change for several reasons. For one thing, our two health care systems—one for disease treatment and cure and one for healing and prevention—rarely bridge the gap and integrate, even in the crisis of cancer. During Susan's first breast cancer, oncologists had made no recommendations on healthy lifestyle during or after her treatment, and some even minimized it. There were few places to find assistance in learning and engaging in these changes. There are no profits to be made from building systems to help people make behavior change, so those systems are minimal. We went on with our lives as before.

During her second breast cancer, twenty-five years later, things were somewhat better. There are now lectures on nutrition, yoga classes, and support groups for cancer patients. There is a Society for Integrative Oncology (SIO), where mainstream oncologists explore the integration of healing practices with the cure-focused treatments in cancer. The role of behavior is now at least acknowledged as important in cancer survivorship—although physicians are not trained in how to use behavior. Advances in the science of healthy behavior are still not integrated into the delivery of cancer care. Our oncologist, one of the best in the region, did not know about SIO. There were no health coaches or coverage for behavior change available to Susan.

The second reason behavior change is hard for Susan is because of her childhood. As Maria discovered, the ability to make behavior change was linked to her childhood experiences, but in a different way. In three major areas of healthy behavior, Susan's childhood was stacked against her. First, while growing up, Susan frequently felt like she did not have enough food. Her family struggled financially, and food was carefully purchased and allocated to feed a family of six. As the "smart and most responsible one" and the oldest girl of four children, she was also expected to help take care of the family. By the time the food for dinner had been passed around, she often did not get enough. Her brother was a competitive swimmer and was constantly hungry, so she intentionally took smaller portions so he could have more. She said nothing about this, but later as an adult the idea of limiting food intake— especially food she could not get as a child—was very challenging to her. She experiences any change in possible food intake as a threat to her well-being, especially when things are stressful. Second, she was not encouraged to participate in sports and exercise. As was true for many girls of her generation, sports was something you watched boys do. She developed no skills or experience in keeping physically fit. Exercise was more difficult for her than for me; I had been involved in many sports. Finally, stress levels were high in her house. Her father had a volatile and unpredictable temper, often flying off the handle, yelling and screaming. She became the peacekeeper of the family, constantly on the alert to anything that might upset him and taking the emotional consequences of his abuse. Susan's stress management tactic for this was to anticipate possible emotional discord and compromise her own needs and desires in order to keep things calm. The only time she was relaxed was when there was social and emotional peace in the family, which was rare. Even today, she still habitually (and automatically) scans the social environment for any developing discord. That makes it hard for her to breathe deeply and induce the relaxation response when awake. Sleep is her only escape, especially when faced with a major assault like chemotherapy and surgery.

These types of adverse childhood experiences (ACE) have been shown to produce lifelong challenges to health and healing for many people. Not only do those with high ACEs have more mental and physical health problems, such experiences establish behavioral, neurological, and physiological patterns that are difficult for people to change. They are a double whammy—producing poor health and inhibiting behavior change to improve that health. If physical or sexual abuse is also involved, these problems are literally beaten into the brain and body of a person, making the induction of healing through behavior especially difficult. Until a person learns to reprogram those automatic emotional and physiological responses, repeated attempts at behavior change often fail, further reinforcing the difficulty. Such reprogramming can be done, but to pull it off requires extra assistance with environmental and social support. This assistance focuses on developing a readiness to change. Once the readiness has been properly prepared, actual behavior change becomes easier.

BRINGING HEALING INTO HEALTH CARE

Just as there is no magic bullet for chronic illness with specific medical treatments—no drug or herb or needle or knife that by itself will make you well—there is also no magic diet or other behavior change that will do this. After my patients and research taught me that most healing was not coming from the treatments I was prescribing, I discovered that the same thing applied to lifestyle. Add to that the paucity of science being applied to understanding lifestyle as therapy, and you can see why we have a plethora of self-care books running the gamut of recommendations. As important as healthy behavior is, if you want to access its healing capacity beyond what you can expect from simply making a change, you must connect that behavior to your life in a unique and meaningful way.

Healing can happen by applying medical treatments like Norma, Aadi, Sergeant Martin, and Xiao did in earlier chapters. It can happen by changing the external environment as Susan and Clara did in chapter 5. It can also happen with behavior changes like those that Jeff, Maria, and Ensign Rogers made. In each case, they found the right combination of approaches for their lives. To do this, however, we needed to focus less on finding a cure—the magic bullet or latest self-improvement fad—and more on how to connect healthy behaviors to our deeper personal dimensions.

One fundamental sign that a medical treatment, physical environment, or lifestyle will tap into the 80% of your healing capacity is the return of joy—a joy that comes from the experience of meaning and purpose. Another sign is an intuitive sense of certainty—a gut feeling that goes beyond belief and superficial desires for things to be a certain way. This gut feeling alone, however, is not sufficient to ensure it's the right healing choice for you. Any treatment or other healing approach should be verified with scientific evidence. What you decide to do should make sense to you and your doctor rationally, feel right to you emotionally, make sense socially, and be doable logistically. It is a committed embrace of the decision and follow-through that comes from your whole being. Many cultures describe this feeling in spiritual terms, but it is rarely seen that way in modern biomedicine. Modern medicine calls this approach by many names, such as person-centered care, precision health, or integrative medicine. The methods used to obtain this may involve personalized care planning, shared decision making, and health coaching. But optimal healing goes beyond the limited concepts of those terms. It involves the whole person and is produced by the meaning response. An emerging field that captures this most completely is called "integrative health."

Whole system sciences is providing powerful tools to more efficiently track when and how healing happens—providing objective ways to check your gut feelings. For example, as part of the million-person NIH Precision Medicine Initiative I described previously, researchers at Stanford University tracked nearly two billion measurements (250,000 a day) on sixty people to see how their day-to-day patterns of behavior correlated with health or illness markers. By analyzing patterns of change in this data over several months, the researchers could predict risk and illness as well as what produced improvements and healing in those people. Currently, this tracking is cumbersome and expensive for a clinic or person to do—but soon it will be relatively easy and some of it is being offered now. Technology is advancing our ability to measure, analyze, and monitor the whole person in ever more rapid and refined ways. Dr. Eric Topol, director of the Scripps Translational Science Institute and editor-in-chief of Medscape, describes this brave new world in his book *The Patient Will See You Now*. Technology is increasingly able to continuously monitor the core components of chronic disease and its risk factors and directly guide patients on how to monitor their own behavioral changes to prevent such disease. Integrative health will take this same technology and flip this monitoring on its head. That is, you will be able to get a continuous "healthy aging" readout and adjust what you do, think, and take to keep in your optimal health and well-being zone. The goal of whole systems science is to see the impact of this whole-person healing approach—be it from conventional or complementary medical treatments, lifestyle medicine or behavior change, social relationships, thoughts and feelings, or maybe even what happens in our soul. That information will be at anyone's fingertips. As this happens, we are creating a true science of whole person healing, and our ability to use it will improve. We will increasingly have precise ways to find the drugs to help each person, provide guidance on the environment to support optimal health, monitor the effect of daily behavior, and interpret a person's intuition.

You don't have to wait for this future, however. Much of this is available to you now—if you seek it and ask for it. There are already clinics and self-care tools delivering integrative health. These clinics and tools coordinate behavioral therapy, nutrition and lifestyle medicine, health coaching, and spirituality along with regular medical treatment. You can find them both inside and outside of medical centers. Those that are part of medical clinics are now delivering healing approaches and merging them with the approaches that seek to cure. I describe them and how you can access or create them at the end of this book.

The gap between our two health systems—between treatment and prevention—is being closed. But the area of behavior and lifestyle is not the widest gap between curing and healing. To understand what is, we must delve even deeper into how healing works—into the dimensions closest to the core of what it means to be human.

Chapter 7

Loving Deeply

How love and fear affect healing.

What are these other fundamental dimensions of being human needed for healing? Simply put, they are the emotions of love and fear—or more precisely, how we experience and manage them. How and what we love is intimately tied to our ability to find deep meaning and stimulate healing. The flip side of love is not hate; it is fear. Fear is the primary emotion alerting us to danger and drives our bodies to react—by fighting, fleeing, or freezing. Our entire brain (and body), with all its complexity, is constantly screening the environment for threats to our survival, asking what we should worry about and act on and what we can let go and relax around. When it thinks it has found a threat, it alerts us with fear and all the psychological and physiological reactions that accompany it.

If there is a single secret to how healing works, it can be found in how we handle our loves and fears. Love and fear are not intangibles— they have a physical effect and are, as we'll explore in this chapter, a matter of life and death. Love opens. Fear contracts. Both of them are needed for healing.

One of the myths about love and fear is that we have no control over them—that they just happen to us. We "fall" in love. We are "seized" by fear. Being subjected to the slings and arrows of emotion is indeed how many people experience their life. But whole systems science has now shown that not only can we learn to manage these emotions, but our health and healing depend on having just the right balance of them in our lives—both to get healthy and to stay healthy. Modern medicine's failure to take advantage of the social and emotional dimensions that help us manage love and fear leaves much of our healing potential untapped. When health systems have made these social and emotional dimensions central to their operations, those systems universally produce better outcomes and reduce costs.

The importance of managing love and fear has actually been shown in the laboratory—using rats and rabbits. Let's start with that.

THE RABBIT EXPERIMENTS

The rabbits were not dying, and that was a problem. How could the scientists find the cure to heart disease if they could not produce it? To study the effects of diet on heart disease, researchers fed different diets to two groups of rabbits and then compared the effects. One group ate a diet very high in fat and cholesterol; a control group ate a normal rabbit diet. Most of the rabbits who ate the high-fat, high-cholesterol diet developed high levels of cholesterol in their blood and blocked arteries in their hearts, putting them at increased risk of heart attack and stroke. It was a standard research test model that reinforced the cholesterol hypothesis of heart disease, a model demonstrated in laboratories all over the world and previously verified in the researchers' own laboratory multiple times.

But this time the results for one group of the fat-eating rabbits were different. Although they developed high levels of blood cholesterol, the rabbits in cages on the lower laboratory shelves had fewer blockages in their arteries and were not dying. The researchers checked and rechecked both the type and the amount of food that the rabbits ate and made sure that these rabbits were identical to the other rabbits used in the experiment. However, they could come up with no explanation for the lower-shelf rabbits' apparent immunity to the unhealthy diets. The researchers were confused. And then they talked to the lab technician.

The lab technician, a short woman, was taking the rabbits in the lower cages out of their cages every day and playing with them. She held them on her lap and petted them. She talked to them. Soothed them. Basically, she loved them. Then she would clean the cages and put them back in. Since she could not reach the higher cages, another technician was taking care of those animals. Those rabbits were not being petted—and they were dying at the normal rates.

The researchers were skeptical that simply soothing and petting an animal could negate the effects of a proven disease-producing diet. To have this effect, the loving touch these rabbits were getting only once a day would have to produce powerful chemicals that reduced the inflammation in the endothelium (lining) and the deposition of cholesterol in their coronary (heart) arteries and reduce blockages.

Most scientists would have not been distracted by the idea of love and simply told the technician to stop petting the rabbits. After all, their grant was funding them to test the diet-heart disease hypothesis, not the love-your-rabbit hypothesis. But the lead investigator was curious. Was love really overcoming diet? To rigorously test that hypothesis, the researchers designed an experiment that randomly divided a new set of rabbits into separate groups. They instructed the technicians to take the rabbits in certain groups out of their cages every day, play with them, stroke them, and love them for different amounts of time. They were to leave the other groups alone, except for routine feeding and care, without taking them out of their cages or touching them, except to transfer them quickly. They then studied the effect of this caring on cholesterol, endothelial function, artery narrowing, and heart disease.

What happened? Despite eating large amounts of fat and cholesterol, and even having elevated blood cholesterol levels, the cuddled rabbits had 60% less plaque in their arteries than the ignored rabbits, even though they were comparable in every other way—genetically, diet, weight, serum cholesterol, and heart rate. The factor that made the difference was love. The researchers were stunned. If only a few minutes of petting each day could reduce heart disease by 60% in a laboratory animal, imagine what power a lifetime of love (or its loss) could have on humans!

One patient in particular showed me clearly the power of love to heal the heart.

MABEL

Mabel was the "grand dame" of a large extended family. At eighty-four, she was the matriarch; for fifty years she had fretted, cared, and cooked for, disciplined, raised, and loved several generations. She was a sister, mother, grandmother, and great-grandmother to a family of nearly sixty—most of them relatives, others having showed up at her door and been "adopted" into the family. This included seven children of her own, nineteen grandchildren, and twenty great and great-great-grandchildren. Every week for three decades, the family had gathered at her house after church on Sundays for food, fellowship, and fun—and some of Mabel's continuously dispensed wisdom. Usually, her advice started with the phrases "Lead with love" or "Love first" or "The Lord loves everyone." If a child misbehaved, she might look at him sternly and say "Child . . ." Then she would advise the person to manage his anger or guilt or attitude better. "The Lord loves all people," she would say—"you and them. It's your job to catch up to the Lord." Not everyone took Mabel's advice, but everyone loved Mabel back.

Mabel's emotional heart may have been healthier than most, but now her physical heart was failing. I had admitted her to the hospital with shortness of breath and a very low cardiac output, a sign that her congestive heart failure—a condition she'd had for more than a decade—had progressed to the end stages. Congestive heart failure (CHF) is one of the leading reasons for hospitalization and has a very high mortality rate—killing more than five million people a year in the United States alone. The death rate from CHF has increased by 35% since the 1990s as the population has aged and our ability to keep people from dying of a sudden heart attack has improved—leaving them to live with damaged hearts that are more likely to fail later. CHF is also one of the most expensive conditions to treat, with more than one million people a year hospitalized—30% to 60% of them more than once. Annual costs of treating CHF in the United States are estimated at $40 billion a year. Mabel had not been hospitalized for more than a year as we had kept her heart functioning, and her overall care improved at home. But that increased home care had a consequence.

Three months before this hospitalization, I had recommended that a home caregiver come in to help her function better in her house. She didn't want that, but the family agreed with me so they found a home health care nurse. In addition, her family began to rotate coming over to be with her and help care for her each day. She didn't like that either. She had always been the one to care for them—not the other way around. Mabel couldn't love others in the way she had done before.

After admitting her to the hospital this time I found her numbers were off—her weight was up, largely from accumulation of water as her heart did not pump effectively. Her ejection fraction—a measure of how weak her heart was—had dropped. Her blood oxygen levels had also dropped—a sign that her lungs were filling up with fluid and not getting sufficient oxygen into the blood. I adjusted her medications and oxygen and diet to help these, and in a few days the numbers were better—but she was not.

One morning when I came in to check on her, she said, "Doc J, I appreciate all you doing for me. Just seems like too much bother, though." She was clearly discouraged.

"No bother, Mabel," I replied as I listened to her lungs and checked her weight. "That's my job—to get you better."

The next day she still complained of shortness of breath and weakness, and her blood oxygen was not quite as good. I prescribed physical therapy, upped her oxygen, and readjusted her medications a bit more. Her numbers improved again. But two days later, she was worse, as were her numbers. I checked a few more things—were her kidneys failing, too? Was her family slipping her salty snacks? Was she on the wrong medications? Was her heart just at the end of its life? Nothing seemed amiss. But this pattern repeated itself. This time I did not adjust any therapy. The numbers improved, then worsened, then improved. Her heart failure was going up and down almost independent of my treatments. I was not sure what was going on.

"Doctor Jonas," the head nurse said to me one morning, "I think you might want to talk to Mabel's family—especially Jason, her grandson. He and the pastor think she wants to die."

Jason, as it turned out, had gone to college and earned a degree in psychology. "My love child," Mabel had once told me about him. "He just sits and listen to me and gives me no grief. Always was that way."

I scheduled a meeting with Jason and the pastor. Indeed, they confirmed that ever since I had prescribed the home nurse and the family came in to care for her, she had complained about being a "burden" and "useless" to her family. "I'm better for you-all dead," she would sometimes blurt out. The family members tried to counter that attitude, imploring her not to say that and insisting that she was still loved. That seemed to make things worse. Jason told me that ever since this hospitalization, she had confessed to him that she was trying to decide whether she should go back home or die right then and there. As family members came and went, she would feel better for a while, but then fall back into her "I'm a burden" attitude. Back and forth this went. I suggested she was depressed, and I prescribed a mood-elevating drug, but it would not become effective for several weeks. Besides, that would not address the core issue that she was struggling with now—the meaning of her life with advanced CHF.

Then the pastor made a suggestion. If we could get the family to agree not to try and "take care of" Mabel on their visits, but to seek out learnings and wisdom from her—let *her* take care of *them*—maybe that would help Mabel feel useful again. Jason agreed. Although he had suggested to individual family members that they not counter Mabel's comments, they had never discussed a coordinated plan for how to receive her love and wisdom. If the doctor and the pastor recommended and helped organize such a plan, he was sure that most of the family would go along.

So, working with the family, we set up a plan to let Mabel love again. Jason and the pastor gathered most of the family together, and they agreed when visiting Mabel to ask her questions related to struggles they were having in life and to seek her wisdom. The basic question they would seek from her was—"What has love got to do with it?"—a question they knew she could answer. The gathering was arranged. I had to transfer the other patient in her room out just to fit in all the family and friends who came—more than thirty in all. The pastor said a prayer, and then the family asked her if she would do this.

"Well," she said between labored breaths, tears in her eyes, "I guess I can try that for a while." The pastor, to my surprise, suggested they sing the old African American spiritual "Ain't Got Time to Die." They all knew the words.

Within three days, Mabel's numbers stabilized—basically back to where they were on the medical regimen I had put her on when she was first admitted to the hospital. She went home with oxygen and hospice. She lived six more months, and she died with her family around her at home. She never entered the hospital again. She had found her healing power through to the end.

THE SCIENCE OF LOVE AND LOSS

From the time we are born to the time we die, life is punctuated by loves—people, places, pets, and passions—that we get deeply attached to. Life is also punctuated by the loss of those same people and passions. Our mind and body are constantly alert to find such loves and on guard against their losses. We instinctively seek the former and avoid the latter. Survival may sometimes depend on it. Yet the world is both ugly and beautiful, inflicting on us trauma and cruelty, and also inducing in us healing and compassion—sometimes all at the same time. How do we find peace in the face of pain and grief? How can we feel whole when we are broken and battered? Why do we try so hard to avoid pain, suffering, and death, even at the risk of not fully living?

It is not an easy task to face suffering, and almost impossible if we are alone. When illness and injury come, when our life is threatened by disease, and our body and soul buried in pain or sadness, it is the presence of a caring person that can often carry us through that suffering into healing. Facing loss is especially difficult if our early experiences with others were not caring, if our first ventures into love were met with rejection or loss or, worse, with anger or violence. If experiences in our childhood involved too much pain or trauma, we may be too afraid to open to the love of others, even when it is offered. Yet it is by sharing our suffering with others—and by its presence as we explore our fears— that healing and wholeness come, because some of the most meaningful experiences humans can have is when we are cared for and care for others. We are social beings; we are not whole without love.

Sociologist Dr. Ian Coulter, chair of integrative health research at the RAND Corporation and a professor at UCLA, described the scientific aspect of this to me in detail. Sociologists define a person as an individual embedded into a social network of mental, physical, and personal interactions. That network not only defines us as a person but also influences what happens to us on all levels of our being—including in our body.

Harvard physician and social scientist Professor Nicholas Christakis and his colleague James Fowler summarized many of these influences in their book *Connected: The Surprising Power of Our Social Networks and How They Shape our Lives.* They say, "As we studied social networks more deeply, we began to think of them as a kind of human superorganism. They grow and evolve. All sorts of things flow and move within them. . . . Seeing ourselves as part of a superorganism allows us to understand our actions, choices, and experiences in a new light." I agree. Who you are connected to—not only your family, but even your "friends' friends' friends"—impacts large swaths of your health and happiness, whether you know it or not. Everything from obesity to smoking to infection to alcohol use and depression are mitigated and influenced by your social network—often in ways you cannot see. Not only does this help us understand and explain how we change along with others, but it also applies to individual healing. If we look at a person as if he has a literal social and emotional body—and treat any injury to this body with the same importance as we treat a cancer or heart attack—we can unleash that aspect of our healing potential. When we do that, this social and emotional dimension of healing provides us with powerful tools for resilience, recovery, and repair.

Extensive evidence shows that social support protects us from disease and death and enhances recovery from illness. In studies with subjects who had similar conditions, strong ties to family and friends reduced the risk of dying by 50% compared to those who were alone. Isolation and loneliness are strong contributors to chronic diseases—both mental and physical—and work primarily through the body's stress and fear responses, inducing inflammation in the walls of blood vessels and in the brain and impairing the immune response. Dr. John Cacioppo, professor of cardiology at the University of Chicago, summarizes much of this research in his book *Loneliness: Human Nature and the Need for Social Connection*. Lonely people have a 45% increased risk of dying from all causes and a 64% increased chance of dementia in later life. The magnitude of increased health risks for people who are socially and emotionally disconnected from others and the comparative protection for people who are well connected are comparable to well-established risk factors such as smoking, obesity, injury, substance abuse, and environmental quality. Here's a specific example: Two studies compared men who had experienced heart attacks. The men who reported being in loving relationships had lower death rates than the men who were not in such relationships. The increased odds of dying after that for those not in loving relationships was as great as if they smoked a pack of cigarettes a day. Research has also shown a significant relationship between a patient's recovery after a heart attack and the extent of the spouse's social support, family stress, marital satisfaction, and sexual comfort. Other studies have found that patients are statistically less likely to die after a serious illness if a nurse simply calls them weekly to check on how they are doing. Several researchers have tested the mental, physical, clinical, and economic impact of making even short but deep emotional connections. Like the rabbits in the study mentioned earlier, connecting to someone who cares for you—even a little—reduces the odds of illness and premature death and helps you heal.

Loneliness is not the same as simply being alone, which for many can be a welcome and enjoyable state. Loneliness refers to the quality and depth of relationships—or lack thereof. It is not about the number of connections, either; rather, it is about how deep those connections are and how happy they make us. When people feel love and safety with others, their stress reactions in the brain and body are diminished and reparative functions improve. Professor Cacioppo points out that in the absence of social safety, stress hormones surge, triggering the release of cardiovascular and inflammatory chemicals and activating genes that lead to damage to mind and body. Socially disconnected people are more prone to arterial stiffening, leading to increased blood pressure—a risk factor for heart disease and stroke. Their bodies are also less efficient at repair and maintenance functions: their wounds heal more slowly, and their sleep—a vital restorative function—is less effective. Connections associated with love and safety increase heart rate variability—a moment-to-moment marker of relaxation and health risk. Increased heart rate variability—that is, a rate that quickens and slows with the cycles of inhalation and exhalation—correlates with resilience, good health, and increased lifespan. Heart rate variability can be tracked minute by minute, making it a good marker of the quality of one's relaxation state, emotional connection, and physical health. Mabel's heart rate variability decreased as her CHF progressed. When she felt love, however, it improved. I smiled as I thought of the science behind social and emotional connection. I could just imagine Mabel saying, "What did I tell you? Love heals with every heartbeat!" It does.

A HEALING PRESENCE

The first time my wife, Susan, went through chemotherapy, she did it largely alone. I was so busy with my job in the military that I often could not be present for her. Like many doctors, I hated feeling helpless, so I was compelled to take action, even when there was no good evidence that any action would help. I didn't know how to feel comfortable just *being* with Susan. It felt like I lost my power and control. So I worked. She found a supportive network to help her through, seeking strength in her spiritual life and the need to care for our young children. She did well.

When she started chemotherapy for cancer the second time around, I told her that this time I would be there—that we were in this together. She believed me and appreciated it, but realized how difficult it would be for me. She also knew that my periodic presence was not enough support for what she was about to go through. After all, she pointed out, I was running a large research organization, had to continue doing my job for our income, and had many demands on my time. Because of that, Susan reached out and gathered helpers around her: our daughters, our son and daughter-in-law, my sister, her sister, her mother, her sisters-in-law, other family members, and friends. Her goal was to take care of herself and help take care of our new grandchild. I didn't realize that she needed more than psychological support from me; she needed my physical presence—with my emotional body.

I should have known this. I had done research showing that the physical presence of a loving person does more than provide psychological support. The physical presence of another person has a direct impact on a person's body and mind. For example, the electromagnetic waves from the beating heart of one person can be detected in the brain of a person standing next to them. The beat of your heart is picked up and produces a sort of reflection in another person's brain. This might partly explain why when you are near a very calm person, you also start to feel calmer. That calming feeling also increases heart rate variability and the activity of the parasympathetic (relaxation response) part of the nervous system and stimulates the vagus nerve. Increased activity in the vagus nerve creates a biochemical and physiological cascade of effects that reduce inflammation and increase resilience to stress at the organ, cellular, and genetic level. Thus a person's physical presence—without her doing anything at all—can influence another person's brain and their other organs, immune system, cells, and genes, as well as bring a feeling of peace. This is probably the underlying reason that some people are said to have a "healing presence." People are probably picking up on the physical emanations from the person's relaxed and calm heart.

There are additional ways in which physical presence influences healing. We know, for example, that electromagnetic waves in the form of heat and infrared radiation emanate from the body, especially the hands. Through meditation, biofeedback, and breathing techniques, people can increase or decrease the amount of this heat and infrared radiation. Infrared radiation, especially in the frequencies of 400 to 800 nanometers, is absorbed by a chemical in our cells called cytochrome c. Stimulation of cytochrome c increases the amount of adenosine triphosphate (ATP)—the energy-producing molecule found in all cells. In dozens of experiments done at Walter Reed Army Institute of Research, investigators found that individuals who put their hands around test tubes containing immune cells while meditating increased the amount of infrared radiation emanating from their hands, which stimulated the immune cells to produce more ATP and energy. After this exposure those cells were more resilient—that is, they survived better when hit with stresses such as heat and chemical shocks. Remarkably, the kind of meditation and visualization that was the most effective for increasing the amount of ATP and resilience of these cells looked like love. Cultivating a feeling of love—such as gratitude, affection, and appreciation—produced the greatest effect. Mental activity such as counting backward or thinking about the weather did not increase ATP or improve cellular resilience.

I knew all this research—had even done some of it—but for some reason I didn't think it was relevant for helping Susan heal. Scientists (including me) are generally skeptical of any research purporting to objectively measure and explain emotional and social interaction or the energy it creates. The area is considered too intangible and subjective to be reliable, so it is dismissed without looking at whether the research is rigorous or relevant. My skeptical doctor side had also dismissed it as an interesting laboratory findings but not relevant for patient care. I wanted something more doable—a medication, supplement, or behavior. I wasn't going to simply wave my hands over her head or take naps with her. What good would that do, I thought? So even as Susan began to lose energy and feel poorly from the chemo infusions, week after week, I didn't think my presence could really make a difference in how she did.

Then one week, I went away on a boating trip through the Grand

Canyon with our daughter. We were off the grid for a while, and I was not with Susan for more than a week. When we got back within cell phone range, I received a call from her. While I was away, her white counts had dropped precipitously and she had developed a fever. The oncologist had given her a shot to boost her white blood counts and put her on antibiotics. If it persisted, she would be hospitalized and isolated.

I came home, fearful that this drop in white blood count was likely to recur the following week, because the effects of chemotherapy tend to be cumulative. But something about just being together started to make her feel better. Then I remembered the research at Walter Reed. Still skeptical, I decided to try a little of this laying on of hands—this healing presence process—myself. I recalled from the research that the technique that affected the immune cells most powerfully involved breathing, imagining a soft white light filled with love being transmitted through the top of my head, down through my arms and hands, and out into her body. After a few minutes of trying this, I could feel warmth coming into my hands from increased blood flow and heat. Susan also said that she could feel something—and then she fell asleep. The session lasted about fifteen minutes.

The next day, her energy was much improved—she was up early and out pulling weeds in the garden, something she had not done for months. Was it from more ATP, I wondered? At her next chemotherapy session two days later, her white blood count had recovered practically back to normal—so she did not need the immune-boosting shot. Were her white blood cells more resistant to the chemo? She was clearly less fatigued, slept less, and was more active during the day. I was stunned. Had the simple physical presence of another loving person produced this response? I decided not to go on any more trips for a while. From then on, my job was to just make sure my body—in all its physical, social, and emotional dimensions—was around.

OPENING UP

Although little research has been done on the therapeutic effect of the physical presence of another person, there is extensive research on the impact of making emotional connections. When our encounter with another person results in connecting to our emotional self—especially to a part we have avoided dealing with because of fear or grief—the healing can be profound. In his book *Opening Up*, social psychologist Dr. James Pennebaker summarizes much of this research. A single sharing of a deep trauma or loss with another can improve health. Some of the most remarkable studies in this area are with Holocaust survivors. Even decades after the war, most Holocaust survivors have never discussed their experiences in concentration camps or the trauma, fear, and losses they endured. In the research, these survivors were asked to write or speak about those experiences to another person who simply listened in a safe and confidential environment. The investigators then measured the impact of this sharing on the survivors' biology (inflammatory response or blood pressure, for example) and health. Compared to those who wrote or spoke about something superficial—the weather or what they had to eat that day—this single deep sharing resulted in significant health improvements. The improvements were wide ranging and lasting—better immune function, less pain, improved mood, and less need for medical care, even a year later.

Other studies have shown that such sharing of deep feelings about trauma and loss can also help heal specific diseases. Patients with rheumatoid arthritis report significant pain reduction after a single episode of such sharing. Patients with asthma have improved lung function—measured objectively with a spirometer—a month after a similar single sharing.

More prolonged or repeated social and emotional exchange has profound and often permanent healing effects, especially if done in an emotionally safe environment and framed and guided in a positive direction with others to witness. An emotionally safe place is a social environment where a person can trust others to stay with them through difficult emotions, to care for and respect them, and to honor their deepest experiences as real and of value. My experience in the military, treating service members and veterans with PTSD and chronic pain, demonstrates this. For example, typical treatments for PTSD with drugs and psychotherapy have a positive but limited effect—usually helping only 20% to 30% of veterans. Exposure therapy—in which the veteran is gradually exposed to his fear triggers—can be a bit better, but it is complicated, and many veterans—especially those who have experienced sexual trauma—will not go through it. But two other approaches that tap into the meaning response have shown larger and often permanent healing.

One approach is a therapeutic retreat, during which veterans are guided to open up to their fears, anger, anguish, and grief in the presence of other veterans who understand, accept, and love them. Dr. Joseph Bobrow describes the profound and prolonged benefit from these retreats in his book *Waking Up from War*. In follow-up assessments of veterans who attend such retreats, a majority experience long-term improvement and restoration in their lives. A second approach is inducing these deep meaningful experiences with hallucinogenic substances. Recent research reports that when even a single dose of such substances is administered, a majority of deeply depressed patients suffering from advanced cancer had major improvement in their mental and emotional state.

ELEMENTS OF THE SOCIAL AND EMOTIONAL DIMENSION

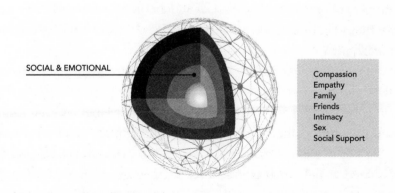

SOCIAL & EMOTIONAL

Compassion
Empathy
Family
Friends
Intimacy
Sex
Social Support

It is important to note that the success of this approach depends on the patients being professionally selected, cared for, and guided to experience deep meaning from the episodes. Simply taking the drug by itself does not produce the healing—and in fact can cause significant harm. The drug isn't key; the meaning is. Healing does not necessarily require a drug—hallucinogenic or not—provided the meaning response occurs. A meaningful experience often occurs spontaneously through what are called exceptional emotional experiences. These occur most often when people are suffering and open up to their emotions. Loss of a loved one—through death, divorce, or another type of separation—increases the risk for disease and death several fold. Between 30% and 50% of people who have experienced a major loss will subsequently have an exceptional experience, often described as spiritual—such as seeing or feeling a deceased person returning or seeming like a ghost, or experiencing a profound sense of the unity of all things. If those experiences are treated respectfully by others and the person is guided toward understanding and acceptance, this can be profoundly healing. If they are dismissed or treated negatively, the experience can damage a person permanently. Healing comes from how meaning is made from those experiences. It involves the social and emotional body.

THE BEAUTY WAY

To help my patients use their social and emotional dimensions to heal, I ask them about their social relationships during a healing-oriented visit with me.

The purpose in exploring these elements is not to do psychotherapy or tell them how to feel. The goal is to help them learn how to use their feelings to find deeper meaning in their lives. Mabel and her family found meaning in her wisdom, love, and teaching—and arranged a way for her to express that. Susan used her social connections and her grandchild to help increase the level of social support and love in her life during a traumatic time that needed enhanced healing. My veteran patients find meaning through deep encounters with their own losses and the support of others who understand and travel with them through their anger, fear, shame, and grief. Whatever the form or method used to create this opening up to deep emotional experiences—groups, drugs, herbs, psychotherapy, energy practices, spiritual encounters, or simply spontaneous acceptance—healing comes from the way meaning is made of those experiences.

Many cultures, both ancient and modern, use the social and emotional dimension to enhance healing capacity. I mentioned how Epidaurus—where the Hippocrates school of medicine in ancient Greece originated—had a theater at its center. In this theater, physicians helped patients learn how to deal with and heal the traumas of life by acting out the drama of emotional connections and disconnections.

Other cultures acknowledge and use this dimension for healing. Consider, for example, the way in which the traditional Navajo culture handles mental illness. Rather than thinking of mental illness as an individual problem, the Navajo consider it a social problem, shared by the whole community. They make no distinction between individual illness and social illness. In their view, we are all swimming in the same body of social "water." Whether we are aware of it or not, we need the water in order to survive, and a disturbance in one part of our individual world affects the world of all the community who "swim" there. The traditional Navajo treatment for mental illness involves the entire community in special healing ceremonies. One is a social ritual called "the Beauty Way," intended to restore beauty, wholeness, and coherence to the community, tribe, and family. There are different versions of the Beauty Way ceremony, but it often consists of a combination of prayers, offerings, rituals and sweat baths, sand paintings, chants, and singing—sometimes for days. The ill person and the community are thought to have lost *hózhó*, the sense of beauty and integration with the universe. By surrounding the ill person with beauty, this appreciation is restored in the social environment, and the individual recovers his sense of meaning and order.

Could incorporation of the social and emotional dimensions as in the Beauty Way ceremony bring healing back into modern medical care? If so, how would that affect the experience of health care and health outcomes, and how much would it cost? Dr. Don Berwick, founder of the Institute for Healthcare Improvement and former director of the Centers for Medicare and Medicaid Services (CMS), pointed me toward one system that has done just that: the Nuka System of Care, developed and run by the Southcentral Foundation (SCF) in Anchorage, Alaska. What attracted me to this system was not just Dr. Berwick's recommendation but also the major impact that SCF produces on the people it serves. In 1982, when the SCF was first formed, the health care services for Alaskan Native peoples provided by the Indian Health Service (IHS) in Anchorage was abysmal. Their rates of alcoholism, diabetes, obesity, domestic violence, suicide, and life expectancy were some of the worst in the country. Premature births and infant mortality were similar to sub-Saharan Africa. It was not that the IHS-provided medical care was bad. In fact, state-of-the-science medical visits, prescription drugs, and specialty care were all available. IHS poured millions of dollars into providing this medical care with costs rising every year. So why was it failing its patients?

From 1982 to 1989, SCF gradually took over health care delivery from the IHS. The results were astonishing. Twenty years after fully taking over health care delivery and after creating its own care approach, the foundation has markedly improved rates of obesity, diabetes, alcoholism, family abuse, and adverse childhood experiences. The need for costly emergency room and urgent care visits has dropped by 36%, primary care by 28%, and hospital admissions by 36%—all while improving the health of the community. Patient satisfaction rates have soared to more than 90%. Employee morale also improved, as shown by steady improvements in workforce commitment and reduction in annual staff turnover and employee satisfaction to 96%. SCF's overall revenue has gone up and, compared to IHS days and to the rest of health care, costs per person have gone down.

What were they doing differently? Had they found some new treatments that science had missed? How had they improved the outcomes of their delivery system so dramatically? I decided to go see for myself.

RELATIONSHIP-CENTERED CARE

When I visited SCF's Anchorage Native Primary Care Center and some of their more remote clinics in 2015, they were running a training program for other health systems on how to improve care and healing. I took the training; talked with employees, health care providers, and patients; and visited with system leaders. SCF had first asked to take over parts of health care for the Alaska Native people from IHS in 1982. From the very beginning, SCF set up "listening circles," in which the people talked about their needs beyond medical care—needs in the physical, behavioral, social, and spiritual dimensions of their lives. The listening circle approach was an adaptation of an Alaskan Native process for social connection and reconciliation traditionally used by many of the tribes. SCF leaders used these circles to directly address the social and emotional dimension. One leader, an employee named Dr. Kathleen Gottlieb, opened up about the deep wounds and adverse childhood experiences in her family. Others followed, revealing the impact of illness and trauma in their lives. Soon these listening circles became Learning Circles, as participants developed deeper relationships and began to help—and challenge—each other to engage in whole-person healing, not just disease treatment. Gradually, this process was embedded into SCF, and, with Ms. Gottlieb as President/CEO, relationship-centered care became part of its standard delivery processes.

The Learning Circle is a safe place where people can address trauma, fear, and grief and deal with their loves and losses with others' support. In the process, they become more whole—more connected to their own social and emotional "bodies"—and healing sets in. One person I spoke with told me she grew up in a family where physical and sexual abuse, alcoholism, suicide, and obesity had been growing problems for more than four generations. By coming to a Learning Circle, she had could break that cycle and raise children who were largely freed from these adverse experiences. She did it by sharing some of the deepest traumas and losses in her own life. Others walked the healing journey with her as she learned to take these behaviors out of her own family and adopt other, healthier behaviors. For those who engaged in this process, life quality improved, and life expectancy jumped by decades—especially for their children. Over the years, this focus on relationships became a core part of the SCF health care operations. Today at SCF the patients are no longer treated as people whose medical services are delivered by strangers. Patients are now treated as customers and are owners of the company. They have continuous input on their own needs and the needs of the community. The use of the social and emotional dimension for healing was incorporated by bringing "behavioral health" into all the clinics. All employees, including physicians, are required to understand and participate in Learning Circles—through SCF's Relationship-based Core Concepts workshop, which is now offered to other health systems.

But I wondered: were the medical treatments provided by SCF somehow more evidence-based, more scientific or state-of-the-art than they had been before they developed the Nuka System of Care? The answer was no. Access to good, evidence-based medical treatments had been part of the IHS before SCF took over care, and that good medical practice had been continually updated for decades by IHS. Yet outcomes had continually worsened. The types of medical treatments and the agents used—drugs, surgery, counseling, emergency, and preventive care—are all part of the current Nuka System of Care and provided by IHS elsewhere. SCF had no unusual medical interventions, no better science, no more magic bullets than other systems. They still make diagnoses and deal with research and medical guidelines, insurance coding, and reimbursement. The doctors and nurses come from standard medical schools and use standard treatment tools. What has changed is relationships and customer ownership. SCF added the social and emotional dimension of healing to their delivery of health care. This allows them to tap into this previously ignored capacity for human healing.

THE FACE OF LOVE

Most of the medical community ignores this data, just as I had. Most physicians and scientists think these dimensions are too intangible, so they seek more material ways to treat illness—preferring to lower cholesterol rather than increase love; to raise brain serotonin rather than deal with grief. Not that lowering cholesterol or raising serotonin are bad things—but they are only a small part of what humans need to heal. Love may be a many-splendored thing—the stuff of poets and songs and mystics—but that splendor does not pay off like a drug or supplement. So, nothing further was ever done with the rabbit data on petting and heart disease, yet we have a multibillion-dollar drug and supplement industry selling you a way to lower cholesterol. Little has been done with the data showing reduced mortality with reduced loneliness, yet we have a multibillion-dollar drug industry to increase serotonin so you can worry less about your loneliness.

After I flew back from Alaska, where I had seen relationship-centered care in full operation, I could not find a health system in our area that integrated this into the care for my own family. When Susan got cancer again, we needed such a system so we had to figure out how build one on our own. Fortunately, we had the awareness and social networks to do so.

After six months of chemotherapy, Susan now faced another, even more traumatic event—the surgery. A double mastectomy and simultaneous DIEP flap reconstruction (deep inferior epigastric perforators, named for the associated blood vessels) this meant a twelve-hour operation involving three surgeons, two anesthesiologists, and four nurses. She would be cut from neck to pelvis, with the top part removed and the bottom part shifted up to the top—her body reorganized. Thank science for anesthesia and antiseptics! The recovery would be long and painful; the physical loss alone would be large. The surgeon said she would bounce back in no time—two weeks. The nurse indicated that she should not lift the grandbaby or even have him on her lap for eight weeks. The risk of suffering would be great; the possibility of falling into sadness and depression was present every day. While Susan had difficulty with the behavioral dimensions of healing that could prepare her for this onslaught—exercise, improved diet and supplements, meditation and visualization—she was good at relationships. During her first cancer she had sought divine love through prayer and meditation and a spiritual meaning for her illness. This time she looked again for love, but not the divine kind of love that spiritual healers describe. This time she sought a different kind of love—the common love of ordinary humans. It was a love that emerged largely from the females in our family, at least in acts and presence. Those who showed up at the door to sit with Susan when she couldn't move were people like our next-door neighbor, Rose Ellen. Rose Ellen doesn't cook, so she didn't bring any meals; she said she couldn't help with the grandchild because she wasn't good with babies. But she came over anyway and said she would be available for anything Susan needed any time, day or night—just let her know. Rose Ellen isn't a romantic type of person, nor is she particularly spiritual or complicated in how she lives her life—but she offered true caring and presence on an as-needed basis.

Others came, too. Susan's friend from college, who'd had a similar procedure a few months before, showed up and stayed for several days cooking, cleaning, and making conversation. Our two daughters came. One, a chaplain—the "analytical one" of the family, who had worked for over a year as a hospital chaplain ministering to the depths of suffering—knew exactly how to be, from lying down in bed with her mother to setting up an online meal chain system that brought food from friends on an organized schedule. Our younger daughter is a singer and teacher, the "creative one" in the family. She recorded a special set of songs for each phase of recovery and brought humor and laughter into the house—sustenance for the soul. Through both chemotherapy and surgery, one person after another showed up—all people Susan had loved and served in her life. Some we had not known well before. Some we had. Our niece from California flew out for ten days to help with the grandbaby and to cook. My sister followed her and did the same thing. I realized from watching this parade of faces—all bringing their physical bodies and human love to our house—that this was also the way that divine love leaked in. No special spiritual healers or waving of hands needed. The support we got from this network of other human beings allowed me to spend time sitting with Susan, helping her to the bathroom and the shower, sleeping next to her when she slept, bringing our new grandbaby up the steps into her room—and going to work. I took periodic breaks to take care of myself, and so I could, with this help from others, be present for her in the long run. We may not have had a Nuka-like health system to deliver relationship-centered care, but Susan used a network of friends and family to bolster the social and emotional dimension of healing on her own. And it worked. Her white count stayed up, her surgery recovery was like clockwork, and the grandbaby brought us joy and thrived. Eight weeks after the end of chemo and surgery not only could Susan lift the grandbaby, but she also had planned a trip for the extended family to Florida during the holiday season. The medical treatments for her cancer may have added only an 7% chance to her ten-year survival, but the quality added to all our lives by the social and emotional dimension of healing was immeasurable. We had found our own Beauty Way.

GLORIA

Not everyone has the network Susan does to tap the social and emotional dimensions of healing. However, that does not mean this dimension can't be used effectively by everyone. Gloria demonstrated that to me. She had retired three years earlier from her job making omelets and doing kitchen work at a local golf club. The club, an old one with an established staff, had been her home for forty years. She started working there when she was twenty-five. It paid reasonably and provided benefits, so she stayed. With that income and her husband's, they raised three children—two of whom had gone to college— something she was very proud of because she had not finished high school. She had retired at age sixty-five, and soon after that, her fatigue and muscle pains became progressively worse. She was diagnosed with fibromyalgia and chronic musculoskeletal back pain. She was told to exercise and rest, given painkillers to take "as needed," and sent to physical therapy and acupuncture. These helped some, but her pain levels hovered "around four to five out of ten all the time," she told me on our first visit, "especially in the morning."

"It is pretty bad. Sometimes it takes me an hour to loosen up and have enough energy to get out of the bedroom"—a common situation with fibromyalgia.

Gloria was referred to me by her primary care doctor because she wanted to do better and heard that I prescribed fewer drugs than other doctors. As we went through her healing-oriented assessment, I found very little amiss in her life. She had a comfortable clean house and a "nice husband who works a lot"; she tried to eat right and walk outside every morning. She went to Catholic mass each Sunday and prayed daily—"for others," she mentioned nonchalantly. Her ten-year-old grandchild (she had five grandchildren who lived some distance from her) had come to stay for the summer. He was a "nice boy, very active, and in camp most of the day." A year previously she had gone to an acupuncturist that her health system covered, which helped her back pain for a while, but then her insurance stopped paying for it. "It did not seem to help my fibromyalgia or my tiredness," she said.

When we got to questions about her social and emotional life, I noticed a shift in her voice. "Do you have good friends you spend time with?" I asked.

Her voice softened as if she did not want me to hear. "Well, doctor," she said slowly, "to be honest, ever since my retirement I have missed everybody. I was at the club for forty years, rarely missed a day. I miss it now. But they are all so busy. I don't want to bother them."

Gloria, it turned out, was lonely. And she was not alone in that. Each year more than sixty million people in the United States suffer from chronic loneliness. It is common after retirement when routine interactions and friendships at work are suddenly stopped. Although her medical diagnosis was fibromyalgia, her problem was loneliness. Was it a coincidence that her chronic pain and frequent visits to the doctors began soon after her retirement? While I had no objective test that could prove this connection, I did know that reconnecting her to a meaningful social network would help her heal. But how to do that? We needed to find a group that Gloria could join.

She seemed to read my mind. "I went to one of those chronic pain support groups, but I didn't like it. Everybody was so sick. I felt worse afterward."

Back to the drawing board, I thought.

"Well, Gloria," I said after a pause. "It seems to me that you would benefit from finding a place to go each day to work with others and do things that are meaningful for you. Let's think about how to do that." She agreed.

Gloria ended up volunteering at a church food pantry and eventually running it. Her pain improved by 80% in about six months. From the day she started, she said she felt better, and gradually her energy returned. My guess is that she was largely cured. Her recovery might have been shortened and even more effective had she access to a clinic like Dr. Jeffery Geller's.

DR. GELLER

Dr. Jeffery Geller is one of the world's experts on healing chronic illness through social connection. He does this through group visits conducted at a community health center in Lawrence, Massachusetts—the poorest county in that state. Some of his groups gather for specific illnesses— like for weight loss, diabetes, cardiovascular disease—or chronic pain, like Gloria had. Some of his groups are to change behavior—like for fitness, cooking, or stress management. Many have no theme other than improving health and well-being in general. But Dr. Geller has a different agenda from all of that.

"What I am really treating," says Dr. Geller, when only slightly pressed, "is loneliness. More people get better, and faster, when I focus on helping them with that than if I only treat their disease or try to change their behavior." He went on to tell me how he came to this. "At first I was using group visits so I could treat more patients. The demand at the clinic is high and our reimbursement is low. Paying for individual instruction in wellness and lifestyle was not possible. Many of them need help with the same things—diet, exercise, stress, medication management—so why not do it as a group?"

At first, Dr. Geller explained, setting up disease-focused groups seemed the right approach. But then he realized that, like Gloria, the majority of people with chronic illness didn't like going to a group where everyone seemed sicker or more depressed than they were. In addition, many were also lonely, and that loneliness was preventing them from healing.

"Even if they were not lonely," Geller said, "connecting with others was not a bad thing for anyone. It's like social exercise. Nobody can pay for psychotherapy or gym membership anyway. The patients who come to this clinic are poor, and life has not been filled with opportunity. Many of them don't even have the five-dollar copay we ask for. So I decided to start a bunch of groups based not on my desires or their medical diagnoses, but on their preferences and friendships. If they join a group they like, they stick with it. If, at the same time, they get guidance from me, our health coaches, or each other to help change to healthier behavior, they get better. And best of all," Dr. Geller noted, "participants become empowered to be healthier because they are supported by others and others need them. They feel important again."

And that is exactly what happened. Groups began to form that did not conform to the usual medical categories the health care system was trying to treat—like weight loss, cancer support, pain, or post–heart attack. Instead, groups were formed around friendships. Often these took the form of youth groups, men's or women's groups, or groups of mothers and seniors. Some combined these categories because the members just got along with each other. Says Dr. Geller, "patients who found and attended a group they liked not only made friends, but their health improved faster than in disease-based groups. Now many of the groups are run by other patients—with help from our staff."

Dr. Geller and his staff have set up a way to tap into the healing power of the social and emotional dimension for people with few other resources than their ability to find friends and the common human love that accompanies it. It would have been the perfect solution for Gloria and many like her.

THE CAKE

The tools used and exact path in a healing journey are different for everyone. Yet the basic processes are the same. Bill gave up seeking cures, then realized the childhood source of his pain and eventually found a path to self-care that kept him largely pain-free and functioning. Jeff continued to smoke after joining a group to help him quit—but he eventually succeeded by substituting a healthy behavior for an unhealthy one. Maria jumped right into the behavioral change without preparation and planning—and suffered from it. Later she found a way to connect it to something more fulfilling in her life. That is when it became a long-term solution and lifted her out of sadness and struggle—and improved her diabetes. Susan and Clara began their journeys in a different dimension: the space they lived in. Susan also added tools from the social and emotional dimension of healing. Accessing the love and care of others helped her recover during her most difficult time in the curing of her cancer—when she felt she could not go on. And it came in an unexpected way.

About the tenth week of Susan's weekly chemotherapy, a deep fatigue hit her. The word *fatigue* does not really describe it adequately. It's hard to describe using any language. It's like having a hundred-pound millstone around your neck and being thrown into the bottom of a river. You can move around a little bit, but you can't get back to the surface. The amount of oxygen is low, and the effort it takes to move is huge. You know you can't get back to the surface, so you are just watching and waiting as the world goes by. Sharks and other scary animals seem to be swimming nearby in the murky water. I too felt her fatigue, especially toward the end of the day when there was a lack of will to even speak. It was more than the fatigue we expected and she'd had from the start of chemotherapy. It kicked in most drastically in the middle of chemotherapy and stretched out for several weeks and into the summer.

On this particular Fourth of July, we had four generations of family with us, including my mother and the grandbaby. But I was worried that she would not be able to participate in one of her favorite family holidays—the Fourth of July and especially the making of The Cake.

This was not just any old cake—it was The Cake. It was a cake Susan prepared for the family gathering every year for over thirty-five years. Everyone looked forward to it. It was, of course, a depiction of the American flag. Susan had been making this cake since before we were married. She usually served it after the family dinner when all were gathered to celebrate Independence Day—a ritual revealed right before the fireworks. Originally, The Cake was made from a cake mix, with thick cream cheese frosting, and decorated with blue and red food coloring and sprinkles. Not the picture of healthy food. Over the years she had substituted healthier ingredients such as blueberries for the starry field and strawberries for the red stripes. She also began to make a light whipping cream frosting with healthier fat and less sugar. I tried to encourage her to use whole grains in the cake mix, but that never quite worked, and I must admit it didn't have the same result as the good old Betty Crocker cake mix, so we ended up sticking with the latter.

But on this particular July Fourth, Susan had just received her tenth weekly chemo treatment and was very tired and anemic. She had not cooked for weeks. Still, despite how she was feeling, she decided to make it.

My ninety-year-old mother, who has moderate dementia, had come to visit, along with my sister and her daughter. We had the core family and more—it was the first July Fourth also for our new grandchild. Despite her dementia, my mother responded with tremendous joy when she saw her great-grandbaby, a reaction that was infectious to us all. Perhaps it was this joy, and that all of her family was together, that motivated my wife to make The Cake. Others helped. Susan made the cake part with the Betty Crocker mix, and our daughter prepared the whipped cream frosting and decorated The Cake while the others played with the baby.

After dinner, Susan placed The Cake on the table to an enthusiastic reaction from everyone. My mother, who had never seen The Cake before, reacted with more great joy.

"It's beautiful!" she said. "I'll have a big piece."

My sister, who usually goes sugar-, gluten-, and dairy-free, ate three pieces. My son, normally not a cake fan, had two; and I—remembering the rabbits—had one myself. The kitchen was cleaned up. We went outside and shot off fireworks and shared music together. When my mother left a couple of days later, her final words were, "Thank you for having me. It was such a joy to see the baby." Then, after a pause that made us think she was confused, she turned to Susan and said "And oh, thank you for that cake!" There was an understanding in her eyes, rarely seen any more with her advancing dementia.

The next day we saw a clear change in Susan. She began to make travel plans. She wanted to go to a wedding we'd been invited to; previously she had been noncommittal, but now she looked at the calendar to plan the trip. She started talking politics again—something she loved. She mentioned walking the Camino de Santiago again, and planning a visit to see her mother and family in Florida the next winter. She spoke of taking care of her grandchild more fully next spring. She considered resuming her volunteer work teaching English as a second language. The Cake had become a healing agent and helped turn things around. It didn't change the physical side effects—she still had the fatigue, her red blood cell count and hemoglobin were still low, and her hair kept falling out—but after The Cake was made and served, she recovered something she had lost during the treatment. It was something even more fundamental than her hair, her toenails (which she also lost) and her white blood cells. Her soul was returning—and along with it, the joys of her life.

Chapter 8

Finding Meaning

How mind and spirit heal.

From birth to death, we humans are constantly trying to understand and make sense of the world. We are meaning-making machines. But unlike machines, we operate in nonrational ways, most of which occurs outside our awareness—even while we sleep. These attempts at sense-making continuously take in information and compare it to both past experience and the current context, determining how to respond. That response is triggered (or not) depending on subtle judgments we make concerning our safety, the social situation, and our very survival. We absorb and integrate that information from many sources at once—our body, sensory perceptions, relationships, memories, beliefs, and hopes—and use that information to create our universe and trigger biological responses.

Meaning is more like a thought field shifting between people and their environments, and it emerges from multiple interacting judgments rather than a single thought. What we believe and expect drives what we see and how our minds and bodies react. Stress, for example, with all its physical, emotional, and mental consequences, often has less to do with an actual threat than with what we believe the threat to be. Meaning is not simply held in the mind; it is constructed in our body by our culture.

The way to access our healing capacity depends on using tools from any of the dimensions of a person to find and construct meaningful responses. We have talked about three of those dimensions—the external environment, our behavior (including lifestyle and medical treatments), and how we use our emotions and social relationships. But the most powerful way we have for making healing work is our own automatic assumptions about whether healing is possible; that is, the story we, our family and friends, and culture tell us about the way things are and can be. In this chapter, I describe patients who have broken out of limiting assumptions and experienced dramatic healing. As in other chapters, I will show you how systems science documents how this healing works and can be enhanced in daily life. My patient Jake showed me how simple and powerful this process can be if we take control of it.

JAKE

Jake was on the edge of death—now for the third time. No one knew why. He had been a tobacco farmer all his life—as had his father and grandfather before him. They did not own the farm; they only worked it. He did not smoke, did not drink, and worked hard every day except Sunday. At eleven years old, he was pulled out of school to work the farm when his family needed extra hands and money to survive. That lasted the rest of his life, even as he grew up and started his own family. Farming, family, and church were the anchors of his life. Jake was a mild-mannered and deeply faithful man. A man of simple needs and little talk. Content with his life. His only major venture outside the farm was a short trip to Vietnam in the military. He was drafted and shipped over with an infantry division just before the end of the war. His unit left six months later and he was discharged back home. That was years ago. He had been healthy all his life, as far as he knew. But he rarely visited a doctor. Then, for reasons neither he or his doctors could explain, he ended up in the intensive care unit (ICU)—not once, but three times—each time on the verge of death.

Each ICU admission had the same pattern. Jake developed a fever and began to get short of breath. X-rays revealed a sudden, severe pneumonia—in both lungs. "A whiteout," they called it. As the doctors watched in frustration, the pneumonia spread, eventually covering his entire lung fields and dropping his blood oxygen to dangerously low levels. The first two times that happened they needed to intubate him (insert a breathing tube) and put him on a breathing machine. Sputum and blood cultures did not reveal a cause. No bacteria were found, and viral levels were also inconclusive. The infectious disease specialist we called in assumed it was a virus and said Jake must have an immune problem. The immunology specialist we called in suspected the same, but no specific immune problem was found. Each of the first two times this happened the pneumonia lasted about six weeks—with two weeks on the breathing machine—and then it gradually cleared up. It took Jake about four months after that to fully recover and get back to work. Now, for the third time in as many years, it was happening again.

When I visited Jake in the ICU, the specialists were debating when to intubate him again. "Probably tonight," said the internist in charge of his hospital care. His pneumonia was spreading as before, and his oxygen levels were beginning to drop. The oxygen by mask was barely keeping him in the range needed for survival. Jake's breathing became more labored by the hour, and he was tired. But the internist wanted to delay as long as possible. Being intubated is never a very good idea unless you absolutely need it. I sat by Jake's bed to see how he was doing and explore what he was thinking of all this.

He was circumspect. "Well, Doc," he said between labored breaths, "I guess . . . the Lord . . . has some purpose in it. . . . Maybe . . . I done somethin' . . . bad or maybe . . . he just wants . . . to test my faith. . . . We all have . . . our cross to bear."

Did he have others pulling for him? I asked

"Oh sure, Doc . . . my family . . . and church prayin' . . . for me every day. . . . I prayin', too. . . . most all day. . . . nothin' else to do . . . I guess."

I was struck by how calm he was, even with his labored breathing, on the edge of intubation and possible death. Could he go through this illness again, having been weakened from the last two times? Then, mostly out of desperation, I had an idea. I tried to frame my proposal in a way he might find meaningful.

"Jake, would you be interested in trying something that might help all that prayer you are having?" I had decided to explore working with Jake's deep faith rather than provide long explanations about mind-body effect, placebo research, the immune system, and visualization.

"Sure, Doc," he responded quickly. "I always want . . . to help the Lord . . . in his will . . . I'm sure he . . . wants me healed . . . I'll help . . . if I can."

I presented Jake with my proposal. "Is there any place in your lungs that you feel is clear? Any place you feel the air goes when you breathe in?" I asked.

Jake thought for a while as I held my breath. Perhaps there was no opportunity to try my idea after all. He took a couple of breaths, deeper than the usual labored ones, and concentrated. Finally, he said, "Sure, Doc . . . air goes right here." He pointed to a place on his lower left chest. "When I take . . . a breath . . . it all . . . goes right there." He pointed again to the same place. An opening.

"Great," I said, seeing a window of hope. "Then here is what I want you to do. As you lie here and pray, I want you to try and relax as much as you can and then imagine in your mind that the air is going into that place and that place is expanding—getting bigger. Imagine that area gradually growing, getting larger and larger, clearer and clearer. Imagine all the love of the Lord and all of those prayers from your family and church and all the air coming into your lungs and clearing away the pneumonia you have—healing your lungs."

We did a few practices sessions in which I encouraged him to visit in his mind a place in his church that he loved, and to feel a sense of peace there. And then to imagine the love and power of the Lord was flowing into that small space in his lung. He got it quickly. Then he smiled. "That be easy, Doc . . . that be real easy . . . to do."

The next morning, I arrived at the hospital to visit Jake, fully expecting him to be on the ventilator. The ICU specialist watching him had thought he would not last the night on his own. Most people tire out and decompensate during the night, and Jake had been on the edge of that the day before. But to my surprise, when I walked into his room, he was sitting up in a chair and still just on the oxygen mask. During the night his oxygen levels had held steady. He smiled when he saw me come in.

"How is it going, Jake?" I asked.

He smiled again. "It goin' fine, Doc. . . . Goin' fine. . . . That thing . . . that thing you taught me . . . works real well. The place for air . . . gettin' bigger." He placed his hand over the left lower chest as he had done before but now using his whole hand to show a larger area. "Got no tube . . . last night." He grinned.

In fact, Jake never got intubated again. The next day his oxygen levels continued to improve, and within a week his pneumonia cleared sufficiently that he was discharged. Jake had healed himself—by using his mind and faith.

THE BODY'S MIND

Coincidence? I wondered. Yes, possibly. Much of healing is coincidence— something statisticians call "regression to the mean." If you go in to see a doctor when you are sickest, what usually happens—no matter what you do—is improve. Doctors mistakenly attribute this improvement to the treatments they prescribe. So do patients. But in this case it didn't seem like regression to the mean was an adequate explanation. Jake had had pneumonia before and recovered, so we knew he could. But he was not yet at the peak of this illness when he turned around. He had never recovered in this short a time—and without intubation.

I didn't know for sure if Jake had really healed himself with his mind and faith. Most patients don't care whether the healing they experience is called "regression to the mean" or a miracle—they are just happy to be better. However, I did know there was rigorous research showing that our mind can influence healing for a number of conditions including pain, anxiety and depression, Parkinson's and Alzheimer's disease, high blood pressure, and heart disease. And it can alter immune function—as it appeared to do in Jake's situation. Professor Alia Crum of Stanford, whose research on "Mind over Milkshakes" I described in chapter 6 (see page 124), has demonstrated how our mind-set, which she defines as our "conscious and embodied expectation to heal," infuses all treatments including those involving drugs, food, exercise, and stress. How we individually and culturally think of and frame a treatment is often the largest contributor to whether and how much that treatment works. Mind-set can also influence the amount of pain and rate of recovery from surgery.

I was in high school when President Nixon visited China in 1972, and the reporter James Reston, who accompanied him, described the amazing power of acupuncture to treat pain, including his own after an emergency operation he underwent there. He described doctors doing full-blown open heart surgery on patients without anesthesia—under the palliative influence of acupuncture alone. I saw similar cases of surgery done without anesthesia using hypnosis during my rotations in psychiatry in the United States. We know the role of the mind in healing is huge, but how it operates is still largely a mystery. At the time I met Jake, studies were just emerging exploring the influence of visualization on biology. Most of these studies involve creating specific images in the mind under relaxed conditions, seeking to influence biological processes. We now know that visualization can influence a number of conditions. This includes reduction of pain, bleeding, and infection after surgery, and acceleration of recovery time. Chronic conditions also benefit from visualization, including high blood pressure, chronic pain, depression, and PTSD. Professional athletes routinely use visualization to enhance endurance and performance. Golf and other skill-based games improve through mental practice.

In 2015, Dr. Mimi Guarneri and Rauni King from Scripps Hospital, along with a colleague, Dr. Shamini Jain from Samueli Institute, conducted a study at Camp Pendleton, California, testing whether mental relaxation in the presence of another combined with mental imagery could help Marines with PTSD. All the Marines in the study had been deployed to Iraq or Afghanistan and suffered significant PTSD on their return. All had received standard treatment with medication and counseling. In the study, half of the Marines were given continued standard treatment and half were given a visualization tape to listen to, along with four treatments of a relaxation method called "healing touch," an approach taught to nurses in which they hold their hands over the patient—similar to what I used with Susan during her chemotherapy. After each of the four deep relaxation sessions, the Marines were asked to listen to a visualization CD once a day for twenty minutes. The CD took them to a safe place of their choosing where the relaxation response was reinforced daily. After three weeks, the Marines were tested again for PTSD. There was more than a 25% drop in PTSD scores in those who used the relaxation sessions and visualization tape compared to usual treatment—an improvement as great as any current PTSD treatment we have with medications or psychotherapy. After the relaxation sessions and visualization practice, the average PTSD scores for the group went below what was considered abnormal. The usual care group improved slightly but was still above the cutoff for PTSD.

JOE

What I found most remarkable about this, however, were the stories service members told about the "coincidental" effects visualization had on them. Joe, a thick-skinned Marine who had been deployed four times, recounted how a buddy, killed next to him in a battle, appeared to him during one of his visualization exercises. The appearance was more than an image, he said. His buddy reached out and touched him—"I felt it," said Joe. His buddy then said that he was fine and that he would always love Joe and be watching over him. "Go on with your life," the phantom buddy said, "you have lots of life left to live, and we did good together."

Joe did not tell his physician about this episode, but broke down in tears at his next healing touch session with the nurse. "Now I know everything will be okay," he said to her after the session. Later, Joe's wife noticed how much less agitated he was. Joe had what is called an "exceptional spiritual experience," meaning one that goes beyond the normal experiences of everyday consciousness. People who have such experiences often describe them as profound, overwhelming, indescribable, and even frightening. They are more than just images—they look, sound, and feel completely real. And the body reacts to them as if they were real. As it turns out, lots of people have these experiences—especially when faced with a life-threatening situation and when they cultivate an open, relaxed mind. They frequently occur during the night and wake people from sleep.

Dr. David Hufford, emeritus professor of sociology and medicine at Penn State University, is one of the world's experts on these exceptional experiences. He told me that between 30% and 40% of people around the world have them at some point in their lives, regardless of the culture they live in. Traumatic experiences increase the likelihood of these experiences. In a study Dr. Hufford did of veterans who returned from the wars in Iraq and Afghanistan, he found that more than 60% of those exposed to combat had these experiences.

"That is a very high rate," he said, "almost double the baseline rate in our culture." These experiences are so profound and sometimes frightening that soldiers rarely talk about them. They are afraid of being labeled "crazy" and put into mental health treatment. Dr. Hufford explained, "If these exceptional experiences are labeled negatively—called hallucinations or a mental illness—that can be damaging. If they are acknowledged as real and treated positively, they can be profoundly healing. Many cultures will use these experiences to help heal a person. Modern medicine usually thinks of them as a sign of illness. We need to reframe how health care deals with these experiences."

In Dr. Guarneri's study, she did not ask how often these experiences occurred in the Marines who did the visualization and healing touch relaxation, so we don't know how common experiences like Joe's were in that group. We do know that hostility scores in the group—something very difficult to improve in war-induced PTSD—dropped markedly in those who did the visualization. They had found a tool and a process to tap into the healing power through their minds and spirits.

BEYOND BELIEF

Belief is a powerful tool for healing. But specific mental practices like those Jake and Joe used do not take optimal advantage of the unconscious processes of meaning-making that occur in the everyday rituals of health care delivery. Research on placebo effects, as described in previous chapters, demonstrates that potential. When ritual and belief are combined with repeated social ritual, they can produce profound effects on chronic illness including pain, mental health, and the immune system. At the time I saw Jake, Dr. Robert Ader, a pioneer in the investigation of conditioned learning and immune function, was demonstrating that by repeatedly pairing the use of an inert substance (a placebo) with an immune-suppressing drug, one could teach the immune system to respond to the inert substance even when the drug was withdrawn. He used rats that had a genetically inbred autoimmune condition— their own immune systems were killing their bodies prematurely, like what goes on in lupus or multiple sclerosis. When this autoimmunity was suppressed with a drug called cyclophosphamide, the rats lived longer. Dr. Ader used a simple process of classical conditioning to train the animals' immune systems to lower their harmful activities. He did this by giving the cyclophosphamide along with a sugar solution. After several pairings of the drug and sugar solution, the drug was gradually reduced but the sugar solution was maintained. Animals who continued to get the sugar solution also continued to have a dampened immune system—and lived almost as long as if they had received the actual drug!

Studies now show that the human immune system can also be taught to do this. Drink Kool-Aid and take an immune-modulating drug a few times together, and soon (within three or four sequences) you can withdraw the drug and get the immune modulation effect—nearly 80% of it—from the Kool-Aid alone. (Don't try this at home! Immune-modulating drugs must be carefully monitored, and this conditioning approach requires precise timing and supervision.) But most people already use the benefit of mental conditioning without even knowing it. Take a headache pill with aspirin in it and you will feel better. Do this a few times, and soon just taking a pill (even without aspirin in it) eases the headache. Meaning influences effect.

When people take an effective brand-name drug for a while, they get used to its working. If they switch to a generic or lower-cost version of the drug, they often report it does not work as well. And it truly won't work as well, but not because the chemicals in the drug have stopped working. Studies have shown that, at least for pain and depression, if a person thinks she is getting a "discounted" drug, rather than the full-priced drug, she will report it as less effective. Another example is that when a "new, improved" drug comes along for an illness (based on hype and advertising), the older drug loses some of its effectiveness as people lose confidence in it. Professor Dan Moerman, the anthropologist from the University of Michigan introduced in chapter 2 (see page 22), demonstrated this dramatically by tracking the effects of established drugs proven to work when a supposedly better drug came along. For example, when a new drug called ranitidine got FDA approval for treatment of stomach ulcers, the company marketed it extensively as better than an established drug called cimetidine. Cimetidine was working well—healing ulcers in about 75% of patients who took it and about 20% more than placebo. However, as excitement grew and use of ranitidine gained popularity, the healing rate of the older drug, cimetidine, diminished—dropping to below 50%. The magnitude of the older drug's effects diminished as the collective mind-set was drawn to the new and "better" drug. So, remarkably, a treatment's healing potency depends not only on how well it actually works, but also on a culture's belief in the relative benefit of alternative treatments for those same conditions. No wonder pharmaceutical companies spend billions pushing new drugs when they first get approved. Not only do the sales go up because of the marketing, but the actual effects are increased if the culture believes they are effective. They are building both conscious and unconscious belief. One of my medical school professors used to admonish his students to "use a new treatment as much as possible when it first comes out, before it loses its effectiveness." Now I know why he said that. Our collective mind affects the magnitude of the meaning. The meaning affects the magnitude of healing.

If this works with rats, how much more effective can it be with humans? Humans have such a powerful mind for making meaning that they can produce this same kind of conditioning with their own words and imagination—no Kool-Aid or pills required. Pediatrician Dr. Karen Olness of Northwest University reported an example of this in a child with an autoimmune disease similar to that of Dr. Ader's rats. The child needed immune-suppressive medications for kidney disease, but they were making her so nauseous that she could not take them anymore. This increased the risk that her disease would flare and threaten her life. Dr. Olness first used a rose fragrance and paired it with the immune-suppressive drugs and nausea-suppressing medications to condition the child's system to react less severely to the immune-suppressing medications. She also taught the child to imagine a rose during these treatments. Soon the side effects of giving the immune-suppressing drugs could be reduced while maintaining the drugs' effectiveness— provided the child imagined the smell and look of a rose when she took them! The child had learned how to control her nausea and immune system with her mind. Like Jake, she used her newfound visualization skills to heal. Children are especially adept at learning to use their minds to heal. A simple visualization CD for children with irritable bowel and stomach pain is more effective and longer lasting than any medication. All the doctor needs to do is give the child the CD and support her in using it.

DANCE OF MINDS

UCLA professor of psychiatry and best-selling author Dr. Daniel Siegel writes about how modern science is revealing a picture of the mind very different from the traditional one currently held by medicine. Rather than think of the mind as emanating from the brain—inside the skull only—he describes the view emerging from whole systems science that the mind operates more as if it resides between individuals, the culture, and the environment. In his book *Mind: A Journey to the Heart of Being Human*, he explains: "Mind is not just what the brain does, not even the social brain. The mind may be something emerging from a higher level of systems functioning than simply what happens inside the skull. This system's basic elements are energy and information flow—and that flow happens inside of us, and between ourselves and others and the world." A growing number of scientists share this view, as more and more evidence accumulates to support it. I am struck by how consistent this view is with the model Dr. Manu drew for me on his whiteboard in rural India as he tried to explain the ancient Ayurveda view of a person. Rather than being separate from others, as our bodies are, the deeper dimensions of our being—in mind and spirit—show that we are all merged together into one inseparable and overlapping mind. Our mind is collective. If this way of understanding the mind is a more accurate description of what we are as humans, then tapping this power of the mind and spirit is essential in order to fully heal and be whole.

Our collective-like mind's influence on healing goes on every day in the clinical encounter. It does not always require long periods of visualization like Jake undertook or the healing touch relaxation given to Joe, the Marine. The meaning response—both good and bad—can come in an instant. The British physician K. B. Thomas demonstrated this in 1987 with a remarkable study entitled "Is there any point to being positive?" He studied two hundred patients who came to the doctor with no specific pathology, only symptoms of illness. This type of patient makes up about half of all visits to a primary care doctor. He divided the two hundred patients into four groups. Two groups got either a positive consultation, in which they were told they had a clear illness that would resolve soon, or a negative consultation, in which they were told that the doctor did not know what they had or if they would get better. Half of each group was then given a placebo pill and the other half nothing. All treatments took the same amount of time.

Two weeks later, the patients were asked by someone new (not the doctor) if they were better and if they needed more treatment. The results showed that 64% of patients who got a positive consultation were better, compared to only 39% of those who got the negative consultation. About 50% in either the placebo or nontreated groups reported being better. In other words, the coincidental healing rate (the "regression to the mean") was about 50%. But a simple shift in the belief and expectations of patients induced by the language and attitude of the doctor could either increase that healing rate by 28% or decrease it by 22%—a total difference of another 50% from the baseline healing rate. The difference in healing rates between those who got a pill and those who did not was only 6%. The shared mind space between doctor and patient significantly enhanced or interfered with the patient's own healing processes—even from a single encounter.

This dance between minds making meaning does not require the doctor to say anything or that it even be consciously perceived by the patient. The late NIH researcher Dr. David D. Price, whose work on placebo I described in chapter 4 (see page 73), demonstrated in several studies that a doctor's belief influences a treatment's effectiveness—even when the patient does not know of that belief. Oral surgeons who had extracted third molars (wisdom teeth) were told that after the extraction their patients would get either a pain killer, a placebo, or naloxone. Naloxone, a drug used to combat narcotic overdose, could increase their pain. The patients were told nothing, but later asked to rate their pain and need for medications. Patients whose surgeons thought their patients had received an effective painkiller reported less pain and had less need for medications, compared to those patients whose surgeons thought their patients had not received an effective pain treatment—either placebo or naloxone. In fact, all patients got placebo. Without any verbal exchanges, patients seemed to read the surgeon's expectations. People surpass rats or rabbits in reading subtle signals and infusing meaning into those signals—even when they don't know they have done so.

This and similar research makes me wonder if it is truly possible to withhold or hide information from a patient or if they read the situation and react on some level no matter what the doctor attempts to do. Indeed, the dance of the mind behaves more like the ebb and flow of energy and information between people and things. Even if we cannot measure it directly, its impact on healing is profound.

NOCEBO

For the most part, patients and physicians are largely oblivious to the healing and the harm that arise from the mind and spiritual dimension. Like the other dimensions of healing, our health care system seems to mostly miss this. We attribute improvements to the specific treatments given rather than to the context and meaning created during the delivery of those treatments. But we do this at our peril. By not acknowledging the more nonlocal view of the human mind described by Dr. Siegel and others, our health care system not only misses a key dimension for healing, but it may be harming us as well. This is seen most clearly in what is called the "nocebo" effect—the negative impact of ritual and belief on health and healing.

For every ritual, belief, conditioning, or social learning process that improves healing, there is the potential for those same processes to harm. In the 1987 study by Dr. Thomas described earlier, patients' recovery rate was cut almost in half by a single negative encounter with their physician. Dr. Price showed how physicians' subtle nonverbal expectations could increase pain. Professor Fabrizio Benedetti, whose research on placebo I described in chapter 2 (see page 25), demonstrated that the pain-relieving effects of our most powerful drugs—such as morphine—can be almost completely negated by delivering the drug with a negative expectation. Morphine works for acute pain, but the ritual and belief surrounding morphine works—or interferes—to an almost equal extent. The endogenous painkillers produced by our mind are just as powerful. Like most physicians trained in the 1980s, I was taught to let the patient know if what I was about to do to them was going to hurt. Before drawing blood, giving a shot, or doing a biopsy, for example, I told them, "This may hurt a little." Then, after the stick, I would try and calm them by saying, "It will get better now" or sometimes, "Now that wasn't so bad, was it?" This happened (and still happens) thousands of times a day in health care. It turns out that by saying this, I was increasing my patient's experience of pain. To add insult to injury, if I tried to reassure them afterward and they were still feeling pain, this made things worse still because my attempt at reassurance was also communicating to them that they should be over it. Now I say nothing to my patients about pain before a procedure. I only describe what I will be doing and then create a mental distraction or have them use a visualization tape or music during the procedure. They can make up their own mind from my description if it will hurt them or not.

The nocebo effect impacts more than pain. And it is also not just transmitted though the clinical encounter. It can be embedded in our cultural beliefs and social communications. Studies by Professor Winfried Rief and colleagues from the University of Marburg, Germany, demonstrate that clinical trials consistently show higher side effects in those receiving placebo when the active drug being tested has higher side effects. These adverse effects are not just from the subjects' baseline symptoms, which they attribute to the drug—although that does happen; the adverse effects produced by giving the placebo actually mimic those of the specific drug being studied. For example, placebo-treated groups in studies of different antidepressants with different side effects will report from two to five times the rate of adverse effects specific to the drug being studied—tricyclic placebos produce tricyclic drug–like side effects, and serotonin-like side effects occur in the placebo groups of the serotonin drug studies. This is often attributed to study subjects being told the potential side effects of a drug before entering a study—part of the process of informed consent. Like Dr. Thomas's patients, these study subjects learn that they might experience specific negative effects—and they do. Unlike Dr. Thomas's patients, however, these side effects continue over the course of the study—often for one to two months—without further communication about the drug. A single encounter with a study coordinator obtaining their informed consent is sufficient to induce negative effects.

The collective mind can influence not only health outcomes, but death outcomes as well. A large study by Dr. David Phillips of the University of California, San Diego, published in the prestigious medical journal *Lancet*, poignantly demonstrates the cultural impact of the meaning response. The study examined the deaths of 28,169 adult Chinese-Americans, and 412,632 randomly selected, matched controls coded "white" on the death certificate. Dr. Phillips showed that: "Chinese-Americans, but not whites, die significantly earlier than normal (1.3–4.9 years) if they have a combination of disease and birth year, which Chinese astrology and [traditional Chinese] medicine consider ill-fated. The more strongly a group is attached to Chinese traditions, the more years of life are lost." He goes on to say, "Our results hold for nearly all major causes of death studied. The reduction in survival cannot be completely explained by a change in the behavior of the Chinese patient, doctor, or death-registrar, but seems to result at least partly from psychosomatic processes." That is, the collective mind.

Chinese astrology assigns one of five elements—fire, earth, metal, water, and wood—to each year (as well as one of the better-known twelve animals), and people born in a metal year, who are expected by the culture to have more lung diseases than people born in other years, actually do have more lung problems—and die earlier than others from lung problems. The same thing is true for lymph problems or immune system problems if people are born in an earth year—thought to be bad luck for the immune system. Major differences in the age at death from lymphatic cancer occurred between those born in earth years and those born in other years. These effects were over and above the impact of other factors, such as smoking, lifestyle, and environmental exposures. Unlike pain, the "side effect" of age at death is a rather hard, objective outcome. The effect was sociocultural—an effect from the collective mind of the culture. The more distant people were generationally from the original Chinese culture, the less this finding held, so that for third-generation Chinese-American people there was no correlation whatsoever—just like non-Chinese Americans.

We do not have to believe in astrology for this to happen; we have only to grow up with a concept that our culture accepts. Stress is often cited as bad for you in Western cultures—thanks to Hans Selye and other scientists of the last century. However, it is also often framed as good for you, as in the phrase "no pain, no gain" used by Joe and his fellow Marines. While both attitudes can harm, people who believe that stress is bad are 43% more likely to die earlier than those who interpret stress as good. Mindset influences mortality.

When Aadi first came to the Ayurvedic hospital to treat his Parkinson's disease, he did not believe in the use of astrology to help him heal. In fact, he had never believed in it, and he told Dr. Manu so each time he came. I think he used the word "poppycock" to describe it. Yet Dr. Manu insisted he get an astrology reading each time anyway.

"He may not personally believe in astrology himself," Manu explained, "but he was raised and lives in a culture that does. He cannot escape its effects, even if they are only psychologically driven. So he might as well try and use information from it to find meaning for his life."

I am not sure whether Aadi ever used that information consciously, but his wife and others in his family commented on how those readings seemed to make sense and described Aadi's life accurately. They, if not he, found them meaningful.

Humans seem to be hardwired to seek out some type of transpersonal or spiritual meaning from illness. This has happened for centuries. When patients arrived at Epidaurus, the ancient Greek center of Hippocrates' medical school, they first consulted with an oracle, who read their spiritual lives to contextualize their illnesses with a deeper meaning before they went on to other treatments. Most indigenous cultures infuse spiritual interpretations and rituals into their diagnoses and treatments. Some of these are clearly harmful—like when a "demon extraction" is substituted for medical treatment in an epileptic. Some can be helpful—like when prayers soothe the anxiety of a patient newly diagnosed with cancer. As with drugs, herbs, lifestyle, and social relationships, our mind-set and spiritual beliefs are simply another tool to use for healing or harm. Short of being hit by a truck or a tornado or an Ebola virus, disease, suffering, and death do not have simple cause-and-effect connections. If we are going to maximize healing from our treatments, we must pay attention to the complex layers of history and traditions, cultural and family influences, and individual beliefs that make meaning in our lives. We need to attend to our collective mind. Until we incorporate an awareness of these forces into health care, they will continue to help or harm us at random, and we will not be able to tap into our full healing potential.

But how can we do that?

PSYKHE

I explore specific mental and spiritual elements of healing with my patients. While there is scientific evidence for the value of each of these elements, the purpose of my exploring these with patients is not to tell them what to believe, but to help them learn how to use their mind and faith to find deeper meaning in their lives. Once we see which elements resonate with them, I look for scientifically validated ways they can enhance those elements' healing power in their lives. This may be a specific mind-body practice, like Jake's visualization, or it may involve helping them link healing behaviors to their spiritual life. I always seek to respect them as they are—with all their wounds and flaws—on a journey to more wholeness and healing.

ELEMENTS OF THE SPIRITUAL AND MENTAL DIMENSION

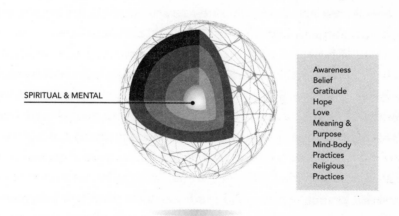

SPIRITUAL & MENTAL

Awareness
Belief
Gratitude
Hope
Love
Meaning &
Purpose
Mind-Body
Practices
Religious
Practices

In ancient times there was no distinction made between what today we call the mind and soul. The Greek word *psykhe,* the root of psyche and psychology, also means "soul, mind, spirit, or the deepest experience people have of themselves." This experience is often "transpersonal" and "transtemporal"—seeming to go beyond the normal boundaries of space and time. This is the dimension of the spirit. While psychologists, clergy, and academics often debate the differences in these terms, I find that when it comes to healing, people use them interchangeably. Those who are atheistic or humanistic will use the terms *mind* or *psyche,* while those with a spiritual or religious preference will add the term *soul* or *spirit.* Whatever they are called, these components provide valuable tools within the inner dimensions of our being for healing. Both disciplines—psychology and religion—tend to be neglected by modern medicine. Thus the role of mind and spirit for healing remains poorly used.

Yet there is substantial evidence that people who engage in spiritual and religious practices stay healthy longer, recover faster, and die with a better quality of life than people who do not. This is, of course, provided those beliefs do not dictate specifically harmful behaviors—such as mutilation, neglect, or violence—or create excessive spiritual (and psychological) distress from guilt, doubt, and dogma. Dr. Harold Koenig, professor of psychiatry at Duke University, has studied, reviewed, and written about the health effects of spiritual and religious practices for decades. In his *Handbook of Religion and Health,* he reviews research showing positive health benefits from participating in faith traditions or spiritual practices. He and others report that the evidence of benefit is particularly strong for mental health conditions such as depression, substance abuse, suicide, dementia, and stress-related disorders. There are also many positive physical health correlations with spiritual and religious practices. Most of the reasons for this make sense. Those who engage in spiritual and religious practices tend to avoid harmful substances (alcohol, tobacco, drugs), engage in social service and support activities, and pray—often in a meditative state—which induces relaxation or catharsis. In addition, some religious beliefs provide soothing explanations for suffering and death accompanied by rituals of forgiveness and reconciliation—further comforting the suffering.

Spiritual-like discussions at the end of life are especially important when we all—regardless of whether we have a faith tradition—seek comfort as we die. Research shows that spiritual rituals and chaplain interactions for those who desire it toward the end of life increase quality of life and satisfaction. As with any medical intervention, negative effects can also occur. Harm is caused by poorly or negatively delivered religious and spiritual beliefs and behaviors, such as blaming the believer for their illness if they remain sick. I have had deeply religious patients admit to me they feel guilty that they have not "prayed deeply enough" if they do not recover. Some religious traditions state that explicitly. Harm also occurs if a religious community on which a person has had lifelong reliance fails to visit and care for the person during serious illness or hospitalization—breaching an unwritten social and moral contract. Whether or not you are religious, if you and your health care professional do not include the mind and spiritual dimension in your conversations—especially toward the end of life—you risk missing out on its use for healing.

THE WOUNDED HEALER

One of the most important effects of a serious illness is its impact not only on the body, but also on the soul (or spirit, or whatever you call your nonphysical inner being). Bodies often heal; souls may not. Sometimes there is a point in an illness when you are not sure if you will ever get better—or if you even want to. It is as if you have lost your will to live. There's no modern medical disease category when a trauma or a stress penetrates your soul. But you feel it nonetheless. You can feel it in some people who suffer from PTSD produced by war, when it is not possible to elicit even a glimmer of hope. You can feel it in the chronic embodied stress of those who have had adverse childhood experiences—when they do not even have a memory of personal power. And you can feel it in the existential threat of a serious disease and its therapy—when a patient asks, "Who am I now?" Soul loss is named in some cultures, especially in Native American and indigenous cultures. They recognize it as a distinct disability separate from any psychological or physical condition. Finding a way back out of such a state is central to recovering one's well-being. Navigating out through that labyrinth is part of the healing journey.

Susan's first cancer changed her view of herself forever. Like many of her colleagues, she had taken a professional life path up to that point—with family in tow. But having cancer at such a young age, along with the triple whammy of surgery, chemotherapy, and radiation, "knocked me out of the path of a normal thirty-five-year-old lawyer," she said. "Even though my body would recover, my spirit had to change. I could never be with my peers or myself in the same way again—pursuing both family and professional careers. After the cure, when they said they got it all, my questions went from 'Why did I get this' to 'Why me?' I realized that I didn't really want to be a lawyer anymore. But then what was I here for, I wondered? Why had I been born?"

For Susan, the illness brought to the forefront what is arguably the most important question in anyone's life: why am I here? Medicine offers chemistry and biology as the answer. People need more than that. They need something more meaningful, something drawn out of the deeper dimensions of who we are—social, emotional, mental, and spiritual. And for most of us, healing requires that we try to answer that question by exploring the mind and spiritual dimensions of our soul.

So here is the irony of healing and what makes it different than curing: the very wound from which we suffer induces the process of healing. To acknowledge and enter that wounding opens the path to wholeness. The priest, writer, and spiritual teacher Henry Nouwen called this "the wounded healer," whereby a person, by accepting and then embracing the fact that he is flawed and wounded, can find a deep peace and joy. He called this the experience of "being beloved"—fully valuing oneself and one's life just as they are. It is an "exceptional spiritual experience" of a different kind. This experience of deep peace and joy can come in a spiritual version, as found by Jake and Joe, or through a different pathway. Aadi found it through Ayurveda, Sergeant Martin through his friends with PTSD, Clara in nature, Mabel with her family, Jeff in running, and Gloria through teaching cooking classes. Each path is unique, yet all lead to the same place of healing and wholeness.

CHAPLAINCY

When my patients seek the spiritual dimension of healing, I may ask if they would like to see a chaplain. Surveys report that most hospitalized patients, and many with serious illness, would like an existential or spiritual discussion with their physician or a visit with a religious professional—but rarely do medical professionals ask patients about their spiritual needs. To help remedy this situation, internist and palliative care physician Dr. Christina Puchalski, founder and director of the George Washington University Institute for Spirituality and Health and author of *Making Health Care Whole: Integrating Spirituality into Patient Care*, trains health care practitioners in how to discuss spirituality in health care. Her yearly course for physicians and other health care professionals teaches them how to integrate patients' spiritual beliefs into their care, address sensitive medical issues that seriously ill patients face, and support health care professionals in providing compassionate care. In other words, it seeks to get health care practitioners and the health care system to take the nonphysical, inner aspects of healing seriously—to recognize and ask patients about the mind and spiritual dimension of their lives.

I am fortunate to be surrounded by people in my family who do look at the spiritual dimension. They have taught me the healing power of attending to the mind and spirit in health care. My father was a chaplain who spent a large part of his career working in hospitals. He was one of the first chaplains to get formal training in hospital chaplaincy—called clinical pastoral education (CPE)—and brought this training into the military. As a young boy, I recall asking him why he, a minister, went to work every day at a hospital, where doctors worked. I thought ministers were supposed to work in churches.

"Why do I work in a hospital?" he replied. "Because that is where a lot of suffering is. I work in a hospital to help alleviate suffering and to heal."

That stuck with me. I wanted to know more. So, before medical school, I decided to do five months of training as a hospital chaplain student. That taught me a lot about healing.

I remember the first patient I was assigned to as a student minister. He was a seventy-three-year-old man dying of metastatic lung cancer and on a morphine drip for pain. He had requested a visit from a chaplain and was willing to see the "student chaplain" first. I was all of twenty-one years old, nervous as a cat, with no idea what I was going to say. When I entered his room, I was relieved to see that he was asleep—apparently sedated by the morphine. Thinking I was off the hook, I sat next to his bed and began to softly read a few prayers. After a few moments, he opened his eyes to look at me. Then he reached his hand over and placed it on my hand and said, "Son, you are going to be okay." Not only was my cover blown, my most basic assumption about healing was flipped on its head—he was healing me! In the spiritual dimension, healing emerges in the space between people—in the collective mind—and its benefits can go either way.

After getting her first breast cancer and recovering from it, my wife also shifted her life focus from being a lawyer to getting a degree in pastoral care. She then worked in a chaplain's counseling center for the military. I was amazed at the stories I heard from her of the spiritual struggles faced by service members and their families. She heard stories with a view of suffering they did not tell me about as a doctor in the clinic. She also told me about healings I had not known were happening to my patients. I looked for the physical causes of their suffering to prescribe a treatment. But with this focus I often totally missed other influences that perpetuated their suffering—influences that my wife was picking up on. The wounding of the cancer and its treatment had awakened her intuitive skills in listening and spiritual care. In recent years our daughter Maeba has enlightened me about the power of the spiritual dimension to heal. After earning her M.Div. degree from Yale Divinity School, she did an additional year of formal CPE training at Yale University Hospital. Prior to becoming a chaplain, she did premedical training and worked in medical research at Johns Hopkins. She also worked in Nepal at a school run by Buddhist nuns and at a clinic in Ethiopia treating children. These experiences and her formal trainings enable her to see the whole person—spiritual, psychological, and physical—and the ways they are linked.

One evening, Maeba was called to visit a man hospitalized for uncontrolled high blood pressure. He was on multiple medications, yet his blood pressure remained dangerously high. After she sat and talked with him for a while, he told her it was the anniversary of the death of his wife, whom he had loved deeply. Maeba prayed with him, holding up the joy of his and his wife's love and the deep sorrow of his loss to clear view. He began to cry, and she sat with him while he mourned. That night his blood pressure returned to normal, and he was discharged the next day. The mechanisms responsible for this are likely explainable. The catharsis of his weeping and the social witness of my daughter likely reduced the stress hormones that were raging through his body and elevating his blood pressure. How often these types of biological healings occur through the spiritual dimension is unknown. Although hospitals with full-time chaplains will chart their visits along with all the other health care professionals, it is rare that those notes are followed or "measured" as drug treatments are. Sources like the *Journal of Pastoral Care & Counseling* are full of case studies like this. How often doctors and nurses read them, much less use these visits in an integrative fashion to heal, is unclear. Thus they remain invisible to most of us health care.

DAVID

Sometimes healing is, as in the Beauty Way, for the collective mind and not just an individual patient. Once Maeba was called to do a baptism of a premature baby born to a drug-addicted mother who, after the birth, walked out of the hospital without a word. The baby was on life support; he was so underdeveloped he could not live on his own. It took social services several days to track the mother down to ask permission to take him off life support after it became apparent he was not going to make it. When they finally got the mother on the phone, she refused to give the baby a name, but did give permission to take him off life support— and then asked that he be baptized. Several of the nurses caring for the abandoned baby were distraught. Not only did he not even have a name, but the mother's only indication of her desire to love the baby—her parting request—was to have the baby baptized. Chaplain Maeba was called in to baptize the baby before he died. The only witnesses were the nurses and one of the doctors who had cared for him and tried to save him. As Maeba prepared the water and the ceremony, she asked the baby's name. The nurses gathered, and, after consulting together, decided to name him David.

The ceremony began. Each caregiver was offered a chance to hold their hands over the water to bless it with their healing touch. "David," Maeba said, "I baptize you in the name of the Father, and of the Son, and of the Holy Spirit," and because of the special circumstances in which she was baptizing a motherless child, she added, "One God: Mother of us all, amen." As the water was placed on the premature infant, the group began to spontaneously weep. This collective catharsis lasted several minutes. The ventilator was then turned off and the baby died. A deep sense of peace emerged, even as everyone grieved David's death. After a silence that under any other circumstances would have seemed long and awkward, but in this context was to be cherished, one of the neonatal ICU nurses commented, "I needed that. For all the little Davids who die here." There was a collective deep breath. She had spoken for all. Despite his short life, his unfortunate circumstances, and his major woundings, David was among the beloved, and it healed them all.

It is not just patients who need mental and spiritual healing. In many ways, the nurse in the neonatal ICU was speaking for all health care—practitioners and patients. Physicians and nurses report the highest rates of burnout of any profession. Nearly half of all physicians have burnout—defined as lack of enthusiasm for work, feeling apathetic, and becoming more callous toward people. The highest rate of burnout is among physicians and nurses in primary care—those at the front lines of health care—where it affects more than 50%. These physicians also have high rates of substance abuse—nearly 15%. Rates of burnout in primary care have risen nearly 20% in the ten years since 2007. As a hospital chaplain, Maeba found that her spiritual care was frequently needed by the staff. This led her to hold a monthly breakfast for the staff of the pediatric ICU.

The causes of burnout are many: excessive workload, clerical burden, inefficiency in our health care system, loss of control over medical decisions, and difficulties in work-life balance. Burnt-out physicians and nurses are not the best healers.

But the primary cause of burnout is, in my opinion, the erosion of meaning. This arises from the lack of opportunity for physicians and nurses to care for themselves and patients in all their dimensions. The imbalanced focus in medicine on the physical aspects of disease, along with the economic and administrative forces dominating medicine, squeeze out the dimensions of healing that they know produce benefit for patients and would allow them to heal the whole person. Those in primary care who see the decline in patients' health and well-being year after year—when they know what could keep them well—bear the heaviest burden. The discouragement of burnout is magnified when they see that the patient's environment, the social and emotional factors, lifestyle and behavior, and the inner dimensions of the mind and spirit also need attention—but they do not have the time or tools to attend to them.

Unfortunately, this discouragement begins in medical school. Medical students in their first year have high levels of altruism and empathy. This empathy drops lower with every year of training, from the time they enter to the time they are licensed four years later. It continues as they get into practice and find that health care is not designed to help patients heal and stay well, and it does not provide the primary tools they need. Our "health care system" is a triple oxymoron—it produces only about 20% of the public's health, it is difficult for those working in it to deliver compassionate care, and it is not an integrated system. No health, no care, and not a system!

Health care needs a new way of thinking and a new design. It needs to shift its economic incentives toward prevention and whole person care, even as the industry profits from doing the opposite. Physicians and nurses need new types of skills and tools for the clinic and hospital. Patients need to expect—even demand—something different from what they are getting from health care. Health care needs to bring healing together with curing. Health care needs a miracle.

MIRACLES

Miracles happen. Most people know this. Many can describe miracles—small or large—that they have seen or experienced in their lives. Miracles in healing are those recoveries that modern science cannot explain. That does not mean they are not explainable. But usually scientists and physicians don't bother to try. They are considered too hard to investigate. Adding the mystery of a miracle to the uncertainties of science makes it even harder. Our research at Walter Reed on how laying on of hands works—through electromagnetic frequencies coming off the hands—explained Susan's boost in energy after I tried it. At least part of why the Marines with PTSD got better with healing touch is explainable—even if from placebo effects. But that does not mean these healings are any less miraculous. In his encyclopedic book *The Future of the Body*, Michael Murphy documents instances of unexplained healing from all over the world—including the meticulous documentation by the Catholic Church of the rare dramatic miracles from visits to Lourdes in France. While more than seven thousand healings from visits to Lourdes have been reported, the church has verified only about seventy as major, unexplained, miraculous healings. These types of miracles are just the dramatic ones that, although they provide evidence that truly mysterious healing can happen, also distract us from the more common and less dramatic miracles seen in health care every day—that is, if we look.

One of the more common "miraculous" events toward the end of life is someone waking up from a coma or sometimes even coming back from the dead to say goodbye to loved ones. My father's death is an example. My father was a Christian minister—Presbyterian. He had served for thirty years in the military and been in three wars—WWII, Korea, and Vietnam. He then spent ten years as a hospital chaplain; ten years as a prison chaplain; five more in service to a poor, rural region in central California; and five more serving the destitute in Las Vegas and San Diego.

He was a man of deep faith who sought to emulate Christ. He believed that God works through people. Once I asked him if he had ever been afraid under fire during the wars. He thought carefully, then told a story about how once bullets passed through the poncho rolled up around his waist. He then said, "No. I was never afraid. I felt Christ next to me."

He and my mother were married nearly sixty years. They had been through the three wars together, moved more than twenty times, and raised four children. They brought their family to Vietnam, Germany, Oklahoma, Texas, California, and New York City—moving almost every two years. They were deeply bonded.

Then, at eighty-six, my dad had a major hemorrhagic (bleeding) stroke and was rapidly dying—falling into a coma within three days. As he lost consciousness, the doctors attempted multiple interventions. They placed intracranial monitors into his head to track the pressure on his brain and catheters to try and drain the blood. "It looks like a crown of thorns," my cousin said. My father had a tube placed down his nose, and they restrained his arms—splayed out to the sides. "Like he is tied to a cross," our son, Chris, said. In this very painful situation and before he went completely unconscious, I asked him if he wanted any pain medication or sedation. He said no. All I could give him was water on a sponge. For me this all evoked the image of Jesus on the cross. Meaning drips thickly over events at the end of life. Gradually, the family came in from all over the country to be with him. He continued to bleed into his head, and the coma became deeper. After about six days, when most people had arrived, he was completely unconscious, not responding even to deep pressure on his sternum. We gathered around him. Our youngest daughter Emily sat at his feet and sang to him for hours. We prayed.

In the evening of the sixth day, my mother came up close and kissed him. Suddenly he woke up and asked, "What happened?" My mother told him he had had a stroke and was in the hospital and the family was all around. They kissed again and each said, "I love you." He then lapsed back into the coma and died the next day. He had come back from a coma to say goodbye to her. A miracle? Perhaps. Explainable? Perhaps. But this kind of happening is not unique. Anyone who has worked in palliative or end-of-life care for a while has witnessed these kinds of miracles. They are more common than the dramatic ones documented in Mr. Murphy's book—and often more meaningful. "It was a miracle for me," my mother recounts, even now, almost ten years later.

Palliative care does not just palliate; it heals—socially, emotionally, mentally, spiritually, and often physically. In a meticulous study published in the *New England Journal of Medicine*, a team led by Dr. Jennifer Temel of the Massachusetts General Hospital randomly divided 150 patients with terminal lung cancer into two groups. One group received standard medical treatment only. The second group was given the option of standard medical treatment plus complete and early palliative care. This care included rapid treatment of pain and distress; psychological, social, and spiritual support, including help with end-of-life decisions; and whole person, integrative care. If the cure-focused treatment was causing more suffering, patients were encouraged to discontinue—the opposite of what usually happens in medicine. Under these circumstances, it was not surprising to find that those in the palliative care group had less pain and less depression and improved quality of life. However, to the surprise of the researchers and the medical profession, when the curative medical treatments were used less often and healing approaches used more often, the patients also lived longer—on average 11.6 months compared to 8.9 months in the curative-only group. It was a small and unexpected miracle. A drug that extended life this long would be rapidly approved. It's still often a struggle to get coverage approved for palliative care.

In America and many other countries, health care does not do dying right. Only about one-third of patients receive formal palliative care, such as the care hospice provides, at the end of life. Few physicians are trained in palliative care, so they don't know what to do once curative treatments are no longer reasonable. Surgeon and author Atul Gawande described this tragedy in his book *Being Mortal*: "This experiment of making mortality a medical experience is just decades old. It is young. And the evidence is, it is failing." The U.S. National Academy of Medicine agrees. In 2014, they published a landmark report, *Death and Dying in America*, recommending that the principles of palliative care be expanded well beyond the end of life and that all physicians be trained in its principles. Those principles include the "frequent assessment of the patient's physical, emotional, social, and spiritual well-being." In other words, healing, as embodied in palliative care, should be part of all health care training.

INTUITION

Mystics describe a state of total unity with the universe, where they see everything connected and have access to all knowledge and wisdom— what they call the mind of God. They also say this knowledge is not unique to them—it is available to all. I learned about this connectivity from my wife, who learned it from her illness and the wounds of her childhood. Susan had always had a spiritual bent and a keen intuition. She went to Yale Divinity School for one year before leaving to go to law school. After being diagnosed with breast cancer the first time at thirty-five years old she returned to spirituality with the hunger of one in mortal crisis and used this dimension to help her decide on treatment and healing. Her father had recently died of lung cancer, and the word *cancer* struck fear into her heart. She thought she would die soon. This drove her into deep introspection and prayer and further cultivated her already skilled intuition. When difficult decisions arose—like whether to do additional chemotherapy for which there was no good scientific evidence of benefit at the time—she would dive into deep thought and prayer until it became clear what to do. This enhanced intuition has served her well. After she was cured, she went back to school to get a pastoral counseling degree and then worked with military couples faced with deployment and war. It is there that we both—I as a doctor and she as a spiritual counselor—saw the kind of "soul loss" that so often impacts service members and veterans, and healing from the soul's restoration. These veterans need spiritual guidance as much or more than medical treatment. Susan has an uncanny ability to know what they need and how to guide them—an intuition she developed out of her own suffering and wounds.

This sixth sense—this intuition—is a way the mind integrates complex information from many sources: from our body, sensory perceptions, relationships, memories, beliefs, and hopes. The response usually occurs below our awareness. Research led by Professor Gerard Hodgkinson, of the Centre for Organizational Strategy, Learning and Change at Leeds University, England, summarized findings from several decades of research on this process. They concluded that intuition is the brain drawing on this tsunami of signals to form a response and decision—but it is a decision made rapidly and unconsciously. That response occurs in the body first—thus the term *gut* feeling. Electrodermal responses—changes in the electrical charge on the skin—usually occur before we are consciously aware of the feeling. All we are usually aware of is a general feeling that something is right or wrong, or that we should turn right or left, go or stop, run or freeze. Often this feeling is right, but not always. Intuition can also mislead. I have had patients who blindly trusted their intuition and abandoned any science- or evidence-based medical treatment, only to suffer and die needlessly. In other words, intuition can be as uncertain as science. Says Professor Hodgkinson, "Humans clearly need both conscious and nonconscious thought processes, but it's likely that neither is intrinsically 'better' than the other." Intuition and science are both imperfect sources of knowledge. Healing requires the integration of both.

For centuries, healers from many cultures have claimed to be able to tap into these spiritual dimensions of healing. But does science show that we interact directly with the collective mind? Is there evidence for spiritual healing? To find out, I led a team in a massive critical summary of the research exploring this type of intuition. I was interested in whether spiritual reality—not just our mental beliefs and social rituals—interacted with material reality. Our goal was to see if there was rigorous evidence—as good as any evidence in modern biological science—that our intentions can interact with the world outside the normal boundaries of time and space: that is, nonlocally. The study was funded by the late Laurance S. Rockefeller three years before he died. It took more than five years to complete and involved dozens of prominent healers and scientists from around the world. We gathered and analyzed hundreds of studies, using state-of-the-art methods for detecting error or bias, and then discussed and synthesized the information in three meetings. The methods and results were published in a book called *Healing, Intention, and Energy Medicine*. We found that, as in other areas of medical research, when scientists tried to isolate the effects of spiritual healing there was uncertainty as to the magnitude of any single outcome. Most results, as in other areas of medicine, showed small effects, difficulty in replication, and bias in publication—all the challenges described by Stanford professor Dr. John Ioannidis in chapter 3 (see page 61) for medical science in general. The best of this research, however, supports the claim by mystics that the connectivity underlying our gut feelings occurs continuously and everywhere. Like electrons, once they touch are always interacting, all living things are always touching. Everything is connected. Susan and many others who, like her, face serious illness, seem to use this mysterious connectivity to navigate the labyrinth of healing through time and space. From this inexplicable connection, the miracles of life arise.

PRAYER

But does this mean that direct spiritual healing—like laying-on-of-hands and prayer—works? It seems it does. And their effects are often about the same magnitude as that of drugs. So far, our understanding of these phenomena remains in the realm of mystery. We do know, however, that the miracles—those unexplained events of healing— probably arise from this mystery and can be tapped if we look for them and use them. Prayer is one tool from the spiritual dimension of healing used by billions. But like other specific approaches to healing, when research attempts to isolate its effects from the other dimensions— the effects shrink and often vanish. Physician and author Dr. Larry Dossey is one of the world's best thinkers and writers about research on healing prayer. He notes the robust but small effects of prayer when studied in randomized controlled trials. In general, he recommends that the spiritual dimensions of healing be left to professional clergy and the physical dimension of healing to physicians. However, he says, just because it does not seem to be as effective as we might wish, it still works and so there are reasons to explore prayer in healing. If prayer works to help us feel whole and loved, it has value. If it contributes to healing, so much the better. As Dossey notes in his book on prayer, *Healing Words*, "The most important reasons for examining the effects of prayer, however, has little to do with its healing effects in illness. The fact that prayer works says something incalculably important about our nature, and how we may be connected with the Absolute." Like any of the dimensions of healing described in this book, the power of specific components of the mind and spirit lies not in their isolated use, but in the meaning response that can be generated with them in our life. Like the other dimensions of healing, mind and spirit provide us with another set of tools for integrative health.

Your Healing Journey

Chapter 9

Integrative Health

The balance of curing and healing.

For millennia, the fundamental nature of the therapeutic encounter has remained largely the same: a person who had been functioning normally and without giving a thought to her health now notices that something is wrong—she doesn't feel well. She seeks someone to help, usually a person with specialized knowledge. In various cultures and eras, this "practitioner" may have been called a shaman, a barber, a priest, or a physician. The ill person hopes the practitioner can help restore her previously normal function. Usually the practitioner does an assessment and makes recommendations, often suggests behavioral change, and then does something to the patient—gives her potions or pills, sticks her with needles or manipulates her body structure, cuts her, or conducts some other ritual. The practitioner administers the healing agent.

The details of this transaction and its rationale have varied from culture to culture and over time. Ancient Greek physicians thought they were manipulating "humors" within the body. Ayurvedic practitioners used the idea of consciousness and *doshas* as the basis for applying their treatments. Ancient Chinese practitioners framed their interventions around the manipulation of "chi" or energy. Shamans and priests sought to divine a spiritual malady and drive out demons or evil spirits.

Then, around the turn of the nineteenth century, about 200 years ago, a new idea arose—a radically different way of understanding the human being and its treatment in health and disease. That new understanding was that all things were made up of small physical substances and parts—chemicals, cells, and other elements that comprise organs and people—and this was best studied with a new approach to knowledge called the scientific process. Modern biomedical science emerged and began breaking the body down into smaller parts and manipulating these, creating theories about how the parts fit together and testing those theories for accuracy. The science of the small and particular—sometimes called "reductionism"—was born. With this came the concept of the human being as a set of mechanical and chemical processes. All biological and psychological processes arose from these chemical interactions, organizing themselves into increasingly complex arrays and manifestations that peaked in the human being. We are, in this view, literately a bag of chemicals elegantly organized to survive and reproduce. Thinking, feeling, and even our very souls are epiphenomena of these chemical interactions. It was a powerful concept.

The value of this thinking soon proved itself in profound and practical ways. The chemical and cellular model of life controlled infectious disease—the number-one killer of humans two hundred years ago. Over time, chemistry produced antiseptics, antibiotics, and analgesic approaches that dramatically alleviated pain and suffering. The physician finally had some tools that were based on more than just magical incantations and historical knowledge. The impact of these discoveries was so dramatic that many of the old ways of thinking—the more holistic views of a person—were discarded. A medical treatment industry grew up around chemistry and physiology and the mechanical manipulation of the body. The pharmaceutical and surgical industries were born. Today, those who have access to this curative approach when they need it are grateful. Those who do not have it want it. The science of the small and particular has been a resounding success—until recently.

By discarding the more holistic, health-promoting, and nonphysical dimensions of what we are as humans, we have lost something essential in health care. While we improved our science and certainty for managing acute disease, we sacrificed what most people value about being alive, and we lost how healing works in chronic illness. Our improvements in health waned. The costs of medical care soared. The value of the mechanical and reductionist model has reached its limits. But by attending to the whole person and integrating this with the scientific process and curative medicine, we can unleash the power of healing and well-being in ways that humanity has never experienced before. In this chapter, I will describe how you can access healing *and* curing and bring them both into your health care and your life with integrative health. Trevor taught me what can happen when we do not integrate these aspects of healing. Mandy taught me what happens when we do.

TREVOR

Trevor began to pray. He was at the end, as far as he knew. He was now back for his fifth visit to the hospital and waiting for a possible kidney transplant. It looked like the possible kidney would not come through again. This was the third time that year and second time in three months that he had been hospitalized to seek a kidney and it had fallen through. It was now 7 am and his wife was packing up to go home. He had a strong feeling that if he did go home now he would never return.

Almost two years to the day he had been in this same hospital after a failed kidney transplant; his body had rejected his wife's donated kidney, and it had to be removed. The prospect of going back on dialysis for another long and indeterminate time, with no functioning kidney, and the knowledge that his wife was living with just one kidney, was devastating. He was finally on the top of the transplant list again, and prepped.

"Give me a few more minutes," he implored his wife. "Something will happen."

His wife sighed. "You are so stubborn," she said. "It's time to go home."

She had always been right before. The pattern of past visits was the same. Hospital personnel called late at night and asked them to come in because they might have a match. He and his wife usually got to the hospital around midnight, which gave him time to be admitted and prepared for surgery. The kidney match would be confirmed about 3 am. It was now 7 am—well past any realistic hope that the transplant would proceed. But he insisted on waiting longer. Trevor went back to praying. He had to believe a miracle would occur. That was all he had left.

But deep down he knew that his wife was right. His "stubborn optimism," as she called it, had gotten him into this mess. It was also what had made him who he was—a successful lawyer and one of the most beloved public servants in his community. A community he had risen out of and returned to help. He was the lucky one, the smart one, the successful one, the one who had escaped a life of poverty and incarceration—and returned to help those who had not escaped. He was one of five children born in a small shack on a dirt road; his father picked fruit and his mother cleaned houses. Neither of his parents had been educated beyond the fifth grade. But they both worked hard and disciplined their kids to do the same. With their love and encouragement, Trevor excelled—in sports, in academics, in popularity. With good grades and an athletic body, he landed a football scholarship to an elite college. He graduated and went on to law school, taking honors and then returning to his community as a public defender—helping those he grew up with get justice and giving back to his community and church. He set up community gatherings where successful members of the community met with children to inspire and mentor them.

When he was growing up, his dad would say that Trevor was always "healthy as a horse." Trevor believed that and never thought about his health. Except for vaccinations as a child and some periodic sports physicals, he never went to a doctor. None of his family ever did. They did not have health insurance and could not afford medical care. If he had an earache or sprained his ankle, his mom would patch it up with home remedies. He always recovered.

When he was hired as public defender, he got health insurance, so he went in for a checkup. That was five years after he left college football and regular athletics. These days, he mostly sat in an office. The doctor was alarmed. Trevor's blood pressure was dangerously high. The doctor prescribed two different medications. "If we can't get it down, we will need to put you in the hospital," he said.

Trevor came back a week later, and while his blood pressure was now out of the alarming range, it was still not normal. The doctor prescribed a third medication. He returned three weeks later. His blood pressure was now under control, but he felt terrible. The medications made him tired, interfered with his sexual function, and made it hard to sleep.

"You will adjust," said the doctor. "The most important thing is, your blood pressure is now down. It was dangerously high." He paused, then emphasized, "You know, it is the silent killer."

Indeed, he was right. Worldwide, untreated or undertreated high blood pressure is the most common risk factor for stroke, heart attack, kidney disease, and heart failure. In the United States, more than seventy-five million people (one in every three adults) has it. More than 30% of people with high blood pressure don't know they have it, and only 50% have it under control. Estimates are that more than one thousand people die each day from high blood pressure. Estimated costs are $50 billion per year. The situation is worse in less economically developed countries. The WHO estimates over one billion people worldwide have high blood pressure—most of it undetected and poorly controlled. Lifestyle is a major risk factor—both for getting it and for controlling it. So is genetics. Over their lifetime, most people will require two or more drugs to control it. The doctors had Trevor on three drugs and were satisfied that it was being adequately treated. From the biological perspective, their job was done. But the job was not done. While they were treating Trevor's disease, they had left out, as often happens in health care today, Trevor. It was this neglect of Trevor as a whole person that would eventually hurt him.

Current guidelines for treatment of high blood pressure recommend more than just drugs. The Joint National Committee on Prevention, Detection, Evaluation, and Treatment of High Blood Pressure (JNC 7) also addresses the behavioral dimensions of healing. Lifestyle modifications are recommended no matter what level of high blood pressure a person has. This includes exercise (which Trevor had stopped doing), a low-salt diet (which Trevor had never even thought to consider), not smoking (Trevor did not smoke), or weight gain (which Trevor had experienced since stopping sports). His doctors asked about these things and suggested he start exercising again and go on a low-salt diet. They gave him a handout of foods to avoid and recommended the DASH diet (Dietary Approaches to Stop Hypertension). But, they emphasized, he would always need the medications. The Joint National Committee also recommends close attention to the social and emotional aspects of healing. The section on "Adherence to Regimens" states: "Motivation improves when patients have positive experiences with and trust in their clinicians. Empathy both builds trust and is a potent motivator. Patient attitudes are greatly influenced by cultural differences, beliefs, and previous experiences with the healthcare system. These attitudes must be understood if the clinician is to build trust and increase communication with patients and families." The committee goes on to list other reasons for "nonadherence," including denial of illness, perception of drugs as symbols of ill health, adverse effects of medications, cost of medications, and lack of patient involvement in the care plan.

Unfortunately, Trevor's doctor had missed the class on empathy and trust, and Trevor had many of these reasons for nonadherence in his life—plus his stubborn optimism. He would be okay, he thought. His doctors never learned all this about Trevor. They did not know him well and did not inquire. They were not able to effectively engage him in behavioral change and found out nothing about his social and emotional background. He needed more than lifelong drugs, with their side effects, which were a key reason for nonadherence. The Joint National Committee Guidelines summary for primary care practitioners covers about twenty-five pages. There are eight pages devoted to drug management, but only one page to lifestyle and one page to nonadherence.

Trevor left his visits with physicians both alarmed and skeptical. He had felt fine before. Now he felt terrible. How had he gone from "healthy as a horse" to an impotent invalid in a matter of weeks? Plus, his insurance did not cover the entire cost of drugs. Some were expensive. Wasn't there a better way? He had read that high blood pressure could be controlled by diet and exercise. He had been an athlete. Why couldn't he use this approach? He inquired around in his community for alternative options to drugs. Several of his friends said they had gotten off medications and felt great by exercising and eating better food. They recommended a local practitioner who used "natural" approaches for treatment of disease. She provided the hope Trevor was looking for. Not only was it possible to treat blood pressure naturally, she said, but diet and supplements could actually replace drugs. The side effects of medications could be avoided. She knew of the DASH diet but said that was just a start. She pointed to a "more effective" diet called the "Rice Diet for Hypertension" that would get people totally off drugs. The diet was developed at a clinic only a few hours from where Trevor lived—at Duke University—and had been "proven" to work for more than seventy-five years. He could go to a private center that delivered this diet or—for less cost—she could help him get on a "cleansing" diet and supplements that would do the same thing. She would help him to make it work with his life.

Trevor, optimistic as always, thought this sounded good and began to work with her. He stopped the medications and started the diet and supplements. He immediately felt better. After three weeks on the diet and supplements he went into a drugstore and had his blood pressure checked. It was almost normal. He was back to his old self—or so he thought.

He didn't see another doctor for ten years—until after his feet began to swell.

THE INTEGRATION GAP

The gap in health care between curing the body and the dimensions of healing is not confined to blood pressure. It is a general gap in health care—one that needs closing. In a recent comprehensive review I took of family medicine, I counted the number of recommendations for the use of drugs and other disease treatments compared to other dimensions described in this book—environmental, behavioral, social/emotional, and mind/spirit. Of the 361 health care management recommendations made during the review, 226 referred to drug management, 87 for behavior and lifestyle, 20 concerned complementary and alternative healing methods (mostly to avoid them), 19 addressed social and emotional counseling, and 9 were for mind-body or spiritual practices. In several lectures on chronic pain, for example, nondrug approaches were recommended as a first-line management in all patients. After one lecture on chronic pain that recommended use of complementary and integrative approaches to pain management, questions from the physicians were focused not on evidence for the effectiveness of these approaches, which ones were covered by insurance, and on how to implement the recommendations. The physicians pointed out that they were not well trained in the delivery of nondrug approaches for pain, that patients did not seek out these practices, and that the health care system did not pay for them. While evidence and a number of recommendations to use these healing dimensions is an improvement over review courses I took a decade ago, there is a lack of integration between curing and healing in our delivery systems. This gap between evidence and practice is difficult to bridge.

STANDARD SYSTEM ALLOWS GAP

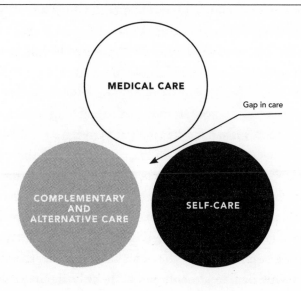

Trevor's doctors treated his numbers but failed to engage him in the lifestyle and social and emotional dimensions required for healing. The alternative practitioner used a diet that can rapidly lower blood pressure in the short run, but has not been shown to be effective in the long run. People cannot stick to it, yet they may think they have eliminated their problem. The herbs and supplements she recommended are not proven to work for high blood pressure. Yet she and Trevor believed in them. The two practitioners—the conventional doctor who addressed Trevor's biology and the alternative practitioner who provided Trevor with what he hoped for—never communicated with each other. Both knew about an effective and proven long-term dietary treatment for high blood pressure—the DASH diet—yet neither could deliver it. Had he followed that diet, Trevor would still have needed drugs, but likely in reduced numbers or doses—and he would have felt better. Despite increasing evidence and recommendations by national organizations to use more behavioral and lifestyle changes, doctors get very little training in nutritional therapy and even less in dealing with the social, emotional, and cultural dimensions of healing. Complementary and alternative practitioners are rarely trained in how to work with serious diseases and have even less training on how to coordinate what they do with physicians. Trevor fell into the gap between evidence-based medicine and person-centered care. The result was fifteen years of "silent" and poorly treated high blood pressure. When he went back to the doctor to see why his legs were swelling, they discovered he had kidney failure produced by poorly controlled high blood pressure. This led to years of kidney dialysis and the abortive attempts to get a transplant.

Trevor needed an integrative health care approach—one that bridged and coordinated the treatments between his biology and the rest of him; between drugs and self-care; between medical treatment and the social and personal determinants of health; between the treatment "agents" and his own "agency"—his inner capacity to heal.

The miracles of modern molecular medicine, with all its success over the last hundred years, have reached a limit when it comes to managing most chronic disease. Extensive research has repeatedly shown that even full access to medical treatments produces only about 15% to 20% of a population's health; the rest depends on lifestyle, environment, and social and personal determinants. This failure to focus on the whole person and delivery systems that address health determinants comes from how medical care is delivered—in silos and directed at discrete parts of people—without empowering them to heal. Modern medicine, so powerful in making miracles around acute disease, is now missing 80% of what's needed for healing chronic disease.

The most recent description of this dilemma was published by leaders at the U.S. National Academy of Medicine in a report called *Vital Directions for Health and Health Care*, edited by Drs. Victor Dzau, Mark McClellan, and Michael McGinnis. They describe how the money spent each year on health care in the United States (the most recent figure then was $3.2 trillion) is no longer providing the value it once did. They find that "an estimated 30% is related to waste, inefficiencies, and excessive price; health disparities are persistent and worsening; and the health and financial burden of chronic illness and disabilities are straining families and communities." They collated expert input in nineteen papers and made four main recommendations: pay for value, empower people, activate communities, and connect care. Had Trevor's physicians been paid to get him better, not to just give him drugs (that is, pay for value); had he been empowered to take responsibility for his health (empower people); had the community he lived in trusted the medical system (activate communities); and had there been an integrated approach between his medical treatment and his more natural approaches (connect care), Trevor would not have been lying in a hospital bed pleading for more time and praying for a donor kidney to appear.

Soon after the publication of *Vital Directions*, Samueli Institute and the Institute for Healthcare Improvement released the Wellbeing in the Nation (WIN) plan, which described how the United States could build an infrastructure to enhance healing in communities across the globe. The report recommends establishing a national well-being index and a community well-being extension service network to facilitate local integration of community well-being efforts. By addressing prevention, health promotion, and well-being, any community and its members can flourish. Both these reports point to local examples. Many communities already have sufficient resources to do this. The integration gap can be filled if we have the will to change our approach and rebalance curing with healing.

FROM SOAP TO HOPE

In the history of medicine, the use of a chemical, cellular science is very new. Our understanding of cell function and the chemistry of cure is only about two centuries old. Oxygen, for example, that essential molecule for survival, was discovered by Joseph Priestley in 1774. The establishment of reductionist science as a basis for medicine is only about a century old—being solidified as the gold standard after the Flexner Report on medical education was published in 1910. The application of this science for human testing in the form of randomized controlled trials (RCTs) is a little more than sixty years old—the first one was done in 1948. The solid establishment of RCTs as the gold standard for what is called evidence-based medicine today is more recent, with a concerted push from academics in Canada and England in the 1970s. The application of technology to further refine and manipulate the body is still more recent. By any metric, the science of medicine is young. So young, in fact, that the downsides and limitations for the prevention and treatment of chronic disease are only now beginning to emerge. As these limitations are more understood, there has been a parallel resurgence of interest in holistic approaches that were dismissed in the last hundred years. As I discovered in my practice, an integrative approach to health was needed—one that merges and coordinates curing and healing. To do that, I had to make a shift from the way I had been taught in medical school and practiced for decades—an approach exclusively focused on finding the disease—to a way of working with patients that enhanced their healing capacity. I had to widen the lens of my practice to reach out of the regular clinic visit to one that touched people in their life-space. I do this by going from what traditional medicine calls a SOAP visit to what I call a HOPE visit. Let me explain.

Most patients don't realize it, but when they visit their physician, he or she already has a specific plan to structure and report on the visit. In almost every visit, a physician will summarize the encounter with something called a SOAP note. SOAP stands for *subjective*, *objective*, *assessment*, and *plan*; it's designed to label the patient with a disease or illness diagnosis and its corresponding treatment.

SOAP is the way that every medical student, resident, and nurse and many other medical care practitioners learn how to organize their thinking around an encounter with a patient. Electronic medical records are built around the SOAP.

Subjective starts with the patient's chief complaint—what he came in for and what he says is bothering him. This complaint is filled in with further questions looking for additional subjective information reported by the patient.

Objective is what the practitioner observes; it includes observations of the body itself and laboratory test results and imaging. While there's no explicit ranking of subjective and objective, most practitioners have a bias toward the objective, giving it more value in the assessment than the subjective or what the patient says.

Assessment is meant to be a succinct summary of what the clinician thinks is the problem and is essentially the diagnosis. This diagnosis is usually attached to a code or a set of terminologies that form the lexicon of all medicine. The assessment is not only how we categorize patients to research them and get new knowledge; it also forms the categories around which we pay the practitioner, and track outcomes for the health care system. Thus it is essential to the livelihood of the health care system and the practitioner.

Finally, the *plan* is what we intend to do about the diagnosis, whether that be the execution of a treatment, the providing of advice, or further assessment and testing. Physicians are taught that the plan needs to align with the assessment and, under ideal circumstances, with at least with the objective part and hopefully, with the subjective part as well. The SOAP note is how we organize the entire experience of the patient visit and follow-up. In most medical encounters, no matter what the patient presents with, they will go out of the office framed in a SOAP. That SOAP is rarely shared with patients; if it is, we rarely ask them whether it makes sense. We don't expect them to know what the diagnostic codes, descriptions, and plans should be or what they mean. Good communication in a clinical encounter entails explaining the assessment and plan in nontechnical terms and the research evidence, with the goal of engaging the patient in clinical decisions. This process is called shared decision making, and it is almost universally espoused as important for every chronic disease decision—yet it is rarely done. Physicians vary considerably in their skill at communicating the assessment and plan to patients, and usually any SOAP discussion remains technical.

The SOAP process happens tens of thousands of time every day around the world; it structures the medical encounter and drives the medical treatment engine. The SOAP note is formulated around a set of basic assumptions that organize all modern medical education, research, and practice. SOAP uses a pathogenic framing: it is about disease and illness, not healing. It is the way modern medicine diagnoses diseases and aligns them with treatment. How much evidence connects the assessment part to the plan part of SOAP determines whether a treatment is judged to be evidence-based or not. This, in turn, structures the way research is done, such as how patients are selected for clinical studies. This then restricts what is allowed in health care. It keeps modern medicine focused on seeking cures. This constant search for cures creates multiple treatments that are "done to" the patient. Because SOAP uses the biomedical, biochemical paradigm, it often misses the dimensions of healing found by and in other parts of patients. The concept of *salutogenesis*—the process of healing—is a concept I and others have expanded on from Aaron Antonovsky, who first coined this term in the 1970s. *Salutogenesis* rarely comes up explicitly in a clinical encounter. Doctors focus on *pathogenesis*—the process of how disease is produced—and how to counteract it. No wonder most clinical encounters are not person-centered or holistic and miss most of healing. We doctors always must fit them into a SOAP! In the medical profession is it called the "tyranny of the chief complaint"—and we are stuck on it.

Doing a SOAP process with each patient visit is important for disease diagnosis and treatment, but if we are to balance curing with whole person healing, we need more than SOAP. We need an encounter focused specifically on healing. So, to balance the standard medical encounter with healing, I follow up the SOAP process with a HOPE note. HOPE stands for healing-oriented practices and environments, and it addresses dimensions of physical, behavioral, social/emotional, and mind/spirit—and so tap into the 80% of how healing works. It involves a set of questions designed to help the person identify and navigate a unique pathway to healing. The HOPE questions probe how the person is already engaged in healing, and then seeks to match that with good evidence to enhance those activities. It highlights what the person has intuitively discovered and adds the rational elements derived from rigorous research. Since both intuition and science are uncertain by themselves, pairing these different ways of knowing maximizes the benefit for both curative treatments and the person's healing capacity. It optimizes the meaning response. By doing a HOPE, I help patients avoid the gap that Trevor had fallen into.

The story of another patient, Mandy, illustrates how SOAP and HOPE together create integrative health and healing.

MANDY

At forty-five years old, Mandy should have been able to maintain a household—but now she could not. Even before the accident, she had struggled to care for two teenaged boys and a nine-year-old daughter, a husband who worked a lot, and a part-time job. Her life consisted of juggling schedules, meals, household chores, phone calls, and social media. There was no time for self-care. She had worked full-time until fifteen years ago. Then, in what she thought was a relatively minor car accident, she sustained a neck whiplash and shoulder ligament tear on her right side. She gave it time to heal and followed all instructions, including physical therapy and taking anti-inflammatories. But the pain never went away. It became chronic. Soon she had major neck stiffness and intractable pain down her shoulder and right arm. A fifteen-year journey with neuropathic pain had begun.

Over that fifteen-year period, she was diagnosed with multiple other conditions, from depression to anxiety to PTSD to neurosis. She continued to try and maintain as healthy a life as possible: exercising as she could, doing physical therapy, eating well, and cultivating relationships with friends and family. As with many patients in chronic pain, these were challenging activities. Most of her encounters with medical professionals resulted in being prescribed more medications. At one point, she was on more than five medications, including the opioid OxyContin, from which she had difficulty freeing herself. The pain would flare up when she tried to taper off of it. Eventually, with the help of an inpatient pain treatment group, she got off the OxyContin and began taking other, less addictive drugs, such as Neurontin and Lyrica, which partially improved both her neuropathic pain and crying episodes. "Let me warn you, Doc—I cry," she said on her first visit with me, tears already welling up in her eyes. "Sometimes I just cry for no reason—sorry." I waited until she stopped.

Her pain was significant. She rated it between five to seven out of ten on a daily basis. It was accompanied by spasms and stiffness in her neck and right shoulder. Over the fifteen years, she had had many other treatments besides drugs: regular physical therapy, steroid injections, and electrical stimulators and psychotherapy, all from conventional pain clinics or her primary care doctor. Like Trevor, she entered into the parallel world of complementary and alternative medicine, seeing chiropractors, acupuncturists, herbalists, homeopaths, and mind-body practitioners. They all seemed to help a bit, some more than others—temporarily. She found that hot baths and meditation helped the most—when she had the time to do them. Sleep was never in the cards, both because of her busy family—the boys were up late doing homework—and because the pain did not ease at night. She woke frequently and never felt rested. Sometimes she would just go into the bathroom and cry.

She came to me because she heard I might help her enhance her own healing capacity. She had heard I had a different approach and would work to integrate it with her regular medical treatments. So we set up a HOPE visit and began to discuss the dimensions of healing in her life. We explored a list of options that science shows helps people with chronic pain heal. I asked her questions like the following:

1. What gave her the greatest joy and well-being in her life? What was her most meaningful activity?

2. Did she have friends and a supportive family—anyone to cry with, to love, who would nurture and support her?

3. What was her daily behavior like? The medical treatments? Her lifestyle—diet, sleep, exercise? What did she do to relax?

4. What was her home like—the physical environment where she spent most of her time? Did she have a special place to give her an escape from the daily chores and hubbub of the day?

These are the main questions I go through with patients during a HOPE assessment, using a chart like the one you see here. Mandy and I made a map to help her navigate toward a healing path, showing these dimensions and the elements in them that we would explore. With patience and persistence, HOPE can often change the trajectory of illness and restore well-being—even if, as in chronic disease, cure is not possible.

THE ELEMENTS OF WHOLE PERSON HEALING ADDRESS IN A HOPE VISIT

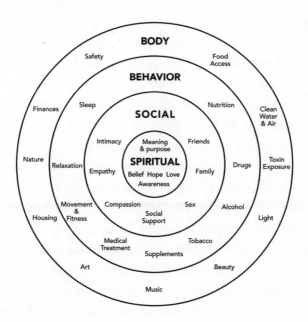

Three things emerged during my dialogue with Mandy. First, many things were right in her life and supported her healing. She had a wonderful family and some good friends. She paid close attention to the food her family ate—lots of fruits and vegetables, fish, whole grains, and minimal sugar. She tried to exercise daily—at least doing her physical therapy each day. But she had challenges in many areas—especially in rest and relaxation. Her schedule, the needs of the household, and her pain made relaxation a challenge. Five years previously, she thought she had been getting better more rapidly, but then was involved in a second car accident. In this one, she struck her head but did not lose consciousness. After evaluating her, the doctors said everything was okay. Soon after that, her crying episodes started. She could not stop thinking of both accidents and that she might never recover. That is when she was diagnosed with PTSD. This was also when the antidepressant medications and counseling were added—providing some relief in her mood but not much for the pain.

I then asked her a question I ask most of my patients: "What do you think is going on?" The timing and setting of this question are key to getting a deep and meaningful response. The purpose of the question is to help patients search their intuition—their heart or gut or soul, depending on how they perceive it. My job is to see if I can match what comes from that intuition with reasonable scientific evidence that might be used to enhance the patient's healing. As it turned out, Mandy's answer held the key to her recovery.

"Well," she said after a slight pause, "it's my brain—there seems to be something wrong with my brain."

"Why do you say that?" I probed and waited.

"Well, I noticed that the first few times I got acupuncture, I had a big relief—like maybe 95% better. Pain down to 1 or 2. But it didn't last. I tried it several times, but after a while it didn't work at all. So I gave up. It was like my brain was trying to heal but could not absorb the treatments. It just wasn't sticking. Like I said, something is wrong with my brain." Mandy started to cry again. "Sorry, doctor."

Our integrative health team got together and looked at the situation. Clearly, the acupuncture was producing endogenous opioids—those internal painkillers that all our brains produce. But after the treatments, her levels of those went down and she was no longer responding. The acupuncturist suggested that she had just not had enough treatments. Repeated acupuncture will not only induce endogenous opioids, but eventually also increase the density of opioid receptors in the brain, making the person more responsive to her own brain's painkillers and prolonging the effect. She just needed more treatments.

The neurologist disagreed. If increases in brain receptors were the problem, they should have shown at least some evidence of effect. Mandy had first done twelve weekly acupuncture treatments, and then an additional four acupuncture treatments spaced once a month. That should have been sufficient for acupuncture to "take," he said. Something else must be going on. He wondered if the head injury she had sustained in her second car accident had caused a problem. I mentioned that her crying episodes—a sign of possible decreased cortical inhibition of her emotions—had begun after the second car accident. This can also happen from brain injury. To see if we could find any evidence for this, we ordered a positron emission tomography (PET) scan.

While neuroimaging technology is advancing by leaps and bounds in medicine, the interpretation of what we see in those images—especially in the brain—is still being worked out. Our interest in this for Mandy was to explore if there was any evidence of brain dysfunction in areas preventing her from responding to the acupuncture. Dr. Daniel Amen is an American psychiatrist who has the most extensive experience in the world in the use of PET scanning to refine our understanding of brain diseases; he has read over twenty-five thousand, including many looking for the effects of subtle brain injury. I had read his book *Change Your Brain, Change Your Life* and wondered if PET imaging would help us in working with Mandy. A PET scan is a rather crude but inexpensive way to look at metabolism in the brain. We hoped that if the PET showed clear changes in the frontal areas of her brain—especially an area of the ventro-medial frontal cortex—this might explain both the crying episodes and the failure of acupuncture to take. It was worth a shot, especially in light of Mandy's own feeling that her brain was not functioning properly.

The PET scan seemed to confirm her feelings and our hypothesis. It demonstrated a reduction in glucose metabolism in the left frontal lobe, not exactly where we had hypothesized, but in an area where some of the executive functions and inhibitory pathways to pain and emotional control might have been damaged. We had no way to know whether this was caused by the car accident or if this explained her ongoing pain and temporary response to opioids and acupuncture. But it seemed to confirm our belief that Mandy needed to try to regrow those areas of the brain. More important, the scan energized Mandy to want to reengage in her own self-care—something she had neglected over the years. The simplest way to regrow the brain is to exercise it. We suggested either biofeedback or an intensive set of relaxation response exercises. Mandy liked that idea, so our next task was to find a method that she enjoyed and could maintain long enough to enhance function in that part of her brain. Mandy decided to try mindfulness meditation.

MIND-BRAIN-BODY

Most of modern biomedicine focuses on treating diseases of the mind—mental and psychosomatic illnesses—by manipulating the brain. But the reverse is also possible. The brain and the rest of the body can be treated through the mind. Mandy needed a way to regrow a part of her brain that had become injured and dysfunctional, even possibly atrophied, by years of pain and treatments to alleviate it. While someday we may be able to regrow parts of brains using stem cells or direct electrical stimulation, those days are not here yet. Our experience with drug and herbal treatments also shows that those methods provide only partial relief in a few and risk producing side effects in many. In the meantime, there are methods to regrow the brain through behavior, social learning, and mind-body practices. Physical exercise can increase neural growth generally. Mandy did some exercise but could not engage in intensive physical training. Also, we could not use exercise to grow the specific areas that seemed to be problematic for her. Biofeedback of brain waves can growth brain areas—often in specific areas. That approach required multiple visits and sophisticated equipment. Virtual reality is another method but is generally not viable for chronic pain. These also cost money and are not easy to incorporate into self-care. We needed an approach Mandy could bring into her daily life. The one that seemed the most practical and meaningful for Mandy was mindfulness meditation training.

For Mandy, this meant creating a process for her to do deep relaxation every day for at least eight weeks. I knew about the research showing that patients who engage in at least eight weeks of mind-body practices such as mindfulness or meditation for thirty minutes a day can grow areas of the frontal lobe that Mandy had lost. She was excited to try this. She had previously tried meditation and found it helped her feel better, and have less anxiety, but she had not kept it up. The challenge now would be integrating it into her daily life. For this, the behavioral medicine and health coach on the team came into play. They worked with her to design—with her family—a process allowing her to engage in thirty minutes of mindfulness meditation every day. She preferred this over the visualization that Jake had done, or heart-rate variability biofeedback—another evidence-based option. The first attempt failed because as long as she was in her house, she felt overwhelmed by responsibilities for her family. She had no place in her house that she could fully relax.

The behaviorist and health coach helped her organize that special place in her house. It turned out to be in her bedroom, where she constructed her own little nurturing corner. The family cooperated to ensure that this place was isolated and not invaded by the rest of them. In her own little corner, she placed some of her favorite sacred symbols and family mementos that she enjoyed. She decorated it with soft cloth and low light. A CD player was set up to deliver favorite music or nature sounds. It was her own optimal healing environment. A set of reminders to both the family members and herself, sent simultaneously through a cell phone app, allowed her to engage in over thirty minutes of mindfulness and breathing practice every day for more than two months. At that point, a repeat PET scan showed improved neurological function in the frontal lobe. This encouraged her to continue. She also noted that her sleep had improved and her pain had dropped from the usual 5 to 7 on a scale of 1 to 10, to a 4 or 5. It was now time to try acupuncture again.

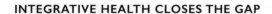

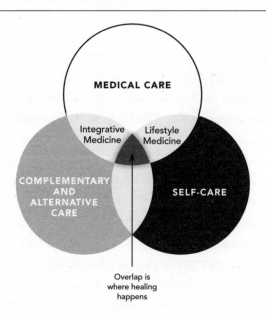

Research shows that it takes between eight and twelve weeks of acupuncture for opioid receptor density to change in the brain. But this had not previously worked for Mandy. We hoped that now that she had the right neurological foundation, the acupuncture would take. Mandy had used her mind to change her brain. So she began a series of twenty acupuncture treatments using a combination of body and ear points. Gradually, over the next two months, the rebound of pain she had previously experienced after acupuncture began to diminish. Within three months, her pain levels were down to 1 or 2 out of 10, and she could scale back her acupuncture to once every month and eventually once every three months. More important, her quality of life, functional capacity, and ability to tap her own healing capacity increased. She learned that when her pain began to increase, it was often because she had not engaged in sufficient self-care, either by not getting enough sleep or by skipping her mindfulness practices or ignoring increased stress in her life. Her medications were now only a low-dose antidepressant, which, along with her restored frontal lobe, prevented most of the crying, and acetaminophen for an occasional pain flare.

Mandy was the beneficiary of integrative health.

I use the term "integrative medicine" in reference to the merger of conventional medicine—as I was trained in—and complementary and alternative medicine, such as acupuncture, chiropractic, or massage. The term "lifestyle medicine" is used in reference to the merger of conventional medicine and behavior in the form of self-care, such as nutrition, exercise, and stress management. "Integrative health" is at the intersection of all three of these fields with good scientific evidence and patient-centered care as the driving principles for its application. This is what Mandy had at her disposal. This is the future of health care for chronic disease.

A SHIFT TOWARD HOLISM

There is a story that around the year 500 BCE, an enlightened ruler in Tibet did a remarkable thing. He invited master healers from all the major healing traditions of the world to a yearlong conference of learning. Physicians came from corners of the known world, including Greece and the Middle East, North Africa, China, and India. Their purpose was to share the best of their craft and synthesize the most effective treatments known to humanity—in other words, to create a truly integrative approach from the world's healing traditions of the time. What emerged was a remarkable system that informed and infused medical thinking for over a thousand years. It was the integrative medicine of its day.

We need a similar effort to integrate the best healing traditions from around the world today. In an age of instant information and global interaction, patients are already exposed to and using practices from multiple healing traditions and nonconventional systems. In 1993, Dr. David Eisenberg of Harvard published a study in the *Journal of the*

American Medical Association showing that over one-third of people in the United States regularly sought out so-called complementary and alternative medicine (CAM) practices and visited alternative healers. A decade later, that number was 40% and climbing. The use of so-called complementary and alternative medicine is even higher in Europe, South America, and Eurasia and up to 80% in the populations of non-Western countries. But rarely do conventional doctors know about these practices. Rarely do patients tell doctors when they are using them, and rarely do doctors ask about or offer them. The gap between curing, healing, and self-care is greater than ever. Patients are the ones saddled with trying to do the proper integration that the profession should be doing. The consequences of this gap can be tragic when people like Trevor, struggling with high blood pressure and eventual kidney failure, seek out more holistic practices but without appropriate scientific input. We need another concerted effort today—like what was done in Tibet a thousand years ago—with the help of modern science and information technology.

Fortunately, there is a shift toward more integration in health care today. The effort is occurring—but with difficulty. In 1948, the WHO came out with a controversial definition of health. The WHO defined health as more than just curing physical disease, but "a state of complete physical, mental, and social well-being and not merely the absence of disease or infirmity." It declared that this definition should be the goal of all health care. However, most of modern medicine went on its reductionist way—looking for finer and finer divisions of the body into the small and particular. The study of DNA was under intense research when WHO published its definition, with the Watson and Crick discovery of its structure published in 1953. The first randomized clinical trial (RCT)—done in the same year as the WHO definition— launched the role of reductionism onto the stage of human testing for medical decision making. As we've discussed, the RCT has become the primary tool for deciding what is good evidence in health care. For the last five decades, this science of the small and particular has continued to dominate biomedical research and clinical practice—being applied everywhere and to everything.

Then, gradually, international groups began to respond to our need for rebalance and more whole person care. In 2001, a landmark report from the Institute of Medicine (now National Academy of Medicine) called *Crossing the Quality Chasm* laid out ten principles for the redesign of health care to provide more patient-centered, holistic care in medicine. The first three recommendations were as follows:

1. Care is based on continuous healing relationships.
2. Care is customized according to patient needs and values.
3. The patient is the source of control.

The report also called for good evidence, shared information, better safety, anticipation of (not just reaction to) patient needs, prevention, and cooperation among clinicians. In other words, team care. In a major effort to live up to these principles, four main primary care associations in the United States—in pediatrics, family medicine, internal medicine, and obstetrics-gynecology—published a joint set of guidelines for the Patient Centered Medical Home in 2007. The idea behind this was to provide care that is the following:

- **PATIENT-CENTERED**: takes into account the needs and preferences of the patient and family
- **COMPREHENSIVE**: covers the whole person, including their physical, mental, prevention, wellness, acute and chronic care
- **COORDINATED**: is organized to integrate all elements of health care delivery
- **ACCESSIBLE**: includes 24/7 care, with telephone and IT communications
- **COMMITTED TO QUALITY AND SAFETY**: ensured thorough continuous improvement

In other words, the call was for medicine to be more responsive to the whole person, be more integrated, and be more focused on prevention and health promotion than our current system. Echoes of *Crossing the Quality Chasm* reverberated throughout the mainstream.

Other groups and other countries too have pushed for more integrative and holistic care. In 2008, the international Institute for Healthcare Improvement (IHI) defined and began to support training for achieving the "Triple Aim" of health care worldwide: (1) improving the patient experience, (2) improving the health of populations, and (3) reducing the per-person cost of health care. The concept of pay for value (rather than for procedure or treatment) emerged from these efforts. The goal was described clearly by visionary leaders such as IHI founder Dr. Don Berwick, who called for an "integrator"—an organization that accepts responsibility for all three aims. Dr. Berwick went on to create the Center for Medicare and Medicaid Innovation, which funded and tested new models of health care, demonstrating how to implement pay for value. Pay for value efforts were already under way in England, Europe, Australia, Singapore, Japan, and other countries. These innovative models are gradually moving more fully toward the type of integrative health care that people like Trevor need to prevent disease and stay healthy, and that Mandy used to heal herself from chronic pain.

But implementing these aspirational principles has been a challenge. Medicine still largely follows individual treatment processes and pays for doing things to a patient rather than supporting healing with a patient. We still spend most of our money and time looking for treatment agents that only incrementally add to overall health, rather than optimizing our own agency for transformational healing. The will is there, but the ways are weak, and the economic drivers are against this when it comes to healing. Recently, the Peterson Foundation funded Stanford's Center for Excellence in Primary Care to find the top 5% of primary care practices that meet the Triple Aim and the patient-centered medical home model, and to describe the characteristics of their success. Not surprisingly, those characteristics were almost identical to those listed in *Crossing the Quality Chasm*. The most effective health care went beyond simply doling out treatments. These practices spent time probing the other dimensions of healing. They addressed the whole person, organized care to make the patient the driver of their own healing, and created teams of caregivers— all processes addressing the behavioral and the social and emotional dimensions of healing. They provide integrative health care at its best.

A NEW WAY TO HEAL

The two missing spheres of integrative health—complementary and alternative practices and lifestyle medicine or self-care—have been growing in research and practice in parallel with the mainstream calls for more person-centered and holistic care. If your physician is interested in learning more about these areas, he or she (and you) can learn more from my description in the next chapter. Many of these resources bring lifestyle and behavioral change into treatment, beyond using them just for the prevention of chronic diseases. Physician pioneer Dr. Dean Ornish has emphasized this point and demonstrated it in rigorous research for decades. In his most recent best-selling book, *The Spectrum,* he brings together the elements of lifestyle medicine to show that we can reverse chronic disease and turn on disease-preventing genes. This is indeed a new way to heal, compared to what most doctors have been learning.

As Trevor and many of my other patients have taught me, behavior is only one dimension needed to tap into the 80% of healing. Almost all patients that I see in my practice know that behavior is important for health. But, as was tragically true for Trevor, having that knowledge is not enough. A recent study published by the Mayo Clinic concluded that only 2.7% of the population engages in the four main behaviors that keep people healthy—not smoking, eating a high vegetable diet, engaging in regular activity, and undertaking adequate stress management. Nor does simply engaging in healthy behaviors address the deeper levels of a person—the social/emotional and mind/spirit dimensions—that are so essential to finding the permanent path to healing. Maria changed her behavior, but wasn't healed until she found a group to teach cooking to. Sergeant Martin was using a treatment—hyperbaric oxygen—proven not to work. Yet by engaging in it with a group of other service members, he improved and healed himself. Had Norma not been enrolled in the clinical study I was running on arthritis, she might never have been motivated enough to move through her pain and return to her volunteer job. For Mabel, as for many seriously ill people and elderly or frail patients, social relationships were the central dimension to her healing and well-being.

We saw in chapter 7 that at least one health care system—the Nuka System of Care in Alaska—could shift their delivery of health care to a relationship and patient-centered paradigm. The success of this system is partially based on anchoring it in Alaskan Native traditions. But the world is increasingly mobile and made up of diverse traditions with multiple cultures and languages. Is it possible to build an integrative healing system flexible enough for our increasingly mobile and multicultural world? To find out, I visited one system that is attempting to do just that.

Dr. Rushika Fernandopulle was born in Sri Lanka, where he found, as I did in Vietnam, that much care still comes from traditional practitioners who use natural substances and conduct ancient rituals—just as Aadi did in the Ayurvedic hospital in nearby India. Infectious disease, lack of sanitation, trauma, and malnutrition were common in Sri Lanka. But Dr. Fernandopulle noticed one thing about people with chronic disease and mental health issues: if they could get clean water and food and had access to the basics of modern medicine, they were happy and generally did well. Their lifestyle and social relationships supported lifelong health. As in the five places in the world identified by author Dan Buettner in his book *Blue Zones*, where people live the longest, healthiest lives, the Sri Lankans had less medicine and less illness than many in Western countries. Traditional practitioners and grandmothers coached people on how to live. There was no gap between the medical space and the life space. The only gap was science.

Then Dr. Fernandopulle came to America and got arguably the best scientific and medical training available at Harvard. Like me, he saw the miracles that modern science could bring to curing. Like me, he had been exposed to both the advantages and the limitations of ancient traditional healing systems. And like me, he saw that for chronic disease, people in the West were not doing better—yet they were paying more. So he set out to try to fill the gaps in the health care system he worked in here. But he found it extremely difficult to change a system that paid for and reinforced only treatment and cure. Like me, he found that the nature of the medical encounter, the payment system, the electronic medical record, and the SOAP note was not designed for healing the whole person. Finally, he gave up trying to change the systems and set out to design and build a new system that could change the nature of health care and fill the gap between curing and healing. He called it Iora, after a small bird in Sri Lanka.

Superficially, the job of an Iora practice is the same as any medical clinic—to prevent and treat illness and disease; to help people get and stay well. However, the second you dig even a little bit deeper, you realize it is indeed very different from typical care. The clinic is filled with specially trained professionals called "health coaches," who work hand in hand with the nurses and doctors to address any area that might impact your health or interfere with your healing. It provides standard treatments like vaccines, medications, minor surgery, and counseling. But it can also provide information on nutrition and behavioral change, stress and social services, and access to financial or legal help, if needed. And it can link you to responsible complementary and alternative practices and integrate that care into the other services. Every member of the health care team and the patient have full access to all information in the health record—which is structured around the patient rather than the payments—and is fully accessible to the patient at all times. The need to worry about the cost of treatment is eliminated, as all care in Iora practices is provided for a flat fee per patient per month (paid for by what Iora calls a sponsor, which could be an insurance health plan or self-insured employer, for instance). Hospital or specialty care is additional, but the Iora team works closely to provide a broader range of care than traditional primary care, improve access, and eliminate unnecessary care (which makes up one-third of medicine), and to facilitate recovery after specialty treatment. Healing and recovery are ever present. Group classes and individual assistance in nutrition and behavioral change are available, and the staff are tuned in to the social/emotional and mental/spiritual lives of the patients. The space is warm and welcoming, without the usual barriers or industrial feel of typical clinics. The health care team knows you. Employees are selected for and trained in listening and empathy. Unlike most clinics in health care, you will not be interrupted within the first sixteen seconds of the encounter. The feel of caring is palpable.

And it heals better. Like the top 5% of primary care practices identified by Stanford, Iora's outcomes are stellar. Data on ten of the clinics open for two years or more shows remarkable results. This includes engagement rates of 85% per year; retention rates of 90% (94% of those engaged); a total medical expense decrease of 14% per year; in-patient admissions and emergency room visits more than 40% below the Medicare fee-for-service average; and a 21% improvement in hypertension outcomes. In addition, Iora has a 90 Net Promoter Score across Medicare markets (this means patients recommend them to others). One hundred percent of patients needing urgent care get a visit within twenty-four hours. Iora's STAR ratings (the Medicare system of quality in five different categories) increase yearly up to 30%.

By the standards of the Triple Aim, the patient-centered medical home, and even the Stanford assessments, Iora meets and exceeds those measures. Equally important, the patients, practitioners, health coaches, and communities enjoy the practice more. Practitioners suffer less burnout, and nurses and physicians feel their skills are well used.

But can this approach be applied in diverse settings with a variety of average people? The answer is that it can. Iora clinics are now up and functioning with good results in areas as diverse as college towns, the Las Vegas strip, and poverty-stricken areas of Queens in New York. "What is needed now," says Dr. Fernandopulle, "is a health care system that truly wants and will pay for this type of integrated care."

HEALING THROUGH PURPOSE

No matter where we start or how we navigate the elements of healing, it is when we can link them to our purpose in life that deep healing happens. This happens more often when the dimensions of healing are aligned. It also happens more often when good science is brought into the process to enhance it. It can happen dramatically when a person finds those elements that induce their greatest meaning response. Then we go beyond the 20% improvement found in cure-based medicine and tap into the 80% of healing potential that lies dormant in everyone.

In his book *Life on Purpose,* Dr. Victor Strecher, professor of public health at the University of Michigan, has summarized the extensive and startling research showing how a life of meaning and purpose prevents and treats chronic disease, reduces suffering, and even prolongs life. When a person feels that they have an important purpose in life, when their values and actions align—especially when that purpose gives back to others—they simply do and are better in all ways. Purpose has been correlated with reduced weight, better sleep, more friends, better sex, faster recovery, less relapse from addictions, less risk of Alzheimer's disease and dementia, less heart disease, lower health care needs, and lower death rates.

We even know the biology of purpose. It increases growth in the ventriculo-medial prefrontal cortex of the brain—the brain location of one's "sense of self"—and it can even maintain and elongate telomeres—the genes that predict your length of life. That individual sense of purpose, when aligned with our family, community, and work, will enhance the health of others in those areas, too. Companies whose employees feel cared for and are aligned with company goals and mission deliver more profits and last longer than companies that don't. Families and communities with purpose have more vibrancy and happiness, less violence and poverty, better health and well-being. Thus the goal in engaging in the HOPE process is to link your healing dimensions to why you are here in the world—your meaning and purpose in life—and to create a meaning response in mind and body.

Once we understand the dimensions of healing and the individual elements of meaning and purpose in creating health and well-being, it changes our perspective on health care and illuminates the path out of the current health care dilemma of higher costs, less satisfaction, and poorer health. My patients who use this approach find that they are no longer victims of a system not designed for them. This understanding becomes the foundation for true health (not just health care) reform.

What is needed now is a willingness to bring healing back into health care. The most effective way to do that is to bring it deliberately and intentionally into your life. You may not have access to integrative health care in a Nuka- or Iora-like system or get your care from one of the top 5% of patient-centered medical facilities. But this should not matter. Remember, only 20% of health comes from the treatments you get by walking into a doctor's office or visiting a medical clinic. The rest—the 80%—comes from you, from using the dimensions of healing already embedded in your life. By engaging in a HOPE-like process, you can unleash that 80%.

In the next, and final, chapter, I provide a simple set of instructions and accompanying tools for doing a HOPE visit. You and your physician can use those tools to access your healing dimensions. In the appendices, I provide a process that you—even without your physician—can use for your own journey to healing. Take this journey into your life; work through the questions yourself; take what you discover to your physician if she is willing to partner with you on that journey. If your doctor is hesitant, give her this book; when she has finished it, ask for impressions. It is my hope that doctors find these principles and tools useful in their own lives. I have. They might even help to ease their burnout and be more patient-centered in their practices. You can be your doctor's healer!

HOPE AND HEALING

The oncologist had unintentionally set my wife up to make The Cake, which was so effective in advancing her recovery. We had tried many other treatments to help her with fatigue, anemia, hair loss, and the risk of heart and nerve damage from chemotherapy. These included both conventional medications and alternative supplements of various types. For most of the alternative treatments, there was little evidence. For a few, there was evidence of harm. The oncologist offered several drugs for dealing with the side effects of therapy. Some worked well, especially for nausea and severe white blood count drops, but again, the evidence for many of them was slim, and nothing helped much for her extreme fatigue.

Then, during one oncologist visit just before the July Fourth holiday, Susan described again her tiredness and shortness of breath. The doctor was headed for the door when I asked about Susan's anemia—low red blood counts. She looked at the labs: "Oh, yes, they are low," she said. "You have anemia." She paused for a bit and then said, "You know, that is most likely what is causing your fatigue. But it is nothing to worry about, Susan. It's expected with chemotherapy. It's not in a dangerous range, so we'll keep an eye on it. It's normal for what you are going through. You will start getting better soon—after the chemotherapy."

Susan told me later that on hearing this, a light went on in her mind. This was "normal," and it was up to her to get through it. After that visit, she said to me, "As I understood it, the doctor basically said to just tough it out. That's what I thought. That is what I am doing and will keep doing. Let's really celebrate the Fourth. It's time to be *normal*."

It was a few days after that Susan mustered the energy to make The Cake. The oncologist, of course, never knew about The Cake or most of the other factors that sustained Susan's healing during the onslaught of the treatment. She didn't have time to. But without The Cake and the hope it engendered in Susan, the healing transformation she had during her cancer treatment might not have occurred. It was a hope the oncologist had given almost as a side comment, thrown out as she put her hand on the door to leave for the next patient. I thought of all the times I had done the same thing with patients. I thought now that it doesn't have to be this way in health care—to focus so much on the treatment and cure that we often miss what induces the healing.

SPIRIT MATTERS

This was the fifth trip to the hospital for Trevor to see if he could get a kidney. When he arrived around midnight, the doctor said that if the possible kidney did not match for him that night, they would discharge him in the morning and start again later in the year. Trevor's wife stayed with him and went to sleep in the chair in his hospital room. In the quiet of the early morning, Trevor reflected on what his wife had said; how his "incorrigible optimism" had gotten him into this mess; how he had not trusted the doctors and believed too much in natural treatments; how he had focused so much on giving back to his community—following his one passion and purpose—that he had neglected himself and his own health. Had there been a system of integrative health to fill the gaps between drugs, diet, and self-care; had the care he received been more person-centered; and had it been better linked to his purpose, he might have avoided years of suffering and expense, prevented the injury his wife endured when she donated her own kidney unsuccessfully, and not had to endure his current almost total dependency on the medical system. Perhaps, he thought quietly to himself, his optimism, his passion, his purpose, his prayer had all been misplaced. He was in a deep despair—hopeless. All he wanted was to be well so he could go back and help his people—young people especially who had been like him. He wanted them to have the opportunity for a full and successful life.

Then he did something he was not supposed to do. He got out of bed without assistance and kneeled to pray. His knees hurt. The IV pole pulled at his arm. He felt dizzy. At the side of the bed he prayed his favorite Bible passage from Isaiah 6:8: "Then I heard the voice of the Lord saying, 'Whom shall I send? And who will go for us?' And I said, 'Here am I. Send me!'" He then got back into bed and thought of the hymn "I Am Here Lord." A deep peace suddenly came over him. At that moment "I knew I was going to get a kidney," said Trevor. He described feeling much more than his usual optimism. It was an overwhelming feeling of release—of giving himself up to whatever God wanted of him and that he was being held in the Lord's loving hands. He fell into a deep sleep—better than he had for weeks.

He awoke at 7 am to his wife packing, getting him ready to be discharged back home. No call for a kidney had come in during the night. When he was fully awake he sat up and reached down to put on his socks—but something held him up.

"Ready?" his wife said, wondering why he was hesitating. It was long past the time they would have called him had the kidney been a match. But he was not ready. All the things that might happen should he leave now raced through this mind. He would have a dialysis treatment. He would go home and get back to work in his law firm and his community—a passion and purpose he would pursue it until the end.

He would go on until it was his time to die, he thought.

"Let's wait a bit," he said to her. They sat in silence, waiting for the doctor to come in to discharge him. He just couldn't bring himself to put his socks on.

When the doctor came in to the room he looked at them with an unusual smile. "Are you ready to go?" the doctor asked, in a strange tone.

"Sure, we are all packed up," said Trevor's wife, ignoring her husband's still bare feet.

"Well, then." The doctor could no longer contain himself; now he was smiling broadly. "You better unpack and get ready for the operating room. We found a kidney. It came in this morning—and it is a match!"

Trevor's wife sat there, stunned. Trevor took a deep breath and broke into a smile to match the doctor's. Finally, he simply said, "Okay then."

He would be healed.

Chapter 10

Creating Healing

Your HOPE consultation.

Doctors don't want frustrated, unhappy patients, and patients don't want burnt-out, unhappy doctors. None of us wants to feel like we are victims of the health care system. But all too often, that is what we get. It does not have to be that way.

To understand why this happens and how to improve it, we need to look beyond the individual doctor, to the health care system and the environment. We then see there are many pressures on the health care system that push it away from the delivery of patient-centered and integrative health, especially for chronic and preventive care. When you as the patient are aware of these pressures, you can counteract them by creating healing relationships with health care professionals and your own healing environment. This chapter describes the forces that can help you and your health care team connect with the inherent healing power in you and in everyone. Let's take a moment to summarize the forces operating on the current health care system.

UNDERSTANDING THE FORCES IN HEALTH CARE

Our modern medical system was originally set up to provide acute care. Problems that require immediate intervention, include injury, trauma, infection, heart attack, and stroke, are much better managed than chronic conditions.

Increasingly, most doctors are subspecialists. Except for those trained in primary care or family medicine, most doctors emerge from medical school well equipped to deal with only part of you—your cardiovascular system, or your bones and muscles, or your digestive organs, or your brain and central nervous system, or your endocrine system (glands and hormones). This is fine if your problems are restricted to these systems, but most health problems—especially those caused by stress and lifestyle—affect the whole person, including body, mind, and spirit. Specialists are not trained to look at health problems in this way.

We are fascinated by technology. Technology has produced tremendous advances in health care and will continue to do so. But there is a downside. The more inventive we get with diagnostic and surgical technology, the more we lose touch with the essential humanity of each patient. Patients are hooked up to blood pressure cuffs and monitors, injected with needles that withdraw blood, operated on through robotic arms attached to tiny cameras, and examined through ultrasound, MRI, and CT scans. Doctors can now peer into our brains, our organs, the very cells and genes of our body and obtain objective information about what is going on there. This is useful, of course, for diagnosis and treatment of disease, but the process tends to reduce people to objects, to depersonalize us. We are treated as if we too are machines, in need of repair, rather than living, breathing people with emotions, fears, and desires, in need of healing.

Doctors live with the potential for mistakes and lawsuits. Given the uncertainty in the science of medicine, the risk for error is high. Doctors don't like this, and many overcompensate with unnecessary care in the hope of overcoming that uncertainty. However, that rarely works. More is not better. In fact, the overuse of medical technologies is one of the main causes of harm to patients. In addition, the risk of malpractice suits or discipline from oversight boards leads many doctors to practice so-called "defensive medicine": ordering extra tests, waiting for specialists to "bless" a diagnosis, and focusing on extra paperwork, which also is often not in the best interest of the patient or based on good research evidence.

Doctors have information and work overload. Once, for my birthday, my father gave me a coffee mug inscribed with the words "Cognitive Overload." The message was clear—slow down and relax. Take time to listen, especially with your heart, not just your brain. We are all flooded with waves of information daily, and it is impossible for any one person (or even a group of people) to extract, synthesize, and make good use of all the information that is now available. In addition, many doctors are overworked. They get paid by volume. Fee-for-service payment systems and reduced fees per patient mean less time per patient. In this system, patients do not always get the best care science has identified, because doctors either do not have time to distill important, evidence-based information; do not know about the latest research; or simply do not have enough time to deliver it. In previous chapters, I have described the consequent rising burnout rate of health professionals. Another consequence is medical error, such as prescribing or delivering the wrong dose of medicine or misreading a test result. The Institute of Medicine reports that preventable human errors in hospitals lead to the deaths of nearly one hundred thousand patients every year in the United States, making it nearly the third leading cause of death. Medical error kills more people than highway accidents, breast cancer, or AIDS. Overload is partly the cause of this.

Managed care increasingly dominates our health care system. Attempts to contain the escalating cost of health care puts treatment decisions into the hands of insurance administrators or government regulators rather than doctors and patients. Both patients and their doctors are frustrated that therapies they consider important or useful are not covered by insurance, or covered only minimally—even when there is sound scientific evidence for their use. This further restricts doctor-patient time together, as reimbursements depend on how many patients are seen and how many procedures are performed. When physicians have only fifteen minutes—or sometimes just five—to devote to a patient, conversations are rushed and patient-doctor relationships don't develop. Patients more often leave with a prescription for a drug rather than a recommendation for lifestyle change, let alone delving into the deeper dimensions of healing. This is not a good environment for prevention, the management of chronic illness, or optimal healing.

The hierarchy in health care puts patients last. The standard medical hierarchy goes like this: doctor, nurse, medical assistant, patient. When you enter the hospital or outpatient system, if you are like most patients, you are dis-eased, dis-robed, dis-empowered, and eventually dis-charged. Such a system prevents a collaborative partnership with your doctor and prevents your doctor from being your advocate within the system.

There is an increasing diversity of patients and practitioners. Patients come into the system from a variety of cultural backgrounds and with personal preferences and beliefs about their health. Too often, doctors and other health professionals are not prepared to provide care that is sensitive to their patients' culture, ethnicity, or belief differences. Witness what happened to Trevor because of this disconnect. In many cases, language may also be a barrier to communication. Even in the alternative medicine world, patients should be wary of "turf" battles among different alternative practitioner groups, each claiming, for example, that their approach—be it naturopathy, chiropractic, or acupuncture—is the best for everyone. No single approach works for everyone or even for the same condition in different people.

SYSTEMS WORKING TOWARD INTEGRATIVE HEALTH

That is the bad news. The good news is that health care systems around the world now implement more integrative health care and are seeking to build a more balanced approach to healing chronic illness. I invite you to seek out these practices, ask for them from your physician, health care system, government, and insurance provider, and bring them into your life. What patients like Trevor could not get twenty years ago is increasingly available today—if you look and ask for it. Integrative health care comes in a variety of forms and names.

In the previous chapter, I provided an overview of policy guidelines and health systems seeking to optimize a patient-centered medical home and other integrated or pay-for-value approaches to health care. I gave several examples, such as the Nuka and Iora systems and the work from the Institute for Healthcare Improvement and Stanford evaluations of the top 5% of primary care in the United States. The Commonwealth Fund reports on such exemplars in integrated care on a regular basis. What most of these systems did not do, however, is integrate complementary and alternative medicine (CAM) approaches into their delivery. Thus, many of them are missing one of the three legs of fully integrative health care: conventional care, complementary care, and self-care. Let me give you a brief overview of groups that are integrating this second leg of integrative health—the Integrative Medicine and Health, traditional, and CAM efforts—around the world.

INTEGRATIVE MEDICINE AND HEALTH

The best global overview of the rise in complementary and alternative approaches to healing is being done by the WHO, whose office of Traditional & Complementary Medicine (T&CM) tracks and advances information, research, and access to non-Western (nonconventional) practices. The use of these practices by patients and physicians is extensive—ranging from between 30% to nearly 90% of the general public in some places. Countries such as Singapore, Japan, China, and Korea provide some or even full coverage of T&CM practices for their populations. Eighty percent of the 129 member countries in the WHO assessment provide acupuncture (originally an approach only in traditional Chinese medicine), including eighteen (14%) with insurance coverage. As of 2012, thirty-nine member countries (30%) had doctoral-level training programs in T&CM, and seventy-three (56%) had government-funded research institutes. The economic output per year in herbal and natural products alone is over $83 billion in China, $7.4 billion in Korea, and $14.8 billion in the United States.

Around the world, the reasons patients give for their use of T&CM are similar to the reasons many of my patients give for seeking complementary and alternative medicine: easier access, dissatisfaction with exclusively conventional care, and a desire for safer and more natural or whole person care. Cost savings were also cited, and there is some data to support this. Reports from WHO and the RAND Corporation (an independent international research group) show lower costs with equal outcomes with some types of T&CM for chronic pain. When integrated into primary care, practices that include T&CM report lower costs for hospitalization and drug use.

The WHO Strategy report and others have found that, as illustrated in Trevor's experience, the two systems of T&CM and conventional medicine often do not integrate with each other—in any country. Usually, T&CM and conventional hospitals and clinics operate separately. A review by RAND researcher Ian Coulter of over seventeen thousand studies on what is called "integrative medicine" around the world showed that only five studies explored full integration between the systems. This means that patients are, unfortunately, caught between these systems and therefore need to become their own integrators. This is challenging, given that the quality of training and products in CAM is often neither regulated nor oriented toward scientific evidence as much as conventional medicine. While some countries, such as Australia, Canada, and certain European countries, closely regulate the quality and use of natural substances such as herbs and supplements, many other countries do not. Supplement and herbal companies can market and sell such products with dubious or inadequate science. The WHO report notes the wide variety and quality of regulations on T&CM compared to conventional medicine worldwide.

While it is not the purpose of this chapter to give a comprehensive summary of global T&CM practices, special mention of a few regions may help readers understand better how to use these systems to achieve their own integrative health. More information is regularly posted on my website at DrWayneJonas.com.

The United States has made outstanding progress in developing integrative medicine in recent years, catalyzed by the NIH, the Office of Alternative Medicine (OAM, which I directed from 1995 to 1999), and then the National Center for Complementary and Integrative Health, which replaced the OAM. This effort facilitated the development of several academic health centers. For those who get their care at academic health centers in the United States, there is a growing group providing integrative medicine and health. The Academic Consortium for Integrative Medicine and Health is made up of over seventy academic health centers and teaching hospitals that provide integrative medicine. In the United States, these include schools such as Harvard, Stanford, Johns Hopkins, Duke, and others, such as the universities of Arizona, Minnesota, Maryland, and California. This effort was supported for several years by a group of private philanthropists, the Bravewell Collaborative. Bravewell, which has since closed, supported not only the academic development of integrative medicine, but also a research network, a movie, and a National Academy of Medicine summit in 2009 called *Integrative Medicine and the Health of the Public*. That summit called for adding the principles of integrative health into health care for more holistic care by incorporating nutrition, mind-body practices, the use of more natural substances, and other complementary treatments into mainstream medical care.

There are many other groups leading the integration of nonconventional medicine into the mainstream. These include the European Society of Integrative Medicine (ESIM) and the International Society for Complementary Medicine Research (ISCMR), which held their tenth and twelfth international congresses, respectively, in 2017. Having followed this field for over three decades, I am struck by how often the philosophies and approaches that begin in these groups get taken up (with or without the same labeling) by mainstream medicine. These groups represent the "stay tuned for what may become the future of prevention and healing." They are the canaries in the coal mine that, instead of alerting to danger in health care, alert to innovations in healing. Most of these organizations seek to better integrate what they do into conventional biomedical health care systems.

One of the pioneers and continued leaders in the area of integrative medical education is Dr. Andrew Weil. His University of Arizona Center for Integrative Medicine has medical education programs and fellowship training—led by Dr. Victoria Maizes—that has taught over 1,500 physicians in the foundations of integrative health, developing a cadre of young doctors with the knowledge and skills for healing. Look up their graduates for a doctor near you. Dr. Weil is a best-selling author whose multiple books describe how you can incorporate integrative medicine in your life. His most recent title, *Mind Over Meds*, is a well-researched book full of practical suggestions for using lifestyle approaches and natural substances to treat many of the conditions, for which most doctors prescribe drugs. This is an especially timely topic as we try to tackle the epidemic of opioid drug overuse and its damaging effects.

Recently, a remarkable experiment in integrative health was launched at the University of California, Irvine (UCI). An entire health sciences college encompassing the schools of medicine, nursing, pharmacy, and public health was formed under the principles of integrative health. The college was launched through a joint partnership of UCI and Susan and Henry Samueli (who also fund the Samueli Integrative Health Programs that I run). The goal of this new college is to "educate the next generation of health science professionals to transcend current boundaries; foster clinical programs with an increased focus on lifestyle, prevention, wellness and optimal health; and promote discovery of an expanded set of tools and platforms that fosters a systems approach to health, inclusive of all forms of evidenced-based healing—conventional and complementary." This will indeed be a new way for health care professionals to learn how to balance curing and healing—and a way to attend to those factors that make healing work.

Other examples include the Cleveland Clinic, one of the top medical centers in the United States. It has started a program in what is called "functional medicine"—a term coined by Dr. Jeffrey Bland over thirty years ago. It seeks to integrate science-based nutritional and lifestyle modifications with mainstream science for delivery in health care. In his recent book *The Disease Delusion*, Dr. Bland describes how the merger of nutrition with genomic medicine is creating a paradigm shift in healing that uses whole systems science and the ancient concept of food as medicine. The Cleveland Clinic program, directed by Dr. Mark Hyman—author of multiple best-selling books on prevention and health promotion—plans to test this approach for its effectiveness in healing several major diseases. Cleveland Clinic also operates an Institute for Integrative Health and Wellness that provides a team approach of CAM and mainstream practitioners. Physicians are gaining greater access to training in nutrition and lifestyle change. The Institute for Functional Medicine (IFM) now offers regular seminars and a certification in functional medicine for physicians. When I last visited the IFM training course, I noticed that they were no longer just preaching to the believers in alternative approaches to medicine. Most of the physicians attending the training were from mainstream organizations like the Veterans Health Administration, Kaiser Permanente, and Providence Health. They were looking for the kind of education in nutrition they did not get in medical school or residency.

The Mayo Clinic—also one of the top health care organizations in the world—has invested heavily in creating new models of healing with both its integrative medicine programs, run for years by Dr. Brent Bauer, and its new multistory Healthy Living Center and programs run by Michael Casey, Dr. Don Hensrud, and others. The Healthy Living Center has taken what we now know from research on health promotion and built a program for facilitating health in everyone, whether healthy or ill. It is this type of integration that is applying what we now know about prevention and the optimal treatment of chronic disease. The Mayo Clinic offers training and delivery to other hospitals and health care centers around the world that seek to adopt these approaches.

The final program to know about is the Center for Spirituality and Healing (CSH) at the University of Minnesota. CSH has been led for thirty years by Mary Jo Kreitzer, a PhD nurse who is a pioneer in the creation of visionary approaches to healing and well-being. Her Model of Well-being has influenced countless patients, professionals, companies, health systems, and policy makers in thinking more clearly about how healing works. It has had a profound influence on my thinking over the years. The course and educational tools from CSH are available to patients and professionals (for more information, see my website, DrWayneJonas.com).

Other organizations offer course in integrative health. While it used to be that many of these courses were taught by practitioners far outside the mainstream, they are now becoming mainstream—just part of good healthcare. I will mention just a few. The Academic Collaborative for Integrative Health (ACIH) is a membership organization for complementary schools, including naturopaths, chiropractors (who also have their own academic membership organization), massage therapists, acupuncturists, and midwives. ACIH represents and advocates for these professions. Recently, the Institute for Lifestyle Medicine, founded and led by Harvard Medical School's Dr. Edward Phillips, is bridging the gap between medical treatment and behavior. Dr. Phillips, along with Yale Professor Dr. David Katz and others, helped organize the American College of Lifestyle Medicine (ACLM), which provides education to licensed health care professionals on how to deliver exercise and nutritional prescriptions. For patients like Trevor, these and other organizations provide physicians with opportunities to acquire knowledge and skills allowing them to bridge conventional care and self-care. While the term *integrative health* is now being used by many organizations—including the NIH National Center for Complementary and Integrative Health—true integration is still rare. What you should look for from those claiming to deliver integrative health are practitioners and health care systems that integrate all three key areas for healing—conventional care, complementary medicine, and self-care. More information on these organizations is also available on my website.

For those who get their care in the U.S. military or Veterans Health Administration (VHA), a radical shift toward more holistic, integrative health is occurring. Admiral Mike Mullen, former Chairman of the Joint Chiefs of Staff, launched a program called Total Force Fitness. This framework incorporated all the elements from the dimensions of healing described in this book, but called it "fitness" rather than health. This included behavioral fitness, social and psychological fitness, and even spiritual fitness. The Total Force Fitness framework is now being implemented throughout the military under various names such as the Healthy Base Initiative and Operation LiveWell. The last two U.S. Army Surgeons General, Lieutenant General Eric Schoomaker and Lieutenant General Patty Horoho, created signature programs in integrative health for pain and performance. The VHA is implementing a personalized health plan program that integrates veteran goals and clinical goals in a holistic manner. Led by Dr. Tracy Gaudet, former director of the Duke Integrative Health Center, and Dr. Ben Kligler, formerly of Beth Israel in New York, it seeks to transform the way the VHA treats patients, from one delivering cure-focused treatments to a system that enhances personalized self-care and healing for every veteran. NATO has also begun to explore use of integrative health in the military in Europe. A recent report by NATO summarized integrative health activities and recommendations in the military in that alliance.

Similar trends toward integrative heath are happening in Europe. While many European countries have long histories of traditional healing—including systems like spa healing, anthroposophical medicine, homeopathy, and herbal treatments—these practices became largely eclipsed with the rise of modern biomedicine early in the twentieth century. A major summary of the current state of complementary medicine was published in 2015 by the European Union (EU). This four-year study, called CAMbrella, described a diversity of CAM practices and regulations in the EU. One challenge in Europe that seems less prominent in many other countries (except perhaps in the United States and Australia) is a strong skeptics movement that challenges CAM, accusing it of being nonscientific. While there is indeed less science in CAM than in conventional care overall, science is challenged to provide certainty in any medical approach, CAM included. We need more and better science in health care all around.

India had a long history of well-developed traditional systems (and some newer CAM systems) before modern Western medicine arrived and quickly dominated national practice and resources. However, the government has recently invested in developing the science and standards for T&CM in India. These systems include Ayurveda, yoga, naturopathy, Unani, Siddha, and homeopathy. Most of these systems are thousands of years old, except for homeopathy, which was exported from Germany in the nineteenth century and then widely adopted around the world. The WHO reports 508 "colleges" in one or more of these systems in India with over 25,000 undergraduate and nearly 2,500 graduate students per year. There is tremendous experience in these systems. However, having visited, examined, and done research on these topics in India, I can say from personal experience that significant improvement in quality is needed before their approaches can be integrated with conventional medicine. Dual-trained physicians like Dr. Manu are still rare. For the time being, they largely remain separate from mainstream conventional medicine and do not provide an integrative health system.

Traditional Chinese medicine (TCM) was the major system in China until the modern era. During and after the Cultural Revolution, TCM was largely ignored and even suppressed. However, China has now made major investments in research and the integration of TCM and modern Western medicine. A 2017 report released by the Chinese government describes the tremendous growth of TCM and an integrated TCM/Western medicine industry in China. They report nearly four thousand TCM hospitals and forty thousand TCM clinics. This includes 446 integrated hospitals and 7,705 integrated clinics, where both TCM and Western medicine are practiced together. There are over twenty-five TCM medical schools and two hundred Western medical schools offering TCM training. They report 11.5% lower outpatient costs and 24% lower inpatient costs in these integrated practices versus conventional Western practices. Over 15% of health care dollars are spent on TCM in the country. The government sees TCM as having an important role in China's socioeconomic influence outside China. The report ends by saying that "The time has come for TCM to experience a renaissance." TCM does seem to be spreading into other countries. Over 183 countries outside China have TCM programs, and 103 countries formally regulate TCM practices, including 18 that pay for acupuncture in health insurance. Acupuncture has largely been accepted as being safe and effective for pain in most countries, including Europe and the United States. However, based on my experience in China, I can say that the quality of clinical TCM research needs improvement before full integration can occur in the West.

WORKING WITH YOUR SYSTEM AND DOCTOR

None of these systems is perfect, but each moves health care in the right direction. Having spent a lot of time in this space, I can say that these systems share a philosophy of healing and self-care, not just curing. As daunting as the list of forces against healing in modern health care sound, you can overcome many of those forces and create healing collaborations that work for you. Start by creating a healing collaboration with your doctor.

Recently, a patient in her late thirties came to me seeking a prescription refill. She was married, worked part-time, and was raising three teenaged boys. She came to see me because her regular doctor was on vacation and she wanted a refill of a muscle relaxant medication for chronic neck pain. She also wanted a prescription for a sleeping pill and an opioid pain medication.

I never automatically refill prescriptions without examining the patient. When I examined her, I found nothing physically wrong with her neck, so I asked her if she had ever had the pain evaluated. She answered, "I know what is causing the neck pain—it is stress." Every time her husband was redeployed to a new military assignment, she would have to sell the house, organize the whole family's move, find new schools for the boys and a new job for herself, and settle into a new community. All of this was giving her, quite literally, a "pain in the neck," she said.

The muscle relaxants gave her some relief, but the pain always flared up at times of major stress. She also commented on what she thought as an unrelated problem: she had to get up in the night to urinate—sometimes as many as six times. Her previous doctor was unable to find any physical reason for this and had prescribed a medication to inhibit her bladder contractions. I explained to her that the number-one cause of frequent urination, when there is no physical explanation, is stress, and that night is a common time for this to occur.

I explained to her that stress stimulates the sympathetic nervous system, which often responds by sending signals to the body that create an urgency to urinate. "All three of the problems you are describing—neck pain, frequent urination, and difficulty sleeping—might well have one cause," I said to her. "It looks like your nervous system is out of balance, with the sympathetic system getting overstimulated. If you could find ways to induce a relaxation response and balance your nervous system, all three of these symptoms might disappear."

She seemed interested, so we talked about some simple ways to induce a relaxation response, including the breathing and relaxation exercises I described in chapter 7 (see page 122) and summarize in the appendices (see page 260). Finally, though, she said with a sigh, "I just don't have the time to myself to do these things." She left with the prescriptions.

About a month later, she was back in my office. "I decided I'd like you to help me induce that relaxation response," she said. I was not sure what motivated her to change her mind, but I was pleased she was ready to take healing into her own hands. We talked about what she might do, and practiced some simple relaxation exercises in the office. To bring that experience more deeply into her life, she decided to take a yoga class three times a week. "I'll tell my family that this is time I need for my health—doctor's orders," she said. She was creating a healing environment for herself by using me as a health collaborator, not just as a pill dispenser. After two months of yoga three days a week, her neck pain, frequent urination, and sleep issues had all resolved.

Find the right doctor for you. If you too are looking for a new doctor who is more of a healing collaborator than a pill dispenser, treat it like a job interview—you want to hire the best health care professional for you and your family. Consider the two reasons to see a doctor: one is to find out if a problem is acute, serious, and needs immediate attention; the other is to find a partner who will help you manage chronic illness and the prevention of disease. There is no other reason to see a doctor.

Acute situations can be handled in either an emergency room, a walk-in clinic, or the same-day unit of a clinic or health plan. But for chronic care and prevention, look for either a primary care doctor, a nurse practitioner, or a physician's assistant (PA) who is licensed to do family medicine, internal medicine, gynecology, or (if you have children) pediatrics. Interview several candidates until you click with one. This is an important relationship, after all, and could become a lifetime—and life-saving—connection. Show candidates the HOPE assessment at the end of this chapter or on my website and see if they will engage with you in that process. Explore to what extent each candidate already asks patients about the healing dimensions. Your goal is to find someone who will develop a collaborative relationship with you for prevention and healing.

There are three key aspects to a good collaborative health relationship: caring, competence, and credibility. Look for this combination in anyone you entrust with your health. Don't be afraid to ask prospective doctors about their education, experience, and special skills. You can also ask about their views on holistic or integrative medicine. If a doctor tells you that all alternative methods are worthless, or that holistic medicine is a waste of time, this may not be the best person for you. However, no matter what a doctor's opinion of complementary and alternative medicine, if he or she is willing to seriously evaluate the medical research for you and not abandon caring for you, he or she can play a valuable role in the collaboration.

I also suggest finding a doctor who works with a team or has access to a network of other kinds of practitioners, including lifestyle experts, health coaches, nutritionists, behaviorists, and other conventional and alternative specialists. These collaborators may be in the community or in the doctor's own health care center or practice. A good indication is if a doctor routinely offers preventive services, integrative medical care, lifestyle and behavioral therapies, and complementary treatments. Ask about the breadth of the candidates' networks. How many practitioners do they regularly work with? Are all practitioners with whom they work licensed by the state? Do they follow up the care their patients receive from these practitioners and regularly collaborate with other providers to find the best combination of care? Do they make recommendations for self-care and provide evidence as part of the treatment decision process? These are all good signs.

As part of your search for a doctor, look at the team with whom he or she works. Prevention and care for chronic conditions require constant communication and teamwork to evaluate changes in your health and the services needed on an ongoing basis. When you visit the office, get a feel for the culture. Do people communicate with each other? Is there a caring, respectful atmosphere? Or do staff members bark commands at each other and appear frenetic, isolated, and disorganized? Those may have burnout and may burn you.

Look also at how the team members treat you. Do they appear competent? Do you trust them? Do you feel cared about and heard? Does a team member, for example, call you prior to or after an office visit to find out any concerns you have? Does the team include you in decision making? Do they prepare you for the best use of the doctor's— and your—time? And, importantly, are they honest with you about what you need—even if it might not be what you want? A colonoscopy is a good example. After the age of fifty, regular colonoscopies and comparable screening tools dramatically reduce the risk of fatal colon cancer, but most people hate to have them done. A good doctor will encourage and remind you to follow recommended prevention and screening guidelines, even if they are unpleasant.

LOOK FOR THE FIVE-P APPROACH

A doctor has five responsibilities in integrative medicine:

1. **PROTECT.** Your doctor should protect you from dangerous, disproven, or toxic practices.
2. **PERMIT.** Your doctor should permit practices that may work and have no harmful side effects—such as mind-body practices, acupuncture, or massage.
3. **PROMOTE.** Your doctor should promote proven conventional practices—such as Pap smears, colonoscopies, and vaccinations—and proven alternative practices, such as

acupuncture, massage, and yoga for chronic back pain, and exercise, mind-body practices, and nutritional changes for many conditions.

4. **PARTNER.** Your doctor should include you as a partner in the health care team and should be willing to research and discuss with you the evidence for all three of the integrative health arms—conventional, complementary, and self-care.

5. **PAYMENT.** Paying for preventive care and health promotion is key to optimizing healing. Whether you have employer-provided health insurance or an individual policy, examine your policy or contact the provider to see what it covers. You can ask your employer to investigate health insurance policies that include complementary and integrative medicine, lifestyle medicine, and health coaching. They can purchase insurance supplements that cover these services. If your claim for alternative services is denied by the insurance company, you should either ask your employer's human resources department to pursue it or have your doctor write to the insurer. Often, contractors who specialize in health care coverage have better success than individuals in pursuing claims approval.

If you like your doctor, enhance the relationship. Have a discussion with him or her about becoming more involved in your health care. This might involve asking your doctor to do some research about the effectiveness of treatments that interest you. Ask your doctor to advise you about prevention and lifestyle changes, including nutrition, exercise, and stress management. Ask how to prevent or minimize the effects of chronic illness and learn about any screening tests you should have. Encourage your doctor to see you as a whole person. During your visits, talk about your family, your work, your interests and hobbies, and any areas in your life that are giving you problems, including your relationships with your spouse, children, or coworkers.

Realize that the doctor's time with you may be limited, so go into the meeting prepared and with an agenda for the visit. Before going into an appointment, think about how your lifestyle affects your health. If you are open to lifestyle changes, ask about available resources. (You could ask, for example, "Do you refer patients to health coaches, nutritionists, or acupuncturists?") Be forthcoming with your health goals. Proactively share what you are hoping to do and how you want to feel. Don't wait until the end to provide key information.

Lastly, make the most of your entire health care team in addition to your physician. If your practice has physician's assistants, nurses, or health coaches, they may be able to supplement the time you spend with your physician. Use their services.

A HOPE CONSULTATION

One of the fastest and most direct ways to engage your health care system in helping you access your own healing capacity is to ask your physician to do a HOPE consultation with you.

We know that both before and after a diagnosis, and between states of health and disease, there are specific health-promoting conditions and actions that can prevent, slow, or reverse chronic disease, strengthen overall health, and improve function, quality of life, and overall well-being. Suffering can be reduced with healing no matter what a person's illness or stage of life—provided those behaviors are meaningful to the person and tap into their inherent healing capacity. Those factors and how they connect to the patient personally are explored during a HOPE consultation and are captured in a HOPE note.

The HOPE consultation is done after a complete medical diagnosis and treatment is completed, including a SOAP note. During the HOPE consultation, the practitioner goes over the core domains of healing with the patient and seeks to reframe the orientation from one of disease treatment to one emphasizing self-healing integrated with medical care. After examining the medical diagnosis and learning about the history and the context in which the patient lives, the HOPE consultation explores the factors that can enhance healing for the individual. These factors are not specific treatments for disease; rather, they focus on activities that complement those treatments to facilitate improvement in symptoms, function, quality of life, happiness, and well-being. Sometimes the disease also resolves during this process. You and your doctor can learn more about how to do a HOPE consultation in the appendix of this book and on my website, DrWayneJonas.com.

THE HOPE OF HEALING

From the minute we are born, we are subjected to the stresses and traumas of life—all of which steadily erode our bodily systems and structures. These onslaughts include fear, anxiety, pain, toxicity in the environment, the need to keep our bodies upright against the force of gravity, the energy it takes to fight off a cold. Even eating and breathing in oxygen causes our cells and tissues to break down.

When you are having a bad day and everything seems to be going wrong, do you sometimes feel that you are battling emotional and physical disintegration? It may be small comfort to know that there is a principle in physics, the second law of thermodynamics, which holds that everything in the universe moves toward entropy—a state of disorder and chaos. Forces of nature *are* constantly acting to dissipate us into the universe, to make us disappear.

But on most days, we do not disintegrate or fall apart—because we also have an inherent capacity to maintain order and repair damage caused by the stresses and traumas of life—to reverse the chaos of the universe and heal. However, when these repair and restoration mechanisms break down, we develop disease or lose our mental, emotional, and/or physical well-being. Of course, there are virulent diseases or traumatic injuries that will initially overwhelm even the most tuned-up repair systems. But by building up and maintaining your inherent healing capacity, you have a better chance of resistance, resilience, and recovery from the onslaughts of life.

I hope that the journey we have taken together through *How Healing Works* will help you find a path filled with courage and hope. You do not have to feel helpless or in despair when things fall apart. The more aware you become of your response to the forces that influence your life, the more you will realize that the conscious decisions you make every moment of every day can change your future for the better. You can influence all the dimensions of your life, surrounding and infusing yourself with the forces of healing.

You can be whole. You can be healed.

The HOPE Consultation

This guide is designed to help you work with health professionals to enhance your own healing capacity. The purpose is to integrate the usual disease treatment, or pathogenic approach, with a health-promoting or salutogenic approach (Aaron Antonovsky, a professor of medical sociology, coined the term *salutogenesis* for this approach, to contrast it with *pathogenesis*, the process of disease).

Every day, often dozens of times a day, hundreds of thousands of physicians and health care professionals around the world write SOAP notes. This behavior is so automatic and engrained that they rarely even consider the implications—how it molds and directs their thinking about every patient they see. SOAP not only extends pathogenic thinking to what's done to the patient, it also creates a set of cultural expectations, frameworks, and behaviors to which all modern medicine conforms.

Healing requires a different type of assessment—an assessment of those behaviors and interactions that facilitate salutogenic thinking, and framework a set of expectations and action focused fostering our inherent healing capacity. A patient's clinical diagnosis may or may not be relevant to the ways in which healing happens. For example, the components of healing are often generic—meaning a process that facilitates healing for one disease also facilitates it for another disease. Therefore, the assessment and the plan in a SOAP note is usually not directly relevant to health promotion and healing. This is where a

HOPE consultation comes in.

The HOPE consultation—the healing-oriented practice and environments visit—consists of a set of questions specifically geared to evaluate aspects of a person's life that facilitates or detracts from healing; that is, it seeks how to enhance the processes of recovery, repair, and the return to wholeness. The goal of the HOPE consultation and HOPE note is to identify those behaviors that stimulate or support healing processes. It involves evaluating a patient in four different dimensions. First is the *inner dimension*—the perceptions, expectations, and awareness held in the mind. Certain types of mental framing around a life can either facilitate and enhance healing, or impair and block it. The second, *interpersonal dimension,* focuses on social relationships and the culture in which we operate. Again, certain types of social connections and relationships, and the nature of those relationships, can either support healing or interfere with it. Third is the *behavioral dimension*—things we do every day to either support and nourish the body's healing capacity or interfere with it and cause further damage. Finally, there is the *external dimension*; that is, the physical environment in which we live. This includes home, work, school, errands, and recreation, including time in nature and exposure to nourishing or toxic elements around them.

THE OPTIMAL HEALING DIMENSIONS

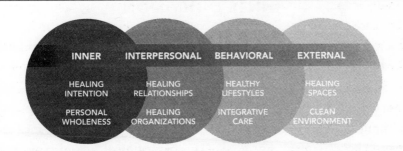

INNER	INTERPERSONAL	BEHAVIORAL	EXTERNAL
HEALING INTENTION	HEALING RELATIONSHIPS	HEALTHY LIFESTYLES	HEALING SPACES
PERSONAL WHOLENESS	HEALING ORGANIZATIONS	INTEGRATIVE CARE	CLEAN ENVIRONMENT

The HOPE note provides a focused, intentional, and systematic way of documenting these healing dimensions, per whole systems science, during a patient visit, providing a tool for addressing each dimension and the elements of healing. The natural overlap of the dimensions enables the patient-practitioner conversation to flow. It complements the disease treatment framework provided by the SOAP. In chronic disease, it fills in dimensions often missed by the SOAP—the environmental, behavioral, social/emotional, and mental/spiritual determinants of health. The HOPE consultation can guide both doctor and patient to improve health and well-being—not simply the treatment of disease. As with any intervention, what happens depends upon the patient's disease and his or her state of health and wellness orientation and readiness. In most patients, the recommendations from a HOPE consultation have a positive impact. It may not cure the disease or improve it significantly, or it may cure the disease or provide major improvement in the illness. In chronic diseases, it can almost always enhance wellness and well-being and improve function, whether the disease is cured or not. However, fully 70% to 80% of what the patient needs from an encounter in the context of a chronic illness is illuminated by the HOPE consultation.

At DrWayneJonas.com, I provide patients and professions with a detailed guide for doing a HOPE consultation. What follows is only a summary of the HOPE elements to familiarize you with the approach. The HOPE consultations four dimensions are: inner, interpersonal, behavioral, and external.

INNER DIMENSION

The inner environment often holds the key to healing and well-being for the patient. This sometimes comes from a spiritual or religious life, or one grounded in meaning and purposeful activities. Often, it involves helping others. It can also be found in a creative pursuit or family activities—any endeavor that brings purpose and meaning beyond the individual. The goal of this part of HOPE is to explore the patient's most profound insight into themselves and see if and how this is connected to their illness, suffering, and healing.

INTERPERSONAL DIMENSION

The social environment is essential to health and healing. Both health and happiness are socially contagious. Social cohesion is not only health enhancing but also essential for sustainable behavioral change in any culture and in any setting. Questions in this part of the HOPE consultation seek to explore the extent of a patient's social connections and support, especially from family and friends.

BEHAVIORAL DIMENSION

Certain behaviors are linked to chronic illness and healing. This section of the HOPE consultation explores what the patient does to help herself or himself heal. Four primary areas are explored; others can be added, as guided by the patient.

STRESS MANAGEMENT: Research has demonstrated the benefits of achieving a deep relaxation capacity, a mind-body state known to counter the stress response and improve receptivity to personal insight and motivation for lifestyle change. These practices can also enhance health and strengthen personal resilience on their own. In the HOPE consultation, the practitioner explores what the patient does to relax and introduces options such as breathing, visualization, mindfulness and meditation, or biofeedback for regular use.

PHYSICAL ACTIVITY: Physical activity can reduce stress, improve pain and brain function, slow aging and heart disease, and help a person reach and maintain an optimum weight. Fitness, along with proper rest and sleep, maintains functioning and productivity of the whole person throughout the lifespan and in any stage of health or illness. The patient is asked about his or her level of activity, and exercise and methods are offered to assist the patient in attaining an appropriate level of movement.

SLEEP: Adequate quantity and quality of sleep improves most symptoms and can reduce stress, relieve pain, improve brain and immune function, slow aging, reduce incidence of heart disease and cancer, and help with achieving an optimum weight. Good sleep helps maintain functioning and productivity of the whole person throughout the lifespan and in any stage of health or illness. The patient is asked about the quantity, quality, and effectiveness of his or her sleep, and the practitioner offers methods to assist in attaining good sleep.

OPTIMUM NUTRITION AND SUBSTANCE USE: Ideal weight and optimal physiological function are best supported through proper nutrition and reduced exposure to toxic substances—nicotine, alcohol, drugs, and environmental toxins—that impair function. Food and substance management requires motivation, environmental controls, food selection training, and family, peer, and community involvement. In the HOPE consultation, the patient is asked about use of these substances, about his or her normal diet, and any symptoms of gastrointestinal dysfunction, such as GERD, excessive gas, IBS, or constipation.

COMPLEMENTARY MEDICAL CARE: The patient is asked about his or her use of and/or interest in practices such as acupuncture, traditional or indigenous medicine, naturopathy, or chiropractic, and use of nutritional supplements and herbs. These practices—sometimes referred to as complementary and alternative medicine (CAM)—can facilitate healing if used appropriately or can harm if used inappropriately. They can be integrated with conventional medicine and self-care based on good evidence.

EXTERNAL DIMENSION

A healthy outer environment affects and supports a healthy person. This dimension attends to the physical structures and settings in which the patient lives and how these facilitate healing and minimize adverse impacts on and from the earth. The patient is asked what his or her home and work environment is like and if she has created a special place in which she feels relaxed and truly at home. Attention to architecture and art, time in nature, sound, smell, and light are key elements in producing such an environment. In addition, the HOPE consultation evaluates and attempts to minimize exposure to toxins that can impair healing and produce disease. I recommend a recent book by Dr. Joe Pizzorno, *The Toxin Solution*, to learn more.

Together, these healing-oriented practices and environments spell "HOPE," for individuals and for society.

SAMPLE QUESTIONS FOR A HOPE CONSULTATION

The following questions are used to guide the conversation between the patient and doctor during the HOPE consultation. Other questions can be added and personalized for each patient, personality, readiness, and circumstances.

Inner

- Why do you seek healing? What is your goal and intention?
- Rate your health (1–10) and what changes you expect can happen (1–10).
- Why are you here in life? What is your purpose? What are your most meaningful daily activities?

Interpersonal

- What are your social connections and relationships?
- How is your social support? Do you have family and friends you can discuss your life events and feelings with? Do you have people you have fun with?
- Tell me about yourself. Tell me about your major traumas in the past.
- What makes you feel happy?

Behavioral

- What do you do during the day? What is your lifestyle like?
- What do you do for stress management? How do you relax, reflect, and recreate?
- Do you smoke or drink alcohol or take drugs?
- How's your diet (describe your last breakfast, lunch, and dinner)?
- Do you exercise? If yes, what types and amounts?
- How is your sleep (quality and hours)? Do you wake refreshed?
- How much water, sugary drinks, and tea or coffee do you drink?
- What is your use of complementary and alternative medicine (CAM)—supplements, herbs, use of other CAM practitioners and healers?

External

- What is your home like? Your work environment?
- Is there a place at home where you can go and feel joyful and relaxed?
- What is your exposure to light, noise, clutter, music, colors, or art?
- What contact with nature do you have?
- What are your exposures to toxins, especially heavy metals or EDCs?

See the illustration on page 221 for the map I use to guide patients toward their own healing path.

THE HOPE NOTE

The answers to these questions form the basis for a HOPE note placed in the medical record. From this assessment, a plan for a meaningful response, to enhance what the patient is already doing to heal, is developed together. The goal of the plan is to match additional evidence-based healing methods to the patient's current activities. That match is summarized in a HOPE list for goal setting and tracking.

After the HOPE consultation, I ask my patients to send me their summary of the top three areas they would like to enhance in the first month and a single goal for that month—expressed in terms of actions or symptom improvement. Usually patients need further assistance in accomplishing their goals. Several tools are available to help with this, including:

- A workbook on healing. I give my patients a workbook called *Optimal Healing Environments: Your Healing Journey*, which is also available free from DrWayneJonas.com.
- **HEALTH COACHING:** If appropriate, I connect the patient with a health coach to help them navigate behavioral change, or further testing.
- **HEALTH PROMOTION GROUPS:** Clinics offer health and well-being groups for general health as well as for specialized populations who need support with managing pain, diabetes, weight loss, cardiovascular problems, and cancer.
- **HEALTH ANALYTICS:** If needed, there are options for science-based testing and artificial intelligence systems to explore specific factors that can increase the probability of health improvements.
- Graphics of the healing dimensions (see page 262) are sometimes provided to help patients visually navigate their many options for healing.

Constructing Your Healing Journey

The following guidelines may seem like simple, even obvious, steps, but they are powerful. Together, they hold the key to 80% of health and healing. As you go through these items, find ones you already enjoy, and then use the ideas and resources in this book to enhance their power. If you find you can incorporate the primary components from each of these dimensions of healing, you will markedly increase the probability of staying well if you are well, or recover if you are under treatment. Working with you doctor or primary care practitioner and a health coach can enhance the effect of these activities.

Many people have told me that they can implement these practices on their own, without professional assistance. The ability to heal is inside you. Making small changes in your day creates large changes over your life. Your hopes, relationships, activities, and places you live and work can spark these healing abilities. As you absorb the ideas described in this book and the summary suggestions in this appendix, note your thoughts, intentions, and expectations. Find the ones that inspire you to live a healthy, vibrant, joyful life with purpose and meaning.

GETTING STARTED

Change is best made in small, thoughtful ways. Start with just one area. As you start to make changes, you'll find that the positive effects will spill into other dimensions of your life.

The following four sets of statements will help you decide where you might want to start. I list the statements in pairs—one pair for each of the four dimensions of healing. Remember that while I have organized these into the four dimensions of HOPE, in reality they are interacting and overlapping dimensions, which is why it doesn't really matter where you start.

First, read the following two statements:

I feel calm and relaxed in my surroundings.

I have a space at work or home for reflection.

If you disagree with these statements, you may want to concentrate on your *physical environment.*

Now consider these two statements:

I avoid behaviors that I know are unhealthy.

I make time for things that bring me joy.

If you disagree with these statements, you may want to focus on the *behavioral dimension.*

Now consider these two statements:

My relationships with others leave me energized.

I feel supported and connected to my family and community.

If you disagree with these statements, you may want to focus on your *social/emotional needs.*

Finally, consider these two statements:

I am fully aware of my body's subtle signs and how they connect to my health.

When I think of my life, I feel hopeful and positive. I like my life.

If you disagree with these statements, you may want to focus on your *mind/spirit connection*.

It does not matter where you begin. Perhaps you want to start with the one you need the most. Or maybe you want to ease in and pick the one that is easiest for you.

Wherever you choose to start, a technique that may help is journaling. This practice can help you heal, grow, become more yourself, and thrive in the following ways:

- Journaling helps bring order to your deepest thoughts and fears.
- Journaling acts as free therapy. It helps you understand the person who knows you best: you.
- You can go back and read what you've written to see how much progress you've made.
- Some find joy in knowing their words help others, so they share their journals. But whether you share your work is up to you.
- Keeping a gratitude journal relieves stress. Exploring what you are thankful for is a powerful reminder of the good in your life.

There are many ways to journal. Grab a notebook, or just pencil your thoughts in the margins of this book. As you turn the pages, know that this is your personal journey to healing. Take it at your own pace. What matters most is that you start!

YOUR PHYSICAL ENVIRONMENT: SURROUNDING YOURSELF WITH BEAUTY AND SIMPLICITY

The places you live, work, play, and receive care affect your ability to find peace, rest, strength, and healing.

Have you ever been somewhere that just makes you feel good and at peace? These healing spaces minimize stress and add joy. They can bring your family and friends together and allow you to be at your best.

Your Home

Of all the places in your life, you probably have the most control over your home. Use this space to support your healing journey. When your home does not bring you joy and peace, you may feel uneasy, disjointed, out of control, unsafe, stressed, and disconnected from yourself and nature.

When you walk in the door after a stressful day at work or school or an appointment, a welcoming home can help return you to a place of peace. Your home's colors, tidiness or clutter, scents, and decor all affect you—continually.

Here are some tips to make your home a place of healing and peace:

- Surround yourself with nature, incorporating natural light, nature views or art, nature sounds, and flowers.
- Decorate with meaning, including photographs of family and friends, meaningful objects, symbols of faith or personal healing, and furniture arranged to encourage interaction.
- Simplify your life by uncluttering and creating quiet spaces for reflection.

Each change in your home is an opportunity to rethink what's in your life. Items that once brought you joy may now make you yearn for the past or evoke feelings of anxiety or anger. Recognize those items and consider replacing them with objects that make you feel good.

A Restful Bedroom

Keeping your bedroom simple, clutter-free, and clean, and ensuring it's dark at night are great ways to help improve your sleep. If streetlights or natural light make your room too bright, purchase inexpensive blackout shades or curtains. Use a clock with a red or blue light, not white or yellow; even better, use a clock that lights up only when you press a button. Surround yourself with comfortable bedding that feels good against your skin. (For more on sleep, see "Recharge at Night," page 280.)

- **COLOR MATTERS.** Choose colors to suit your mood. Warm reds, oranges, and yellows energize and stimulate, while cool blue, green, and violet evoke feelings of peace and restfulness.
- **EXPERIMENT WITH SCENTS.** The sense of smell has a powerful connection to the brain. What you smell can stimulate feelings of well-being, improve your mood, relieve stress, and clear your mind. What makes you breathe more deeply when you enter a room?

Talk to your care provider about using aromatherapy. Note: If someone in your home is pregnant or has asthma or a chronic lung disease, your doctor may want you to avoid certain essential oils.

- **MUFFLE SOUNDS.** Most people now live in loud urban environments. Sounds can be stressful (noise pollution) or soothing. Experiment with playing music to set a mood or to block out noises like street traffic. Carpets, curtains, and soft fabrics absorb sound; hard surfaces amplify them. White noise and simple soft earplugs also help to reduce the decibels.
- **LIGHT YOUR DAY AND NIGHT.** Warm, natural light is soothing, while fluorescent or overhead lighting can be harsh. To create a feeling of warmth and intimacy, try lower, warmer lights. Put ceiling fixtures on a dimmer, especially over a dining table. Wall sconces and side lamps can help. Indirect light is more soothing than direct. Windows and skylights bring in natural light.

On the Road

If you feel like you live in your car or in hotels, make those spaces positive places. Small changes, like keeping the inside of your car trash-free, might make a traffic jam less stressful. Music can sooth and carry you with the traffic rather than against it. Here are a few more ideas for making car rides more pleasant:

- Consider adding an air freshener or car diffuser. Scents of lavender or vanilla relax; orange or eucalyptus scents energize.
- Turn car time into a time of learning or rejuvenation. Books on tape! Podcasts! But don't email or text while driving!
- Take a few minutes to repeat a positive or motivating thought to focus attention and interrupt the stress response.

At the Hospital or Other Care Facility

It's important to make the most of your interactions with the medical care space. This includes taking steps to reduce your anxiety during appointments. When you need to be hospitalized, ask for a single room and a room with a natural view; this has been shown to speed recovery.

Connect with Nature

The restorative quality of nature has been well documented. Take time out to watch a sunset or find a green space to eat lunch in during your day. Working in a community garden or simply enjoying it can help you connect to the earth. If gardening is not an option for you, try walking in a local park or green space. Walk on earth with your bare feet if you are in a safe and sanitary place to do so.

Whether you live in the city, the country, or somewhere in between, be aware of the life around you. You can do this through enjoying artwork that depicts scenes of nature, getting to know local flora and fauna, viewing of green and sky through a window or an online video of waves crashing along the shore.

Track how changes in nature affect your mood, your body, and your energy level. If you find yourself becoming depressed or sad during rainy weekends, try to see the beauty in the raindrops, or reserve an activity you love for rainy days. Or if it's not too cold, go outside and enjoy the feel of the rain.

Set an Environment Self-Care Goal

Wherever you spend your time, make sure that the spaces around you don't add unnecessary stress to your days and nights. Focus on the spaces in which you spend the most time first and then move on to improve the others.

What is one improvement that you can make at home, work, or school today?

HEALTHY BEHAVIOR

Living a healthy life is one of the key things you can do to stay or become well. How you eat, move, relax, and connect to others—all of these play major roles in healing your body, mind, and spirit. The choices you make today matter. And today's choices determine the choices available to you tomorrow.

How to Change

The problem lies not in knowing what you should be doing, but rather in making these changes habitual and meaningful to you. Link the behavior to the meaning and joy in your life. This will prepare you emotionally and mentally to sustain the behavior in the long run.

Before you consider which behaviors are right for you to change now, read the following list on how change happens. These are ten effective ways to make any healthy behavior change stick:

1. **DEVELOP A PLAN.** Pick one or two small changes that feel manageable and that give you pleasure: two yoga postures, switching from white to whole grain bread, starting tango lessons, going on a picnic, or joining a book club or a volunteer group.
2. **PICK SOMETHING YOU CAN DO.** Choose a small, realistic, attainable change. Do that first. Don't pick something you just think you should do. If needed, break it into small parts and do part of it first.
3. **TELL SOMEBODY.** Have them ask you about it monthly.
4. **FIND A GROUP.** Look for or create social situations that encourage healing behaviors: a walking club, a healthy cooking class, a family or friend to monitor you.
5. **PLAN FOR A SLIP.** Times when you are not doing the

behavior or even intentional slips are important for long-term change. Build in occasional times when you do not do the new behavior.

6. **KNOW THE REAL REASON FOR MAKING THE CHANGE.** The most effective reasons for sustained behavior change are intrinsic (I want to feel better) rather than extrinsic (I want to be liked).

7. **IT MAY BE HARD.** Prepare to be uncomfortable for a while. Change is not easy. Your plan should include how to deal with that.

8. **BE READY.** Sometimes the time is not right to make a change. Maybe today is not the day to start. If so, admit that and take more time to prepare.

9. **START.** Are you a chronic procrastinator (about 20% of people are) or just procrastinating on this one behavior? If chronic, seek help to deal with that first.

10. **ASK YOUR DOCTOR.** Discuss lifestyle and prevention behaviors with your medical team and ask about any helpful resources your health care services offer—such as behaviorists, health coaches, nutritionists, fitness trainers, or rehabilitation specialists.

EATING, DRINKING, AND COOKING

The rituals of cooking and sharing meals and the effects of eating wholesome food in healthful quantities are profoundly important to prevention, recovery, wellness, and well-being.

Why We Eat

Food is loaded with meaning and emotion. Food is family, tradition, and comfort; sometimes we even use food to self-medicate. When we use food and/or alcohol to fill an emotional void or to quiet or dull negative emotions, this may lead to overeating or unhealthy choices. Some of us overeat or consume alcohol out of stress, anger, depression, anxiety, frustration, or loneliness. Know why you eat, and make eating to fill physical hunger or to enjoy taste—not to dispel sadness or treat pain.

Build a Positive Relationship with Food

As with other relationships in your life, it's important that your relationship with food be a healthy one. This involves some key shifts in thoughts and behaviors:

- Accept that the food rules or family traditions of your past may no longer be needed or helpful for you. For example, give yourself the okay to no longer need to finish everything on your plate.
- Understand that you are a unique person with your own needs and challenges. Learn to trust your hunger and listen to your sense of fullness.
- What you see in magazines, over the internet, and on TV is not always true. If you struggle with a healthy body image, it may help to limit your exposure to unhealthy body images in the media.
- Mind-set matters when it comes to food. Remember the mind over milkshake experiment. Be positive, even in how you talk about food. Thinking of your food as either a diet or bad adds judgment. Changing your language can help. Instead of seeing sweets as bad, see them as a treat.

Eat Mindfully

Too often we eat food without even a thought. It's easy to eat what's in front of you without paying attention to whether you are hungry or when you become full.

Keep these tips in mind:

- Eat slowly. Most meals are consumed in an average of seven to eleven minutes. Fast eating can lead to overeating. The body doesn't have time to cue your brain that you are full. If you struggle with eating speed, try to focus more on enjoying the meal rather than just slowing down.

- Eating includes all the senses—taste, touch, smell, sound, and sight. Paying attention to the multisensory experience of eating is called "eating mindfully." Eating mindfully requires learning your sense of fullness. Be alert to your body's subtle clues rather than waiting for a bellyache. If something is so delicious that you want to keep eating, try saying, "I can have more later if I'm full. I don't have to eat it now."

- Use a smaller plate. Most people will eat everything on the plate in front of them. Research shows that people automatically cut down on how much they eat if they simply use a smaller plate.

Remember that Food is Your Fuel

Instead of depriving yourself, focus on adding good whole foods. And because vegetables and fruits contain mostly water, eating more of them will increase your hydration levels.

Consider the following when focusing on food:

- Keep a food journal, either on your phone or on paper, to track what you eat throughout the day. We are often not aware of what and how much we eat. Some mobile apps help with this and offer motivation to choose a healthier diet.

- Foods with sugar, high-fructose corn syrup, artificial sweeteners, and unhealthy fats have been linked to heart disease, cancer, and diabetes. High-fiber diets can lessen some of these effects.

- Eating too much and not exercising are the usual causes of obesity, but they are not the only ones. Especially in times of stress, the problem may be not eating enough or not eating the right foods. Some people react to certain foods, like gluten or milk protein. Ask your integrative physician how to determine if there are certain foods you should avoid.

- Your health care provider or a dietitian may be able to help you design a healthy eating plan and set realistic weight goals to keep you healthy.

Drink Water, Always

Water affects weight loss, muscle fatigue, skin health (including fewer wrinkles), kidney and bowel function, and more. Carrying a (refillable) bottle of water with you everywhere you go may help you remember to drink more often. Also, try to drink a glass of water instead of another type of beverage with every snack and meal. Flavored sweet drinks contribute little to better health. Fruit juice should be diluted by at least half.

Recognize Your Patterns and Hurdles

Are you so hungry that you grab a snack on your way home before mealtime? Eat a piece of fruit, a bag of healthy (unbuttered) popcorn, or a handful of (roasted, unsalted) nuts on the way home so you aren't ravenous when you walk in the door.

Are you too tired to make the healthy meal you'd planned, so you find yourself ordering pizza? Try having more easy meals like sandwiches or soup. Make a week's worth of healthy meals and freeze them in small packets to pull out and defrost.

Meal Planning and Mealtimes

Meal planning can be good for your budget, your stress level, and your waistline. Have ingredients on hand for easy pantry or freezer meals if you don't have time to buy fresh ingredients. Know where you can stop for a healthier takeout option if an appointment or workday runs long. Try these meal-planning tips:

- Aim to shop only once a week. Fewer trips to the grocery store and drive-through can save time. Running into the store to pick up an item can lead to overbuying and more stress.
- Eat before you shop for food. If you go to the grocery store hungry, you are likely to buy more than you would if you were full.
- Keep healthy food on hand. It is easier to eat healthy when your pantry, fridge, freezer, and cabinets are well stocked with healthy food. Get rid of what you don't want around.

- Involve your children so they will be more likely to eat healthy and help with meal prep. If they can see the meal plan, it will cut down on the questions of "What's for dinner?" or "What can I eat?"
- Don't start the plan with all new foods. Begin with a two-week rotation of your favorite recipes. Occasionally add a new recipe.
- Make sure your plan is realistic. If you're accustomed to relying on takeout meals, plan for the occasional takeout.
- Meals planned, prepared, and shared together at home tend to be healthier and more balanced than meals eaten at restaurants or on the go. Meals eaten out are often fried or highly salted. Plus, soda and other sweetened beverages are consumed more often when eating out.
- Meals bring families together. When you can, making time for a family dinner is good for the mind, body, and spirit. Family meals help foster family bonds, feelings of belonging, security, and love. This is especially important during times of change. Eating together builds a sense of tradition that can last a lifetime. A study showed that health promoting genes are turned on before people even eat if they prepare the food together.

Move More

Motion is a lotion. Exercise can help both your body and your mind work more smoothly.

It's important to get least thirty minutes of exercise a day. Ask your doctor to suggest ways to move more. Learn how much exercise is right for you, especially if you are trying to lose weight or have certain physical conditions like heart disease or asthma. Research now shows that it is more important to simply move more often during the day than to do thirty straight minutes of exercise and then sit for the rest of the day.

Look at movement as something to include throughout your day. Your doctor or a physical therapist may give you a list of exercises and stretches you can do whenever you have a few minutes. Can you do leg lifts or ankle circles while waiting or at your desk? I got rid of my sitting desk at the office and now have only a standing and treadmill desk. I do walking meetings whenever possible. Might you park farther from the store to get a few more steps in? Use the stairs instead of the elevator. These activities add up.

Walking provides many of the same health benefits as running and can be done more often with loved ones.

Recharge at Night

Sleep impacts many areas of life—your overall health, pain level, memory, weight control, and even your mood and outlook. Sleep problems can be caused by a host of issues, including light or noise intruding on your bedroom; a mind run amok; breathing problems; medications; pain; depression; stress; substances such as alcohol, caffeine, and nicotine; heart and lung diseases; and even simple inactivity. That's why it's important to talk to your care provider about any issues you are experiencing. Your provider may also help you optimize the hours of sleep that you do get.

Consider these common tips for better sleep:

- Establish a winding-down routine with quiet, soothing activities in the hour before bedtime.
- Go to bed and wake up at the same time each day—even on weekends.
- Maintain a dark, electronics-free bedroom.
- Avoid caffeine, nicotine, alcohol, and sugar for several hours before bed.
- Exercise during the morning or early afternoon.

When these tips aren't enough, it may be time to reach out for professional help.

Make Time for Joy

Even in the most difficult situations, choosing to feel grateful can help you cope. Focusing on gratitude prevents helplessness and hopelessness from taking over.

Instead of worrying about what you can't control, use your mental energy to find moments of joy in ways you can, like these:

- Dream new dreams. You may have had to put past dreams aside, but that doesn't mean you can't come up with new ones. Focus on new goals and dreams that you can work toward.
- Tap into a creative outlet to release emotions and experience the joy of art. Try music, crafting, sewing, drawing, journaling, scrapbooking, birding, or photography.
- Look forward to the future. Maintaining a sense of hopefulness is critical. Finding meaning and purpose in life can lead to happiness. Have something to look forward to. Plan.
- Keep inspiration on hand to help you get through the rough patches. Phone a friend, visit a place of worship, or carry uplifting quotes or readings in your wallet or purse. Inspirational music is literally at everyone's fingertips now with their phone.
- Say yes to things that make you happy. Stay connected with people who recharge your battery and make you feel good.
- Laugh and play. Try a game night at home, play fetch with your pet, do a crossword puzzle, or listen to a comedian on TV. Laughter, humor, and play can reduce stress, boost your energy, and help you connect with others.
- Don't compare your life to others'. Allow your life to be uniquely yours.

Decrease Anxiety

You may not be able to control the stressors in your life, but you can learn skills that will prevent the stressors from controlling you. Be aware of your breathing. Shallow, upper chest breathing is a sign of stress. Taking thirty seconds to do a deep breathing exercise will trigger your body's natural relaxation response. Remember, people who saw stress as strengthening them improved much more than those who saw the same stress as hurting them. Stress, when well handled, can help in healing. Mind-set matters.

Nourish Your Spiritual Self

Focus on love and forgiveness—and start with yourself. If you don't love and forgive yourself, it's hard to inspire, motivate, and encourage others.

Meditation techniques, such as loving-kindness meditation, can help address anger and emotional pain. This practice is used to address feelings such as shame, guilt, fear, chronic pain, a lack of support, and difficulties with other people.

Breathe

Breathing techniques and mobile apps can teach you to use your breath to self-calm. The breath triggers changes in the body's nervous system that help you better manage stress. Deep breathing techniques help reduce feelings of anxiety and stress by blunting the expression of genes turned on during stress and lowers blood pressure.

Put one hand on your chest and another on your stomach. As you inhale and exhale, your abdomen should rise and fall. This is called "belly breathing." If your belly is not involved, your breathing may be too shallow. You can benefit greatly from learning and practicing belly breathing.

Deal with Unhealthy Behaviors

Let's face it, we all do things that we know are not healthy. In fact, allowing ourselves occasional unhealthy behaviors—when we build them into life intentionally—can help us maintain healthy behaviors most of the other times. They are that spot of yang in the yin and vice versa. But it is important that these behaviors don't become your main habits. Once they do, they are hard to break and sometimes require professional help.

Social groups can help—your community center, church, and online support groups. The important thing is to develop awareness of your behaviors and seek help. If you are a very private person, hesitant to share personal issues, that first step you take to seek help is the most difficult. Having someone you trust join with you will make it easier. A group of two is still a community.

Use your healthy relationships to find support to manage unhealthy behaviors before they become a habit. Break bad habits so they do not become addictions. Or turn them into positive addictions. Find healthy habits to fill the void left when ending the bad habits.

Dealing with medical care systems is also a learned behavior. Here are some principles to allow you to keep those encounters focused on healing.

Focus on Prevention

Without proper care, a cough can become pneumonia, a strain can become a fracture, and a muscle pull can become a tear. Early detection of many cancers and heart disease can prevent progression, complications, and death. Maintaining your health care is important to prevent chronic problems and keep you at the top of your game in body, mind, and spirit.

Access Integrative Health Care

Integrative medicine includes the best of conventional medicine, such as procedures and medications, and the best of nonconventional medicine, such as mind-body practices, acupuncture, massage, chiropractic care, energy medicine (like Reiki or healing touch), and supplements.

Integrative health balances this medical and illness treatment with self-care and health creation—fully integrating preventative care and lifestyle with the treatment of disease, illness, and injury. While there are many models for delivering integrative health care, here are a few key clues you can look for in a primary care practice to determine if you are receiving integrative health care:

1. **TEAM-BASED:** Integrative health care is best delivered by a team of providers, which can include your physician, physician's assistants, and nurses, as well as other health care professionals with expertise in behavioral change, such as counseling, health coaching, nutrition, massage, acupuncture, or energy medicine.
2. **TRANSPARENT:** The team makes available all your health records and test results so that you can track your progress and be an informed part of the decision making about your health and well-being.

3. **AWARE:** The team is knowledgeable about you and aware of your health, well-being, and life goals so that they can best support you in your healing journey.
4. **ACCESSIBLE:** Members of the team are available by phone, text, or email when you have a question or need clarification, so you can stay on track toward your health goals.

Make the Most of an Appointment

Depending on where you are on your healing journey, you may spend considerable time in the hospital or doctor's office. Making the most of health care appointments can help improve care and lessen stress. Consider the following:

- **PREPARE FOR THE VISIT:** Recognize that it's okay to talk about embarrassing or upsetting symptoms. Write down what needs to be covered during the appointment to ensure you don't forget something important. Bring a list of medications and their use to the appointment.
- **DURING THE VISIT:** Advocate for yourself when needed. Clearly express what you need from the doctor. It can be helpful to use a tape recorder for important consults to prevent confusion. Many smartphones have a record function. Taking notes can also help you remember what was said. If you end up confused, ask for a follow-up consult.
- **AFTER THE VISIT:** Check in with a loved one. How do you think the appointment went? What do you wish had gone differently? Are you missing any important information?
- **SEE CHAPTER 10:** Creating Healing (pages 252–259) for an in-depth review of how to work with your doctor and the health care system.

FOCUS ON THE SOCIAL-EMOTIONAL DIMENSION

People are social beings. Relationships provide a sense of belonging, care, and support. Positive relationships can also be good for your health. Love and support reduce stress, boost your immune system, improve quality of life, and prevent feeling lonely or depressed. And they prolong life.

Positive relationships refuel you, especially when your tank is low. These are healing relationships; they are characterized by trust, honesty, compassion, and safety.

By using this checklist, you can decide which relationships are healing and which can be improved. For each relationship, ask yourself if the following statements are true:

- **TRUST:** I feel emotionally and physically safe. I don't have to guard against being hurt.
- **HONESTY:** Both the other person and I can reveal true feelings without harm to either of us.
- **COMPASSION:** Both the other person and I have the ability and willingness to understand one another and express kindness.
- **SAFETY:** Both the other person and I feel safe with each other—physically and emotionally.

If a relationship leaves you running on fumes, consider options to protect yourself and change the relationship. It is possible to learn skills that improve the relationship's quality and boost its ability to heal. If not, get out of the relationship.

Communicating Is Key

Honest and open communication is key to the healing relationships you are working to build. It can be important to voice feelings or fears that seem unthinkable. When they go unspoken, they can lead to angry outbursts, withdrawal, resentment, and guilt trips that drive a wedge into the relationship.

Most communication has little to do with what you say. Your

stance, posture, breathing, and even your muscle tightness all relay a message—as do the tone, speed, and volume of your voice.

Here are some tips for speaking your mind mindfully:

- Relax and breathe.
- Go into difficult conversations with a goal. Example goals include the following: Be honest and direct; express feelings and thoughts; find common ground; create harmony.
- Ask if it's a good time to talk, so you begin the conversation on the right foot.
- Treat the individual with dignity, respect, and courtesy.

Focus on active listening. When you listen, focus on both verbal and nonverbal messages. Here are some tips for active listening:

- Maintain appropriate eye contact for your culture.
- Paraphrase and repeat to confirm that you understand what the other person is saying. Don't jump to conclusions.
- Ask questions to clarify.
- Try not to think about what you are going to say next; it's more important to be attentive, even if it means there is a pause before you talk. Pause and take a breath before you talk.
- Affirm the other person's comments and offer encouragement by nodding, saying yes, or using phrases such as "Tell me more" or "I understand."
- Listen for disclaimers and qualifiers (maybe, but, mostly, usually, probably), as they are typically followed by new information.
- Avoid distractions, such as TV, pets, or other people, so you don't have to compete for attention.
- The more you can encourage the other person to talk, especially in high-stress situations, the more you can understand what they are trying to share with you.

Focus on "I" communication. "I" messages (rather than "you" messages) are the foundation of positive communication. "You" messages may make the other person feel uncomfortable and attacked. They may make the person stop listening, withdraw, or fight back—none of which resolve the question or concern. "I" messages achieve the following:

- Help you take ownership of your own thoughts and feelings.
- Make you explore what you think and feel.
- Increase your chances of being heard.
- Help keep conversations positive.

For example:
"I feel overwhelmed and need help with the chores." (I message) versus "You never help around the house."

Set Goals for Success

Each family or individual defines success differently. Paying attention to goals and celebrating achievements may be helpful on your journey. It is powerful to say, "We hit the goal we were reaching for!" Goals may be small or incremental, but they lead to feelings of pride and motivation for the next step. The recovery process is a careful balance of accepting reality and working toward change.

Some symptoms, conditions, and circumstances lessen with time and treatment. But for others, learning to cope with what is there is a more helpful approach. When recovery isn't possible, shift your focus to discovery. You and your partner may discover steps, self-care strategies, and behaviors that reduce daily challenges and improve quality of life.

Your medical team—especially the behaviorist—may provide advice about what is practical to make sure your expectations are realistic.

Go Ahead and Vent

Venting your emotions is appropriate at times to release tension rather than bottling it up inside. However, there are some ways and places to vent that are more helpful than others. See if any of these work for you:

- **WRITE.** Get out a piece of paper and write for ten minutes without stopping. You can even pretend that you are talking with another person or another part of yourself. See what that person has to say, in your own words.
- **TALK.** When venting to a person, be sure to do so with someone you trust and with whom you are on good terms. Choose someone who is supportive and helpful rather than enabling negative emotions. Tell the person that you just need to vent first, and ask if it is okay.
- **EXERCISE.** Physical activity can release chemicals in the brain that relieve stress and tension. Consider yoga, qigong, and tai chi as well as other personal self-care practices.
- **BREATHE.** Since it's impossible to be stressed and relaxed at the same time, use breathing techniques to calm down.

Set Boundaries

Part of maintaining healthy relationships involves setting boundaries—an important part of self-care. A boundary controls how much access others have to your heart, time, and energies. It is a protective fence you build around yourself that allows you to monitor the impact others have on you.

Leaving yourself too open can leave you bruised and battered by the comments, moods, and opinions of others. But staying too closed can leave you isolated and locked inside yourself. Finding the right balance takes time. Set boundaries in your own time frame, and only when you are ready. Counselors can help you with protecting your heart, freeing yourself from the need to please others, and saying no when appropriate.

Learning to establish healthy boundaries can help you in all your relationships, whether with your family, friends, neighbors, or coworkers.

Create Healing Groups and Get Involved

You are part of many groups that influence your life: school, workplace, church, community organizations. Being involved in healthy groups with healing qualities supports your health and well-being. These types of healing groups allow you to participate in making decisions that affect you. They promote open and honest communication, create a climate of trust and personal responsibility, and inspire a sense of belonging. They are fun!

Are you actively involved in an organization? Getting involved is critical if you want the organization to develop a healing culture. Opportunities such as PTA, clubs, committees, and volunteer activities are ways to inspire change. As a part of these groups, set a good example for others. Build healing relationships with your coworkers. This can provide you with opportunities to practice your own self-care and to share with others ways to support greater personal well-being—in family, school, and work environments and in other social situations.

Foster a Culture of Healing

Groups that foster a culture of healing have the following in common:

- Respect for individuals, including their inner lives
- A system of values that is present at all levels
- Honest and open communication
- A climate of trust
- A focus on learning rather than blame
- Opportunities for self-care, like exercise and yoga

Do the groups that you belong to help you to heal or impede you?

Lead or Follow

Ask yourself: Am I a good leader? Am I a good follower? Good leaders and good followers walk their talk. They work on improving their communication skills, they treat others as they would like to be treated, and they are good team players. Examine your role in the groups that you are a part of and explore shifting them toward a healing culture. The best way to do this is to lead by example.

Set a Social/Emotional Dimension Self-Care Goal

Part of any relationship includes dealing with the moods and feelings of others. Self-care is important because it can be easier to deal with the emotions of others when you are taking good care of yourself. Once you are in a strong and healthy place, you will be better able to cocreate a healthy relationship.

What is one thing you can do to improve a relationship in your life today?

YOUR MIND-SPIRIT CONNECTIONS

Who you are at the deepest level includes the thoughts, feelings, and wishes that come from your mind. It also includes your spiritual life and having a sense of meaning or purpose.

The healing that arises from an experience of personal wholeness happens only when the mind, body, and spirit are in balance. A weakness or imbalance in one of these can negatively affect the others. For example, severe emotional stress can cause high blood pressure and other illnesses in an otherwise healthy body. Likewise, a physical illness or injury can cause depression in a usually healthy mind.

Two elements are key to your healing journey:

- Developing an intention and expectation for healing
- Feeling the wholeness that comes from mind, body, and spirit practices

Develop Healing Intention

Healing intention is a conscious choice to improve your health or the health of another. It includes belief in improved well-being and the hope that a goal can be reached. Belief and hope set the stage for healing to occur. As we saw from the research on placebo, belief itself is a powerful healer.

If you don't truly believe that you can be healed, or if some part of you is holding onto the disease or condition, you might disrupt or limit your own healing on a subconscious level. Don't underestimate yourself! By developing healing intention, you set the stage for healing to occur.

Developing healing intention includes awareness, intention, and reflection.

Build Your Self-Awareness

Awareness addresses the question: "How do I feel?" It helps you learn what your body is telling you and to connect to what you think about to who you are.

You can become aware of your body's subtle signals, such as changes in energy level or mood. Bring these feelings to your conscious mind. This allows you to change behaviors that don't contribute to your health and learn new skills to change your automatic responses. Physical symptoms are often messages from your body telling you how it is doing and what it needs.

Some turn to active practices like walking, yoga, or repeating a centering word. Others use religious prayer, rituals, and services. You can also just take a few moments to be quiet or to meditate.

This awareness of how the mind, body, and spirit work together gives you the information you need to guide you on a healing path.

Once you know how you feel, it's essential to know what you want. For those whose lives have diverged from what they had planned, this can be a challenge. But it's key to rebuild this knowledge so you can create new goals and plans that may be different, but are also meaningful and fulfilling.

On a spiritual level, once you connect with your inner self, you can direct your intention to bring this sense of peace and healing in your life.

Take Time to Reflect

The story you tell yourself about your life is powerful. It creates a mind-set that impacts your physical response to any stimulus or situation. This self-story can be a way to help you grasp the themes of your life and find meaning in them. When your sense of meaning in life is altered, it can lead to feelings of distress. Regaining that sense of purpose—even in suffering, or despite suffering—is vital for health and well-being.

Meaning and purpose help you deal with loss and grief, create hope and dispel despair, and find joy and stop sadness. They allow you to accept a new normal, find a sense of well-being within it, and control your outlook.

Journaling, creative writing, art therapy, and peer mentoring may be helpful as you reflect on questions of who you are and what role your illness has played in your life. Also important to your self-story are the questions: What is my purpose? How do I fit into my family, my community, my life? What are my values or spiritual beliefs?

For many, spirituality, faith, and religion are central parts of who they are. They can influence how you cope with trauma, fear, or loss. They may help you find happiness and meaning within rather than from external influences such as wealth, belongings, work, fame, or fancy food, which may leave you feeling empty, lost, and alone.

Experience Personal Wholeness

Personal wholeness is the feeling of well-being that occurs when your body, mind, and spirit are aligned and moving in harmony and balance.

Think about a time when you felt most authentic, most whole, most complete and happy. Perhaps you were doing something that you felt was important and meaningful. It could include reaching a major milestone or completing a difficult task. It could also be something from daily life, like cooking a tasty meal or teaching a child to ride a bike. When the experience of complete wholeness arises, a healing presence or unity occurs.

Activities that connect your physical body with your nonphysical mind and spirit help to integrate your biological responses with your psychological responses. From these practices, you can experience a sense of wholeness that enhances recovery and resilience.

Add a Mind-Body Practice to Your Toolbox

The same mind-body practices that help you develop a sense of self can counteract stress and its harmful effects. The most important thing to know about mind-body practices is that there is no single right way. These practices go through cycles of popularity. However, all have the same intended effect of breaking the train of everyday thoughts and inducing deep relaxation. What doesn't work for someone else may work for you.

Consider these factors when picking a mind-body practice:

- **PHYSICAL ENERGY:** Do you enjoy being physically active? If yes, consider a moving meditation like tai chi, qigong, yoga, walking, and running, or an active meditation like art therapy or journaling. If no, consider breathing techniques, meditation, or mindfulness-based stress reduction, loving-kindness meditation, or progressive muscle relaxation.
- **SELF-BASED OR PRACTITIONER-BASED:** Practices such as acupuncture, chiropractic or osteopathic manipulation, massage, and other bodywork require making time to see an outside practitioner. For some, that time out can be relaxing, while others may find it stressful. Some practices require nothing more than your attention and a few seconds (breathing, mantra repetition). And there are various others that, once learned, can be practiced on your own, such as acupressure, Reiki, yoga, or tai chi.
- **TIME:** Consider what fits into your schedule. Do you have thirty seconds? Five minutes? An hour? There is a mind-body practice for every time frame.
- **BELIEF AND CONVICTION:** Choose a practice and terminology that fits into your belief system. Whether it's making time for prayer, meditation, or quiet reflection, you are practicing self-care. It is not important to be convinced that the practice will work for you. However, it is important to stay open and to do it. Approach it in a spirit of experimentation. Check it out.

Schedule this time regularly. Just knowing that you have time set aside just for you can be helpful.

Think Positive

Positive thinking is a mind-set that turns anxiety into opportunity. It builds healthy self-esteem and self-value. Remember the experiments of Stanford Professor Crum showing that how one framed stress—either as resilience building or draining—produced the dominant effect that stress had on a person. These skills can keep you from doubting yourself during the ups and downs of life:

- Start each day with the intent to learn something new.
- Give yourself permission to be wrong.
- Start with "thanks" or a gratitude practice.

Self-talk is the stream of thoughts running through your head from the moment you wake up until you fall asleep. If your thoughts are mostly negative, it's more difficult to cope with stressful situations.

Instead of expecting the worst outcome of any situation, focus on the best. When you deal with life's difficulties in a positive and productive way, you'll reap health benefits including a longer life span, greater resistance to illness, and better mental and physical well-being.

Live in the Moment

Notice how much of your day you spend thinking about the past or the future. Thoughts of the past can keep you from being present and making the most of this day—distracting you from the present joy.

Many people think of mindfulness as being in a calm, Zen state. And it can be. But more realistically, it's about being present to your best self. Mindfulness means being aware of what your mind is up to in each moment but not getting caught up in or controlled by your thoughts. It can help to remind yourself: "My thoughts do not control me."

Trust Your Inner Guidance

How often do you ignore what your gut is telling you? You may think, "I should call a friend for support," but decide not to because it's late. Or you may think, "I wish I could reschedule those plans," but attend to them anyway and regret it later.

Over time, as you become mindful of your thoughts and feelings, you will begin to trust your inner guidance. You may notice that when you follow your instinct, you feel better. On the other hand, when you fall back into old patterns of holding back and doing what you think you should, you feel worse.

PAUSE AND TAKE A STEP BACK

Now that you've seen how the four dimensions of your life can affect your self-healing abilities, pause and take a step back. See where your journey began and where it has taken you.

You have seen that self-care means:

- Surrounding yourself with healing spaces (physical environment)
- Making healthy life choices (behavioral dimension)
- Maintaining strong social connections (social/emotional needs)
- Building a strong sense of identity (mind/spirit-connection)

I hope this book has inspired you to begin your healing journey. Perhaps you've already taken your first steps. When you've had time to make some progress, I invite you to return to consider these questions and observations, and reflect on how far you've come and what you've learned. If you have kept a journal, go back and read your first few entries. Have you learned anything about yourself or others along the way?

Note how a change in one area of your life impacts other areas. If you resolved conflicts with others, how did that make you feel about yourself? If you started taking walks, how did it affect your sleep or stress levels or pain?

You might have noticed that some of the changes you made affected those around you in a positive way. By looking deeply into your life and relationships with others, you can work toward peace and healing. That peace and healing will spread to those around you.

Amplify your healing by sharing your experiences with others along the path of life. As I learned from my first patient as a student chaplain before medical school—a 74-year-old man dying of lung cancer—the healer and healee share one goal and one mutually beneficial process. The healing process benefits both and all others with whom they are connected. And that, on the greater human scale, is how healing works.

Additional Reading on Integrative Health

The Cochrane Collaboration: cochrane.org
A respected international online resource for evidence about health care practices. They have an integrative medicine (CAM) section.

The National Institutes of Health (NIH) National Center for Complementary and Integrative Health: nccih.nih.gov
A good source for information on complementary and integrative practices.

Natural Medicines: naturalmedicines.therapeuticresearch.com
A good source of information on natural products—their effectiveness, safety, and quality.

Choosing Wisely: choosingwisely.org/
A good source of information on what you and your doctor should *not* be doing and what does not work.

Notes

Introduction

The concepts and data in this book have been drawn from hundreds of readings and references—mostly from the peer-reviewed medical literature. However, because of space limitations, I have selected key references for readers, choosing to include those that illustrate the main points made in each chapter, support some of the lesser-known facts, or provide readers with information and concepts that meaningfully supplement the text. For readers interested in more references on specific topics such as placebo, optimal healing environments, evidence-based medicine, whole systems science, complementary and integrative medicine, the HOPE note, or healing in general, please go to my website: DrWayneJonas.com.

Chapter 1: The Paradox of Healing

One of the most striking observations about healing practices is their tremendous diversity of models, beliefs, practices, and traditions around the world, from spiritual healing to herbal treatments, physical manipulation, surgery, and drugs. Theories of disease are equally diverse, ranging from spirits to consciousness to energy to chemicals. Despite this diversity, all claim to work, and observational studies often support those claims. For further reading about this, I suggest a classic in medical anthropology by Arthur Kleinman and a clear comparative review of different healing systems by Stanley Krippner. These can be found at:

Kleinman, Arthur. *Patients and Healers in the Context of Culture.* Berkeley: University of California Press, 1980.

Krippner, S. "Common Aspects of Traditional Healing Systems Across Cultures," in *Essentials of Complementary and Alternative Medicine.* Jonas, W. B. and J. S. Levin (eds.). Philadelphia: Lippincott Williams & Wilkins, 1999.

I was startled by Norma's response to the placebo. However, this is common in patients—and research studies. Some useful information sources mentioned in this chapter are the following:

Many treatments that have produced 60% to 80% improvement when delivered under normal practice conditions are found later to work no better than placebo when studied in randomized controlled studies. For a good summary, see Roberts, A. H., D. G. Kewman, L. Mercier, and M. Hovell (1993)."The power of nonspecific effects in healing: Implications for psychosocial and biological treatments." *Clinical Psychology Review* 13(5): 375–391.

At the time I was treating Bill, the best data showed that acupuncture was no more effective than placebo acupuncture. That was true until Andrew Vickers and colleagues from Sloan Kettering collected individual data from all the top studies in the world and pooled this data for analysis. This proved that the effects from acupuncture were not all due to placebo—something still not known by most physicians. See Vickers, A. J., A. M. Cronin, A. C. Maschino, et al. (2012). "Acupuncture for chronic pain: Individual patient data meta-analysis." *Archives of Internal Medicine* 172(19): 1444–1453; and, Vickers, A. J. and K. Linde (2014). "Acupuncture for chronic pain." *Journal of the American Medical Association* 311(9): 955–956.

It is hard for people to imagine that most of the effects from surgery might be due to factors other than the surgery, so studies are rarely done to test those other factors. In chronic pain, data shows that 87% of the effect of surgery is coming from factors other than the surgery itself. For summaries of surgery studies and why it heals see Beecher, H. K. (1961). "Surgery as placebo. A quantitative study of bias." *Journal of the American Medical Association* 176: 1102–1107; and, Johnson, A. G. (1994). "Surgery as a placebo." *The Lancet* 344(8930): 1140–1142; and, Jonas, W. B., C. Crawford, L. Colloca, T. J. Kaptchuk, B. Moseley, F. G. Miller, L. Kriston, K. Linde, and K. Meissner (2015). "To what extent are surgery and invasive procedures effective beyond a placebo response? A systematic review with meta-analysis of randomized, sham controlled trials." BMJ Open: e009655. doi:10.1136/bmjopen-2015-009655; Jonas, W. B., C. C. Crawford, K. Meissner, and L. Colloca. "The Wound that Heals: Placebo, Pain and Surgery," *Placebo and Pain*. L. Colloca, M. A. Flaten, and K. Meissner (eds.). Boston: Elsevier, 2013; 227–233.

People with brain injury like Sergeant Martin get better during hyperbaric oxygen treatments, but not from the oxygen. See Miller, R., L. K. Weaver, N. Bahraini, et al. (2015). "Effects of hyperbaric oxygen on symptoms and quality of life among service members with persistent post-concussion symptoms: A randomized clinical trial." *Journal of the American Medical Association Internal Medicine* 175(1): 43–52; and, Hoge, C. W. and W. B. Jonas, (2015). "The Ritual of Hyperbaric Oxygen and Lessons for the Treatment of Persistent Post-concussion Symptoms in Military Personnel." *Journal of the American Medical Association Internal Medicine* 175(1): 53–54; and, Crawford, C., L. Teo, E. M. Yang, C. Isbister, and K. Berry (2016). "Is Hyperbaric Oxygen Therapy Effective for Traumatic Brain Injury? A Rapid Evidence Assessment of the Literature and Recommendations for the Field." *Journal of Head Trauma Rehabilitation* (Open Access) doi:10.1097/HTR.0000000000000256.

Chapter 2: How We Heal

Over the last twenty to thirty years, researchers and practitioners have been repeatedly surprised at how large the improvement is in groups who are not getting an active treatment. Research on this effect—often called the "placebo effect" or "placebo response"—has grown tremendously. The best source of information on this sleeping giant in medicine is the database that is supported and maintained by the Society for Interdisciplinary Placebo Studies (SIPS). You can access this database (updated monthly) at: jips.online/.

A nice single summary of key research findings on the placebo response and its implications for healing can be found in the special journal issue: Meissner, K., N. Niko Kohls, and C. Luana (June 27, 2011). "Introduction to placebo effects in medicine: mechanisms and clinical implications." *Philosophical Transactions of the Royal Society of London Biological Sciences* 366(1572): 1783–1789.

Other selected references readers may find of interest mentioned in this chapter include (in the order they are described):

Jonas, W. B., C. P. Rapoza, and W. F. Blair (1996). "The effect of niacinamide on osteoarthritis: A pilot study." *Inflammation Research* 45(7): 330–334.

Franklin, B., Majault, L. Roy, Sallin, J. S. Bailly, D'Arcet, de Bory, J. I. Guillotin, and A. Lavoisier (2002). "Report of the commissioners charged by the king with the examination of animal magnetism." *International Journal of Clinical and Experimental Hypnosis* 50(4): 332–363. A summary of Franklin's investigation of Mesmerism—using blinded methods.

Beecher, H. K. (1955). "The powerful placebo." *Journal of the American Medical Association* 159(17): 1602–1606. Posited that placebo accounts for about one-third of all outcomes.

Moerman, D. E. (2000). "Cultural Variations in the Placebo Effect: Ulcers, Anxiety, and Blood Pressure." *Medical Anthropology Quarterly* 14(1): 51–72. Showed that placebo responses varied from 0% to 100% for the same treatment depending on the context, and not one-third, as Beecher claimed.

Kaptchuk, T. J., et. al. (2008). "Components of placebo effect: a randomized controlled trial in patients with irritable bowel syndrome." *The British Medical Journal* 336(7651): 999–1003. Elegant study showing how the ritual delivers much of the placebo response.

Kaptchuk, T. J., E. Friedlander, J. M. Kelley, M. N. Sanchez, E. Kokkotou, J. P. Singer, M. Kowalczykowski, F. G. Miller, I. Kirsch, and A. J. Lembo (2010). "Placebos without deception: a randomized controlled trial in irritable bowel syndrome." *PLoS One* 5(12): e15591. One of the first studies to show that telling people they were getting placebos did not significantly reduce their response.

Carvalho, C., J. M. Caetano, L. Cunha, P. Rebouta, T. J. Kaptchuk, and I. Kirsch (2016). "Open-label placebo treatment in chronic low back pain: a randomized controlled trial." *Pain* 157(12): 2766. Confirmation of the above and showing clinically significant improvement for a major public health problem (back pain) from the placebo response—even when patients knew they were taking placebo.

For information about how placebo works in the brain, see the following three articles: Benedetti, F., H. S. Mayberg, T. D. Wager, C. S. Stohler, and J. K. Zubieta (2005). "Neurobiological mechanisms of the placebo effect." *Journal of Neuroscience* 25(45): 10390–10402; and, Amanzio, M., et al. (2001). "Response variability to analgesics: a role for non-specific activation of endogenous opioids." *Pain* 90(3): 205–215; and, Wager, T. D. and L. Y. Atlas (2015). "The neuroscience of placebo effects: connecting context, learning and health." *National Review of Neuroscience* 16(7): 403–418. I also highly recommend the book by Professor Fabrizio Benedetti of the University of Turin, Italy, who is one of the world's most renowned researchers on placebo. See Benedetti, Fabrizio. *Placebo Effects*. London: Oxford University Press, 2014.

It is not the placebo (the fake pill or treatment) that produces healing; it is the meaning that the ritual of treatment produces. See Moerman, D. E. and W. B. Jonas (March 19, 2002). "Deconstructing the placebo effect and finding the meaning response." *Annals of Internal Medicine* 136(6): 471–476; and Jonas, W. B. (June 27, 2011). "Reframing placebo in research and practice." *Philosophical Transactions of the Royal Society of London Biological Sciences*. 366(1572): 1896–1904.

There are now good sources for evidence summaries comparing treatments. These sources include the Cochrane Collaboration database, which can be found at cochrane.org. While Cochrane is an important site for finding evidence summaries from randomized controlled studies, they rarely do comparative reviews across treatments. Some good sources for comparative evidence reviews across treatments like the ones I did for Bill are *BMJ Clinical Evidence Updates* at clinicalevidence.bmj. com/x/set/static/cms/citations-updates.html; and *The Agency for Healthcare Research and Quality EPC Evidence-Based Reports* at www.ahrq.gov/research/findings/evidence-based-reports/index.html. Make sure your doctor has consulted one or more of these sources before he or she prescribes a treatment.

Personal engagement with the deeper aspect of yourself (especially social and emotional traumas) is profoundly healing. See, for example: Pennebaker, J. W. *Opening Up: The Healing Power of Expressing Emotions*. New York: Guildford Press, 1997; and, Smyth, J. M., A. A. Stone, A. Hurewitz, and A. Kaell (1999). "Effects of writing about stressful experiences on symptom reduction in patients with asthma or rheumatoid arthritis: a randomized trial." *Journal of the American Medical Association* 281(14): 1304–1309.

Nondrug approaches to healing are gradually gaining evidence and mainstream emphasis, especially for pain. See, for example: Qaseem, A., T. J. Wilt, R. M. McLean, and M. A. Forciea (2017). "Noninvasive Treatments for Acute, Subacute, and Chronic Low Back Pain: A Clinical Practice Guideline from the American College of Physicians." *Annals of Internal Medicine* 166(7): 514–530; and, Jonas, W. B., E. Schoomaker, K. Berry, and C. Buckenmaier III (2016). "A Time for Massage." *Pain Medicine* 17(8): 1389–1390. doi:10.1093/pm/pnw086. Published online May 9, 2016; and, Crawford, C., C. Lee, C. Buckenmaier, E. Schoomaker, R. Petri, W. B. Jonas, and the Active Self-Care Therapies for Pain (PACT) Working Group (April 2014). "The Current State of the Science for Active Self-Care Complementary and Integrative Medicine Therapies in the Management of Chronic Pain Symptoms: Lessons Learned, Directions for the Future." *Pain Medicine* 15: S104–S113. doi:10.1111/pme.12406.

Chapter 3: How Science Misses Healing

There is an ongoing debate in biomedical research about the role of what is called "reductionist" science, using approaches such as randomized, placebo-controlled trials (RCTs) as the primary type of evidence needed before accepting, using, and paying for treatments in practice. The importance of RCTs is clear, but their limitations are becoming more evident. Medical science is seeking better ways to collect evidence. For a good overall framing of the debate, see Federoff, H. J. and L. O. Gostin (2009). "Evolving from Reductionism to Holism: Is There a Future for Systems Medicine?" *Journal of Internal Medicine* 302(9): 994–996. See also notes for chapter 4 on systems science.

Other selected citations readers may find of interest mentioned in this chapter include the following (in the order they are described):

Ayurveda is one of the oldest systems of healing in the world. The following chapter gives an excellent overview by one of the world's leading practitioners. Lad, V. D. "Ayurvedic Medicine," in Jonas, W. B. and J. S. Levin (eds.) *Essentials of Complementary and Alternative Medicine.* Philadelphia: Lippincott Williams & Wilkins, 1999; also see Chopra, A. and V. V. Doiphode (2002). "Ayurvedic medicine. Core concepts, therapeutic principles, and current relevance." *Medical Clinics of North America* 86(1):75–89. Recent research at University of California, San Diego, and Chopra Center hints at the mechanisms that might explain Aadi's recovery. See Mills, P. J., et al. (2016). "The Self-Directed Biological Transformation Initiative and Well-Being." *The Journal of Alternative and Complementary Medicine* 22(8): 627–634.

Information on the global use of complementary, traditional, and integrative practices comes from the World Health Organization's Office of Traditional Medicine at who.int/medicines/areas/traditional/en. The WHO defines traditional medicine as "the sum total of the knowledge, skills, and practices based on the theories, beliefs, and experiences indigenous to different cultures, whether explicable or not, used in the maintenance of health as well as in the prevention, diagnosis, improvement, or treatment of physical and mental illness."

Cousins, Norman. *Anatomy of an Illness as Perceived by the Patient: Reflections on Healing and Regeneration.* New York: W. W. Norton & Co., 1979. One of the most clear and touching descriptions of how one man constructed his own healing journey.

The three-armed study led by Professor Jonathan Davidson of Duke, which showed that an herb, a proven drug, and placebo all worked the same for depression, can be found in Hypericum Depression Trial Study Group (2002). "Effect of hypericum perforatum (St. John's Wort) in major depressive disorder: A randomized controlled trial." *Journal of Internal Medicine* 287(14): 1807–1814. My commentary on how both professionals and the public missed the key issue for healing that this study revealed can be found in: Jonas, W. B. (2002). "St. John's Wort and depression." *Journal of Internal Medicine* 288: 446.

Little known to most people, replicability of scientific findings is a major problem in biology, psychology, and medicine. Most findings cannot be independently replicated. For a discussion and data on this issue see the following: Ioannidis, J. P. A. (2005). "Why most published research findings are false." *PLoS Med* 2(8): e124; and, Ioannidis, J. P. (2017). "Acknowledging and Overcoming Non-reproducibility in Basic and Preclinical Research." *Journal of Internal Medicine* 317(10): 1019–1020; and, Wallach, J. D., P. G. Sullivan, J. F. Trepanowski, K. L. Sainani, E. W. Steyerberg, and J. P. Ioannidis (2017). "Evaluation of Evidence of Statistical Support and Corroboration of Subgroup Claims in Randomized Clinical Trials." *Journal of Internal Medicine* 177(4): 554–560; and, Prasad, V., A. Cifu, and J. P. A. Ioannidis (2012). "Reversals of Established Medical Practices: Evidence to

Abandon Ship." *Journal of Internal Medicine* 307(1): 37–38. Several groups are trying to address this issue. See a summary of those efforts in Yong, E. (August 27, 2015). "How Reliable are Psychology Studies?" *The Atlantic*.

Partly because of the above, the overuse of unproven treatments and treatments proven not to work is large—likely one-third of everything done in medicine. To remedy this, guidelines for stopping treatments that are often used but known to harm or not help can be found at choosingwisely.org/about-us. I suggest reviewing any treatments you are doing with your doctor using this site to see what you can stop doing.

For a nice summary of the decline effect and problems with scientific validity see Lehrer, J. (December 13, 2010). "The truth wears off: Is there something wrong with the scientific method?" *The New Yorker*. For even more detail on why this happens, see the book by Richard Harris, science reporter for PBS, called *Rigor Mortis: How Sloppy Science Creates Worthless Cures, Crushes Hope, and Wastes Billions*. New York: Basic Books, 2017.

The information for the statin graphic in this chapter comes from Redberg, R. F. and M. H. Katz (2016). "Statins for Primary Prevention: The Debate Is Intense, but the Data Are Weak." *Journal of Internal Medicine* 316(19): 1979–1981.

Evidence-based medicine is not as accurate as most people think. Pulitzer Prize–winning author Siddhartha Mukherjee eloquently describes the uncertainty of science and the challenge of using science for making decisions in medicine. See Mukherjee, Siddhartha. *The Laws of Medicine: Field Notes from an Uncertain Science*. New York: Simon and Schuster, 2015.

Chapter 4: A Science for Healing

There is a need to build better science and information models to address the limitations of the reductionist approach described in chapter 3. In the 1960s, this was called the "biopsychosocial" model of medicine and became the foundation for the specialty of family medicine—the specialty I practice. More recently, what I call "whole systems science" is being fed by large-scale efforts for using "big data" sets drawn from daily health care delivery and linking this data with the basic biomarkers of disease and health—at cellular, chemical, and genetic levels—and then linking that to people's activities, experiences, and long-term health outcomes. It is a big task. The largest ongoing scientific effort in this is the one-million person study by the National Institutes of Health called the Precision Medicine Initiative. See allofus.nih.gov/. For summaries of whole systems and complexity science in primary care, complementary medicine, and implementation science, see the following three references:

On primary care: Sturmberg, J. P., C. M. Martin, and D. A. Katerndahl (2014). "Systems and Complexity Thinking in the General Practice Literature: An Integrative, Historical Narrative Review." *Annals of Family Medicine* 66–74.

On complementary medicine: Verhoef, M., M. Koithan, I. R. Bell, J. Ives, and W. B. Jonas (2012). "Whole Complementary and Alternative Medical Systems and Complexity: Creating Collaborative Relationships." *Forschende Komplementärmedizin* 19(Suppl 1): 3–6. This entire issue is about the application of whole systems science to complementary medicine.

On health care delivery: Leykum, L. K., H. J. Lanham, J. A. Pugh, M. Parchman, R. A. Anderson, B. F. Crabtree, P. A. Nutting, W. L. Miller, K. C. Stange, and R. R. McDanie (2014). "Manifestations and implications of uncertainty for improving healthcare systems: an analysis of observational and interventional studies grounded in complexity science." *Implementation Science* 9(165): 2–13.

Other selected references of interest include (in the order topics are addressed):

Price, D. D. (2015). "Unconscious and conscious mediation of analgesia and hyperalgesia." *Proceedings of the National Academy of Sciences of the United States of America* 112(25): 7624–7625. What your doctor believes influences your healing response.

Frank, Jerome and Julia Frank. *Persuasion & Healing.* Baltimore: Johns Hopkins University Press, 1961. A classic on the influence of healers on those seeking treatment.

Walach, H. and Jonas W. B. (2004). "Placebo research: The evidence base for harnessing self-healing capacities." *The Journal of Alternative and Complementary Medicine* 10(Suppl 1): S103–S112. Outlines a roadmap for healing by examining placebo research.

de Craen, A. J., D. E. Moerman, S. H. Heisterkamp, G. N. Tytgat, J. G. Tijssen, and J. Kleijnen (1999). "Placebo effect in the treatment of duodenal ulcer." *British Journal of Clinical Pharmacology* 48(6): 853–860. Outcomes vary for the same treatment depending on where the treatment is delivered (home or hospital), the number of pills (two or four per day), and the color of the pills.

Ader, R. and N. Cohen (1975). "Behaviorally conditioned immunosuppression." *Psychosomatic Medicine* 37(4): 333–340. Professor Ader's breakthrough work showed that animals could learn how to alter their own immune system and live longer. This has also now been shown in humans.

The idea that small doses of toxins (or any stimulant) can induce healing is extensively documented in science but not widely known or applied in medicine. The best source of information on this is the International Dose-Response Society led by Edward Calabrese and colleagues at the University of Massachusetts, Amherst. See the peer-reviewed journal *Dose-Response* at dose-response.org for access to this extensive scientific field. Professor Calabrese's database is an encyclopedic source of scientific information showing how toxic substances from oxygen to stressful behaviors such as fasting and exercise can induce protective and reparative responses that lead to healing. See the three articles below for summaries on general mechanisms and how this works in exercise and fasting.

On the biological mechanisms: Calabrese, E. J. (2013). "Hormetic mechanisms." *Critical Reviews in Toxicology* 43(7): 580–606.

On exercise: Ji, L. L., J. R. Dickman, C. Kang, and R. Koenig (2010). "Exercise-induced hormesis may help healthy aging." *Dose-Response* 8: 73–79.

On fasting: Mattson, M. P. and R. Wan (2005). "Beneficial effects of intermittent fasting and caloric restriction on the cardiovascular and cerebrovascular systems." *The Journal of Nutritional Biochemistry* 16(3): 129–137.

Since most of us are overstimulated psychologically, removal of that stimulation through relaxation allows healing on the clinical, physiological, and genetic levels: See the classic work by Benson, Herbert and Miriam Z. Klipper. *The Relaxation Response.* New York: HarperCollins, 1992. Also see Dusek, J. A., H. H. Otu, A. L. Wohlhueter, M. Bhasin, L. F. Zerbini, M. G. Joseph, H. Benson, and T. A. Libermann (2008). "Genomic counter-stress changes induced by the relaxation response." *PloS One* 3(7): e2576; and, Bhasin, M. K., J. A. Dusek, B. H. Chang, M. G. Joseph, J. W. Denninger, G. L. Fricchione, H. Benson, and T. A. Libermann (2013). "Relaxation response induces temporal transcriptome changes in energy metabolism, insulin secretion and inflammatory pathways." *PLoS One* 8(5): e62817.

Chapter 5: Coming Home

Detecting disease early is a double-edged sword. The benefits of early detection depend primarily on whether there is a safe and effective treatment for the diseases found. This is nowhere more evident than in cancer, where new technologies are finding the disease earlier and earlier. While it is usually good to catch cancer early, what if our body would have normally taken care of an early cancer on its own? Then treatment might do more harm than good. Even as Susan went through one of the harshest treatments for breast cancer there is—three types of chemotherapy, major surgery, antihormonal therapy—the debate heated up about overtreatment and harm from the type of treatments she was getting. See the following opinion and two studies about this ongoing debate:

Narod, S. A., J. Iqbal, and V. Giannakeas (2015). "Breast cancer mortality after a diagnosis of ductal carcinoma in situ." *Journal of the American Medical Association Oncology* 1(7): 888–896. See also Winer, E. (May 17, 2017). "Breast Cancer: When is Less Treatment Better?" Dana-Farber Cancer Institute, blog.dana-farber.org/insight/2016/10/eric-winer-less-breast-cancer-treatment. And see also Welch, H. G., P. C. Prorok, A. J. O'Malley, and B. S. Kramer (2016). "Breast-Cancer Tumor Size, Overdiagnosis, and Mammography Screening Effectiveness." *New England Journal of Medicine* 375: 1438–1447. Also of concern for Susan was whether treatment might increase the spread of cancer. See Karagiannis, G. S., J. M. Pastoriza, Y. Wang, A. S. Harney, D. Entenberg, J. Pignatelli, V. P. Sharma, E. A. Xue, E. Cheng, T. M. D'Alfonso, J. G. Jones, J. Anampa, T. E. Rohan, J. A. Sparano, J. S. Condeelis, and M. H. Oktay (2017). "Neoadjuvant chemotherapy induces breast cancer metastasis through a TMEM-mediated mechanism." *Science Translational Medicine* 9(397).

Other selected references readers may find of interest mentioned in this chapter include (in the order topics are described):

Sternberg, Esther M. *Healing Spaces: The Science of Place and Well-being.* Cambridge, MA: Harvard University Press, 2009. Already a classic on how space affects our biology and health.

Ulrich, Roger (1984). "View through a window may influence recovery." *Science* 4647: 224–225. If you have to go into the hospital, make sure you can see natural views from the window.

Park, B. J., Y. Tsunetsugu, T. Kasetani, T. Kagawa, and Y. Miyazaki (2010). "The physiological effects of Shinrin-yoku (taking in the forest atmosphere or forest bathing): evidence from field experiments in 24 forests across Japan." *Environmental Health and Preventive Medicine* 15(1): 18. A traditional Japanese healing method now opening to the light of science.

Schweitzer, M., L. Gilpin, and S. Frampton (2004). "Healing spaces: elements of environmental design that make an impact on health." *The Journal of Alternative Complementary Medicine* 10(Suppl 1): S71–83.

Louv, Richard. *Last Child in the Woods: Saving Our Children from Nature-Deficit Disorder.* New York: Algonquin Books, 2008. Children need immersion in nature.

The model and components of an optimal healing environment (OHE) were developed by Samueli Institute over a decade and have been researched and described in several articles and books. Some of the main ones are the following:

Jonas, W. B. and R. A. Chez (2004). "Toward optimal healing environments in health care." *The Journal of Alternative Complementary Medicine* 10(Suppl 1): S1–S6. The entire issue is on OHE in various specialties.

Sakallaris, B. R., L. MacAllister, M. Voss, K. Smith, and W. B. Jonas (May 2015). "Optimal healing environments." *Global Advances in Health and Medicine* 4(3):40–45. doi:10.7453/gahmj.2015.043. An update on healing environments.

Christianson, J., M. Finch, B. Findlay, C. Goertz, and W. B. Jonas. *Reinventing the Patient Experience: Strategies for Hospital Leaders.* Chicago: Health Administration Press, 2007. Case studies of seven different hospitals and how they created optimal healing environments.

Kashman, Scott and Joan Odorizzi. *Transforming Healthcare: Healthy Team, Healthy Business.* Cape Coral, FL: Book in a Box. An in-depth study of how one hospital went from a "D" rating to "top of class" by following the optimal healing environment model.

Chapter 6: Acting Right

The importance of a healthy lifestyle is perhaps the most emphasized and familiar aspect of health and healing to readers. We are, in fact, bombarded with self-help books and advice saying don't smoke, don't stress, drink moderately, exercise daily, and eat healthier food. For ongoing information about the therapeutic aspects of lifestyle, follow the American College of Lifestyle Medicine, which tracks and summarizes this literature constantly at lifestylemedicine.org. I summarize the essence of this literature in this chapter and in the appendices. The main purpose of this chapter is to show that sustainable healthy behavior is more complicated than just knowing the facts. Behavior must be infused with meaning and the right mind-set to be optimally effective.

Selected references readers may find of interest mentioned in this chapter include (in the order topics are described):

Loprinzi, P. D., A. Branscum, J. Hanks, and E. Smit (2016). "Healthy Lifestyle Characteristics and Their Joint Association with Cardiovascular Disease Biomarkers in U.S. Adults." *Mayo Clinic Proceedings* 91(4): 432–442. Less than 3% of the population follows even the top four recommendations for a healthy lifestyle.

Mehta, N. and M. Myrskylä (2017). "The Population Health Benefits of a Healthy Lifestyle: Life Expectancy Increased and Onset of Disability Delayed." *Health Affairs* 36(8): 1495–1502. A nice summary of the key healthy behaviors for population health.

Bradley, E., M. Canavan, E. Rogan, K. Talbert-Slagle, C. Ndumele, L. Taylor, and L. Curry (2016). "Variation in Health Outcomes: The Role of Spending on Social Services, Public Health and Healthcare, 2000–2009." *Health Affairs* 35(3): 760–768. How priorities in spending that enable healthy behavior compared to health care treatments differentially impact actual health.

Squires, D. and C. Anderson (2015). "U.S. Health Care from a Global Perspective: Spending, Use of Services, Prices, and Health in 13 Countries." The Commonwealth Fund. Includes comparisons across developed countries.

Multiple foundations and nations are seeking better ways to deliver health. Here are only a few of the more developed and documented approaches to moving from health care to health and well-being:

Chatterjee, A., S. Kubendran, J. King, and R. DeVol (2014). "Checkup Time: Chronic Disease and Wellness in America—Measuring the Economic Burden in a Changing Nation." Milken Institute. milkeninstitute.org/publications/view/618.

Robert Wood Johnson Foundation (2013). "Return on Investments in Public Health: Saving Lives and Money." rwjf.org/content/dam/farm/reports/issue_briefs/2013/rwjf72446.

National Prevention Council (2011). "National Prevention Strategy." Washington, D.C., U.S. Department of Health and Human Services. Office of the Surgeon General.

National Center for Chronic Disease Prevention and Health Promotion (2009). "The Power of Prevention: Chronic Disease . . . the Public Health Challenge of the 21st Century." Centers for Disease Control and Prevention. See cdc.gov/chronicdisease/pdf/2009-power-of- prevention.pdf.

The Vitality Institute (2014). "Investing in Prevention: A National Imperative." thevitalityinstitute. org/site/wp-content/uploads/2014/06/Vitality_Recommendations2014.pdf.

Scottish Government (2016). "Creating a Healthier Scotland." scdc.org.uk/news/article/ creating-healthier-scotland-summary-report.

Singapore is one of the most progressive and effective health promotion cities in the world and includes traditional and integrative health care delivery. See hpb.gov.sg/article/ singapore-comes-together-to-celebrate-20-years-of-healthy-lifestyle.

You don't see what you don't measure. One of the most comprehensive ways to measure well-being in a country has been done in Canada, and it is paying off. Outcomes are better and costs of health care are significantly lower than its neighbor to the south. See uwaterloo.ca/canadian-index-wellbeing/ for how they measure health and well-being.

For a summary of the impact of the community health movement in the United States see Norris, T. (2013). "Healthy Communities at Twenty-Five." *National Civic Review* 102: 4–9.

For plans for advancing nonconventional medicine globally, see "WHO Traditional Medicine Strategy: 2014–2013." World Health Organization. See who.int/medicines/publications/traditional/trm_strategy14_23/en.

WHO plans for addressing chronic disease in general is well summarized in Alwan, A. (2011). "Global Status Report on Noncommunicable Diseases 2010." World Health Organization. See www.who.int/nmh/publications/wha_resolution53_14/en.

The United Nations is also working to address community health globally. See Beaglehole, R., R. Bonita, G. Alleyne, R. Horton, L. Li, P. Lincoln, J. C. Mbanya, M. McKee, R. Moodie, S. Nishtar, P. Piot, K. S. Reddy, and D. Stuckler (2011). "UN High-Level Meeting on Non-Communicable Diseases: addressing four questions." *The Lancet* 378(9789): 449–455.

Other key sources of lifestyle and healing information as mentioned in the chapter are the following:

Metzl, Jordan. *The Exercise Cure: A Doctor's All-Natural, No-Pill Prescription for Better Health and Longer Life.* Emmaus, PA: Rodale, 2013. Exercise induces healing and keeps us functional and alive.

Johnston, B. C., S. Kanters, K. Bandayrel, et al. (2014). "Comparison of weight loss among named diet programs in overweight and obese adults: A meta-analysis." *Journal of the American Medical Association* 312(9): 923–933. It is more important to pay attention that your diet is primarily whole foods and not full of additives or toxins—and that you believe it is healthy—than to worry about its exact composition. This study showed that all the current commercial diets were basically the same when it comes to weight loss.

Studies by Stanford Professor Alia Crum have examined the impact of mind-set on the impact of lifestyle and behavior on health. Mind-set influences all aspect[s] of lifestyle and healthy behavior. See Crum, A. J. and E. J. Langer (2007). "Mind-set matters: exercise and the placebo effect." *Psychological Science* 18(2): 165–171; and, Crum, Alia J., et al. (2011). "Mind over milkshakes: mind-sets, not just nutrients, determine ghrelin response." *Health Psychology* 30(4): 424l; and, Crum, Alia, et al. (2017). "De-stressing stress: The power of mindsets and the art of stressing mindfully." *The Wiley Blackwell Handbook of Mindfulness*, 948–963; and, Crum, A. J., K. A. Leibowitz, and A. Verghese (2017). "Making mindset matter." *British Medical Journal* 356: j674.

Do gene changes come from the food we eat or the social environment of the eating? See Ordovas, J. M. (2008). "Genotype-phenotype associations: modulation by diet and obesity." *Obesity* 16(Suppl 3): S40–S46. doi:10.1038/oby.2008.515.

Giordano J. and W. B. Jonas (2007). "Asclepius and hygieia in dialectic: Philosophical, ethical and educational foundations of an integrative medicine." *Integrative Medicine Insights* 2: 53–60. A description of the ancient Greek Hippocratic school of medicine and how it addressed all the dimensions of healing.

Jonas, W. B., P. Deuster, F. O'Connor, and C. Macedonia (2010). "Total Force Fitness for the 21st Century: A New Paradigm." *Military Medicine* (Suppl). 175(8). The United States military's framework for whole systems health and well-being.

Mission: Readiness, Military Leaders for Kids. Report: "Too Fat to Fight: Retired Military Leaders Want Junk Food Out of America's Schools." Washington, D.C., Mission: Readiness, 2010. Obesity is a threat to national security.

For current training in healthy cooking for health professionals, see the Harvard program Healthy Kitchens, Healthy Lives at hms.harvard.edu/news/harvard-medical-school-and- culinary-institute-america-launch-healthy-kitchens-healthy-lives-4-20-07.

For information on complementary, lifestyle, and integrative approaches in cancer, see the Society for Integrative Oncology at integrativeonc.org; and, also the book by Block, Keith I. *Life Over Cancer*. New York: Bantam/Random House, 2009. Dr. Block's book is the best and most comprehensive overview on evidence-based integrative oncology available for patients.

Pletcher, M. J. and C. E. McCulloch (2017). "The Challenges of Generating Evidence to Support Precision Medicine." *Journal of the American Medical Association Internal Medicine* 177(4): 561–562. The NIH needs you to join their whole systems science initiative called Precision Medicine.

Topol, Eric. *The Patient Will See You Now: The Future of Medicine Is in Your Hands*. New York: Basic Books, 2016. How technology is democratizing health care and putting patients in charge of their health.

Chapter 7: Loving Deeply

We often think of love and fear as solely psychological—all in the mind—and as having little impact on the body. This is not true, but the myth persists in the modern mind. When we finally break this misperception, it will crack open whole new dimensions for healing. I use this remarkable but little known experiment on rabbits to show how, despite the objective demonstration that love is as power-ful as cholesterol-lowering drugs in preventing heart disease, we have largely ignored the former and made an industry of the latter.

Selected references readers may find of interest mentioned in this chapter include the following:

Nerem, R. M., M. J. Levesque, and J. F. Cornhill (1980). "Social environment as a factor in diet-in-duced atherosclerosis." *Science* 208(4451): 1475–1476. The formal "love your rabbit" experiment described in the chapter.

Titler, M. G., G. A. Jensen, J. M. Dochterman, X-J M. Xie, D. Reed, and L. L. Shever (April 2008). "Cost of Hospital Care for Older Adults with Heart Failure: Medical, Pharmaceutical, and Nursing Costs." *Health Services Research Journal* 43(2): 635–655. Heart failure is costly, and the costs are rising.

Berwick, D. M., T. W. Nolan, and J. Whittington (2008). "The triple aim: care, health, and cost." *Health Affairs* (Millwood) 27(3): 759–769. The triple aim—simultaneously improving health out-comes, and the quality of patient experience and lowering costs—has become the mantra for value in health care.

Christakis, Nicholas. A. and James H. Fowler. *Connected: The Surprising Power of Our Social Networks and How They Shape Our Lives*. New York: Little Brown, 2009. Research shows that your friend, their friends, and their friends all have an impact on your health and healing capacity.

Cacioppo, John T. and William Patrick. *Loneliness: Human Nature and the Need for Social Connection*. New York: W.W. Norton & Company, 2008. One of the best overviews of the science of loneliness and its impact on health.

Farmer, I. P., P. S. Meyer, D. J. Ramsey, D. C. Goff, M. L. Wear, D. R. Labarthe, and M. Z. Nichaman (1996). "Higher levels of social support predict greater survival following acute myocardial infarction: The Corpus Christi Heart Project." *Behavioral Medicine* 22(2): 59–66.

How does the physical presence of a person affect the other? The studies on how electromagnetic waves of the heart impact the electromagnetic waves of the brain of persons standing next to each other can be found in McCraty, Rollin. *The Science of the Heart*. Boulder Creek, CA: HeartMath Institute, 2015. Available at heartmath.org.

Two studies we conducted at Walter Reed Army Institute of Research demonstrated that electromagnetic waves coming off the hands of a healer can increase the energy molecules of cells. See Kiang, J. G., J. A. Ives, and W. B. Jonas (2005). "External bioenergy-induced increases in intracellular free calcium concentrations are mediated by Na+/Ca 2+ exchanger and L-type calcium channel." *Molecular and Cellular Biochemistry* 271(1): 51–59; and, Kiang, J. G., D. Marotta, M. Wirkus, and Jonas, W. B. (2002). "External Bioenergy Increases Intracellular Free Calcium Concentration and Reduces Cellular Response to Heat Stress." *Journal of Investigative Medicine* 50(1): 38–45. This might be the mechanism for the ancient method of laying-on of hands. More research is needed.

Kemper, K. J. *Authentic Healing: A Practical Guide for Caregivers*. Minneapolis, MN: Two Harbors Press, 2016. In this book, Dr. Kemper, professor of pediatrics at The Ohio State University College of Medicine, describes how to use bioenergy healing in day-to-day practice.

Pennebaker, J. W. *Opening Up: The Healing Power of Expressing Emotions*. New York: Guildford Press, 1997. (Second edition published in 2012.) This book summarizes decades of research showing that by engaging past areas of deep personal and emotional trauma, such as through therapeutic writing, the brain, immune system, physiological function, and even health care needs improve.

Even a single episode of therapeutic writing improves pain (in rheumatoid arthritis) and lung function (in asthma). See Smyth, J. M., A. A. Stone, A. Hurewitz, and A. Kaell (1999). "Effects of writing about stressful experiences on symptom reduction in patients with asthma or rheumatoid arthritis: a randomized trial." *Journal of the American Medical Association* 281(14): 1304–1309.

Facing your past traumatic experiences in the presence of loving persons can heal the effects of past trauma in veterans who have gone to war. See Bobrow, Joseph. *Waking Up from War: A Better Way Home for Veterans and Nations*. Durham, NC: Pitchstone Publishing, 2015. And about those who have not gone to war but experienced trauma nonetheless, see van de Kolk, Bessel. *The Body Keeps the Score: Brain, Mind, and Body in the Healing of Trauma*. New York: Penguin, 2014. New discoveries in the healing of trauma are helping to us to understand the fundamental dynamics of healing in general.

Griffiths, R. R., M. W. Johnson, M. A. Carducci, A. Umbricht, W. A. Richards, B. D. Richards, M. P. Cosimano, and M. A. Klinedinst (2016). "Psilocybin produces substantial and sustained decreases in depression and anxiety in patients with life-threatening cancer: A randomized double-blind trial." *Journal of Psychopharmacology* 30(12): 1181–1197. It appears that psychoactive drugs can open people to their fears, which if then reexperienced in a positive manner can permanently heal anxiety, depression, and other emotional ills. Research is ongoing to see if this approach will also work for veterans with refractory PTSD. I predict it will work.

For a description of the social approach to healing individuals in the Navajo Beauty Way and other similar ceremonies, see gonativeamericanconcepts.wordpress.com/the-blessing-way/ and gonativeamerica.com/10-NavajoBeautyway.html.

Moerman, D. E. *Meaning, Medicine, and the 'Placebo Effect'*. Cambridge, MA: Cambridge University Press, 2002. The definitive summary of how meaning and context work across cultures to explain the placebo response.

For a description on how relationship-centered care improved the health of a community of people and became a demonstration model for using the social and emotional dimensions of healing health care, see Gottlieb, K. (2013). "The Nuka System of Care: improving health through ownership and relationships." *International Journal of Circumpolar Health* 72(1): 211–218; and, Driscoll, D. L., V. Hiratsuka, J. M. Johnston, S. Norman, K. M. Reilly, J. Shaw, and D. Dillard (2013). "Process and outcomes of patient-centered medical care with Alaska Native people at South Central Foundation." *The Annals of Family Medicine* 11(Suppl 1): S41–S49.

Group care not only can address loneliness but also facilitate behavioral change and impact health care costs. For a description of the approach taken by Dr. Jeffery Geller, see Geller, J., P. Janson, E. McGovern, and A. Valdini (1999). "Loneliness as a predictor of hospital emergency department use." *Journal of Family Practice* 48(10): 801–807; and, Geller, J. S., A. Orkaby, and G. D. Cleghorn (2011). "Impact of a group medical visit program on Latino health–related quality of life." *EXPLORE: The Journal of Science and Healing* 7(2): 94–99.

Chapter 8: Finding Meaning

It is difficult for scientists and physicians to believe that the subtle and largely immeasurable aspects of our mind and spirit are important for healing. But they are. They need to be considered and used in health care. I have spent a considerable part of my research career exploring this area, seeking to increase the scientific rigor and amount of evidence in the mental and spiritual dimensions of healing. Of course, more research is needed. While the role of mind-body practices, mindfulness, and mind-set is increasingly accepted in medicine, the subtler spiritual aspects of our lives is still largely taboo in medicine.

One of the most thoughtful writers in this area is Dr. Larry Dossey, whose books explore these areas. I recommend starting with his classic, *Healing Words: Power of Prayer and the Practice of Medicine* (San Francisco: Harper Collins, 1993), and also his *Healing Beyond the Body: Medicine and the Infinite Reach of the Mind* (Boulder, CO: Shambhala Publications, 2003).

Daniel Benor's *Healing Research* (Munich: Helix Verlag, 1993) contains a detailed summary of research. A criteria-based, critical evaluation of these areas can be found in Jonas, W. B. and C. C. Crawford (eds.). *Healing, Intention and Energy Medicine: Science, Methodology and Clinical Implications.* London: Churchill Livingston, 2003.

For extensive summaries of the health effects from religious and spiritual practices, see Koenig, H., D. King, and V. B. Carson, *Handbook of Religion and Health, 2nd Edition.* New York: Oxford University Press, 2012; especially for nurses, see Carson, V. B. and H. Koenig *Spiritual Dimensions of Nursing Practice.* West Conshohocken, PA: Templeton Foundation Press, 2008; and especially for physicians, see Puchalski, C. and B. Ferrell *Making Health Care Whole: Integrating Spirituality into Patient Care.* West Conshohocken, PA: Templeton Foundation Press, 2011. Professor Puchalski conducts an annual training at George Washington University on spiritual issues in medicine.

Other selected references readers may find of interest mentioned in this chapter include (in order of their description):

Classics in the use of guided imagery for healing are the books by Jeanne Achtenberg (*Imagery in Healing*, Boston: Shambhala, 1985) and Carl Simonton (*The Healing Journey*, New York: Bantam, 1992) and Belleruth Naprastek (*Staying Well with Guided Imagery*, New York: Warner, 1994).

Newer, practical sites for getting both information and downloads of guided imagery for use in life can be obtained from the Academy for Guided Imagery (acadgi.com) and the website of Dr. Naprastek at healthjourneys.com. I have been involved in clinical studies with veterans using the work of Dr. Naprastek and found it useful and effective.

The remarkable effects of imagery and healing touch when used with Marines for PTSD can be found in Jain, S., G. F. McMahon, P. Hasen, M. P. Kozub, V. Porter, R. King, and E. M. Guarneri (2012). "Healing Touch with Guided Imagery for PTSD in returning active duty military: a random-ized controlled trial." *Military Medicine* 177(9): 1015–1021.

Veterans deployed to war have almost twice the rate of exceptional and spiritual experiences than the general population. See Hufford, David. "Spiritual experiences in Veterans deployed to Iraq and

Afghanistan." Personal communication; and, Hufford, D. J., M. J. Fritts, and J. E. Rhodes (2010). "Spiritual fitness." *Military Medicine* 175(8S): 73–87.

We can teach the body to respond in specific ways to inert substances or other signals through the process of classical conditioning. For examples of this, see the classic study of immune suppression in rats by Ader, R. and N. Cohen (1975). "Behaviorally conditioned immunosuppression." *Psychosomatic Medicine* 37(4): 333–340; and, in humans by Goebel, M. U., et al. (2002). "Behavioral conditioning of immunosuppression is possible in humans." *Federation of American Studies for Experimental Biology Journal* 16:1869–1873; and, in other conditions, see Kroes, M. C. W., J. E. Dunsmoor, W. E. Mackey, M. McClay, and E. A. Phelps (2017). "Context conditioning in humans using commercially available immersive Virtual Reality." *Scientific Reports* 7:8640. doi:/10.1038/s41598-017-08184-7; and, Colloca, L., L. Lopiano, M. Lanotte and F. Benedetti (2004). "Overt versus covert treatment for pain, anxiety, and Parkinson's disease." *The Lancet Neurology* 3: 679–684.

Branding (the label on the pill) and price (expensive or cheap) make a difference in the effectiveness of treatments. See Margo, C. E. (1999). "The Placebo Effect." *Survey of Ophthalmology* 44: 31–44, for an example of branding; and, Waber, R. L., B. Shiv, Z. Carmon, and D. Ariely (2008). "Commercial features of placebo and therapeutics." *Journal of the American Medical Association* 299(9): 1016–7 for an example of how price impacts effectiveness. Drug companies know about these effects. How much of the fluctuation in branding and drug prices is to impact their perceived effectiveness rather than because of their real effects?

Moerman, D. E. *Meaning, Medicine, and the 'Placebo Effect'*. Cambridge, MA: Cambridge University Press, 2002. The definitive summary of how meaning and context work across cultures to explain the placebo response.

For a detailed description of the use of conditioned immunosuppression in an eleven-year-old child with a life-threatening disease by Dr. Karen Olness, professor of pediatrics at Case Western Reserve, see Marchant, J. "You can train your body into thinking it's had medicine." *Mosaic: The Science of Life*. mosaicscience.com/story/medicine-without-the-medicine-how-to-train-your-immune-system-placebo.

Siegel, Daniel J. *Mind: A Journey to The Heart of Being Human*. New York: W.W. Norton & Company, 2016. A visionary book by a University of California, Los Angeles, psychiatrist on how the mind works, both inside and outside the body.

For a study on how expectations can be established during a single clinical visit and profoundly affect outcomes in primary care, see Thomas, K. B. (1987). "General practice consultations: is there any point in being positive?" *British Medical Journal* (Clinical Research Edition) 294(6581): 1200–1202.

Gracely, R. H. (1979). "Physicians expectations for pain relief." *Society for Neuroscience Abstracts* 5: 609; also in Levine, J., N. Gordon, and H. Fields (1978). "The mechanism of placebo analgesia." *The Lancet* 312(8091): 654–657. It matters what your physician believes will work, not just what you believe. Ask your doctor about his or her belief in a treatment.

Lang, E. V., O. Hatisopoulou, T. Koch, K. Berbaum, S. Lutgendorf, E. Kettenmann, L. Henrietta, T. J. Kaptchuk (2005). "Can words hurt? Patient-provider interactions during invasive procedures." *Pain* 114: 303–309. Don't let your doctor say "This will hurt," because it will if he does.

Schedlowski, M., P. Enck, W. Rief, and U. Bingel (2015). "Neuro-bio-behavioral mechanisms of placebo and nocebo responses: implications for clinical trials and clinical practice." *Pharmacological Reviews* 67(3): 697–730. The side effects of drugs increase the more we expect them to.

The study on death in China, related to astrology, is found in Phillips, D. P., T. E. Ruth, and L. M. Wagner (1993). "Psychology and survival." *The Lancet* 342(8880): 1142–1145.

A spiritual view of healing through and because of trauma: Nouwen, Henri J. M. *The Wounded Healer: Ministry in Contemporary Society*. New York: Image/Doubleday Books, 1979.

Shanafelt, T. D., L. N. Dyrbye, and C. P. West (2017). "Addressing Physician Burnout: The Way Forward." *Journal of the American Medical Association* 317(9): 901–902. Up to 50% of doctors are burnt out and say they have lost their passion for medical practice and empathy for patients.

Murphy, Robin. *The Future of the Body: Explorations into the Further Evolution of Human Nature*. New York: Tarcher/Putnam, 1992. Mr. Murphy has provided an encyclopedic review of our body's remarkable ability to heal.

Temel, J. S., J. A. Greer, A. Muzikansky, E. R. Gallagher, S. Admane, V. A. Jackson, et al. (2010). "Early palliative care for patients with metastatic non–small-cell lung cancer." *New England Journal of Medicine* 363(8): 733–742. By providing less treatment and more comfort and caring for patients with advanced lung cancer, they felt better and lived longer.

Doctors and our health care system do not deal well with death and dying. See Institute of Medicine. *Dying in America: Improving Quality and Honoring Individual Preferences Near the End of Life*. Washington, D. C.: National Academies Press, 2015 and Gawande, Atul. *Being Mortal: Medicine and What Matters in the End*. New York: Metropolitan Books, 2014. Dr. Gawande writes about the need to extend healing into times of death and dying. I write about the need to extend healing into routine medical care at all times.

For studies on the value and limitation of intuition, see the extensive work by Professor Gerard Hodgkinson and his team of the Centre for Organizational Strategy, Learning and Change at Leeds University, England. Their findings are summarized at leeds.ac.uk/news/article/367/ go_with_your_gut__intuition_is_more_than_just_a_hunch_says_leeds_research.

For a rigorous evaluation, using three types of validity, of the research done on mind and spirit for healing, see Jonas, W. B. and C.C. Crawford (eds.). *Healing, Intention and Energy Medicine: Science, Methodology and Clinical Implications*. London: Churchill Livingston, 2003.

For a review and statistical comparison of the outcomes of prayer-like (psychic intention) activity, showing that the effects are similar to that of aspirin in preventing heart disease, see the 1995 study "An Assessment of the Evidence for Psychic Functioning" by Professor Jessica Utts, who chairs the Department of Statistics, University of California, Irvine, and is the past president of the American Statistical Association. Find the study online at citeseerx.ist.psu.edu/viewdoc/ download?doi=10.1.1.40.8219&rep=rep1&type=pdf.

Chapter 9: Integrative Health

Leaders in medical education and practice regularly call for more holistic, humanistic, personalized care. Unfortunately, technology, economics, politics, or tradition often subvert these recommendations. Then, calls for more healing reassert themselves under various names—biopsychosocial, patient-centered, relationship-centered, personalized, humanistic, proactive, holistic, or sharing medicine, for example. Integrative health is the most recent and comprehensive attempt to return healing to health care. We cannot afford a health care system that does not value health, healing, and well-being. If I were to recommend just one book about these dynamics, it would be Kenneth Ludmerer's *A Time to Heal* (New York: Oxford University Press, 1999), which is an encyclopedic history of the forces and dynamics facing a more holistic, humanistic, caring medical system.

Hypertension, like Trevor had, is one of the most important individual and public health conditions in the world. It is treatable, and its complications, which are myriad and include heart disease, stroke, and kidney failure, are top causes of death and disability. For a summary, see the World Health Organization (2013). "A global brief on hypertension: silent killer, global public health crisis: World Health Day 2013." who.int/cardiovascular_diseases/publications/global_brief_hypertension/en.

At the time that Trevor went to the doctor, the major guidelines for treating and managing hypertension were in The Seventh Report of the Joint National Committee on Prevention, Detection, Evaluation, and Treatment of High Blood Pressure (JNC7). See nhlbi.nih.gov/files/docs/guidelines/jnc7full.pdf. The more recent guidelines (called JNC8) have even less detail on integration of the social and nondrug approaches to hypertension, saying it is "beyond the scope" of the recommendations. Without integration of these dimensions into practice, however, more patients like Trevor may fall through the gap.

Other references of interest mentioned in this chapter include the following:

Steinberg, D., G. G. Bennett, and L. Svetkey (2017). "The DASH diet, 20 years later." *Journal of the American Medical Association* 317(15): 1529–1530.

Trevor's "natural medicine" practitioner may have been influenced by a popular book on the Rice Diet. See Rosati, Kitty Gurkin and Robert Rosati. *The Rice Diet Solution: The World-famous Low-sodium, Good-carb, Detox Diet for Quick and Lasting Weight Loss.* New York: Simon and Schuster, 2006. However, what Trevor did not understand was that the original diet, developed by Duke physician Walter Kempner in 1939, was for a very different type of patient than he was. See Klemmer, P., et al. (2014). "Who and what drove Walter Kempner? The rice diet revisited." *Hypertension* 64(4): 684–688.

For summaries of the factors that contribute most to population health and how our health care systems can better address those factors and close the gap see: Kindig, D. A., B. C. Booske, and P. L. Remington (2010). "Mobilizing Action Toward Community Health (MATCH): metrics, incentives, and partnerships for population health." *Preventing Chronic Disease* 7(4): A68; and, Dzau, V. J., M. B. McClellan, J. M. McGinnis, S. P. Burke, M. J. Coye, A. Diaz, T. A. Daschle, W. H. Frist, M. Gaines, M. A. Hamburg, J. E. Henney, S. Kumanyika, M. O. Leavitt, R. M. Parker, L. G. Sandy, L. D. Schaeffer, G. D. Steele, P. Thompson, and E. Zerhouni (2017). "Vital Directions for Health and Health Care: Priorities from a National Academy of Medicine Initiative." *Journal of the American Medical Association* 317(14): 1461–1470; and, Samueli Institute's *"Wellbeing in the Nation: A Plan to Strengthen and Sustain our Nation's Wellbeing, Community by Community"* available at wellbeinginthenation.org.

For information about evidence-based medicine and why it has become so important, see Belsey, Jonathan and Tony Snell (1997). "What is evidence-based medicine?" *Hayward Medical Communications*; and, Jaeschke, R. and G. H. Guyatt (October 1999). "What is evidence-based medicine?" *Seminars in Medical Practice* 2(3): 3–7.

The term *salutogenesis* meaning "the generation of health" was first coined by psychologist Aaron Antonovsky. See Antonovsky, Aaron. *Unraveling the Mystery of Health.* San Francisco: Jossey-Bass, 1987. I have expanded the use of the term salutogenesis beyond psychology into medicine and use it to complement the concept of *pathogenesis* meaning "the generation of disease." See Jonas, W. B., R. A. Chez, K. Smith, B. Sakallaris, and C. Crawford (2014). "Salutogenesis: The Defining Concept for a New Healthcare System." *Global Advances in Health Medicine* 3: 82–91.

Hölzel, Britta K., et al. (2011). "Mindfulness practice leads to increases in regional brain gray matter density." *Psychiatry Research: Neuroimaging* 191(1): 36–43. This research is what made us think that Mandy would benefit from an eight-week session of mindfulness before we resumed acupuncture treatment for her chronic pain.

While the story about the origins of Tibetan medicine as an intentional synthesis from multiple traditions did not likely occur exactly like this, the story does speak to the fact that Tibetan medicine is a tradition that intentionally draws from the multiple healing approaches from India, China, and the Middle East—and, more recently, the West.

For serial data on the growing popularity and use of complementary and alternative medicine in the United States, see Eisenberg, D. M., R. B. Davis, S. L. Ettner, S. Appel, S. Wilkey, M. Van Rompay,

R. C. Kessler (1998). "Trends in alternative medicine use in the United State 1990–1997: Results of a follow-up national survey." *Journal of the American Medical Association* 280(18): 1569–1575; and, Nahin, R. L., P. M. Barnes, B. J. Stussman, and B. Bloom (2009). "Costs of complementary and alternative medicine (CAM) and frequency of visits to CAM practitioners: United States, 2007." *National Health Statistics Reports* 18: 1–14; and, Clarke, T. C., L. I. Black, B. J. Stussman, P. M. Barnes, and R. L. Nahin (2015). "Trends in the Use of Complementary Health Approaches Among Adults: United States, 2002–2012." *National Health Statistics Reports* 79:1–16.

World Health Organization (1948). "Definition of health" see who.int/suggestions/faq/en/; also, see "Constitution of WHO: principles." who.int/about/mission/en.

Institute of Medicine. *Crossing the Quality Chasm: A New Health System for the 21st Century.* Washington, D.C.: National Academy of Sciences Press, 2001. A landmark study in which person-centered care is clearly defined and called for.

Ornish, Dean. *The Spectrum: A Scientifically Proven Program to Feel Better, Live Longer, Lose Weight, and Gain Health.* New York: Ballantine Books, 2008. Dr. Ornish is a pioneer in health promotion and lifestyle medicine and this is his most holistic view yet.

Buettner, Dan. *The Blue Zones: 9 Lessons for Living Longer from the People Who've Lived the Longest.* Washington, D.C.: National Geographic Books, 2012. Readers are often surprised by how simple actions can have a significant influence on well-being and mentality.

For information on Iora Health System, see iorahealth.com. Team-based, patient-centered care in action.

For a report on the top-five percent of primary care clinics, see Petersen Health Foundation (2013). "America's Most Valuable Care: Primary Care Snapshots." petersonhealthcare.org/identification-uncovering-americas-most-valuable-care/primary-care-snapshots.

Strecher, Victor J. *Life on Purpose: How Living for What Matters Most Changes Everything.* San Francisco: HarperCollins, 2016. Summarizes data on how meaning creates health and healing and how to bring purpose into your life. Developer of the JOOL app for purpose in life.

Chapter 10: Creating Healing

There are a number of health care leaders and systems redesigning the way health care and healing is delivered along the lines of integrative health. I describe some of them in this chapter; see the following for more information.

Burnt-out providers can't heal. Yet the problem of burnout is growing (and now estimated at nearly 50% in primary care physicians and nurses). See Shanafelt, T. D., L. N. Dyrbye, and C. P. West (2017). "Addressing Physician Burnout: The Way Forward." *Journal of the American Medical Association* 317(9): 901–902; and, Dyrbye, L. N., T. D. Shanafelt, C. A. Sinsky, P. F. Cipriano, J. Bhatt, A. Ommaya, C. P. West, and D. Meyers (2017). "Burnout among health-care professionals: A call to explore and address this underrecognized threat to safe, high-quality care." *NAM Perspectives.* Discussion Paper, National Academy of Medicine, Washington, D.C. nam.edu/Burnout-Among-Health-Care-Professionals.

The Commonwealth Fund's link to "exemplars" in health care: commonwealthfund.org/grants-and-fellowships/grants/2012/jul/exemplars-of-local-health-care-delivery-reform.

The World Health Organization has an office of traditional medicine that tracks its use and advances research and application globally. See World Health Organization (2005). "National policy on traditional medicine and regulation of herbal medicines: Report of a WHO global survey" at apps.who.int/iris/bitstream/10665/43229/1/9241593237.pdf; and, World Health Organization (2014). "WHO

Traditional Medicine Strategy 2014–2023. Geneva; 2013" at who.int/medicines/publications/traditional/trm_strategy14_23/en.

Herman, Patricia M., et al. (2012). "Are complementary therapies and integrative care cost-effective? A systematic review of economic evaluations." *BMJ Open* 2(5): e001046. Does adding complementary medicine save money? Apparently so, if done appropriately.

Khorsan, R., I. D. Coulter, C. Crawford, and A. F. Hsiao (2011). "Systematic review of integrative health-care research: randomized control trials, clinical controlled trials, and meta-analysis." *Evidence-Based Complementary and Alternative Medicine* 2011(pii): 636134. Most research evaluates CAM practices with little exploration of the true integration of conventional and CAM practices.

National Academy of Medicine. *Integrative Medicine and the Health of the Public: A Summary of February 2009 Summit.* Washington, D.C.: The National Academies Press, 2009. The United States National Academy of Medicine calls for more integration in 2009. This echoed a White House Commission report from nearly a decade earlier. See Dean, Karen L. (2001). "White House Commission on Complementary and Alternative Medicine Policy Town Hall Meeting: Practitioners and Patients Speak Up." *Alternative & Complementary Therapies* 7(2): 108–111.

Information on medical and health education schools with integrative health activities can be found at The Academic Consortium for Integrative Health and Medicine, imconsortium.org.

For integrative medical information in Europe, see The European Society of Integrative Medicine (ESIM) at european-society-integrative-medicine.org.

Information on research in complementary and integrative medicine globally can be obtained from the International Society for Complementary Medicine Research (ISCMR) at iscmr.org.

University of Arizona Center for Integrative Medicine, founded by Dr. Andrew Weil (integrative-medicine.arizona.edu/), is one of the first and premier university centers for integrative medicine. They have taught over 1,500 health care providers and are expanding their services. This is one of the first places physicians go for training when they want to do more integrative medicine.

Weil, Andrew. *Mind Over Meds.* Boston: Little, Brown and Company, 2017. The latest book by a pioneer in natural medicine who popularized the term *integrative medicine.*

Information on the Susan and Henry Samueli College of Health Sciences and University of California, Irvine can be found at uci.edu. This unique college will consist of four schools—medicine, nursing, pharmacy, and public (or population) health—all oriented toward providing education in integrative health at a major public university.

Cleveland Clinic has two major efforts on integrative health. They are Integrative Health and Wellness Institute at my.clevelandclinic.org/departments/wellness/integrative, and the Center for Functional Medicine at my.clevelandclinic.org/departments/functional-medicine.

Bland, Jeffrey. *The Disease Delusion.* New York: HarperCollins, 2014. The latest book by a pioneer of applied nutritional therapy, using systems science approaches. Dr. Bland coined the term *functional medicine.*

Information and training in functional medicine can be obtained from the Institute for Functional Medicine at ifm.org.

The Mayo Clinic also two major efforts in integrative health housed in their Center for Integrative Health (mayoclinic.org/departments-centers/integrative-medicine-health) and their Healthy Living Center (healthyliving.mayoclinic.org/the-mayo-clinic-difference.php).

Notes

Tools for self-care and integrative health can be found at the Center for Spirituality and Healing at the University of Minnesota. See csh.umn.edu. Led by nurse researcher Dr. Mary Jo Kreitzer, many of these tools are free or available at minimal cost to the public.

Also available to the public at minimal cost are tools for self-care and integrative health developed by pediatrician Dr. Kathi Kemper at The Ohio State University College of Medicine. I recommend her courses on herbs and dietary supplements (herbs-supplements.osu.edu) and, in mind-body skills training for resilience (mind-bodyhealth.osu.edu). For parents, Dr. Kemper has written the definitive guide to holistic health for children, *The Holistic Pediatrician* (San Francisco: HarperCollins, 2016), originally published in 1996.

The Academic Collaborative for Integrative Health (ACIH) is an association of higher education schools in the complementary health professions—acupuncture, massage, naturopathy, and midwifery. They can be found at integrativehealth.org.

Information on chiropractic medicine education and practice can be found at two sites: the World Federation of Chiropractic, an advocate for a broad role in health care rather than solely spinal manipulation (wfc.org) and the World Chiropractic Alliance, a chiropractic medicine organization primarily advocating for spinal manipulation (worldchiropracticalliance.org). Chiropractic medical education is overseen by the Councils on Chiropractic Education International, but each country regulates their educational and licensing requirements. In the United States, this is the Council on Chiropractic Education (cce-usa.org).

Information on integration of conventional medicine and lifestyle can be obtained from the Institute for Lifestyle Medicine (instituteoflifestylemedicine.org).

Acknowledgments

So many people deserve thanks for assisting with this work that it would take another book to acknowledge them.

I need to start with my wife, Susan, who let me tell her story of multiple cancer survivals, including the most recent. She keeps me connected to the spirit. She is also my first editor and best critic!

Our children are now my teachers. Our son, Chris, and daughter-in-law, Marzia, and their beautiful child, show me how to thrive. Our daughter Maeba is always taking me deeper into life, and our other daughter Emily "E. J." shows me how to always love learning. Thanks to you all.

My father, Henry, and mother, Joan, still show me their wisdom. I hope I have transmitted a bit of that through this book.

The insights in this book would not have happened without the friendship and long-standing support of Henry and Susan Samueli. Their vision for evidence-based, integrative health has been steadfast. I am confident their impact has only begun. Thanks also to Mike Schulman, who leads the Samueli office, and Gerald Solomon, who heads the Samueli Foundation.

My colleague and coworker Doug Cavarocchi saw the value of this book long before I did and made it happen. He found our agent, Jim Levine, who has been instrumental in molding its message and contributing his passion and expertise continuously. He also found our publisher, Lorena Jones, who has taken a gamble on this vision of the future of health care. She and her team understand the urgency of the message and necessity for its widespread distribution. My co worker Jennifer Dorr helped write the practical appendices and continues to contribute to my website (DrWayneJonas.com). Thanks also to Lexie Robinson, who has supported the production at every turn.

My former colleagues at Samueli Institute have helped shape the movement from health care to health. Joan Walter is a get-it-done professional with tremendous integrity and commitment to healing. Ron Chez taught me how to take healing into the mainstream. John Ives brought insights to

Acknowledgments

the science. Thanks also to Kevin Berry, Bonnie Sakallaris, Mac Beckner, Katherine Smith, Dawn Bellanti, Barbara Findley, Alex York, Shamini Jain, Raheleh Khorsan, Kelly Gourdin, Linda Honig, Viviane Enslein, Courtney Lee, Chris Baur, Brian Thiel, and David Eisenberg, who all still carry the work of healing forward in research, action, and writing. A special call-out to Cindy Crawford, who learned evidence-based medicine from me and then took it to the new heights used in this book and elsewhere.

There are many leaders in health care, research, health policy, and practice from whom I have learned and drawn on for this book. A heartfelt thanks to Daniel Amen, Cathy Baase, Brent Bauer, Berkeley and Elinor Bedell, Iris Bell, Brian and Susan Berman, Herb Benson, Don Berwick, Clem Bezold, Keith Block, Robert Bonakdar, Josie Briggs, Ed Calabrese, Barrie Cassileth, Richard Carmona, Vint Cerf, Bill Chatfield, Margaret Chesney, Christine Choate, Deepak Chopra, Gail Christopher, Luana Colloca, Ian Coulter, Regan Crump, Jonathan Davidson, Larry and Barbie Dossey, Bob Duggan, Howard Federoff, Mimi Guarneri, Tracy Gaudet, Mary Guerrera, Paul Funk, Jeff Geller, Bill and Penny George, Jim Giordano, Andrea Gordon, Jim Gordon, Stephen Groft, Patrick Hanaway, Adi Haramati, Larry Hardaway, Tom Harkin, Mark Hyman, Kurt and Lori Henry, George Isham, Charlotte Rose Kerr, Ruth Kirschstein, Ben Kligler, Fredi Kronenberg, David Jones, Sam Jones, Kathi Kemper, Mary Jo Kreitzer, Linnea Larson, Jeff Levi, George Lewith, Klaus Linde, Michael Lerner, Victoria Maizes, Shaista Malik, Robert Marsten, Barbara Mikulski, Will Miller, Jim Moran, Mike and Deb Mullen, Richard Neimtzow, Bill Novelli, Fran O'Connor, Dean Ornish, Mehmet Oz, Jonathan Peck, Joe Pizzorno, Bill and Frances Purkert, David Rakel, Henri Roca, Stefan Schmidt, Stephen Schmidt, Eric and Audrey Schoomaker, Eric and Patty Shinseki, Esther Sternberg, Soma Stout, Gene Thin Elk, John Umhau, Harald Walach, John Weeks, Andy Weil, Jeffrey White, David Williams, Jim Zimble, and many others. Thanks also to the people of the Bayview Marriott in Newport Beach, California, where about half of this book was written.

And, finally, thanks to all my patients. You are the true healers. When we sit together and see together, we all heal together.

Index

Academic Collaborative for Integrative Health (ACIH), 249

Academic Consortium for Integrative Medicine and Health, 246

Active listening, 286

Acupuncture, 7, 14, 20–21, 23, 34, 177, 222–224, 226, 251

Ader, Robert, 180

Adverse childhood experiences (ACE), 138–39

Alcohol, 264

Amen, Daniel, 223

American College of Lifestyle Medicine (ACLM), 249

American College of Physicians, 38

Amygdala, 100

Ankylosing spondylitis (AK), 49–52

Antiarrhythmic drugs, 12–13

Antonovsky, Aaron, 218, 260

Anxiety, 281

Appointments
  making the most of, 257, 284
  reducing anxiety during, 272

Aromatherapy, 271–72

Arthritis, 5–6, 17–18, 75–76, 156

Astrology, 186–88

Autoimmune diseases, 180, 182

Ayurveda, 42–48, 83–86, 89, 127

Ayyadurai, V. A. Shiva, 89

Back pain, 19–21, 30–39, 81–83, 165

Bauer, Brent, 248

Beauty Way ceremony, 159–60, 195

Bedroom, 111, 271–72

Beecher, Henry, 22

Behavioral dimension, 108, 126, 261, 263–64, 265–66

Behavior and lifestyle
  changing, 116–17, 118, 136–38, 274–75, 282–83
  childhood experiences and, 138–39
  disease and, 117–18
  healthy, 113, 120, 125–27
  importance of, 108, 113
  meaning and, 136–39
  monitoring, 141–42
  placebo effect and, 122–23

Belief
  doctor's, 174
  importance of, 17–18, 180
  nocebo effect and, 185–88

Belly breathing, 282

Benedetti, Fabrizio, 26, 27, 33, 80, 185

Benson, Herbert, 84, 121

Berwick, Don, 160, 230

Bland, Jeffrey, 247
Bobrow, Joseph, 157
Boundaries, setting, 288–89
Brain injury, 8–12, 29, 78–81,
223–25
Bravewell Collaborative, 246
Breast cancer, 93–99, 136–39,
162–65, 192
Breathing, 282
Buettner, Dan, 232
Building Healthy Military
Communities program, 130
Burnout, 196–97

Cacioppo, John, 151, 152
CAMbrella, 250
Cancer, 93–99, 117, 136–39,
162–65, 192, 198
Car rides, 272
Casey, Michael, 248
Center for Integrative Medicine,
246–47
Center for Medicare and Medicaid
Innovation, 230
Center for Spirituality and Healing
(CSH), 248
Chaplaincy, 192–95
Chemotherapy, 97–98, 169, 236
Chen, Yu, 51
Christakis, Nicholas, 150
Cimetidine, 181
Cleveland Clinic, 247–48
Clinical pastoral education (CPE), 193
Collaborative medicine, 108
Color, effects of, 271–72
Coma, waking up from, 198–99
Communication
importance of, 285
tips for, 286–87

Complementary and alternative
medicine (CAM), 228, 244–45,
264
Conditioning, 76, 123, 180
Congestive heart failure (CHF), 146–47
Coulter, Ian, 150, 245
Cousins, Norman, 49, 51–52
Crossing the Quality Chasm, 229, 230
Crum, Alia, 122, 176, 294
Curing vs. healing, 32–33
Cytochrome c, 154

DASH (Dietary Approaches to Stop
Hypertension) diet, 211, 212
Davidson, Jonathan, 58–59, 60
Death
causes of, 117
meaning response and, 186–87
palliative care and, 198–200
Decline effect, 60–61
Depression, 53–59, 62, 177
Diabetes, 15, 114–17, 118, 134
Diabetes Prevention Study, 115
Disease
chronic, 74, 215, 227
-focused approach, 71
from whole systems science
perspective, 69–70
Doctors. See Physicians
Dopamine, 41, 45–46, 47, 48, 120
Doshas, 44–45, 206
Dossey, Larry, 203–4
Drugs
efficacy of, 15
frequent dosing, 76–77
meaning and, 180–81
side effects of, 34, 62–63
testing of, 57, 60–61, 64
use of, 264

See also individual drugs
Dzau, Victor, 215

Eating
  effects of, 87
  mindfully, 276
  patterns, 122, 278
  reasons for, 275
  See also Fasting; Food
Eisenberg, David, 227
Emotional connections, importance
  of, 156–58
Emotions
  sharing, 156–58
  venting, 288
Entropy, 258
Environment
  ideal, 110
  importance of, 92, 99–101, 264,
    270
  setting self-care goals for, 273
  tips for, 270–73
  See also Healing environments
Epidaurus, 127, 159, 188
Errors, medical, 12, 241, 242
European Society of Integrative
  Medicine (ESIM), 246
Exceptional spiritual experiences,
  157–58, 178–79
Exercise
  benefits of, 75, 123, 263, 279
  mind-set and, 123
  research on, 121
  tips for, 279
Exposure therapy, 157
External dimension, 108, 109, 261,
  264, 266

Family Empowerment program, 131

Fast food, 133
Fasting, 86–87
Fear, 143–44
Feng shui, 109
Fernandopulle, Rushika, 232–34
Fibromyalgia, 165–67
Fight, flight, or freeze response,
  100, 143
Flexner Report, 216
Followers vs. leaders, 290
Food
  building positive relationship
    with, 276
  fast, 133
  as fuel, 276–77
  journal, 277
  labeling, 124
  management, 264
  meal planning, 278–79
  meaning response and, 123–25
  military and, 132–35
  See also Eating
Forgiveness, 282
Fowler, James, 150
Frank, Jerome, 75
Franklin, Benjamin, 17

Gaudet, Tracy, 250
Gawande, Atul, 200
Geller, Jeffery, 167–68
Gelsemium, 55–56
Ghrelin, 124
Goals, setting, 287–88, 290
Gottlieb, Kathleen, 161
Gratitude, 280–81
Great Wall Hospital, 49–51, 109
Grief, 149, 161
Guarneri, Mimi, 177, 179

Hands, laying on of, 155, 198, 203
Healing
  bringing, into health care, 140–42
  curing vs., 31–33
  dimensions of, 261, 262–64
  etymology of, 47
  fear and, 143–44
  -focused approach, 72
  fostering culture of, 289–90
  groups and organizations, 107, 289
  intention, 107, 291
  joy and, 139–41
  love and, 143–44
  meaning response and, 71–74
  paradox of, 1–15
  physical presence and, 152–55
  principles of, 89–90
  through purpose, 234–36
  relationships and, 107
  rituals and, 23–26, 28, 37, 53
  spiritual, 202–4
  unexplained, 198–201
  wholeness and, 46–47
Healing environments
  examples of, 92
  home as, 270–71
  hospitals as, 101–2
  optimal, 102, 106–8
Healing journey
  guidelines for, 268–95
  reviewing, 295–96
  starting, 268–70
Healing touch, 178, 198
Health, definition of, 228
Health care system, structure of, 240–43
Healthy Base Initiative, 130–31, 250
Healthy Kitchen, Healthy Lives, 131

Heart disease, 63, 117, 131–32, 144–45, 146, 151, 152
Hensrud, Don, 248
Herbal remedies, 14
High blood pressure. See Hypertension
Hippocampus, 100
Hippocrates, 127, 159, 188
Hodgkinson, Gerard, 202
Home, as healing environment, 108, 270–71
Homeopathy, 14, 17, 55
Hope, false vs. true, 9
HOPE consultation
  asking for, 257
  benefits of, 262
  example of, 219–24
  factors explored by, 258
  followup after, 266–67
  goal of, 235, 261
  healing dimensions and, 221, 261, 262–64
  sample questions for, 221–22, 265–66
HOPE note, 261, 262, 266
Horoho, Patty, 250
Hospitals, 101–2, 106, 108, 272
Hufford, David, 179
Hyman, Mark, 248
Hyperbaric oxygen (HBO) therapy, 10–12, 28, 78–80
Hypericin, 57
Hypertension, 15, 134, 177, 210–12, 214

"I" messages, 287
Indian Health Service (IHS), 160, 161
Infrared radiation, 154
Inner dimension, 107, 261, 262, 265

Inner guidance, trusting, 295

Institute for Functional Medicine (IFM), 248

Institute for Healthcare Improvement, 215, 230

Institute for Integrative Health and Wellness, 248

Institute for Lifestyle Medicine, 249

Institute of Medicine, 242

Integrative health
  accessing, 283–84
  definition of, 141, 283
  gap closed by, 226
  need for, 214–16
  trend toward, 229–31, 243–52

Integrative medicine
  definition of, 227
  history of, 227
  physicians' responsibilities in, 255–57

International Society for Complementary Medicine Research (ISCMR), 246

Interpersonal dimension, 107, 261, 263, 265, 285

Intuition, 201–3

Ioannidis, John, 60, 203

Iora, 233–34

Isolation, 151

Jain, Shamini, 177

Journaling, 35, 269–70, 277

Joy
  healing and, 140–41
  making time for, 280–81

Kaptchuk, Ted J., 23–26, 33

Katz, David, 249

Kaufman, William, 5, 76

King, Rauni, 177

Kligler, Ben, 250

Koenig, Harold, 190

Kreitzer, Mary Jo, 248

Laughter therapy, 49, 52

Leaders vs. followers, 289

Learning Circles, 161–62

Legend, John, 99

Lifestyle. *See* Behavior and lifestyle

Lifestyle medicine, definition of, 227

Light, 102, 272

Listening
  active, 286
  circles, 161

Loneliness, 151–52, 166–68

Loss
  exceptional experiences after, 157–58
  facing, 149

Louv, Richard, 106

Love
  control and, 143
  focusing on, 281
  healing and, 143–44
  loss and, 149–52
  power of, 144–49, 152

Maizes, Victoria, 247

Massage, 38, 85–86

Mattson, Mark, 87, 121

Mayo Clinic, 231, 248

McClellan, Mark, 215

McGinnis, Michael, 215

Meal planning, 278–79

Meaning
  constructing, 172
  erosion of, 197
  influence of, on effect, 180–81

Meaning response
  death and, 186–87
  definition of, 71–72
  food and, 123–25
  individualized healing journey
    and, 72
  size of, 61
Meditation, 282. *See also*
  Mindfulness
Mediterranean diet, 122, 124
Mesmer, Anton, 17
Metabolically Optimized Brain, 131
Metzl, Jordan D., 121
Mind
  -body practices, 293–94
  brain and, 224
  collective nature of, 182–84, 186,
    195
  of God, 201
  -set, role of, 122–23, 176–77, 187
Mindfulness, 84, 225, 276, 294
Miracles, 198–201
Moerman, Dan, 22, 29, 33, 181
Morphine, 185
Moxa, 3
Mukherjee, Siddhartha, 63
Mullen, Mike, 130, 249
Murphy, Michael, 198
Music therapy, 78

National Academy of Medicine, 215,
  229, 246
Nature
  connecting with, 272–73
  exposure to, 102, 106, 109–10
Navajo, 159
Niacinamide, 5–7, 18, 76
Nicotine, 264
Nightingale, Florence, 109

NIH (National Institutes of Health),
  14, 49, 57, 58, 59, 73, 140
Nocebo response, 16, 185–88
Nouwen, Henry, 192
Nuka System of Care, 160, 162, 232
Number needed to treat (NNT), 77
Nurses, burnout of, 196–97
Nutrition, 264

Obesity, 133–35
OHEs (optimal healing
  environments)
  benefits of, 102, 106
  definition of, 106
  domains of, 107–8
Olness, Karen, 182
Operation Live Well, 130
Ordovás, José, 124, 125
Ornish, Dean, 231

Padimadi, Manu, 44–48, 68, 84, 86,
  183, 188, 251
Pain
  back, 19–21, 30–39, 81–83, 165
  chronic, 24, 39, 177, 213, 220–21
  drugs for, 15, 185
  nocebo effect and, 185
Palliative care, 199–200
Parkinson's disease, 41–43, 45–47,
  48, 83–88, 126, 188
Pathogenesis, 218, 260
Patient Centered Medical Home
  model, 229, 230
Pennebaker, James, 37, 156
Persuasion and Healing, 75
Peterson Foundation, 230
PET (positron emission
  tomography) scanning, 223–24
Phillips, David, 186

Phillips, Edward, 249
Physicians
    burnout of, 196–97
    impact of beliefs of, 174–75
    integrative medicine and, 255–57
    relationship with, 252–55, 256
    role of, in health care system,
        240–42
    selecting, 253
    See also Appointments
Phytoncides, 110
Pizzorno, Joe, 265
Placebo response
    context and, 22–24
    examples of, 6, 12, 16–21
    importance of, 16
    magnitude of, 26–27
    nocebo effect and, 186
    prevalence of, 7, 22
    renaming, 29, 61
    rituals and, 23–26, 28
    underlying mechanisms of, 29
    variability of, 22–24
    See also Meaning response
Pneumonia, 174–76
Positive thinking, 294
Prayer, 174–75, 203–4, 238
Precision Medicine Initiative (PMI),
    73, 140
Prevention
    focusing on, 129, 283
    treatment vs., 127–29
Price, David D., 74, 184, 185
Priestley, Joseph, 216
Procrastination, 274
PTSD, 8, 9, 78–81, 157, 177–78,
    179, 191, 198
Puchalski, Christina, 193
Purpose, healing through, 234–36

Randomized controlled trials
    (RCTs), 216, 228–29
Ranitidine, 181
Regression to the mean, 176
Relationship-centered care, 161–65
Relationships
    boundaries and, 288–89
    communication and, 285–87
    healing and, 107
    importance of, 285
    improving, 285–90
Relaxation response, 84, 122, 153,
    253
Religious practices, impact of,
    189–92
Reston, James, 177
Retreats, therapeutic, 157
Rice Diet for Hypertension, 212
Rief, Winfried, 186
Rituals
    creating individualized, 37
    effects of, 23–26, 28, 53, 74
    nocebo effect and, 185–88
Rockefeller, Laurance S., 202

Salutogenesis, 218, 260
Samueli, Susan and Henry, 247
Samueli Institute, 11, 12, 14, 106,
    130–31, 215
Sattvic mind, 84
Schoomaker, Eric, 250
Schweitzer, Marc, 105
Science
    limitations of reductionist, 40–41,
        63–64, 66, 207–8
    whole systems, 67–71, 73, 89–90,
        121, 141
Self-awareness, building, 291
Self-story, importance of, 291–92

Self-talk, 294
Selye, Hans, 187
Serotonin, 57, 119, 163
Shinrin-yoku, 110
Shirodhara, 86
Side effects, 34, 35, 62–63, 186
Siegel, Daniel, 182
Sleep
  benefits of, 263–64
  problems, 280
  tips for, 280
Smoking, 118–20
SOAP (subjective, objective,
    assessment, and plan) notes,
    216–19, 260, 262
Social support, 151, 158
Society for Integrative Oncology
    (SIO), 137
Society for Interdisciplinary Placebo
    Science (SIPS), 26
Soul loss, 191, 201
Sounds, 271–72
Southcentral Foundation (SCF),
    160–62
Spiritual healing, 202–4
Spirituality, discussing, 193
Spiritual practices, impact of,
    189–92
Spiritual self, nourishing, 282
SSRIs (selective serotonin reuptake
    inhibitors), 54, 57, 62
Starvation, periodic, 86–87
Statin drugs, 63
Sternberg, Esther, 100
Sthapatya ved, 109
St. John's wort, 55–62
Strecher, Victor, 235
Stress management
  approaches to, 121–22

  benefits of, 263
  meaning and, 187
  tips for, 282
Suggestibility, 18–19
Supplements, 14
Surgery
  efficacy of, 7, 15, 82
  fake, 7
  ritual of, 31
Systematic reviews, 12

TCM (traditional Chinese
    medicine), 251–52
Technology, 241
Temel, Jennifer, 200
Temple, Bob, 57
Thomas, K. B., 183, 185, 186
Topol, Eric, 141
Total Force Fitness, 129–31, 135,
    249
Toxins, environmental, 264
Trauma, 36–37, 161, 179, 191
Travel, 272
Triple Aim, 230, 234
Tui na, 50

Ulcers, 15, 181
Ulrich, Roger, 101–2
University of Arizona, 246–47
University of California, Irvine
    (UCI), 247
University of Minnesota, 248
U.S. Army, 129–31

Vagus nerve, 153
Veterans Health Administration
    (VHA), 248, 249
Visualization, 177–78

*Vital Directions for Health and Health
      Care*, 215
Vitamin C, 49, 52

Walter Reed Army Institute of
      Research, 14, 154
Water, 278
Weight, 134–35, 264, 277
Weil, Andrew, 247
Wellbeing in the Nation (WIN)
      plan, 215–16
WHO (World Health
      Organization), 14, 49, 228, 244,
      251
Wholeness, personal, 45, 46–47,
      68–69, 107, 293
Whole systems science, 67–71,
      73–74, 89–90, 121, 141
"Wounded healer," 191–92

Yoga, 38, 85

6/21 ART £2

Ency
of m
architecture

San I Cassels 2

Edited by   Wolfgang Pehnt

Contributors   Kyösti Alander, Helsinki
Reyner Banham, London
Maurice Besset, Paris
Peter Blake, New York
Max Cetto, Mexico City
G. F. Chadwick, Hale Barns, Cheshire
Alexandre Cirici-Pellicer, Barcelona
Robert L. Delevoy, Brussels
Tobias Faber, Copenhagen
Giuseppe Giordanino, Turin
Vittorio Gregotti, Novara
Henry-Russell Hitchcock, Northampton, Mass.
Hubert Hoffmann, Graz
John M. Jacobus Jr., Berkeley, Calif.
Jürgen Joedicke, Stuttgart
William H. Jordy, Providence, R.I.
Shinji Koike, Tokio
Björn Linn, Bromma
Harold Meek, Belfast
Henrique E. Mindlin, Rio de Janeiro
Leonardo Mosso, Turin
Herbert Ohl, Ulm
Margit Staber, Zurich
Klaus-Jakob Thiele, Berlin
Mark Hartland Thomas, Sittingbourne, Kent
Giuseppe Varaldo, Turin
Giulia Veronesi, Milan
J. J. Vriend, Amsterdam
Arnold Whittick, Crawley, Sussex
Gian Pio Zuccotti, Turin

Encyclopaedia
of modern
architecture

General editor: Gerd Hatje

446 illustrations

Thames and Hudson London

Translations from the German
by Irene and Harold Meek
from the French, Spanish and Italian
by Harold Meek
from the Danish by G. D. Liversage
from the Dutch by E. van Daalen

Asterisks preceding names in the text indicate that separate entries devoted to them appear elsewhere in the book.

Originally published as
Knaurs lexikon der modernen architektur
© Droemersche Verlagsanstalt Th. Knaur Nachf.
Munich and Zurich 1963
This edition © Thames and Hudson London 1963
Reprinted 1971
Printed by Jarrold and Sons Limited, Norwich

ISBN 0 500 18025 3 Cloth bound
ISBN 0 500 20023 8 Paper bound

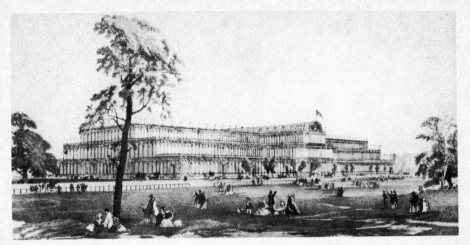

Joseph Paxton. Crystal Palace. London, 1851

Introduction

In the year 1850, Prince Albert delivered a remarkable speech at a banquet for the chief magistrates of the City of London. His Royal Highness attempted to secure the support of the representatives of this thriving metropolis for his pet scheme for a Great International Exhibition; and the plan he unfolded testified to no mean optimism: 'Nobody who has paid any attention to the peculiar features of our present era will doubt for a moment that we are living at a period of most wonderful transition, which tends rapidly to accomplish that great end, to which indeed, all history points—the realization of the unity of mankind. . . .' Distances between continents were vanishing, scholarship and knowledge were becoming common property, and the products of all nations were available to the citizens to choose from. Gratitude to the Almighty would overwhelm the viewer of this vast exhibition, concluded the Prince.

As amazing as the exhibition itself, the first ever of such proportions, was the building in which it was housed: Joseph *Paxton's Crystal Palace. This huge building, erected in the breathtakingly short period of nine months, seized on the imagination of its contemporaries as did few structures of the 19th century before the Eiffel Tower. The delicate filigree of the metalwork, filled in by glass panes, the immensity of the boundless interior, and

the transparency and weightlessness of the walls seemed to the public of the day to herald the arrival of a new style—unless, like Ruskin, they were of the opinion that the Crystal Palace was a greenhouse like others, only larger. Glass and iron were the building materials which made a new aesthetic conception of architecture possible. It was not these materials that were new. The tradition of iron construction went back to the 18th century and had already produced some excellent schemes in the first half of the century. After all, the prize-winning competition design for the Crystal Palace by Hector Horeau, which was not actually used, also envisaged a light iron structure. But the conquest of this vast space by a seemingly insubstantial and unreal tracery of walls and the apparent merging of interior and exterior were new. Contemporary prints prefer to show an interior partly suffused by sunlight and yet shaded in turn by clouds, a hazy light that seems to abolish the limitations of space. New, too, was the impression of a labyrinth without narrowness and weight, similar to the three-dimensional openwork effect of the Eiffel Tower's steel frame three decades later.

The Crystal Palace was no bolt from the blue. As early as 1832, the French social reformer and sectarian Barthélemy Prosper Enfantin unfolded the vision of a new architecture which assigns a principal rôle

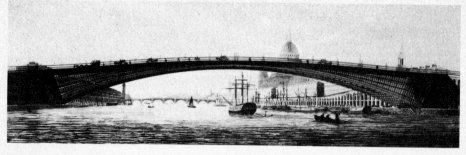

Thomas Telford. Design for a bridge over the Thames. London, 1801

to iron, compares parts of the structure with the molecular composition of the body, and speaks of the 'open form' of such an architecture of the future. The 'metallurgical architecture' demanded by an only recently rediscovered architectural theorist, William Vose Pickett, in a book published in 1845 seems to have anticipated modern architecture with its framed and suspended structures and its *brise-soleil*. Paxton's Crystal Palace was not such an unqualified

William Le Baron Jenney. Home Insurance Building. Chicago, 1883–5

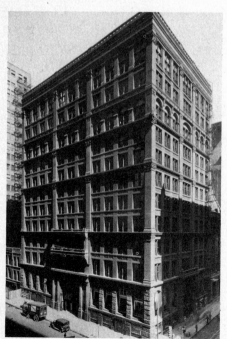

success because it surprised and amazed its generation but because it had fulfilled their secret hopes and ambitions.

Architectural historians have investigated the 19th century for its pioneer works such as the Crystal Palace, and have long seen in these undoubtedly bold achievements the first steps towards modern architecture. They have pointed to early examples of bridge-building, cast- and wrought-iron vaulting and suspension and girder type bridges, which were already achieving astonishing spans in England and North America. In high structures there were buildings that combined load-bearing masonry and iron frames. The aesthetic charm that emanates from such factory and warehouse buildings with their heavy, solid outer walls and light, internal columns of iron may not have been obvious to contemporaries, but buildings to which the public had access such as Henri *Labrouste's Sainte-Geneviève Library in Paris (1843–50) already display it. American firms were experimenting with façades made up of prefabricated cast-iron units as early as the middle of the century, and these permitted extensive penetration of the outer walls too.

But materials alone do not create a new style. A new style is born only when an individual genius such as Paxton or Eiffel or an ambitious group such as the architects of the so-called *Chicago School after 1880, adopt the new building materials. *Burnham, *Root and *Sullivan arrived at their imposing, clear and withal lively designs for multi-storey buildings, not, in the first place, thanks to the new system of framed structures, but mainly due to their notions of style derived from the great *Richardson. William Le Baron *Jenney did not know himself that he had created the first steel-frame structure with his Home Insurance Building (1883–5)—that was only discovered when it was later pulled down; and one of the main examples of this school, the Monadnock Building (1889–91) is structurally a traditional solid masonry building. The Chicago School was a special case; it did not found a tradition. Until the advent of the department stores around 1900, the new steel structures were hardly noticeable in the townscape; the façades of the city stations only rarely betrayed the bold lines of the halls hidden beyond the entrance lobbies. Reinforced concrete structures became aesthetically attractive only in the new century, although the effective patents were taken out in the sixties of the 19th century. Despite the Crystal Palace, despite the Machinery Hall and the Eiffel Tower of the World Exhibition of 1889, the type of architecture in which the taste of the age was expressed did not make use of the new opportunities. The Paris Opera by Charles Garnier (1861–74) was more a symptom of its times than the elliptical exhibition galleries (1867) of Frédéric Le Play.

If Prince Albert in his speech before the city fathers praised the availability of all the world's merchandise, his generation exercised this sovereignty with regard to history. The 19th century was the century of stylistic imitations. The boundless availability of forms, which history had taken several thousand years to develop, was at the ready disposal of this well-informed century. The reversion to a distant past had in the first instance a concrete significance. The memory of Greek forms was a memory of classicism, Greek intellect, simplicity, nobility and greatness. Behind the protagonists of the Gothic Revival, too, there were ideas other than simply the reawakening of dead history, for most European countries connected reminiscences of their first national glory with the Gothic epoch. Disregarding the fact that English and German Gothic were unthinkable without Saint-Denis and Chartres, neo-Gothic buildings like the Houses of Parliament in London (1840–65) and the reconstructed Cologne Cathedral became memorials to a national consciousness which had grown stronger during the romantic age. Karl Friedrich von *Schinkel's design for a Prussian national

Ferdinand Dutert and Contamin. Machinery Hall at the International Exhibition. Paris, 1889

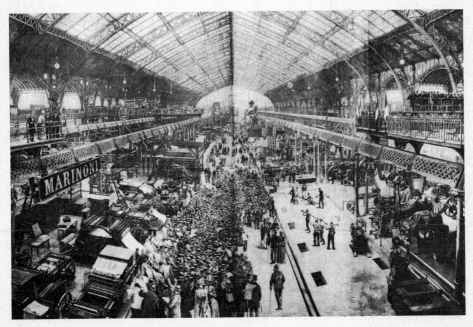

cathedral, of course, is in the most romantic fairy-tale Gothic.

Such arguments did not apply to the attempts to revive the other styles. The town became a populated museum, a permanent exhibition. The great architects of the century already built in heterogeneous styles. John *Nash was not only responsible for magnificent Ionic columns but also for the bizarre effects of the Brighton Pavilion (1815–23) with its oriental trappings.

John Nash. Brighton Pavilion, 1815–23

John Nash and James Thomson. Cumberland Terrace, Regents Park. London, 1826–7

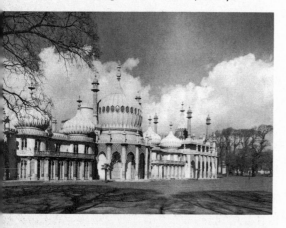

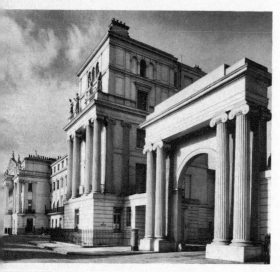

Schinkel supplied Gothic and Renaissance schemes to choose from for his Werdersche Church in Berlin (built from 1825 to 1831). Eventually not only were alternative proposals such as these possible, but even the combination of different styles in the same building. Friedrich Schmidt, architect of the Vienna Town Hall (started 1872) declared in reply to the question whether the building was conceived more in the Gothic or the Renaissance vein: 'It is the accomplishment of an artist who has absorbed the architecture of past centuries.' The 'cold synthesis', in which the elements do not merge but remain separate and recognizable with their different origins, became the ideal. It was typical of the arrogance of the age to force successive periods to exist side by side.

The 19th century not only had styles, it had a style—*its* style. Development may appear to have resolved itself into an endless reprise of architectural fashions, but in reality this carnival of imitation followed consistent rules. The 18th century bequeathed its successors an architecture that loved large stereometric buildings, used decoration with restraint and tried to preserve continuity of surfaces. The classical motifs of column, entablature and arch were set off by plain wall surfaces or confronted by them. The pillars on John *Soane's Bank of England (1803) look like cut-out vertical wall panels. On twin-tower façades of churches (The Ludwigskirche in Munich by Friedrich von Gärtner, 1829–40; Saint-Vincent-de-Paul, Paris, 1824–44, by Lepère and Hittorff) the individual towers remain tied in by surface continuity and only appear as separate parts of the building in the upper storeys.

The historic styles employed by architects at this time were interpreted in this sense. Klenze and his contemporaries at Munich at the time of Ludwig I built Renaissance palaces in the new Ludwigsviertel part of the town, but they took as their model the Early Florentine Renaissance, not the Roman High Renaissance with its strongly accentuated wall relief. And Gothic examples fascinated them not primarily by their spatial interpenetration. A late building by Schinkel, the neo-Gothic castle of Kamenz in Silesia (1838–65) still shows an unsurpassed refinement in its treatment of wall surfaces. The unpierced walls make up a sculptural whole—the purer and more

severe in style the earlier the masters are of
this romantic classicism. It was not without reason that the twenties and early
thirties of this century, with their inclina-
tion to stereometric form, discovered an
affinity with Ledoux, Boullée, Durand,
Sobre, Lequeu, Soane, Gilly, Weinbrenner,
Haller von Hallerstein and partly even
with Schinkel! It is significant that a
book by Emil Kaufmann which came
out in 1933 was called *From Ledoux to Le
Corbusier.*

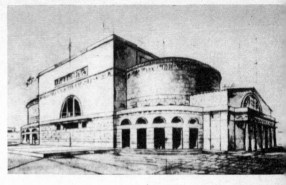

As the century progressed, so did the tendency to carve up surfaces. Architecture
became picturesque. Clearly defined massing gave way to something that looked as
if it had been nibbled at from outside, and
plebeian wealth replaced noble poverty.
Details that were formerly precise and
clearly legible became clumsy, complicated
and restless, and could only be understood
as part of the whole building—and sometimes not even then. Picturesque arrange-
ments took over from the—still valid—
symmetrical plan. A large structure was
now subdivided into so many main and
subsidiary parts that the orderly effect of
symmetry, especially as seen from a narrow
street, was considerably weakened. What
applies to the exterior also applies to the
inside. Niches and bays hived off the draw-
ing-rooms to conform with late-bourgeois
notions of comfort and ease. If multiplicity
of forms was a tacit demand, then the mixture of heterogeneous forms was its consequence. At the beginning of the 19th
century architects selected their models
from the stylistic conceptions of their time.

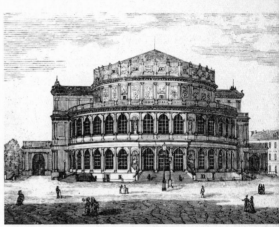

In the second half of the century anything
goes: distinguished antique, heavy Romanesque, riven Gothic, opulent Renaissance
and, finally, Baroque, whose hour struck
only when the plastic treatment and spatial
exploitation of the walls had sufficiently
progressed.
In the field of town planning 19th-century
architecture failed almost completely. The
romantic classicism prevalent around 1800
already had a tendency to break down the
walls of the 'place' and isolate buildings
that were of any significance in the design
of the town. Open space was no longer

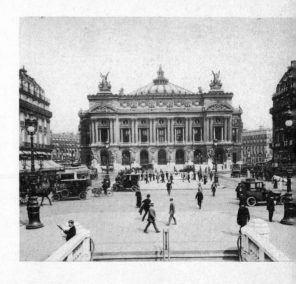

Friedrich Gilly. Theatre. Berlin, 1800. Project

Gottfried Semper. Opera House. Dresden, 1837–41

Charles Garnier. Opera House. Paris, 1861–74

considered as a positive shape, a spatial concept, which created its own limits as it
were, in the way the Baroque squares had
done so admirably. Open space was now
an element pressing in from an undefined
distance, which was framed by architectural
shapes, but was not moulded by them.

The transition to such town planning layouts was an early development. Already
the Place de la Concorde in Paris (since
1753) is no longer formed by its peripheral
buildings, by its architectural frame, but
is open in several directions. A generously
proportioned plan like that by Ludwig
Förster for the Vienna Ringstrasse (1857–
8)—the highest level of spatial luxury that
town planning afforded itself in this economical century—strings together a series
of open spaces and groups of buildings.
The open spaces are arranged axially about
each part of the polygonal *Ring*-Strasse,
but are not in any relationship to each other,

nor do they set each other off. Undefined
open space surrounds the prominent buildings, which are grouped as though at an
exhibition. This scheme, dismantled ram-
parts done up as boulevards with prestige
buildings strung out alongside, was a customary town-planning recipe of the 19th
century and in line with the contemporary
need for display. More rigorous measures,
such as the breaches driven by Baron
Haussmann at the time of Napoleon III
through the chaos that was Paris, are
among the few effective solutions. These
sanitary measures, however, did not develop any new conception of town life, and
behind the new façades everything remained the same. The outer peripheries of
the towns were completely left to look
after themselves and spread along the
traffic arteries.

The rapid growth of cities was the worst
problem. In 1860, the USA had nine

Ludwig Förster. Project for the Ringstrasse. Vienna, 1857–8

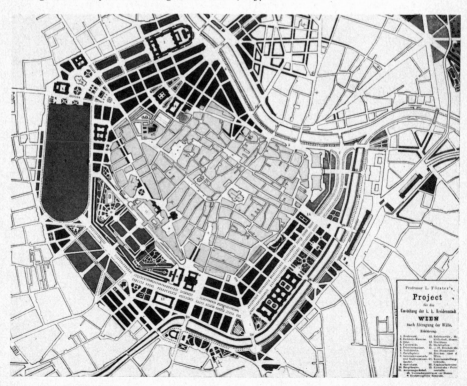

cities with more than 100,000 inhabitants; by 1910 there were fifty. London increased its size eightfold within a hundred and fifty years, Mannheim and Düsseldorf went up by more than fourfold in forty years, while Chicago doubled its size in a single decade from 1880 to 1890. Building regulations were restricted to a minimum. The Berlin by-laws allowed any height of building in streets over fifty feet wide and permitted back yards seventeen feet square! The old town centres had to assume the civic functions of vastly increased living conglomerations. The attention of architects was focused on the monumental buildings; for the decorative treatment of apartment house façades there existed pattern books. Structural engineers were kept fully occupied with the enormous task of maintaining the services for this mammoth organization. When the buildings they erected needed an architect's touch, details familiar from other types of edifice were employed to meet the new requirements as far as was practical. But for factories, abattoirs, power stations, market halls, and water towers the academies had no models.

The reaction to these circumstances, which was especially marked in England in the *Arts and Crafts movement, was as heroic as it was helpless. Especially as the understandable discontent with the industrial age often went together with an antagonism towards machinery and thus seemed to rule out in advance any hopes of far-reaching efficiency. The diagnosis was correct, the cure imperfect. The furniture, furnishing materials and wallpapers made by William *Morris in his workshops with the help of his Pre-Raphaelite friends were new and original creations which contrasted favourably with the stylistic imitations of the eclectics. But the era of the machine could only be successfully combated by the use of machinery—not without it. The distrust of the division of labour and the manufacturing methods of industry survived until late in the present century; it echoes still in the slogan of the early *Bauhaus days: 'Architects, sculptors, painters, we must all return to handicraft!'

A great change in attitude to the machine had by no means yet occurred around 1900 when enthusiasm for 'the beauty in the tremendous force of its vast but calm outlines' and 'the clean, smooth, polish of the machine' inspired progressive spirits.

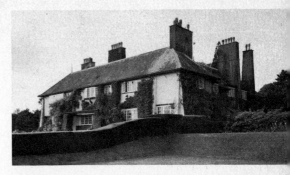

Charles Annesley Voysey. Perrycroft House. Colwall, 1893

Obrist and van de *Velde praised the 'wonderful fitness for purpose' of ocean liners, locomotives, and aeroplanes, and yet Obrist's embroideries and van de Velde's silver service were not intended for mass production by machinery but required the tools of a craftsman. *Le Corbusier, for example, talked of *prefabrication early on in his career, but when he called the house 'a machine for living in' he was not only thinking of the smooth functioning of these buildings but of the formal properties of the machine as well. What fascinated him in the motor-car to such an extent that he called his projects after motor-car marques, and what he tried to achieve in his houses, was not least the 'simple shell, which creates space for manifold organs'. The smooth and perfect shapes, the dynamic appearance and the sound of speed appealed to his aesthetic senses, which carefully selected the objects of his admiration. A typewriter or a sewing-machine with their visually complex mechanisms had to wait for the Surrealists before they were aesthetically acceptable. And it was but one step further from aesthetic appraisal to the recognition that the new and rational methods of construction, already long employed by structural engineers, were eminently compatible with 'great' architecture, the architecture of architects.

This step was not yet taken by the *Art Nouveau. But at least it combined the various tendencies towards a new architecture within a consistent style. Scant justice is done to the era between 1880 and 1910 when it is merely looked on as a transitional period to modern art and architecture, for within it lay the presuppositions of the

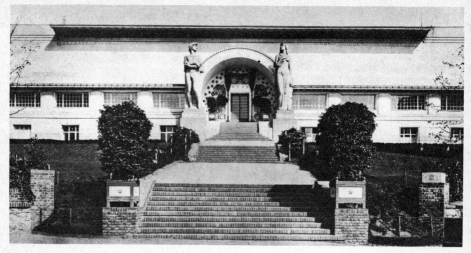

Joseph Olbrich. Ernst-Ludwig-Haus. Darmstadt, 1901

20th century. The awareness of what the functions of a house should be that characterized the pioneers of the Arts and Crafts movement, led to the epoch-making houses of *Voysey and *Mackintosh; parallel development in North America was due to the work of the young Frank Lloyd *Wright and a number of Californian architects. The elegant surface treatment which the anonymous London town house had preserved since the beginning of the 19th century entered into a fascinating combination with the idiosyncratic sense of proportion of the nineties (Ashbee, Godwin, *Shaw, Voysey). The cubic building fantasies of the time of Soane and the architects of the French Revolution were echoed in the Late Art Nouveau period, by Viennese practitioners in particular. Iron and glass, which structural engineers had boldly introduced into their designs time and again in the course of the century, were made to serve the new style's need for ornamental expression, and employed to perform tricks of decoration (*Horta, *Guimard).

But above all Art Nouveau starting from

Frank Lloyd Wright. Martin House. Buffalo, N.Y., 1904

Page 13. Antoni Gaudí. Casa Milà. Barcelona, 1905–10

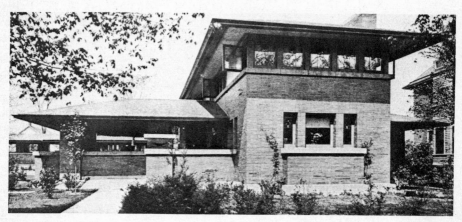

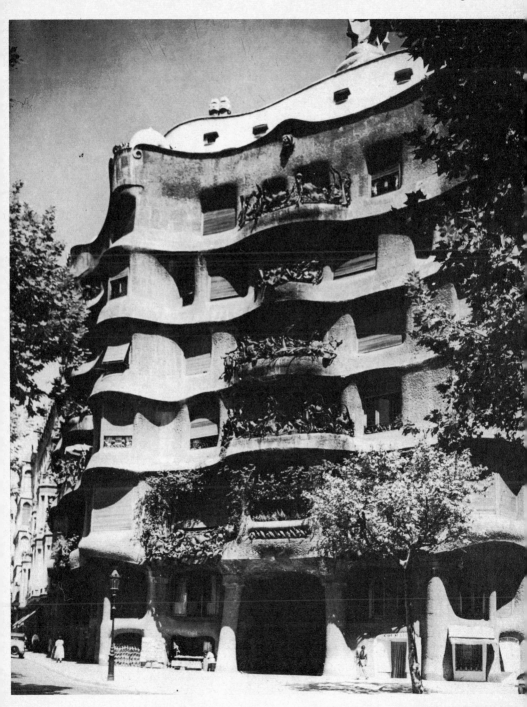

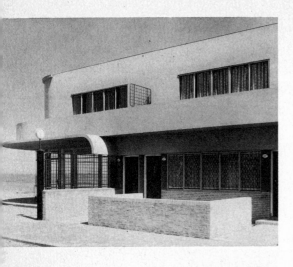

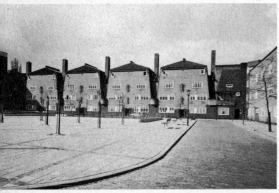

Jacobus Johannes Pieter Oud. Workers' housing.
Hook of Holland, 1924

Michael de Klerk. De Dageraad housing estate.
Amsterdam, 1920–2

mere surface decoration advanced to a fully
three-dimensional expression of architecture which formed a direct link with
*Expressionism. The transition from Art
Nouveau to Expressionism is everywhere
fluid. Expression was aimed at by both
movements, even if Expressionism hardly
took over the flowing contours and the
ostensibly soft masses of Art Nouveau,
with its manifold reminiscences of and
associations with the organic world of
nature. But the darkly menacing cubic
forms of Mackintosh's Glasgow School of
Art (1893–1909), the unadorned blocks of

Adolf *Loos, betraying so much of Art
Nouveau proportions, Rudolf Steiner's
Goetheanum at Dornach near Basle
(1925–8) or the phantasmagoria of Antoni
*Gaudí's late work can be interpreted both
as products of Art Nouveau and as manifestations of Expressionism.
It is much more difficult to find connections
between Expressionism and the style of the
twenties, although they were close and
manifold. Only in the *Netherlands was
the situation sharpened by controversy as
the School of *Amsterdam opposed the
Rotterdam Group. *Wendingen on the
one side, De *Stijl on the other; picturesque individual homes here and rows of
whitewashed disciplined houses there; pic-
turesque-plastic thinking as against fascination with objective form; this was the
sharply defined antithesis despite a common derivation from the forerunner of
modern Dutch architecture, Hendrik
Petrus *Berlage, and despite the great impact made by Frank Lloyd *Wright on both
*Wendingen and De Stijl.
But in Central Europe, the fronts overlapped, just as did Art Nouveau and Expressionism. Nearly every great architect of
the twenties went through an Expressionist
phase. Peter Behrens's Turbine Factory in
Berlin (1908–9), which is looked on as the
manifesto of functional architecture, has
massive corner piers, a huge cornice formed
by the side windows canting inwards, and
a heavy roof, features dictated by an urge
for Expressionism—not by structural necessity. The glazed façades of the factories
by Walter *Gropius have exerted a
revolutionary effect. They did not preclude
the fact that the model factory at the
Cologne Werkbund Exhibition of 1914 was
built on a strictly axial plan and confronts

Adolf Loos. Small house. 1923. Model

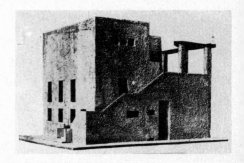

the viewer with a heavy Egyptian-type façade, properties that seem to be out of keeping with the modernity of the staircase towers. Bruno *Taut's pavilions at various exhibitions set out to demonstrate not so much the practicality as the poetic magic of the new building materials, steel and glass. The first *Bauhaus Manifesto is decorated with a woodcut by Lyonel Feininger, which idealizes the Gothic cathedral and expresses the affinity of the Bauhaus idea with the thinking of medieval building craftsmen—Expressionism of the purest water. In the years immediately after the First World War, when commissions were hard to come by, visionary drawings were made by numerous architects who later played a part in the Berlin association *Der Ring*, and these, together with those of *Sant'Elia are among the most beautiful architectural esquisses of our time. *Mies van der Rohe's glass-house projects with their poetic quality are a part of this trend no less than the avowed expressiveness of *Poelzig's space caverns and *Mendelsohn's architectural sculpture.

A new development in the twenties, which affected Expressionism as well, is the involvement of time in the experience of a

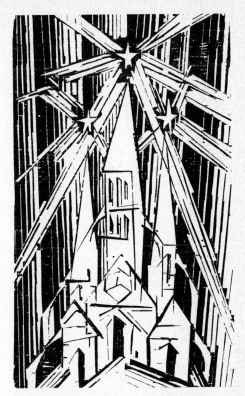

Lyonel Feininger. Woodcut from the first Bauhaus manifesto. 1919

Walter Gropius and Adolf Meyer. Model factory at the Werkbund Exhibition. Cologne, 1914

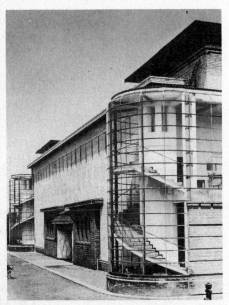

work of architecture. Three-dimensional shapes, whether sculpture or architecture, are only revealed in all their aspects when the viewer moves around them, i.e. after the passage of a certain time. But the plastic buildings of Expressionism were uniformly constructed; Gaudí's Casa Milà does not reveal new vistas from whatever side it is looked at. An outstanding building of the twenties, on the other hand, such as the Bauhaus at Dessau (1925) or Le Corbusier's project for the League of Nations (1927), is only fully appreciated if the observer constantly changes his viewing position. The intersections of different parts of the building, the ever-changing perspectives, the constant variations in visual scale, and the alternation from high to low, large to small, nearness to distance, horizontal to vertical have been carefully worked out in the design. As the eye can only make what is meant to be a three-dimensional

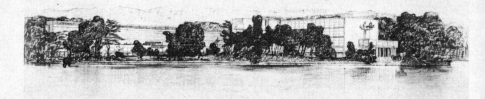

Le Corbusier. League of Nations Palace. Geneva, 1927. Project

composition into a flat picture from a fixed viewpoint, the original aesthetic intent of the building can only be fulfilled by a person in motion. 'It is essential to walk round a building in order to grasp its shape and the function of its parts' writes Gropius in relation to the Bauhaus scheme.

From this a new vocabulary of shapes emerged: in particular the dissolution of the mass into slender members of changing dimensions; asymmetry of plan; locating individual wings at angles apart; and the creation of vistas by means of ground floor columns or space-spanning bridges. No part of the building demands prior attention, so special features and wall reliefs are dispensed with. The eye travels over white, smooth walls and is led on by horizontal strips of window, rows of columns or wall openings. Baroque architecture also 'led the eye', but by means of intersecting streets which revealed a building at right angles or diagonally; oval or circular open spaces, parterres or fountains were obstacles on the prescribed route. The architecture of the twenties knows no such routes. The spectator goes his own way, and the building is meant to be seen from any angle.

Already the 'Città Nuova' by the Italian Sant'Elia had included movement as part of its architectural and urbanistic conception, in conformity with the Futurist delight in the dynamics of modern city traffic. But Sant' Elia was not so much concerned with the movement of the spectator and not at all with the free rhythm and calmness of tempo which are the prerequisites of such building schemes of the twenties as the Bauhaus or the Weissenhof housing estate at Stuttgart. Sant'Elia was concerned with the movement of the object, not of the beholder: the rushing

traffic on several levels, arriving and departing trains, escalators and elevators, motor cars, and aeroplanes landing and taking off. Sant'Elia, and not Le Corbusier, first wrote of the modern house that was to resemble a gigantic machine. Sant' Elia's architectural shapes are compact and monumental, as though rooted in the ground; they are often symmetrical, and can be grasped from one viewpoint.

Many practitioners of modern architecture were only concerned with the new aesthetic inasfar as it served a new social attitude. 'We know no problems of form, only problems of building', Mies van der Rohe said in 1923. There have probably seldom been times in which architects were less aware of an aesthetic ideal. The aims of the spatial organization of a house were correct exploitation of the site, appropriate orientation, sound insulation, short, time-saving circulation for the housewife, and clear distinctions between individual zones of function. The preoccupation with these basic problems of human habitation was accompanied by growing scientific precision, and by no means only in Europe but in South America, for example, too.

The key word of this era is a concept whose history reaches back into the 19th century but which ultimately lies behind every type of architecture in some form or other: *Functionalism. The relationship of building to function has been the subject of many interpretations, in the light of the purpose for which the building is to be used, its materials, structure and environment. The opinion has often been voiced that the expression of function is beautiful in itself. As Bruno Taut said in 1929: 'Serviceability becomes the actual content of aesthetics.' The second assumption, which remained unspoken at the time, was that the factors determining functional architecture are themselves unchangeable and are not for their part postulated by any one style. Philip *Johnson recounted to students at Harvard University the reaction of visitors to his Barcelona chairs, designed by Mies van der Rohe: 'When people come who like them, they exclaim "What wonderful chairs!" Which they really are. And when they sit down, they remark ". . . and how comfortable!" But if someone comes who dislikes chairs made from strips of curved steel, he will generally say: "How uncomfortable!"'

In the twenties we find numerous examples of people thinking their chairs comfortable because they liked their design. Architecture was then expressing functions founded on aesthetic ideals. Thus extensive use of glass walls met the demand for well-lit living and working areas and for close contact between interior and exterior, but the practice was unwisely introduced before the problem of protection from the sun had been solved. Sun louvres only appeared again during the thirties in the wake of new aesthetic ideas for enlivening façades three-dimensionally.

The twenties were a great Utopian period. The new architecture had to be quite different from the historical styles of the past. Divorced from art-historical development, this architecture was meant to be timeless and valid in the encounter between purpose and material. That is why the functional argument carried such weight. It seemed to guarantee that architecture was now orientated towards viewpoints that were constant and lay within the nature of man or the characteristics of materials. 'The objectivization of personal and national features is clearly recognizable in modern architecture' (Gropius, 1924). An international agreement seemed possible. For the attribute 'international' also appears among the designations which the period conferred upon itself. Gropius called his 'picture book of modern architecture' in 1924 *Internationale Architektur*, and the tag *International Style*, coined in a publication of the year 1932 by Hitchcock and Johnson, took its place beside Rationalism or *Neue Sachlichkeit*. Regional variations of this general canon were permissible, but only as voices that were part of a polyphonic harmony. Team-work like the Weissenhof housing estate of the *Deutscher Werkbund, to which sixteen architects from different countries contributed, the founding of the architectural organization *CIAM and the work submitted in the large international competitions of the twenties, forcefully demonstrated the new spirit of unity, even if the judges themselves still awarded the prizes to reactionaries.

It was not only Central Europe—the *Netherlands, *Germany and *Switzerland —that was in the throes of the new movement. When Gropius compiled the first Bauhaus book in 1924, the *Internationale Architektur*, more than half of the eighty-five examples of the new style were designs or models only. But in the course of one decade, the International Style established itself. In *Italy, the young *gruppo 7 was formed. In *France an avant-garde emerged whose clients were generally private patrons. In *Finland there were promising beginnings. *Sweden's eminent architect Erik Gunnar *Asplund wheeled round and openly joined the new movement with the Stockholm Exhibition of 1930. Modern architecture emerged in Hungary, Poland and above all in Czechoslovakia.

But already the two enormous reservoirs of power were considered to be the United States and the Soviet Union. The *United States had silos and factories whose sober pathos delighted Gropius, Le Corbusier and Mendelsohn. Even though architects such as *Schindler or *Neutra only concerned themselves with private building, the victory of the new idea was only a question of time in this land of phenomenal activity. Russia made such remarkable contributions as *Constructivism. With his 'Suprematist architektona' Malevich created abstract compositions in which the interplay and spatial relationship between rectangular shapes is explored; the Bauhaus published his work in the Bauhaus Books series which as a rule were reserved for their own products.

The ideas of the Russian architects at this time were informed by a technological mystique. Structure is exposed. El *Lissitzky projected multi-storey buildings as 'Cloud Props'; in a scheme for the Lenin Institute, Moscow, in 1927, J. J. Leonidov designed a glass sphere suspended by steel ropes to house an auditorium for 4,000 people. Even the less ambitious designs for offices and industrial plants show a graphic

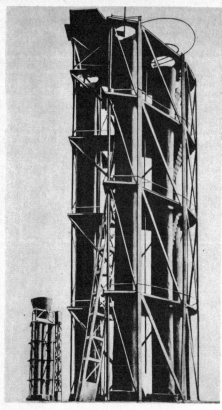

Chemical works. Detail. Moscow, before 1929.
Project

Palace of the Soviets in Moscow (1931) on
the other, stemmed from similar considerations! America and Russia were the lands
of promise for modern architecture.

But this ideal of international unity was
impossible without some simplifications.
Already two of the greatest exponents did
not fit into the picture which the new
movement had of itself. Frank Lloyd
Wright, who had been of great influence
since the turn of the century, possessed too
much poetry, pathos and stubbornness to
allow his work to be derived from 'utilitarian elements'. *Oud, the Dutch pro-
tagonist of the new architecture, called
Wright one of the greatest architects of his
time. But he also gave a warning that the
'lyric enchantment that sounded from the
pipes of this architectural pied piper was
at the same time damaging the purity of
tone' of the new architecture. How little
inspiration Wright's work derived from
the strict and disciplined architecture of
that period is borne out by the fact that
there is a temporary falling off in his industry in the twenties. Le Corbusier, too,
aroused some misgivings, although his
individual forms (the features on his villa

Alvar Aalto. Sanatorium. Paimio, 1929–33

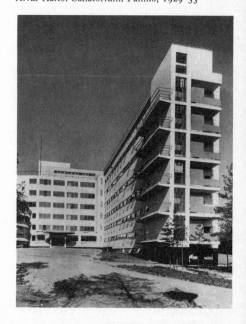

brilliance and precision which betray a
fascination for all that is technical. The
defeat of the huge but badly equipped
Russian army in the First World War had
relentlessly revealed the need for technology: now technology was looked on as the
means of salvation that would safeguard the
future of the new order. Erich Mendelsohn,
who knew the architecture of the USSR
and the USA at first hand, saw the problem
as a need to create a synthesis of America's
'rational intelligence' and Russia's 'vehe-
ment feeling', and he thought such a
task was capable of achievement. Perhaps
the attraction which big competitions
had for the world's greatest architects,
like the one for the Chicago Tribune Skyscraper (1922) on the one hand and those
for the Kharkov Theatre (1930) and the

roofs) at this time could not yet be understood as anticipations of his later sculptural play with forms. Bruno Taut wrote that it was Le Corbusier's greatest weakness that 'he was an abstract painter as well and that he mixed up architectural problems with those of painting', and Mendelsohn reproached him with lack of economy in his Weissenhof flats.

To the extent that the architecture of smooth white surfaces, rectangles, clearly articulated groupings, lightness and transparency, encountered new and hitherto unexplored fields, it changed. Alvar *Aalto's early buildings indicate already how design determined by function leads to a new style image, as soon as stylistic attitude is freer and gesture more liberal. For example, Le Corbusier's design for the League of Nations Building at Geneva (1927) envisaged a curved ceiling above the auditorium descending in great waves, clearly breaking back from each other, to the speaker's desk. The lecture hall in Aalto's library at Viipuri (1927–35) also has a ceiling suspended from the structural roof for the same acoustic reasons, but it is now developed in a freely undulating flow, sometimes rising, sometimes flat, a shape that only a few years earlier would not have been acceptable in the citadels of the International Style.

Aalto's architecture with its organic materials, its adaptation to the surrounding countryside and its avoidance of all dogma is the most conspicuous example of this change, because it is the work of a great architect. The new relationship to nature, as shown by his buildings, is not confined to him. The architects of the twenties had a preference for unadorned precise technological shapes. Their buildings, too, showed a fruitful relationship to exterior space and to nature; the opening up of the wall, the way a building's parts reach out to the open air and the invasion of the living areas by nature (Le Corbusier's buildings on *pilotis*, and his roof gardens!) all bear witness to it. But this relationship was one of contrasts. Here stood the man-made structure with its taut, clean lines and pure homogeneous surfaces, while there lay luxuriant untamed nature. As Oud put it in 1921: 'Instead of the natural charm of uncultivated material, the broken effect of glass, intricately textured surfaces, clouded colours, fused enamels and the weathering of walls

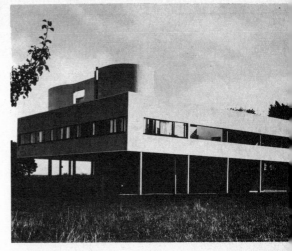

Le Corbusier. Villa Savoye. Poissy, 1927–31

we now have the attraction of cultivated material, clear glass, shining curved surfaces, the sparkling and brilliance of colour and the glitter of steel.' After 1930 and again after 1950 'natural charm' began to break through again.

Frank Lloyd Wright. Offices for S. C. Johnson and Son. Racine, Wis., 1936–9

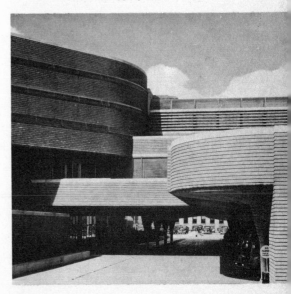

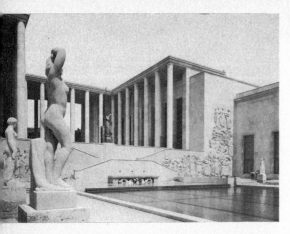

A. Aubert, J. C. Dondel, M. Dastugue, P. Viard.
Museum of Modern Art. Paris, 1937

A new appreciation of the lively rather than
the stylized surface, as expressed by Aalto's
choice of building materials, gained ground
in many places. In southern countries the
necessity for protection from sun and glare
provides a functional reason for this. Le
Corbusier put honeycombed screens on the
elevations in his designs for multi-storey
blocks. In *Denmark, the new University
at Aarhus founded in 1932 affords an
example of the effects that can be achieved

Frank Lloyd Wright. Kalita Humphreys Theater.
Dallas, Texas, 1960

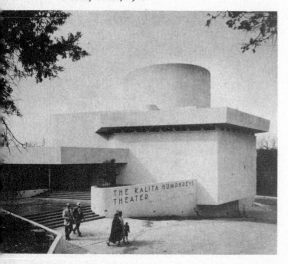

by the use of bricks without any detriment
to the modernity of its idiom. Lively surface textures are featured at *Gardella's
elegant clinic at Alessandria (1936–8) and
at the entrance to the Finsbury Health
Centre, London (1938). The aptitude of
Brazilian architects in the field of plastic
and free-form inventions first revealed
itself before a great public at the New York
World's Fair of 1939 in the pavilion by
*Costa and *Niemeyer. Modern architec-
ture was no longer essentially confined to
a small area in Central Europe but made
its appearance now all along the periphery
of its former centre.
The geographic decentralization coincided
with a stylistic one. Architecture in the
thirties is more divided, perhaps richer in
possibilities, but also less grandiose than
in the preceding period. The stylistic
formula of the twenties would no longer
wear. Frank Lloyd Wright's individual
type of art, which had derived little benefit
from a climate of spiritual sobriety and
ascetic poetry, now flourished, but concerned itself with the large-scale disposition
of masses and with less detailed ornament.
The other great architects of the older
generation did not build much, mainly for
reasons beyond their creative powers. Le
Corbusier received only a few commissions,
as measured against the wealth of his ideas.
Gropius, forced into exile after 1933, had
to adapt himself twice to new surroundings,
once in England and once in America.
Finally, Mies van der Rohe did not succeed
in building a single large project between
his Tugendhat House at Brno in 1930 and
the Illinois Institute in Chicago, started in
1940!
Just as in the 19th century, the architecture
of the engineers was separate from that of
the architects. *Shell constructions, which
have played an important part since the
end of the Second World War, were mainly
used for industrial schemes, and not as yet
for public buildings except by *Torroja.
*Nervi's large-span steel or reinforced con-
crete halls were at first only used as aircraft hangars; his world-wide reputation
was only established after the war.
Periods of modern architecture when the
contemporary style's powers of expansion
flag for a while, are usually characterized
by an emergence of classicism. Classicism
is the temptation of the century. Architects
of all generations gave in to it: Peter Beh-

rens as well as Walter Gropius, and both with buildings of national prestige to their credit, the German Embassy in St Petersburg (1911–12) and the United States Embassy in Athens (1961). Fascists everywhere under the sun encouraged this more or less secret leaning, and made classicism the official style of architecture. The accessories of the style such as columns, pillars, pilasters, cornices, and flights of steps were raised to an imperial pseudo-grandeur and, in their violation of human scale, personified the inhuman power that raised these buildings. Fascist, National Socialist, and Soviet types of government architectures were presented at the Paris International Exhibition of 1937; their declamatory gesticulations laid bare the ideology behind the style. Even nations that had no need of such hollow forms of self-assertion succumbed to the attractive force of neoclassicism. The buildings which were put up in Paris at the same time on the opposite bank of the Seine, the Musée d'Art Moderne and the Palais Chaillot, were close behind the concrete pamphlets of the dictatorships for dreary amplitude.

Classicism was not only a temptation but also a legitimate possibility. Nobody will deny the respect due to Asplund's Stockholm Crematorium (1935–40) which the quiet dignity of this building deserves. The Lincoln Memorial in Washington (1914–22) and the National Gallery of Art there (1937) are honest examples which are all the more justified as the first public buildings of the newly created country were in this style at the very beginning of the North American tradition in building. Classicism in America meant memories of independence and the wars of liberation.

Apart from the imitation of column and pillar, gable and abacus, latent classicism is evident in more than one important modern building (*neoclassicism). Mies van der Rohe has built in an unmistakable idiom, free of all imitation, after his early villas with their reminiscences of Schinkel. But the way he places steel sections in front of a wall in order to reveal the play of forces in the framework hidden in the wall, recalls the symbolism of forces expressed by the individual parts of a building in classical architecture. In the designs for the layout of the Illinois Institute of Technology in Chicago, which preceded the final scheme of 1940, there is an axial

arrangement of the architecture—and hence also of the people it serves—which corresponds to the clear orientation and axial stress of classical architecture. The Seagram Building in New York (1958) has remained the most clearly defined expression of this style so far. Related tendencies, albeit less strongly marked, are to be found in the decorative variants of current North American architecture.

What is modern architecture? Is it architecture based on the latest possibilities of building technique, from the earliest cast-iron structures to prestressed reinforced concrete? Architecture that aims at realizing a new style of living, perhaps in the manner of CIAM's ideals? Architecture which believes in a new spatial conception, the open plan that links indoors and outdoors and combines both in a single continuum? Or is modern architecture a provisional expression that will pass away by itself, because only after a period of time can clear and precise notions of style develop?

The situation became clear four or five years after the end of the Second World War. Around 1950, Olympus was unanimous and the gods distributed their gifts. Walter Gropius had trained himself a team of young American architects. Mies van der Rohe's ideal of the clear and crystalline

Ludwig Mies van der Rohe. Alumni Memorial Hall, Illinois Institute of Technology. Chicago, 1945–6. Detail

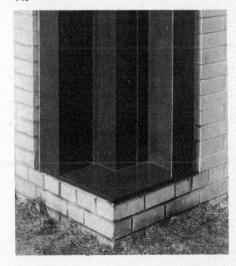

cube was accepted by the great American architectural firms and eventually by post-war European architects also. An unpleasant episode, that of the erection of the United Nations Building in New York (1950–1), indicates how effortlessly the conceptions of the great authorities—in this case Le Corbusier's—could be carried out, even if association with the great masters of modern architecture was uncomfortable, as association with genius has always been. International Style, Functionalism, Rationalism or whatever they were called, were of equal importance in 1950. This kind of architecture, however, was no longer as dogmatic as it had been in the twenties, and regional and personal variations were admitted in considerably greater measure. Surfaces were more lively and textured and natural materials held their ground against the smooth white planes of the twenties—tendencies that continued from the thirties into the fifties. Colour began to assume a greater importance; but after all Le Corbusier and

Bruno Taut had already pleaded for colour in building in the twenties.

In all, there was a mandatory stock of forms in 1950, which could be summarized, as they had been twenty-five years before, under headings such as transparency, visual lightness, and apparent weightlessness. Only a few years after the middle of the century the scene changed. There are times that favour the formation of traditions and those that react with neurotic vehemence to its every onset. Wright, Gropius, Mies van der Rohe, Le Corbusier: at what time did a new generation have the opportunity to build alongside their own forebears and to debate with their living exemplars? Frank Lloyd Wright, however much he had acted as a motive force at decisive moments, was no teacher in the sense of being a schoolmaster; his protean individualism did not lend itself to ready transference. Le Corbusier, in his Unité d'Habitation at Marseilles (under construction in 1950), created the type of the slab-shaped high apartment block, with

Ludwig Mies van der Rohe. Chemotechnics and Metallurgy Building, Illinois Institute of Technology. Chicago, 1946

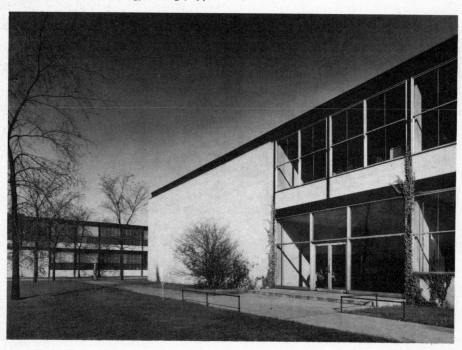

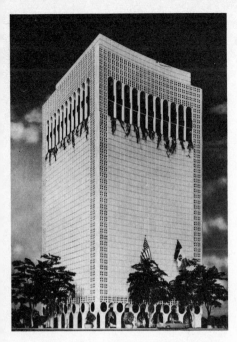

Edward Durell Stone. Gallery of Modern Art.
New York, c. 1957. Model

and Merrill, which has an exceptional feeling for the trends of the time, completed Lever House, the model prototype of the multi-storey office block in which the load-bearing frame remains concealed and a fully glazed outer skin forms a *curtain wall. With its precise rectilinear shape in the thoroughgoing Miesian tradition, and free of all decoration, this building proved the starting point of a new tendency in architectural decoration. Verticals and horizontals are equally distributed in the treatment of the glass façade; the surfaces which envelop Lever House are completely devoid of directionality. The division by storeys is shown up clearly and the structural frame is discernible through the transparent panes. More recent buildings play decorative tricks with the curtain walling. The walls, which are not load-bearing, consist of pressed aluminium panels, handicraft-type metal grilles, or prefabricated concrete or plastic units which are assembled in monumental patterns. In

Skidmore, Owings and Merrill. Lever House.
New York, 1952

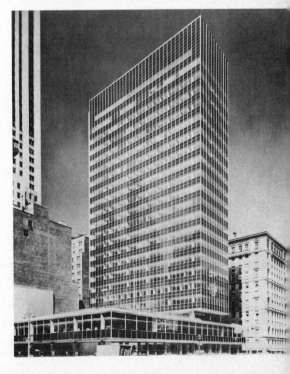

internal service passages and two-storey flats; a building that had, or could have had, the force of a model. But since Ronchamp (1950–4) at the latest, his architecture has assumed an individual look, even to the untrained eye, that is unrepeatable. Gropius seems to have become a victim of his own pedagogic virtue in giving his pupils and collaborators a clear field for their own development; the University at Bagdad (under construction), which he designed with his *TAC team, is not likely to become such an important example as the Dessau Bauhaus (1926) and the Harvard Graduate Center at Cambridge, Mass. (1949–50) had been.

The most spectacular is the decline of van der Rohe's pupils. Mies himself has probably built more since 1950 than during the first four decades of his creative life. Each year, these apparently simple structures spring up, standing or reclining boxes of sublime proportions and finely modelled profile. But his former disciples have long since renounced his ideal of ascetic nobility. In 1952 the large firm of Skidmore, Owings

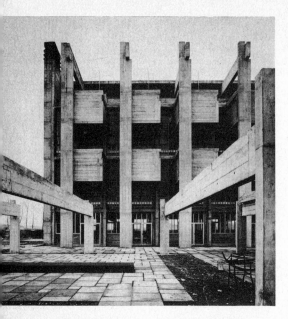

Vittoriano Viganò. Istituto Marchiandi. Milan, 1957

the American Pavilion at the Brussels International Exhibition by Edward D. *Stone (1958) this divagation received the accolade of official prestige.

The excessively smooth form of this boneless type of decorative architecture is confronted by the rugged forms of a number of others, mainly the work of Italian architects. This faction, to which the architecture of *Japan and the later Le Corbusier also belongs, has declared its opposition to the jewel-like wall mem-

Eero Saarinen. TWA Airport Terminal Building. Idlewild, New York, 1962. Model

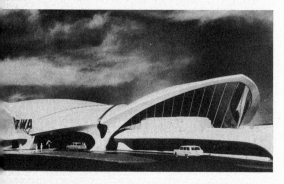

branes of the Americans. The wall becomes heavy and solid even where it is not load-bearing. Building materials are preferred with rough, granular, and contrasty textures such as brick and exposed concrete with the shuttering marks showing up as coarsely as possible. The predilection for weighty loads is carried to such extremes that the Torre Velasca in Milan (1957) has been provided with a huge crown-like top. Acute or obtuse angles reign supreme, with a tendency to hard, dissonant articulation of the individual parts of a building. The visual scale is constantly jumping and small units are abruptly confronted with large ones. Detail, like overall form, is block-shaped and heavy in appearance. The cultivated elegance of the decorator-architects is faced with brutal Expression, while the hedonists confront men wrestling with problems.

In all this antagonism between the two camps, a form of unity subsists in more than just the affront towards the classical concept of balance between load and support found in the creations of a Mies van der Rohe. Both parties exist in a deeply thought-out relationship to the history of architecture. Even the classic phase of modern architecture, the twenties, was not divorced from history, however much its protest against the style-imitations of the 19th century would have us believe it. Gropius sold Napoleon's table linen which his family had owned, in order to acquire building land for the Bauhaus in Weimar: an act which has its symbolic overtones. At least the twenties did not sell history completely for the sake of the present. Then, too, there was a historic revival but it was, so to say, ahistoric: it preferred those periods of time that had an anonymous character: the classical temples of Greece, which Le Corbusier had learnt to admire on his travels, the grain silos of the 19th century in North America, the farmhouse.

In the architecture of 1960, on the other hand, the past is admitted in almost every shape. In Italy, silhouettes appear that recall the baptistries of Parma and Cremona, and office blocks which recall medieval fortress towers. The Americans build semicircular structures amid gardens which invite comparison with the English 18th-century 'crescents', and there is constant borrowing from various exotic styles, mainly the Islamic ones but also from late

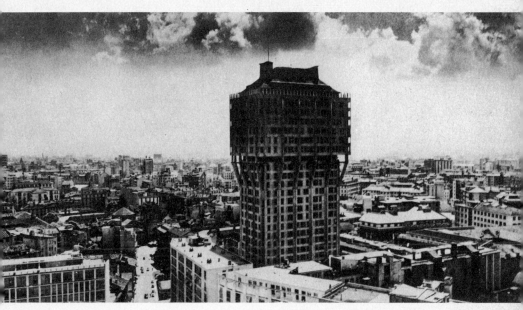

BBPR. Torre Velasca. Milan, 1957

Gothic. *Yamasaki attempted to combine 'the typical English character of the Palace of Westminster with the elegant lightness of the Doge's Palace' in his design for the American Embassy in London. His project was completely in accord with the ideas behind the huge building programme of the United States. A decade earlier, a country that erected prestige buildings abroad would have wanted these to reflect its own way of living and building. As a matter of fact, the American consulates in post-war Germany were images of what had just manifested itself in the Lever Building, New York, as the most recent tendency in United States architecture. The new buildings of the US State Department, over fifty diplomatic missions, reflect on the contrary the environment in which they are erected; a case of applied diplomacy. The competition for the Embassy in London explicitly demanded 'an architectural style which creates an atmosphere of good will by its intelligent appreciation and consideration of the site and by its adaptation of the architecture to its surroundings'.

The relationship of modern architecture to itself is already being reflected on—a situation that is alien to the historic styles. High and Late Renaissance knew no reversions to Early Renaissance; but modern architecture reminds itself with verbal quotations of Art Nouveau ('neo-Liberty'), De Stijl ('neo-neoplasticism') or the functionalism of the twenties, an

Minoru Yamasaki. McGregor Memorial Community Conference Center. Detroit, Mich., 1959

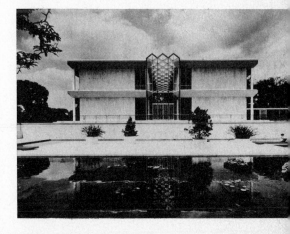

important phase of its own evolution. A new eclecticism is in the air.

The tendency to a literary programme is hence boundless. It stretches from an expression of certain psychological states to pure symbolism of form. Paul *Rudolph, one of the most talented of the younger American architects, demands that architects should concern themselves 'with considerations of vision, symbolism, and content'. Yamasaki advocated a 'friendly, more gentle kind of building', and attacks 'muscular boasting' in architecture; Edward D. Stone talks of a 'need for richness, exuberance and pure unadulterated freshness'. A picturesque character has been more and more demanded for buildings in recent years. The famous south-east

Carlos Raúl Villanueva. Building for the Faculty of Architecture and Town Planning, University City, Caracas, 1957

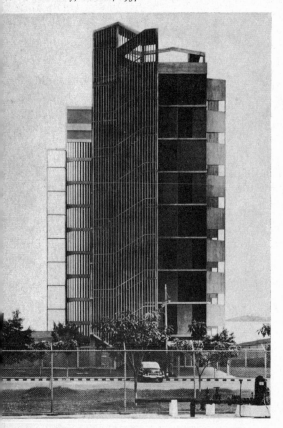

corner of Le Corbusier's Ronchamp Chapel (1950–4) suggests the bold curve of a ship's bow by legitimate means, i.e. through the expressiveness of its abstract shape. Eero *Saarinen's Idlewild Airport Terminal Building (1962) must have been inspired by the thought of a bird in flight. But it is pushing architecture too far if it has to express freedom of speech (*Stubbins's Congress Hall, Berlin, 1957) or if the pools on the model of a Capitol for the fiftieth State of the USA are meant to represent the sea surrounding the Hawaiian Islands.

It is the eternal privilege of contemporaries to think of their own times as being particularly complex and involved. Hence modern architecture, too, is a mass of contradictions. A revaluation of the historic styles has led to a plurality of expression that would have been unthinkable even as recently as 1950. Countries that were on the periphery of architectural development before, now offer individual and unmistakable solutions of their own—South America, Japan. The great architects have lost much of their power to serve as models. Art form seems to triumph over residential form, and architecture as formal expression over architecture as social design. At the same time the problem of the modern city is becoming ever more pressing, while the demand for prefabrication and the industrialization of building is undeniable.

Architectural critics from all over the world have their say in this book. They would probably not agree on all points as regards matter, method and even basic conceptions if they came together round a table. But they would be unanimous in their belief that the forms and problems of contemporary architecture must be debated passionately. It is right to take an interest in the history of modern architecture not only because modern architecture has arrived at a stage in its development where architects themselves have again become interested in history, but above all because modern times have lasted long enough to provide the answers to many questions.

WOLFGANG PEHNT

Page 27. Le Corbusier. Notre-Dame du Haut, South-east Angle. Ronchamp, 1950–4

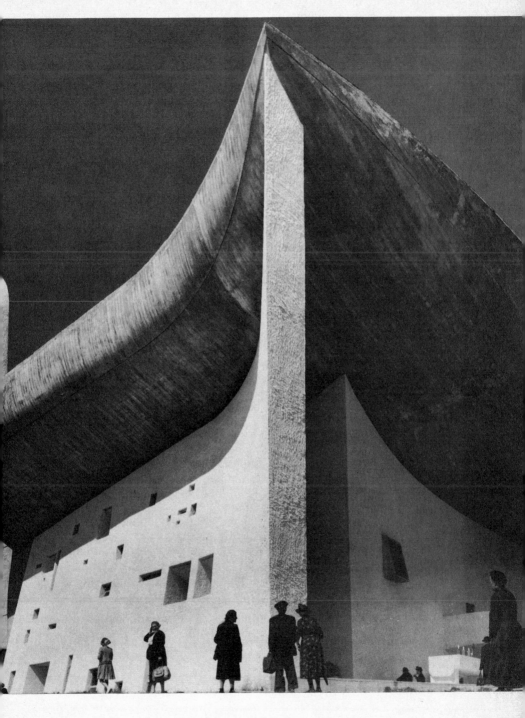

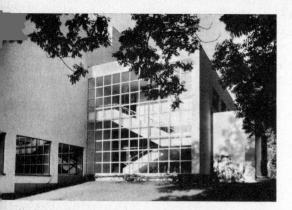

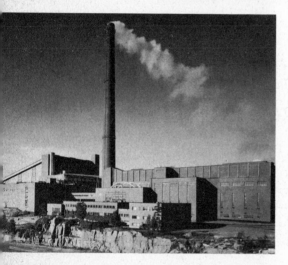

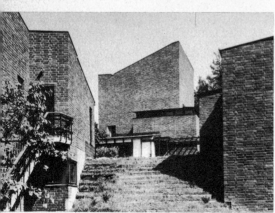

Aalto, Hugo Henrik Alvar, b. Kuortane, Finland, 1898. Aalto studied under Sigurd Frosterus at Helsinki Polytechnic, where he graduated in architecture in 1921. In the years immediately following he travelled in Scandinavia and Central Europe, worked for a short time in the planning office of the 1923 Gothenburg Fair, and made his official début with the Tampere Industrial Exhibition of 1922, though his first work was really the remodelling of his mother's house, the Mammula of Alajärvi, carried out when he was still a student. He opened his first office in Jyväskylä, and in 1925 married Aino Marsio, who until her death in 1949 was his principal collaborator, especially in the work connected with the organization and production of Artek timber furniture, first designed in 1928 for Paimio Sanatorium.

In Jyväskylä Aalto erected a number of 'pre-functionalist' buildings including the Trade Union Theatre (1923–5). He moved to Turku in 1927, and collaborated with Erik *Bryggman in 1929 on the Jubilee Exhibition organized to celebrate the seventh centenary of the city. This exhibition displayed an exemplary feeling of coherence, and considerable originality as a graphic structure. It also marks an important stage in the history of Finnish architecture, for with it both Aalto and Bryggman reached the culmination of their development towards *Functionalism, abandoning the decorative elements of their former classic style to produce the first expression of modern architecture in Scandinavia.

The works which Alvar Aalto carried out over these years already reveal the fully developed character of his art, which may be set beside that of the greatest artists, because it succeeds both in being of its time and, simultaneously, timeless. They include the Library at Viipuri (1927–35), newspaper offices for the Turun Sanomat (1929–30), and Paimio Sanatorium (1929–33). This first 'white' period continued right up to the Second World War, and is

Alvar Aalto. Municipal Library. Viipuri, 1927–35

Alvar Aalto. Cellulose factory. Sunila, 1936–9

Alvar Aalto. Town Hall. Säynätsalo, 1950–2

Page 29. Alvar Aalto. Church. Vuoksenniska, near Imatra, 1956–8

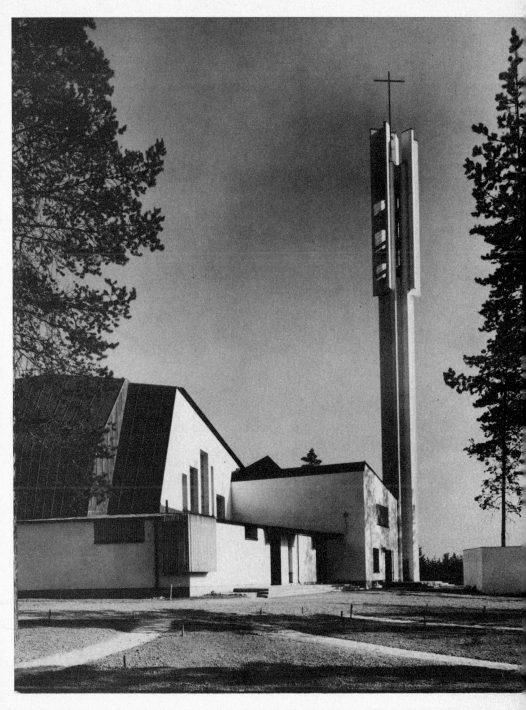

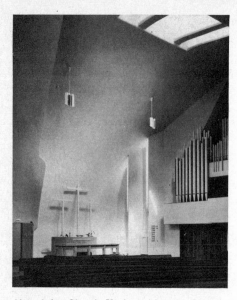

Alvar Aalto. Church. Vuoksenniska, near Imatra, 1956–8

rich in projects such as those at Paimio and Viipuri, which will always be considered among the classics of modern architecture: the architect's own house at Riihitie 10, Helsinki (1935–6), a delightful and little-known masterpiece; the Finnish Pavilions at the International Exhibitions in Paris (1937) and New York (1939); the terraced house of Kauttua and the Villa Mairea (1938–9); and a number of industrial buildings such as the cellulose factory at Toppila (1930–1), and the huge industrial

Alvar Aalto. Maison Carré. Bazoches, 1956–8

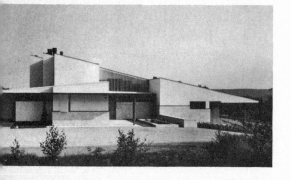

and residential Sunila complex (1936–9, completed 1951–4).

After the intermission of the war years, Alvar Aalto applied himself to rebuilding his native land. In 1944–5 he drew up a master-plan for the development of Rovaniemi, the capital of Finnish Lapland, in conjunction with Y. Lindegren, B. Saarnio, M. Tavio, and K. Simberg. The works built or projected in the first ten years after the war may be ascribed to what we shall call the artist's middle or mature period. It may also be referred to as his 'red' or 'Cézanne' period, from the intense hues of the bricks he employed and his manner of handling volumes, but above all from the way that light is broken into facets in the manner of Cézanne; or his 'Italian' period, from the affectionate memories that are embodied of the severe Tuscan contours of towers and strongholds, and from the way he contrives internal courtyards, often raised at a higher level, where the explicit feeling of authority is tempered to a human scale. The work which embodies and concludes the structural and spatial experiments of this period, while constituting its highest and most perfect expression, is the Town Hall at Säynätsalo (1950–2). Mention should also be made of the imposing campus of Jyväskylä Teachers' Training College (1952–7), and the Funeral Chapel for Malmi, near Helsinki, a fine design that has remained unbuilt.

It was at this time that Alvar Aalto's intense work on civic schemes began, which are altering the face of Helsinki. His buildings of the fifties, such as the Rautatalo office block, 1952–4, one of his greatest projects; the Engineers' Institute, 1952; the National Pensions Institution, 1952–6; and the Cultural Centre, 1955–8, are of an intermediate stage between his 'red' and second 'white' periods, which may be literally referred to as 'bronze'. Aalto's command of plastic design had become enriched to an extraordinary degree, backed as it was by thirty years of building experience. The butterfly roof of Säynätsalo Town Hall and the great hull of the Stadium at Otaniemi may serve as symbols of this supreme mastery of technology and three-dimensional design in the handling of wood: Finland's most typical and traditional, if modest, building material. The following schemes date from the same years: the design for Seinajoki Episcopalian

Church (1952), completed in 1958 as part of a more extensive town-planning layout currently in course of realization; the Enso-Gutzeit paper mill at Summa (1953); the cemetery and chapels for Kongens Lyngby, near Copenhagen, in collaboration with Jean-Jacques Baruel (not built); the design for Vienna Municipal Hall (1953, not built); the Oulu Theatre project (1955); Otaniemi Polytechnic (1955, under construction); the development plan for Imatra (1947–53) and the regional plan for Lapland (1950–7).

Meanwhile, Aalto's second 'white' period begins in 1953, with the country house he built himself, of a somewhat experimental character, on the island of Muuratsalo. In 1955 came his masterly studio, completely in white, where Aalto's habitual attention to the psychological effects of colour reaches its ultimate stage in surroundings with no colour at all, intended to be conducive to work and quiet meditation. His eight-storey block of flats for the Berlin Interbau dates from 1955–7; then came the project for the Municipal Centre at Gothenburg (1956), the Church at Vuoksenniska near Imatra, and the Maison Carré, in the neighbourhood of Paris (both between 1956 and 1958). The latter work was carried out in collaboration with Elissa Makkinheimo, whom Aalto married in 1952. The almost 'Mycenaean' articulation of spaces gives the interiors of these buildings less volumetric definition, as grouping becomes ever more complex. Space is no longer simply fluid in the way it was at Viipuri, but grows, and, as it were, breathes in every direction around man. This treatment characterizes Aalto's most recent works, in course of construction or projected: the museums for Aalborg (Denmark) and Bagdad; Kiruna Town Hall; the Volkswagen Cultural Centre at Wolfsburg, and the tower house at Bremen. All these schemes were drawn up in 1958, and the last two are under construction. Later works include the Enso-Gutzeit office block at Helsinki (1959–62), the Opera House at Essen, and the Cultural Centre in Helsinki. Numerous other schemes are at the planning stage.

No other architecture of the present day exerts quite the same fascination as Alvar Aalto's: rich in allegory, unforeseeable, at once mystical and sensual, rationalist and anti-rationalist. As an outstanding prac-

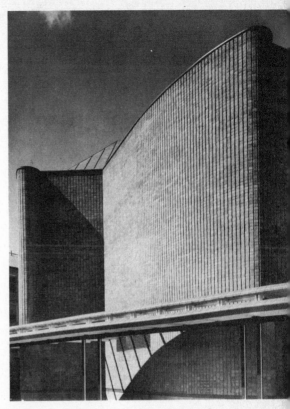

Alvar Aalto. Cultural Centre. Helsinki, 1955–8

titioner of *organic architecture, he is aristocratically remote from all the mannerisms that have appeared due to a misunderstanding of this term. In the present state of architecture, where the need to provide accommodation for ever-increasing masses of people has led, and too often still leads to a frightful deterioration in the human and psychological qualities of housing and urban environments, to say nothing of the aesthetic considerations involved, the work of this poet amongst architects, so rich in affectionate attention to all human needs, expressed and latent, recognized or forgotten, is a source of comfort and hope. With the current spread of 'new' materials, whether used with greater commercial brashness or more barbarous insipidity it is difficult to say, Aalto's lamps and chairs, and the materials he employs, speak to us with an ancient wisdom whose very memory we seem to have lost. His work is a protest against everything stupid, unnatural and impoverished that goes under the name of 'modern', against fashionable clichés and trick photography. It is the contradictory and coherent work of a genius who does not adapt himself to the conventions of today or yesterday, because he is one of the men of our time who understands with the greatest clarity what the word tradition really means, and how, having grasped its spirit perfectly, one becomes part of it: without nostalgia, or complexes, though with all the respect due to it: in fine, a free man.

Bibliography: Alvar Aalto, 'Zwischen Humanismus und Materialismus', in *Der Bau*, No. 7/8, Vienna 1955; reprinted in *Baukunst und Werkform*, Volume IX, No. 6, Darmstadt 1956; Alvar Aalto, 'Problemi di architettura', in *Quaderni* ACJ, Turin 1956; Alvar Aalto, RIBA Annual Discourse, London in *RIBA Journal*, May 1957; Ed. and Cl. Neuenschwander, *Alvar Aalto and Finnish Architecture*, London 1954; Pier Carlo Santini and Göran Schildt, 'Alvar Aalto from Sunila to Imatra: Ideas, Projects and Buildings' in *Zodiac 3*, Milan 1958; Frederick Gutheim, *Alvar Aalto*, New York 1960; Göran Schildt and Leonardo Mosso, *Alvar Aalto*, Jyväskylä 1962; *Alvar Aalto*, ed. K. Fleig, Zurich and London 1963 (complete works 1922–1962).

LEONARDO MOSSO

Aberdeen, David du Rieu, b. 1913. Studied at Bartlett School of Architecture, London University; later lecturer at the Atelier of Advanced Design there (1947–53). Won the open competition for the TUC Memorial Building, London (1953–56). Housing at Basildon, Harlow and N. Southgate (London), the latter featuring a thirteen-storey point block. Redevelopment of Paddington Hospital; commercial buildings; aircraft hangars.

Abramovitz, Max, b. Chicago 1908. Studied at the University of Illinois and at Columbia University. In partnership with Wallace K. *Harrison.

Adler, Dankmar, b. near Weimar, Saxony 1844, d. Chicago 1900. Central Music Hall in Chicago (1879). In 1879 Louis *Sullivan joined Adler's firm and became a partner

two years later. Their collaboration, in which Sullivan was responsible for the formal design of projects, lasted till 1895.

Albini, Franco, b. Robbiate, Como 1905. Graduated 1929 at Milan, where he now lives. His first essays in architecture were made during the thirties, in connection with the Milan Triennali and Trade Fairs. The fine pavilion for the Istituto Nazionale delle Assicurazioni dates from 1935. It was the first of his designs to be built, and already unmistakable. Having come to maturity of outlook and architectural practice during the years when Persico and Pagano were conducting their polemics in the pages of *Casabella* on behalf of a rationalist architecture in the European manner, and against the current of the *Novecento Italiano*, Albini has kept faith with those distant premisses to a greater degree than perhaps any other of his companions. This will be readily perceived if his entire work is analysed; in this way it would be seen how he likes thinking of architecture in essentially rational terms, to which he restricts the emotions of fantasy. Of course, there is more to it than that: there is his consciousness of profound underlying reasons, social and historic order and architectural rationalism.

For many years Albini's fantasy played on the contrast between his lively, spatial intuitions (as expressed by his frequent clever use of transparent, i.e. luminous, diaphragms, and reticulated panels, i.e. openwork panels which let the light flow in) and the clear orthogonal geometry of his structures. The contrast was finally resolved by identifying the formal element in the structure itself and from then onwards Albini's style has been more strongly expressed. This is exemplified in the field of architecture from his first villa in Milan, 1938, and his workers' flats there, 1936–8, to the Palazzo INA at Parma, 1951, the new municipal offices at Genoa, 1959 and on through to the large department store La Rinascente in Rome, 1961, his most recent and most discussed work. In the field of town planning, it may be traced from his first studies and projects, produced in conjunction with Pagano, Camus and Palanti before the war, down to the development plan for Reggio Emilia (1947–8, in collaboration); in industrial design: from the metal chair, in whose design he collaborated for the 1936 Triennale, to the circular armchair, designed in collaboration with Franca Helg for the Triennale of 1960; in the fitting out of shops, houses and museums: from the Museo di Palazzo Bianco at Genoa in 1951, a high-water mark in international museology, to the Museo del Tesoro di San Lorenzo at Genoa, 1954–6, which is one of the most intense and interesting works of recent Italian architecture, starting from its plan, laid out with a pure organic geometry, like that of a crystal.

Albini, who has attained world stature as a museum architect, has been entrusted with the project for the great new museums of Egyptian art at Cairo, currently under construction. He was a member of the executive committee of the 1951 Triennale; has lectured for some years at the Venice Istituto Universitario di Architettura; and was awarded the Olivetti national prize for architecture in 1957.

Bibliography: Giuseppe Samonà, 'Franco Albini e la cultura architettonica in Italia', in *Zodiac 3*, Milan 1958; G. C. Argan, *Franco Albini*, Milan 1962. See also: *Architectural Review*, March 1957 and December 1960.

GIULIA VERONESI

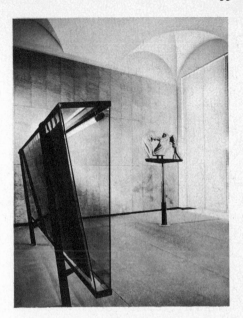

Franco Albini. Museo di Palazzo Bianco. Genoa, 1951

Almqvist, Osvald, b. Trankil near Karlstad 1884, d. Stockholm 1950. Studied at Stockholm Technical College. The 'first Swedish functionalist'. He founded a School of Architecture in 1910, together with *Asplund, Bergsten, *Lewerentz, and other young architects, which lasted only a short time but contributed to a clarification of the situation in Sweden. Housing, power stations.

Amsterdam, School of. Group of architects that started from the break with *Berlage and provided a parallel movement in the twenties and thirties of this century to contemporary German *Expressionism. Their mouthpiece was the journal *Wendingen*. The plastically conceived shapes of their brick buildings were in sharp contrast to the buildings of De *Stijl. Most eminent exponents were Kramer, van der Mey, and Michael de *Klerk.

Antonelli, Alessandro, b. Ghemme, Novara 1798, d. Turin 1888. Professor at the Accademia di Belle Arti at Turin. He built the multi-shell cupolas of St Gaudenzio at

Novara (1841–81) and of the Mole Antonelliana built, but not completed, as a synagogue, now municipal museum at Turin (1863–88); bold feats of engineering, which relied in the main on Classic Revival forms of decoration.

Franco Albini. La Rinascente department store. Rome, 1958–61. Model (first version)

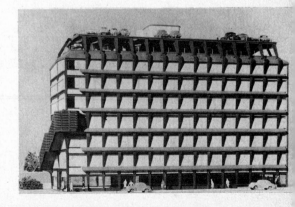

Architects' Co-Partnership. Practice originally founded by C. K. Capon, P. L. Cocke, M. H. Cooke-Yarborough, L. M. de Syllas, J. M. Grice and M. A. R. Powers. Their rubber factory at Brynmawr, South Wales (1949) with its repetition of simple but powerful shapes gave the first indication of the feeling for sculptural effect which characterizes the firm's style. This has been displayed since in a series of educational buildings, including schools in London, Warwickshire, Hertfordshire and Dorsetshire, and university premises at Leicester, Carmarthen and Cambridge. Their hall of residence for undergraduates at St John's College, Oxford has an ingenious plan comprising a series of related hexagons, whose cellular character provides an interesting silhouette in sympathy with the existing medieval building.

HAROLD MEEK

Aronco, Raimondo d', b. Gemona, Udine 1857, d. Naples 1932. Graduate of Venice Academy. Together with *Basile and *Sommaruga he was the most important exponent of *Art Nouveau in Italy. D'Aronco designed the main building of the Turin Industrial Exhibition (1902), a bizarre mixture of the most varying influences including the Viennese. Worked in Turkey. Later, like *Horta and partly also *Behrens, he turned to designing in the Classic Revival style.

Art Nouveau. Extensive romantic, individualist and anti-historical movement which affected the whole of Europe between 1890 and 1910. It was known in England at the time as the 'modern style'; in Belgium as the *coup de fouet* (whiplash) or *paling* (eel) style (from the flexible line introduced by *Horta), or the *style des Vingt* (in view of the important part played by a group of this name led by Octave Maus); in Germany it was called the *Jugendstil*, from the Munich periodical *Jugend*; in France the *style nouille* (noodle style) or *style Guimard* (after the architect Henri *Guimard, who designed the decorative entrances to the Paris Métro in 1899). The Austrians named it the *Sezessionsstil* (after the Viennese *Sezession* group, led from 1897 on by the painter Klimt and the architects *Hoffmann and *Olbrich); in Italy it was the *stile Liberty* or *stile floreale*, and in Spain *modernismo*.

Known more generally as the *style 1900*, Art Nouveau expresses an essentially decorative trend that aims to highlight the ornamental value of the curved line, which may be floral in origin (Belgium, France) or geometric (Scotland, Austria). This line gives rise to two-dimensional, slender, sinuous, undulating and invariably asymmetrical forms. The applied arts were the first to be affected (textiles by William Morris, 1880; wood-engraved title page to *Wren's City Churches* by Arthur H. Mackmurdo, 1883; vases by Émile Gallé, 1884; ornamental lettering by Fernand Khnopff and Georges Lemmen, 1890–1; mural tapestry *The Angels' Vigil* by Henry van de Velde, 1891; furniture by Gustave Serrurier-Bovy, 1891; title page for *Dominical* by van de Velde, 1892).

Next came architecture, represented by the house which the architect Victor *Horta built at Brussels in 1892 for the engineer Tassel, a key-work of the new style, which was to find a dazzling counterpart a few years later in the Elvira studio at Munich by August *Endell (1897–8, destroyed). Among the most characteristic architectural products of Art Nouveau, albeit widely differing in purpose and plastic expression, may be counted the houses built by Paul *Hankar in Brussels (1893–1900); the works of Willem Kromhout (1864–1940), Th. Sluyterman (1863–1931) and L. A. H. Wolf in the Netherlands; Guimard's Castel Béranger (1897–8), Métro stations and the auditorium of the Humbert de Romans building (1902, destroyed) at Paris; Horta's Maison du Peuple (1896–99) and the former Hôtel Solvay (1895–1900) in Brussels; the overhead Stadtbahn station at the Karlsplatz, Vienna (1897) by Otto *Wagner; and the Folkwang Museum laid out by van de Velde at Hagen (1900–2). All these works are the result of a deliberate attempt to put an end to imitations of past styles; in its place is offered a florid type of architecture which exploits craft skills, using coloured materials (faience cabochons, stoneware, terracotta panels, stained glass), exotic veneers, moulded stonework, grilles, balconies, and tapered brackets in wrought-iron; and burgeoning with asymmetrical door- and window-frames, bow and horse-shoe windows, etc. We are in the presence of a type of architecture which is seeking a relationship between surface and ornament, rather than a spatial expression of plan. An exception to this may be found in buildings designed in the tradition of the English country house (*Voysey, *Mackintosh), with their principle of building from inside to out; and the Continental examples based on them (Olbrich's houses on the Mathildenhöhe at Darmstadt). In the later phases of Art Nouveau, façade decoration was accompanied by a powerful plastic treatment of the whole building, either by the dramatic accentuation of individual parts of the structure (Glasgow Art School, 1898–1909, by Mackintosh) or by the sculptural modelling of the whole building mass (Werkbundtheater, Cologne, 1914 by van de Velde; Casa Milà, Barcelona, 1905–10, by *Gaudí).

Art Nouveau was first and foremost an aesthetic undertaking, based on social theories and inspired by aesthetes such as Ruskin, Morris and Oscar Wilde. It was born from a panic fear of the rise of industrialism, and from a determination to create a new style, in view of the 19th century's stylistic bankruptcy, which would affect the design of objects of everyday use and leave its mark ultimately on the décor and surroundings of daily life.

In theory, from the ethical and political point of view, it appears as an attempt to integrate art with social life; in practice, and from the cultural point of view, it assumes the manner of a reactionary bourgeois movement. Art Nouveau tried, in effect, to relieve man from the pressures of a technological milieu. Faced with the machine, which it regarded as the work of the devil, it aimed at renewing contact with nature and rehabilitating the tool in its rôle of the 'lengthener of the hand': by the same token, it obliged the artist to express himself in the margin of the living forces of technology. On the other hand, it claimed to be able to fashion a three-dimensional universe, independent of the fundamental support of the true creators of the epoch (Cézanne, Gauguin, Van Gogh, Munch) or rather, only borrowing the most external trappings of their inspiration. The point may thus be seen at which Art Nouveau (in the midst of its romantic, sentimental and social outbursts) posed in contradictory terms the problem of the social relations of art. It may also be seen how it brought about, in all fields, a real severance between life and thought, and partially destroyed the 'relation between plant and soil'.

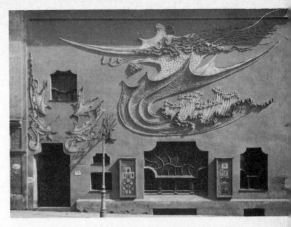

August Endell. Elvira photographic studio. Munich, 1897–8

Art Nouveau may thus be compared to a short circuit; by confounding style and surface ornament, and by basing all its efforts on theories of decoration, it appeared as a parenthesis in the organic development of history. At a time of the most prodigious industrial development, which saw the works of *Eiffel, Contamin and Dutert, and the early *Gropius, Art Nouveau kept painters, sculptors and architects at a respectful distance from the complex of technology, and inveigled them into a concern for virtuous craftsmanship rather than for machines and machine

Hector Guimard. Entrance to a Métro station. Paris, 1900

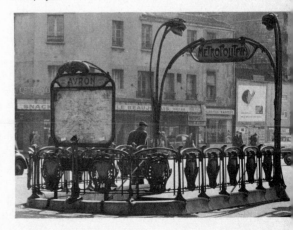

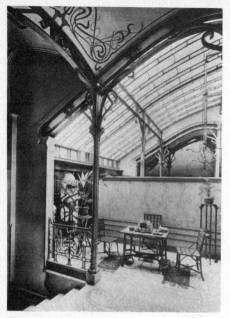

Victor Horta. Hôtel Tassel. Brussels, 1892–3

products. Hence, despite the ever-increasing tempo of human life, Art Nouveau wished to protect the quiet little world dreamt of by Ruskin, Morris, Tolstoy, Dickens, Renan, Zola and many others. Distinguished architects of the Art Nouveau style, such as Mackintosh, *Behrens and the Viennese masters became pioneers of modern architecture, it is true, but with their forward-looking buildings they overstepped the frontiers which the style had imposed upon its adherents.

Bibliography: Fritz Schmalenbach, *Jugendstil. Ein Beitrag zu Theorie und Geschichte der Flächenkunst*, Würzburg 1934; Stephan Tschudi Madsen, *Sources of Art Nouveau*, New York 1956; Helmut Seling (editor), *Jugendstil. Der Weg ins 20. Jahrhundert*, Heidelberg 1959; Peter Selz and Mildred Constantine (editors) *Art Nouveau. Art and Design at the Turn of the Century*, New York 1959; Louis Gans, *Nieuwe Kunst. De Nederlandse Bijtrage tot de 'Art Nouveau'*, Utrecht 1960; Jean Cassou, Emil Langui, Nikolaus Pevsner, *Durchbruch zum 20. Jahrhundert, Kunst und Kultur der Jahrhundertwende*, Munich 1962; Robert Schmutzler, *Jugendstil-Art Nouveau*, Stuttgart 1962.

ROBERT L. DELEVOY

Arts and Crafts. In 1861 William *Morris, together with a group of Pre-Raphaelite painters and architects in London, founded the firm of Morris, Marshall and Faulkner, Fine Art Workmen in Painting, Carving, Furniture and the Metals. He thus took the first step in a movement that was to lead over the next thirty years to an ultimate crystallization in C. R. Ashbee's Arts and Crafts Exhibition Society of 1888. The route was marked by a series of experiments, researches and battles, including the foundation of various other associations for the purpose of reviving craft production and fighting the encroachments of machinery on life. In its progress, the movement was to exercise a profound influence on the development of new ideas, tastes and methods of work over the whole of Europe. Inspired by the example of medieval craftsmen, Morris conducted a passionate campaign throughout these years to restore a genuine feeling of creativity to the decorative arts (i.e. those pertaining to domestic interiors), and indirectly to architecture as well. He fought against the

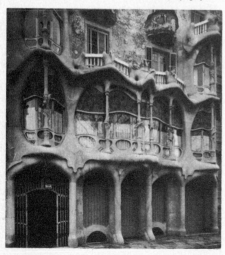

Antoni Gaudí. Casa Batlló. Barcelona, 1905–7

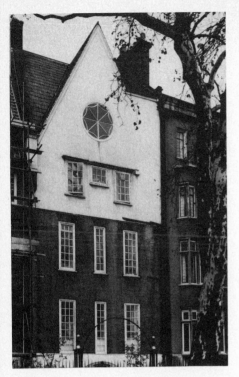

Charles Robert Ashbee. House in Cheyne Walk. London, 1904

lowering of standards that had been brought about when the market was flooded with cheap mass-produced goods which brought not truth and beauty, but falsehood and ugliness into everyday life. Behind this attitude lay the moralizing aesthetics of John Ruskin.

But in the years that had passed since Morris & Co. was founded, the rise of industrial mass-production methods and the abhorred machine were facts that could no longer be suppressed or ignored. Ashbee, indeed, took account of them, and accepted, at least in theory, the need for collaboration with industry. In this may be seen the beginnings of industrial design, which ever since the time of the Crystal Palace had been a desideratum of the machine age.

The social, or even Socialist, presuppositions of this process are clear: to raise to the dignity of art the cheap, widely distributed, mass-produced standard product.

Its influence is clear, too, especially on van de Velde's work in this sphere, and in the developments which gave rise to the *Deutscher Werkbund. An important rôle in this respect was played by the German architect Hermann *Muthesius, who spread the knowledge of modern English domestic architecture throughout Germany in the early years of this century with his numerous well-documented books on the English house and the exhibitions he organized abroad of English furniture and decorative schemes.

With the question of taste, however, things were more complex and difficult, not least because Walter Crane, the first president of the Arts and Crafts Society was still personally bound up with the old Pre-Raphaelite aesthetic, and sometimes opposed a greater 'opening-up' of the movement, although some of the most advanced architects of the day were to be found amongst the first members and exhibitors, men such as C. F. A. *Voysey, C. R. Ashbee, W. R. Lethaby, George Walton and E. L. Lutyens. Crane, in fact, always categorically excluded from the Society's exhibitions the works of the young C. R. *Mackintosh, and the whole Glasgow School, which was to exert such an influence on the Continent, particularly in Vienna.

It may nevertheless be affirmed that the Arts and Crafts movement made a lasting impression in both the aesthetic and technical spheres. Its abandonment of the

Philip Webb. Red House. Bexley Heath, Kent, 1859

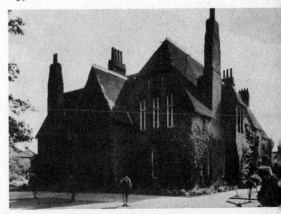

stylistic imitations of the 19th century, its disavowal of illusionistic patterns and its preference for continuous forms laid the basis for the creative fantasies of *Art Nouveau and Jugendstil, and for the break with the aesthetic outlook of the 19th century, which the art of the present century was to consummate.

Bibliography: Nikolaus Pevsner, *An Enquiry into Industrial Art in England*, New York 1937; Nikolaus Pevsner, *Pioneers of Modern Design from William Morris to Walter Gropius*, New York 1949; Jean Cassou, Emil Langui, and Nikolaus Pevsner, *Durchbruch zum 20. Jahrhundert, Kunst und Kultur der Jahrhundertwende*, Munich 1962.

GIULIA VERONESI

Aslin, Charles Herbert, b. Sheffield 1893, d. 1959. Studied at Sheffield University Department of Architecture. After a career in various local authority offices Aslin became County Architect for Hertfordshire in 1945, where he stayed till his retirement in 1958.

At the end of the Second World War, acute shortage of school places in Hertfordshire, together with lack of manpower and craftsmen in the building trade moved Aslin to tackle the problem as a quasi-military 'planned operation'. Taking advantage of the production potential of light industry, built up during the war, he organized a system of school *prefabrication from factory-made parts, of sufficient flexibility to allow each school to be treated individually.

Erik Gunnar Asplund. Law Courts Extension. Gothenburg, 1934–7

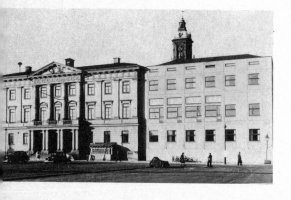

The prototype was Cheshunt Primary School, built in 1946 on an 8 foot 3 inch grid. In 1947, eleven schools were projected on a serial production basis, with flat roofs, solid floors, and standardized stanchions and beam connections; in 1948–49, development proceeded on twenty-one primary schools, while the 1947 schools were being completed. Development on these lines has continued ever since, with the 8 foot 3 inch grid successfully applied to multi-storey buildings, though a later development has led to the introduction of a 2 foot 8 inch planning module. The hundredth school of this type was opened in 1955.

Aslin also pioneered the use of bold clear colours in schools. He was President of the RIBA in 1954–6.

Bibliography: C. H. Aslin, 'Specialized developments in school construction' in *Journal of the RIBA*, November 1950; K. C. Twist, J. T. Redpath and K. C. Evans, 'Hertfordshire Schools Development' in *Architects' Journal* (London), 12 and 26.5.1955, 11.8.1955, 19.4.1956 and 2.8.1956.

HAROLD MEEK

Asplund, Erik Gunnar, b. Stockholm 1885, d. Stockholm 1940. The architecture of Erik Gunnar Asplund, one of the most prominent of Swedish architects of the first half of the twentieth century, is of historical significance because it shows the transition from traditional to modern architecture. Asplund received his architectural training at the Technical High School and the Academy of Art, Stockholm. He completed his training and began practice in 1909. His early work consisted mainly of houses. In 1913–14 he went to Italy and Greece to study the architecture of these countries; the visit made a profound impression on him and the influence of classical architecture can be discerned in almost all his work.

Among the buildings for which he was responsible on his return, from about 1914 to 1928 which represents his early period, were the layout of the Stockholm South Cemetery in collaboration with Sigurd Lewerentz, the Woodland Chapel in the same cemetery (1918–20), the Snellman villa, Djursholm (1917), the Skandia Cinema (1922–3) and the Stockholm City Library (1924–7). The last two mentioned are among Asplund's most important works, and they are both strongly classical in design. The Skandia Cinema, which was much admired at the time it was built, is rectangular in shape with side balconies and a design that depends for its aesthetic effect on a balance of verticals and horizontals, with a restrained use of classical decoration. The City Library is symmetrical in plan with a large cylindrical lending hall enclosed on three sides by rectangular blocks containing reading and study rooms and offices. The central part was originally designed to be surmounted by a dome, but this was abandoned for a flat roof over the cylinder. The whole work is a classical conception with an accent on simplicity and severity which was a trend of the time. If Asplund had continued designing in the style of the Skandia Cinema and the Stockholm City Library, he would have been regarded as another competent traditional architect, but with the buildings of the Stockholm Exhibition of 1930, for which he was responsible, he showed himself a modern architect expressively handling glass and steel with the lightness of effect that these materials create. This is seen especially in the Paradise Restaurant with its slender supports, its glass walls, its circular glass tower, and large coloured sun blinds, the very epitomization of the new architecture in Europe.

After this exhibition Asplund designed the Bredenberg store in Stockholm (1933–5), which has something of the lightness of the exhibition buildings; the State Bacteriological Laboratory, Stockholm (1933–7); the Gothenburg Law Courts Extension (1934–7), the design of which is modern in spirit yet harmonizes in scale with the original building in the classical style; and lastly the Forest Crematorium, Stockholm South Cemetery, begun in 1935 and completed in 1940. This building is generally regarded as his masterpiece. The work involved the remoulding of the site: the transformation of a gravel pit to a wind-swept hill on the summit of which the crematorium was built. Near it is a large pool, to reflect the sky, and a large marble cross. The group of buildings consists of three chapels, the crematorium and the columbarium; at the main entrance is a large portico with numerous plain shafts. Simple, dramatic and original as is the

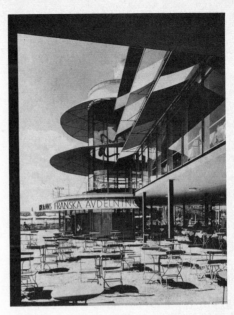

Erik Gunnar Asplund. Stockholm Exhibition, 1930

Erik Gunnar Asplund. Forest Crematorium. Stockholm, 1935–40

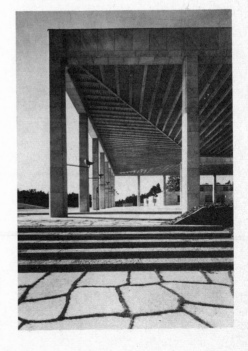

design for a purpose of this kind it is essentially Greek in conception, the feeling of repose that it creates depending on the relation of verticals and horizontals; it demonstrates how Greek architectural feeling can live in architecture that seems to be imbued with the modern spirit.

Bibliography: Bruno Zevi, *E. Gunnar Asplund*, Milan 1948; Holmdahl and Odeen (eds), *Gunnar Asplund, Architect*, Stockholm 1950; Eric de Maré, *Gunnar Asplund —A great modern architect*, London 1955.

ARNOLD WHITTICK

Athens Charter. A manifesto published by the international architectural organization *CIAM in 1933, setting out data and requirements connected with the problem of the modern city under five main headings (Dwellings, Recreation, Work, Transportation, Historic Buildings).

Austria. The wealth and power of the old monarchy on the Danube found its chief expression in the concentration of culture at Vienna, which reached a climax around 1900 in *Art Nouveau. The extensive diffusion of Austrian architecture, arts and crafts to other countries has never been achieved again. *Wagner, *Hoffmann, *Olbrich and *Loos triumphed over senseless eclecticism and produced outstanding examples of new conceptions of space. It is characteristic of the Vienna School that it never quite cut itself loose from tradition, whether it condemned

Adolf Loos. Steiner House. Vienna, 1910

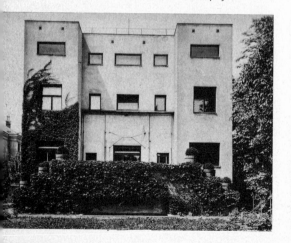

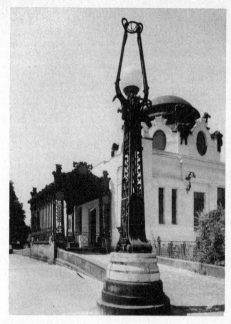

Otto Wagner. Station building for the Vienna Stadtbahn. Vienna, 1896–7

ornament radically like Loos, or sought to give it a new purpose like Hoffmann. It always adhered to the native tradition, especially to Kornhäusel.

Decimated Austria was hit harder by the consequences of the First World War than any other country. The new style in building, that second great attempt to do away with the influences of the past, had only met with a weak response in Austria. Furthermore, the puritanical and ascetic features of the movement, of the kind the Bauhaus embodies for example, are properties that are alien to the Austrian mentality. That is why significant Austrian architects became successful only when they went abroad: *Schindler, *Neutra, Bieber, Brenner, Schuster, Gottwald, Steinbüschel, *Seidler and Petschnigg.

Others transformed the influences entering from the north and west to achieve a charming compromise, as did Lichtblau and Haertl, or Strnad, who started off with classical shapes and modified them subjectively. Frank produced typical examples with a clear directness and cultivated the Viennese arts and crafts in new shapes.

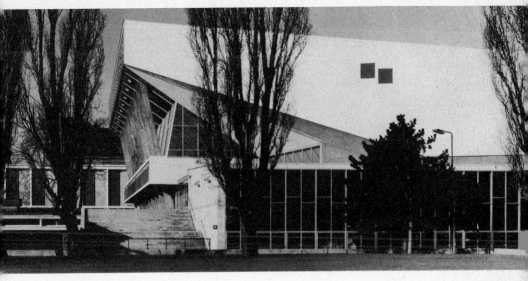

Roland Rainer. Municipal Hall. Vienna, 1954–8

Schuster revived the Biedermeier tradition. *Holzmeister, too, starting off in the traditional idiom, developed strong and capricious forms (churches and Salzburg Festival Theatre).

After the Second World War, economic stagnation was even more paralysing than between the wars. It is largely due to the vitality of Roland *Rainer and his school that this lethargy has been overcome.

Karl Schwanzer. Austrian Pavilion at the International Exhibition. Brussels, 1958

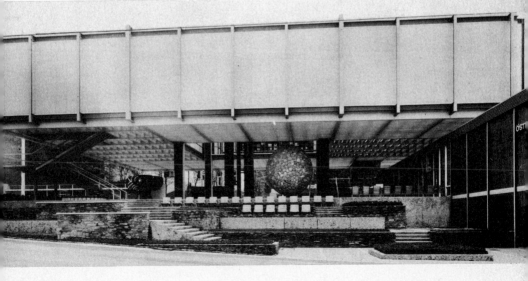

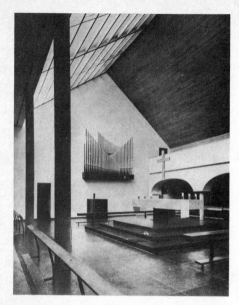

Arbeitsgruppe 4. Parish Church. Salzburg-Parsch, 1955–6

Rainer combines strict economy and rationality with a sure feeling for the expression of any building function. His Vienna Municipal Hall (1954–8) for 16,000 people, a steel structure with aluminium cladding, is of a new type for this class of building; one which he has employed again for halls at Bremen and Ludwigsburg. In conscious contrast to the fortress-like blocks of flats built in Vienna during the twenties, Rainer, in conjunction with Auböck, put up an experimental estate of detached prefabricated houses adjoining the old Vienna Werkbund estate. These examples, like others inspired by him in housing estates by younger architects (Windbrechtinger/Ketterer, Sekler, Freyler), propagate his theories on low buildings in cities. Only after a hard struggle has Rainer been able to carry into effect his general plan for rebuilding in Vienna.

A characteristic combination of the principles of modern architecture with the traditions of the Vienna School of 1900 has been achieved by architects such as Lorenz, who combines restraint in outer shape with a three-dimensional feeling for space, or Gottwald, a typical engineer-architect who

has built some remarkable schools and industrial buildings in Germany. His four-storey block of flats in the Hansa district of Berlin is an interesting solution of the problem of flexibility in the provision of dwelling space. A lucid demonstration of Austrian architecture is afforded by the exhibition pavilion at Brussels (1958) by Schwanzer which was re-erected in Vienna for the Museum of the Twentieth Century. Strict logicality in the manner of Loos is perpetuated in the work of Arbeitsgruppe 4 (Holzbauer, Kurrent, Spalt): church near Salzburg, shops. There are also manifestations of individuality in sports buildings such as the Gänshäufel Baths, Vienna, by Fellerer and Wörle, and in the simple and clear shapes of the airport buildings at Schwechat by the architects Klaudy, Pfeffer, Hoch and Schimka.

HUBERT HOFFMANN

Bakema, Jacob B., b. Groningen 1914. Studied architecture and hydraulic engineering in his home town, graduated at evening classes in advanced architecture in Amsterdam (HBO), and attended lectures part-time at the Delft Technical College. After that he worked for a few years under

J. H. van den Broek and Jacob B. Bakema. Lijnbaan pedestrian precinct. Rotterdam, 1953

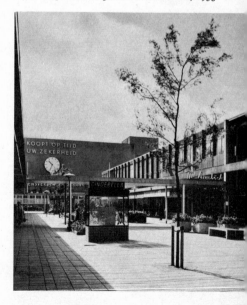

Professor Cor van *Eesteren, in the town-planning department of the City Architect's office in Amsterdam, and in the office of Van Tijen and Maaskant. Went into partnership with J. H. van den *Broek in 1948. Solely responsible for the art centre 't Venster in Rotterdam (1947) and the Civic Centre Plan for St Louis, Missouri (1955).

J. J. VRIEND

Baldessari, Luciano, b. Rovereto near Trento 1896. Graduated Milan 1922. Architect, painter, stage designer. Exhibition architecture, including the free forms of the Breda Pavilion, Milan (1951).

Bartning, Otto, b. Karlsruhe 1883, d. Darmstadt 1959. Studied at the Technical Colleges of Berlin and Karlsruhe. Industrial, administrative, domestic and hospital buildings and, in particular, Protestant churches. Steel church on the Pressa, Cologne (1928); Church of the Resurrection, Essen, on a circular plan (1930); emergency churches of prefabricated timber construction for the German Evangelical Relief Organization (designed 1946).

Basile, Ernesto, b. Palermo 1857, d. Palermo 1932. Built shortly after the turn of the century in the Italian *Art Nouveau style (Casa Basile, 1904; Casa Frassini, 1906, both at Palermo). Later changed over to a Classic Revival style and opposed the *Functionalist architecture of the twenties.

Baudot, Anatole de, b. Saarburg 1834, d. Paris 1915. Pupil of *Labrouste and *Viollet-le-Duc. De Baudot, 'Romantic of Reinforced Concrete', introduced the new building material to ecclesiastical architecture (St Jean-de-Montmartre, Paris, 1894–7). Besides designing buildings he carried out restorations and worked as an architectural writer.

Bauhaus. The Bauhaus was a school of design, building, and craftsmanship founded by Walter *Gropius in Weimar in 1919. It was transferred to Dessau in 1925, where it continued until 1928, and then transferred to Berlin, ultimately closing in 1933. The ideas and teaching of the Bauhaus have exercised a profound influence throughout the world.

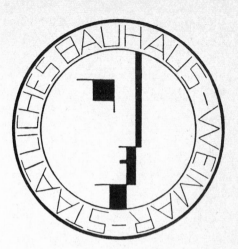

Oskar Schlemmer. Bauhaus symbol, 1922

Before the First World War the Belgian architect Henry van de *Velde had been director of the Grossherzogliche Sächsische Kunstgewerbeschule and the Grossherzogliche Sächsische Hochschule für Bildende Kunst at Weimar, and he had recommended to the Grand Duke of Saxe-Weimar that Walter Gropius should be his successor. The Grand Duke summoned Gropius for an interview in 1915, and Gropius asked for and was given full powers to reorganize the schools; when he took up his appointment in 1919 he united the two schools under the name of Das Staatliche Bauhaus Weimar. This was of profound significance because it made clear at the outset that one of the main purposes of the new school was to unite art and craft which had for too long been divorced from each other. Gropius contended that the artist or architect should also be a craftsman, that he should have experience of working in various materials so that he knew their qualities and that he should at the same time study theories of form and design. The traditional distinction between artist and craftsman should, Gropius thought, be eliminated. He also believed that a building should be the result of collective effort, and that each artist-craftsman should contribute his part with a full awareness of its purpose in relation to the whole building. Gropius was therefore an advocate of team-work in the creation of a building and in the production of furniture,

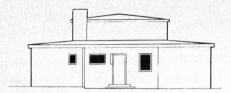

Georg Muche. Bauhaus experimental house.
Weimar, 1923. Elevation and plan

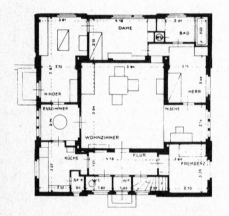

pottery, and all the various architectural arts.

The teaching thus comprehended industrial production. Gropius was not opposed, as was William *Morris, to the increasing use of machinery in the production of well-designed objects, but he believed that the machine should be made absolutely subservient to the will of the creative designer. This part of Gropius's teaching has perhaps been most difficult for many people to understand. Many critics have asked why it is necessary for students to master a craft in a material and yet acquiesce in industrial production. But Gropius regarded machinery merely as an elaboration of the hand tool of the craftsman, and thought it was necessary to know the nature of the material and all its potentialities before the tool or machine could be used to the best advantage.

There is obviously a correlation of teamwork in building and the necessary division of labour in industrial production, but the best results are likely to be obtained in both if members of the team not only master their own particular part but grasp its relation to the complete building or indus-

trial product. By thus using the machine to the best advantage the training at the Bauhaus was directed not to works of hand craftsmanship but to the creation of type-forms which could serve as models for mass production. And in the creation of this type-form the artist himself produces the prototype, that is if it is a teapot he makes this in the clay with his own hands as the model for mass production; he is no longer merely the drawing-board designer, but the designer-craftsman.

The curriculum of training consisted of two parallel courses of instruction, one devoted to the study of materials and craft (Werklehre) and the other to the theories of form and design (Formlehre). In the early years of the school it was necessary for the student to be taught by two masters, one in each section, an artist and a craftsman, because of the difficulty at that time of finding teachers who were sufficiently masters of both. These two teachers worked in close collaboration. Instruction at the school began with a preliminary course of six months, during which period the student worked with various materials— stone, wood, metal, clay, glass, pigments, and textiles—while he received elementary instruction in the theory of form. The purpose of working and experimenting with materials was to discover with which particular material the student had naturally the most creative aptitude, for it was an essential purpose to bring out the latent creative faculties of the individual. It might be that one student had a strong feeling for wood, another for the harder materials, stone and metal, another for textiles, another for pigments and colour. He was instructed in the use of tools and later in the use of machines that in industry have supplanted these tools. In the school devoted to form and design, instruction was given in the study and representation of natural form, in geometry and principles of building construction, in composition and the theories of volume, colour, and design.

Gropius was fortunate in gathering together some very able teachers, many of whom afterwards became famous in their various spheres. Among the first was Johannes Itten, who joined the school in 1919 and whom Gropius had first met a year earlier teaching in a private school in Vienna. Gropius was impressed with Itten's methods of education and invited him to the Bauhaus to direct the preliminary course. Itten's teaching included the study of the physical character of natural materials by representation and experiment, for it was contended that representing a material intelligently was one way of appreciating its structure. And in working in a particular material the student must not only develop a feeling for it in all its aspects, but he must appreciate its relation to other materials so as to be aware of its qualities by comparison and contrast. Other teachers at the Bauhaus at Weimar were Lyonel Feininger, printer and graphic artist, and Gerhard Marcks, sculptor and potter, both of whom joined in 1919; Georg Muche, painter and writer, who joined in 1920; Paul Klee, painter, graphic artist, and writer; and Oskar Schlemmer, painter and stage designer, who joined in 1921; Wassily Kandinsky, painter and graphic artist, who joined in 1922; and László Moholy-Nagy, painter, theatrical designer, photographer, and typographer, who joined in 1923.

In 1923, at the request of the Thuringian Legislative Assembly, the Bauhaus held an exhibition of its work which was to serve as a report on the four years of the life of the Bauhaus. Gropius felt that this was a bit premature; he would have preferred to wait until more mature results could be presented. The theme of the exhibition was 'Art and Technics, a New Unity', and included in the exhibition were designs in various materials, various products of the different workshops, examples of theoretical studies, and a one-family house called 'Am Horn' which was built and furnished by the Bauhaus workshops. This house was planned as a large square with several small rooms arranged round a central larger one; it was enthusiastically acclaimed by many critics, among them Dr E. Redslob, the National Art Director of Germany, who praised its organic unity.

In spite of the progress and success of the Bauhaus it met with much local opposition from the more conservative members of the community, while the whole enterprise was associated with Socialism in the minds of many because it happened to be established at a time when there was a Socialist régime. It also met with considerable hostility from the Thuringian Government, which more or less forced Gropius to a decision at the end of 1924 to close the

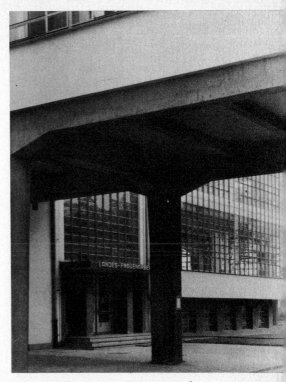

Walter Gropius. Bauhaus. Dessau, 1925–6

school. Both teachers and students wholeheartedly supported Gropius; the Director and masters notified the Government of Thuringia on 26 December of their decision to close the institution, created by them, on the expiration of their contracts on 1 April 1925.

Various cities discussed the possibility of transplanting the Bauhaus, among them Frankfurt, Hagen, Mannheim, Darmstadt and Dessau. The Mayor of Dessau succeeded in securing the transfer of the Bauhaus to his town. He appropriated seven houses for the use of the school while a new building was being erected. This building, designed by Gropius in response to the request of the City Council, was begun in the autumn of 1925 and completed in December 1926. It consisted of three principal wings, a school of design occupying one, workshops another, and a students' hostel a third. The first two were linked by a bridge over a roadway, and in

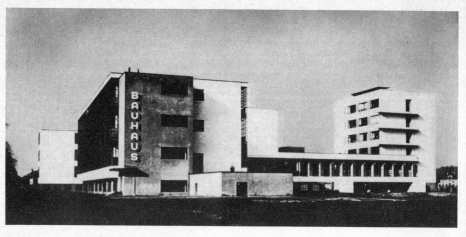

Walter Gropius. Bauhaus. Dessau, 1925–6

this bridge were administrative rooms, club rooms, and a private atelier for Professor Gropius. The students' hostel was a six-storey building consisting of twenty-eight studio-dormitory rooms. The building was constructed partly of *reinforced concrete. In the workshops' wing reinforced concrete floor slabs and supporting mushroom posts were employed with the supports set well back to allow a large uninterrupted *glass screen on the façade extending for three storeys. This was probably the first time so ambitious a use of glass screen was employed in an industrial building, and it helped to lead the way to similar constructions throughout Europe and America.

With the re-establishment of the Bauhaus at Dessau, the opportunity was taken to revise the curriculum. The earlier method of joint instruction by two masters, an artist and a craftsman, was abandoned and was supplanted by that of one master who was trained as both. This was becoming increasingly possible because several former Bauhaus students were now appointed masters: Josef Albers, Herbert Bayer, Marcel *Breuer, Hinnerk Scheper, and Joost Schmidt. Seven of the masters who had been with the Bauhaus at Weimar continued at Dessau. Gerhard Marcks left because there were not sufficient funds to install his pottery workshop at Dessau. Johannes Itten had left in the spring of 1923 owing to differences of opinion on

the conduct of the preliminary course, and his work was continued by Moholy-Nagy and Josef Albers, who jointly broadened its scope. In revising the course at Dessau the opportunity was also taken to reaffirm the principles which guided the Bauhaus system of education: these could be summarized as training in design, technics, and craftsmanship for all kinds of creative work, especially building; the execution of experimental work, especially building and interior decoration; the development of models or type-forms for industrial production and the sale of such models to industry. As a general doctrine the Bauhaus sought to establish the common citizenship of all forms of creative work and their interdependence on each other.

The Bauhaus continued at Dessau under the direction of Walter Gropius until early in 1928, when he resigned because he wished to devote himself more freely to his creative work without being restricted by official duties; on his recommendation Hannes *Meyer, the Swiss architect, who had been head of the department of architecture, became director. Meyer resigned in June 1930 as the result of differences with the municipal authority, who then tried to persuade Gropius to take over again. Instead, Gropius recommended the appointment of Ludwig *Mies van der Rohe, who accepted the position. In October 1932, after the National Socialist party had taken over the Government of

Anhalt, the Bauhaus moved to Berlin; in April 1933 it was closed by the National Socialists. From April 1933 the building at Dessau was used for the training of political leaders.

Although the school was closed, its teaching and methods were by no means dead, and they continued to exercise a wide influence throughout the world. Indeed, it may be said that its influence has been strongest since it ceased to exist, probably because it takes time for such ideas to spread. Many art schools in Europe and America have adopted in part its methods of teaching, especially as many of its masters and students have taken positions in art schools and institutes throughout Europe and America. For example, Moholy-Nagy became director of the New Bauhaus—now the Institute of Design—at Chicago, where Bauhaus methods were employed. They have also been introduced partially at the school of architecture at Harvard University, the Laboratory School of Industrial Design in New York, and in the School of Design in southern California. It would be a mistake to think that the ideas that prompted Bauhaus training are universally accepted, but it is doubtful whether any method of art teaching of the century has had quite the same impact.

Bibliography: Walter Gropius, *Idee und Aufbau des Staatlichen Bauhauses*, Weimar 1923; *Neue Arbeiten der Bauhauswerkstatten*, 1925 (English translation, *The New Architecture and the Bauhaus*, London 1935, reprinted 1955); Herbert Bayer, Walter Gropius, and Ise Gropius, *Bauhaus 1919–1928* (London 1939, Boston 1952); Hans Maria Wingler, *Das Bauhaus*, *Weimar*, *Dessau, Berlin*, Cologne 1962.

ARNOLD WHITTICK

BBPR. Partnership of architects Lodovico Barbiano di Belgioioso, Enrico Peressutti, Ernesto N. *Rogers, and (until his death in 1945) Gian Luigi Banfi. The team achieved international fame with its Sanatorium at Legnano (1937–8); more recent buildings such as the Torre Velasca, Milan (1957), endeavour to establish a poetic style by reference to tradition and local atmosphere. Housing and industrial buildings; exhibition architecture (children's maze at the Milan Triennale 1954); restoration work; interior decoration (Museum at the Castello Sforzesco, Milan, 1952–6).

Beaudouin, Eugène, b. Paris 1898. Student at the French Academy in Rome. In collaboration with Marcel *Lods he designed, in 1933, the Cité de la Muette at Drancy, near Paris, a mixed development estate where prefabricated reinforced concrete units were used; the Pavilion School at Suresnes (1932–5); and the Maison du Peuple at Clichy (1939). Cité Rotterdam suburb at Strasbourg (1951–3). Town and regional planning.

Beaux-Arts. *École des Beaux-Arts.

Behrens, Peter, b. Hamburg 1868, d. Berlin 1940. In a society torn between archaic mental attitudes and a blind faith in the lightning progress of technology, Behrens was one of the first architects of the 20th century to develop a form of architectural thought that would answer to the demands of an industrialized civilization. At a period when the moral and social demands put forward by the Expressionist painters of Dresden (*Die Brücke*) were leading to new directions in the graphic arts, he was in at the birth of modern architecture in Germany, where he exerted a leading influence between 1900 and 1914. Furthermore, the sidelines derived from architecture in which he engaged inaugurated (1907) a form of specialization that has become widely known in our times under the name of Industrial Design. Here, too, he deeply influenced the development of technology and style at a time when the propagation of craft-derived forms by the exponents of *Art Nouveau was threatening to undermine any attempts to formulate design principles in conformity with new ways of living.

Behrens did not discover his true vocation from the first. Like *van de Velde and *Le Corbusier, he was a painter at first, and came to architecture via the so-called applied arts. From 1886 to 1889 he attended painting classes at the art schools of Karlsruhe and Düsseldorf. In 1890 he was impressed by the work of the *luministes* (Israels) in Holland, and the work of painters such as Leibl in Munich; he was a founder-member of the Münchner Sezession in 1893. Already interested in the graphic arts, his early compositions (coloured woodcuts, frontispieces for books, etc.) are still permeated by the decorative influence of Art Nouveau.

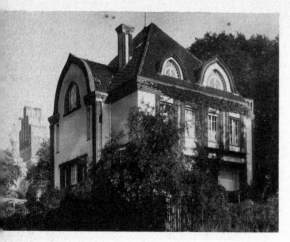

Peter Behrens. Behrens House. Darmstadt, 1901

After travelling in Italy (1896), Behrens turned in 1898 to problems of industrial production and designed a number of prototype flasks for mass production by a large glass works; these are already notable for their plain, straightforward shapes. In 1899 the Grand Duke Ernst Ludwig invited him to stay at Darmstadt and join a group of young artists (the architects J. M. *Olbrich and P. Huber, the painters and interior decorators H. Christiansen and P. Bürck, and the sculptors L. Habich and R. Bosselt) who under the name of *Die Sieben* (The Seven) had as their aim the establishment of effective relationships between all the plastic arts. It was then that

Peter Behrens. AEG Turbine Factory. Berlin, 1908–9

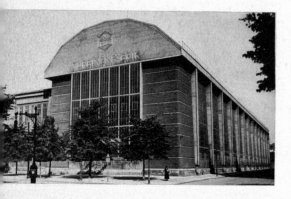

Behrens took up architecture and, as van de Velde had done at Uccle five years before, he built his own house and fitted it out completely in a unitary style that betrayed the influence of both van de Velde and *Mackintosh. At the instance of *Muthesius, he was appointed head of the Düsseldorf School of Art in 1903, a post he held until 1907. From this period onwards his classical temperament led him to design sober, powerful and massive works, of mathematical severity and uncompromisingly functionalist in style. The houses he built for Obenauer (Saarbrücken, 1905–06), Cuno and Schroeder (Eppenhausen near Hagen, 1908–10) express this rationalistic tendency, that was ultimately to distinguish the work of Behrens from the plastic dynamism and lyricism of *Poelzig and *Mendelsohn.

In 1907, the year the Deutscher Werkbund was founded, Behrens was summoned to Berlin by the AEG (the German General Electrical Company). His duties comprised the design not only of pieces of electrical equipment (cookers, radiators, ventilators, lamps, etc.) but also of the firm's packaging, catalogues, leaflets, posters, letterheads, showrooms, shops, and, to boot, factories and workshops. The circumstance is of much importance: it marks the emergence, in the midst of industry, of a desire to humanize technology. By employing an architect to ensure a good visual appearance for their products, the AEG was bringing objects into daily life that were not only functionally efficient, but were harmoniously and sensitively designed as well, permeated as they were by an authentically creative style which, in the last analysis, projected the brand image of an industrial power. At the same time, and under the same auspices, Behrens introduced a new expression of monumentality to European architecture with his turbine factory for the AEG (Berlin, 1908–9)—the first German building in glass and steel—the high tension plant (1910) and the factory for small motors (1910–11), etc. Behrens also built a complete district of flats for AEG workers at Henningsdorf, near Berlin (1910–11). Apart from numerous factories which he erected throughout his career, mention should be made of certain other

Page 49. Peter Behrens. Entrance hall of the Hoechst Dyeworks offices. 1920–5

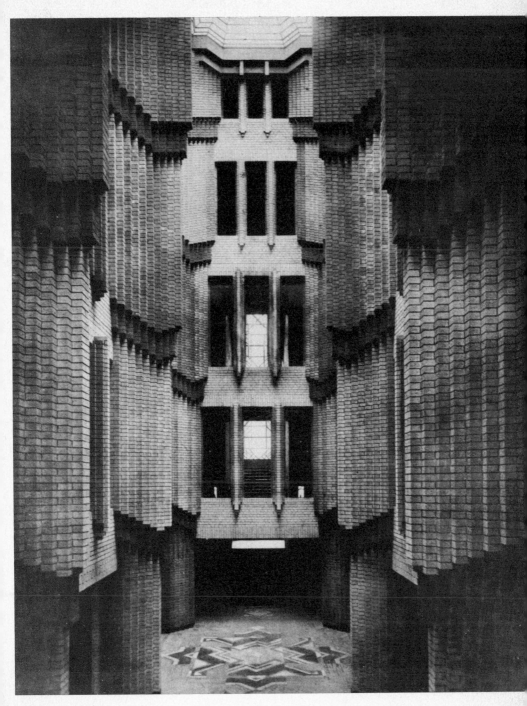

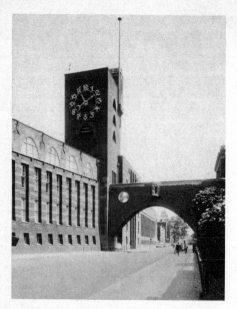

Peter Behrens. Offices of the Hoechst Dyeworks, 1920–5

major works of his, designed in a neo-classic style that expressed their owners' need for prestige. These include the Mannesmann offices at Düsseldorf (1913–23), those for the Continental Rubber Company at Hanover (1911–12), and the German Embassy in St Petersburg (1911–12).

In 1922 Behrens was appointed director of the School of Architecture at the Vienna Academy; some of the buildings he designed in the following years may be considered as examples of German *Expressionism (Hoechst Dyeworks, 1920–5). In 1936 he became head of the department of architecture at the Prussian Academy of Arts, Berlin. His most outstanding pupils are: Le Corbusier, who worked in his Berlin office from 1910 to 1911; Gropius, from 1907 to 1910; and Mies van der Rohe, from 1908 to 1911.

Bibliography: Peter Behrens, *Feste des Lebens und der Kunst*, Jena 1900; Fritz Hoeber, *Peter Behrens*, Munich 1913; Paul Joseph Cremers, *Peter Behrens, Sein Werk von 1909 bis zur Gegenwart*, Essen 1928; K. M. Grimme, *Peter Behrens und seine Wiener akademische Meisterschule*, Vienna 1930

ROBERT L. DELEVOY

Belluschi, Pietro, b. Ancona 1899. From 1927 chief designer in an architect's office at Portland, Oregon; since 1943 has intermittently run an office of his own. Now mainly a consultant and designer in collaboration with other architects. Residential and office buildings, shopping centres, ecclesiastical buildings. Equitable Savings Building at Portland, Oregon (1948), in which all façade units together with the aluminium-clad stanchions are arranged flush with the wall plane.

Berg, Max, b. Stettin 1870. Studied at Technical College, Berlin-Charlottenburg. City Architect, Breslau (1912–13). His Centenary Hall at Breslau, a huge cupola with exposed ribs, was one of the boldest reinforced concrete structures of its time. Exhibition Hall Messehof (1925) and hydro-electric station at Breslau.

Berlage, Hendrik Petrus, b. Amsterdam 1856, d. The Hague 1934. Berlage studied at Zurich, and had his own practice in Amsterdam from 1889 onwards; he is regarded as one of the great innovators of architecture around the year 1900. Reacting against 19th-century eclecticism, he aimed at an 'honest awareness of the problems of architecture' and a craftsmanlike approach to materials and construction. Berlage revealed once more to his contemporaries the meaning and magic of brickwork. Plastering a wall was tantamount to falsification in his eyes, and he eschewed its use even in the rooms of private houses. Berlage's 'moral' outlook was in harmony with the social climate of the times, which since *c.* 1895 was strongly influenced by the rising labour movement.

Despite his rejection of all historic styles, Berlage felt attracted by the massive gravity of the Romanesque, which is reflected in his semicircular arches and his large unbroken wall surfaces. These features also recall the work of the American architect H. H. *Richardson, who probably influenced him during his trip to America. Characteristic works of his include the Diamond-workers' House, Amsterdam (1899–1900), Holland House, London (1914), and above all Amsterdam Stock Exchange, completed in 1903. The Stock Exchange was the outcome of a competition held in 1897, which Berlage won with a design he subsequently altered in many details. In this monumental work, Berlage used a light-coloured stone for special features, in addition to brick. The steel roof structure over the main hall is left exposed. There is a certain aridity of conception here which cannot be overlooked; it appears also in Berlage's earliest designs for furniture.

As an architectural writer, Berlage exerted great influence through his numerous publications and lectures. Many buildings, especially in the *Netherlands, are based on Berlage's work, even though they differ formally from it. He himself, in

Bill, Max, b. Winterthur 1908. Painter, sculptor, exhibition designer, architect. Studied at Zurich Art School and (1927–9) at the *Bauhaus. From 1951 to 1956 rector of the Hochschule für Gestaltung at Ulm and head of the departments of architecture and industrial design. Private houses, offices. The buildings of the Ulm Hochschule (1953–5) embody a complex scheme in an open, easily graspable layout, which harmonizes well with its setting.

Bibliography: Tomás Maldonado, *Max Bill,* Stuttgart 1956; Margit Staber, 'Max Bill und die Umweltgestaltung', in *Zodiac 9,* Milan 1962.

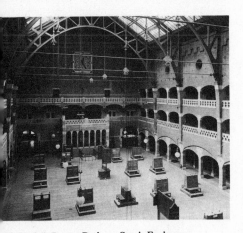

Hendrik Petrus Berlage. Stock Exchange. Amsterdam, 1897–1903

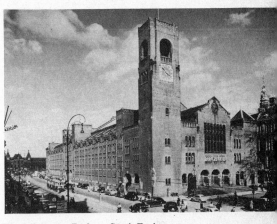

Hendrik Petrus Berlage. Stock Exchange. Amsterdam, 1897–1903

his later years came under the influence of the young *Expressionist architects. In 1928 he attended the first congress of *CIAM at La Sarraz, but felt himself too committed to a more traditional conception of architecture to be able to join the CIAM.

Bibliography: Hendrik Petrus Berlage, *Gedanken über den Stil in der Baukunst,* Leipzig 1905; Hendrik Petrus Berlage, *Grundlagen und Entwicklung der Architektur,* Berlin 1908; Hendrik Petrus Berlage, *Studies over Bouwkunst, Stijl en Samenleving,* Rotterdam 1910; Jan Gratama, *Dr. H. P. Berlage Bouwmeester,* Rotterdam 1925.

J. J. VRIEND

Bogardus, James, b. Catskill, New York 1800, d. New York 1874. Manufacturer and inventor, who built multi-storeyed factory buildings in the mid-19th century, where the outer walls were assembled from cast-iron units (his own factory in New York, 1848–9; Harper and Brothers Building, New York, 1854). The publicity Bogardus gave his buildings resulted in the widespread adoption of cast-iron façades, which paved the way for steel-frame structures (*Steel).

Böhm, Dominikus, b. Jettingen, Bavaria 1880, d. Cologne 1955. Studied at Stuttgart Technical College under Theodor *Fischer. Catholic ecclesiastical buildings

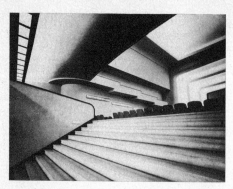

Rino Levi. Art Palacio Cinema. São Paulo, 1936

(e.g. Church at Mainz-Bischoffsheim, 1926; St Engelbert at Cologne-Riehl, 1930; St Maria Königin at Cologne-Marienburg, 1954).
Bibliography: August Hoff and H. Muck, *Böhm, Leben und Werk*, Munich and Zurich 1962.

Bonatz, Paul, b. Solgne, Lorraine 1877, d. Berlin 1951. Pupil and successor of Theodor *Fischer at Stuttgart Technical College. Main station at Stuttgart (1913–27, together with F. E. Scholer). Cultural, commercial, and industrial buildings.

Bourgeois, Victor, b. Charleroi 1897, d. Brussels 1962; 1914–19 student at the Académie Royale des Beaux-Arts, Brussels. His conception of architecture as the mirror of society led him early in his career to the problem of municipal housing. The

Attilio Correia Lima. Santos Dumont de Hidros Airport. Rio de Janeiro, 1938

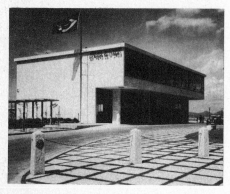

Cité Moderne at Berchem-Ste-Agathe near Brussels (1922–5) seeks to relieve the monotonous character of the estate by varying the articulation of terraced housing and by the use of open squares and courtyards and lively façade elements. Social buildings, schools, estates, town planning. Professor at the École Nationale Supérieure d'Architecture.
Bibliography: Georges Linze, *Victor Bourgeois*, Brussels 1961.

Brazil. When in 1943 the Museum of Modern Art of New York presented its exhibition on old and new architecture in Brazil, the world was suddenly made aware that in a faraway country the International Architecture of the 1920s had blossomed into a tropical version. Characterized by its daring formal expression, its lyrical content, and its regional connotations, it also had strong spiritual links with the colonial past of the country. As a matter of fact, it had sprung up in the wake of two rebel movements, the Modern Art Week in São Paulo, 1922, and the Regionalist movement in Recife, 1926, led by Gilberto Freyre, which aimed at giving new shape to Brazilian intellectual and artistic life, not only by bringing it up to a truly contemporary outlook, rooted in the most genuine sources of Brazilian life, but also by attempting to destroy the alien influences which had dominated the country since the arrival in 1806 of the King of Portugal, D. João VI, when he fled the Napoleonic invasion and transferred his court to Rio de Janeiro. In 1816 D. João VI invited a French mission of painters, sculptors, and architects to 'civilize' the country, with the result that the organic development of a local architecture, brought about throughout the colonial period by an ecological assimilation of the Portuguese Baroque style, was disrupted, and all kinds of foreign pseudo-styles were introduced, turning the 19th century into an uncharacteristic interval, chiefly taken up by copies of whatever might be done abroad—not only in architecture but in all the arts.

Page 53. Lúcio Costa, Oscar Niemeyer, Jorge Machado Moreira, Affonso Eduardo Reidy, Ernani Vasconcellos and Carlos Leão; consultant architect, Le Corbusier. Ministry of Education. Rio de Janeiro, 1937–43

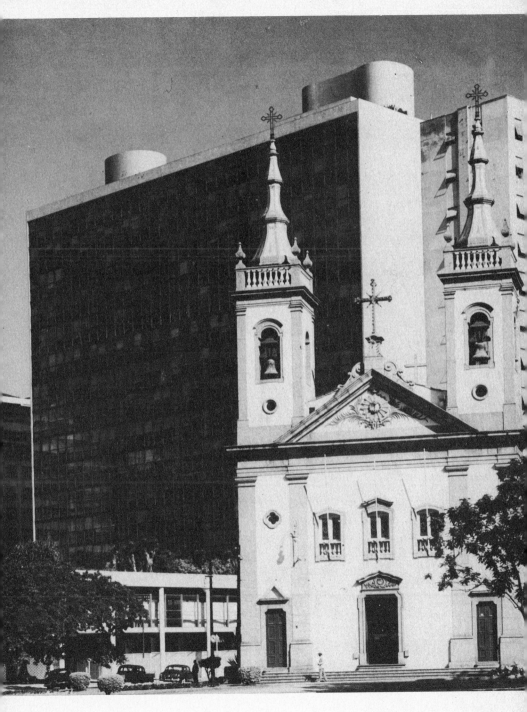

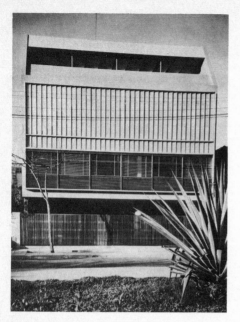

Jorge Machado Moreira. House for Antonio
Ceppa. Rio de Janeiro, 1958

A few years before these two movements,
scientific studies of the effect of sunlight
on buildings had been started by Alexandre
Albuquerque, who in 1916 succeeded in
incorporating into the Building Code of
the city of São Paulo precise requirements
as to the minimum provision of sunlight in
a new building. There existed thus in the
1920s not only an intellectual atmosphere
receptive to the new ideas in architecture
but also a sound regional approach to the
basic problem of the exposure of buildings,
both in order to assure a minimum of sunlight and also to control its excess. In 1927
in São Paulo, G. *Warchavchik, a new-
comer from Russia, presented his first
cube-like houses to the public, and was
later joined in partnership by Lúcio *Costa.
When the Revolution of 1930, led by
Getulio Vargas, upset all the conventional
political and cultural values of the country
and launched a programme of important
new public works, the younger architects
were in a way prepared for the decisive, if
paradoxical, episode of the new building
for the Ministry of Education and Health.
A competition was held for the design of
this building, and all the modern projects

were disqualified by a conservative jury.
But the Minister of Education, Gustavo
Capenema, who was surrounded by a
group of far-seeing collaborators, had the
daring, after paying the prizes awarded by
the jury, to invite Lúcio Costa, one of the
disqualified competitors, to design the final
project. Lúcio Costa insisted on a team of
all the other rejected candidates being
formed, and this was done. Lúcio Costa,
Oscar *Niemeyer, Jorge Machado Moreira,
Affonso Eduardo *Reidy, Ernani Vasconcellos, and Carlos Leão were thus responsible for the development of the final design.
In 1936, *Le Corbusier was invited as a
consultant on this project, as well as on one
for the new University City. He stayed in
Brazil only three weeks, working with the
group and giving a few public lectures, but
during this short stay the turning-point
was reached and modern architecture was
irrevocably established. Le Corbusier's
main ideas fell on fertile ground. The
concept of pilotis was especially good for
the Brazilian climate, the brise-soleil were
in many cases an absolute necessity, and
his basically lyrical formal approach was
thoroughly suited to the Brazilian spirit.
A local version of International Architecture thus emerged. Prior to this, Warchavchik's houses, from 1928 on, and Rino
Levi's outstandingly direct Art Palacio
Cinema in São Paulo (1936) must of course
be mentioned.
In the years that followed, i.e. from 1937
to 1943, an impressive number of distin-
guished jobs show how quickly maturity
was achieved. They include: Oscar Nie-
meyer's Day Nursery in Rio (1937), his
Ouro Preto Hotel (1940), his Casino, Yacht
Club and Dance Hall (1943), and the São
Francisco Chapel (1944) at Pampúlha; Luiz
Nunes's (with Fernando Saturnio de Brito)
Water Tower at Olinda (1937); Attilio
Correia Lima's Santos Dumont de Hidros
Airport in Rio (1938), with Jorge Ferreira,
Thomaz Estrella, Renato Mesquita dos
Santos and Renato Soeiro; Lúcio Costa's
and Oscar Niemeyer's (with Paul Lester
Wiener) Brazilian Pavilion at the New York
World's Fair (1939); Marcelo and Milton
Roberto's ABI—the Brazilian Press Asso-
ciation Building (1938), the Instituto de
Resseguros Building (1942), and the Santos
Dumont Airport Building (1944), all in
Rio; Alvaro Vital Brasil's Edificio Esther
apartment building (with Adhemar Marin-

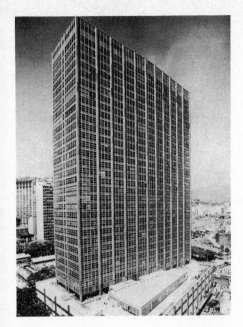

Henrique E. Mindlin. Avenida Central Building.
Rio de Janeiro, 1961

Garcia Roza, Henrique E. Mindlin, and
Giancarlo Palanti. The most important
events in the history of Brazilian architec-
ture since 1950 are Oscar Niemeyer's
Ibirapuéra Exhibition Pavilions in São
Paulo (1953); in Rio, Lúcio Costa's Parque
Guinle apartment buildings (1948–50–54);
Affonso Eduardo Reidy's Pedregulho
Housing Estate and his Museum of
Modern Art in Rio de Janeiro (1954 –);
Jorge Machado Moreira's University City
(1953–), as well as, of course, Niemeyer's
superb buildings in Brasilia.

In spite of obvious individual differences,
there is in most Brazilian work a deliberate
formal research, an attempt at lightness
and airiness and, in many cases, a trans-
literation into contemporary terms of old
elements from the colonial past (such as
open ceramic tile work, various forms of
'jalousies', or the renewed use of ceramic
murals in tiles, i.e. *azulejos*, or in mosaic)
which give it a common character. There
is in general, however, much less use of
colour in the exterior than might be
expected by the foreign visitor. It is

Oscar Niemeyer, Zenon Lotufo, Helio Uchôa
and Eduardo Kneese de Mello. Palace of
Industry, Ibirapuéra Park. São Paulo, 1951–4

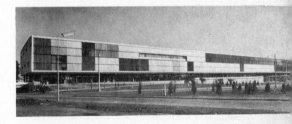

ho) in São Paulo (1938) and his Vital
Brasil Institute, in Niteroi (1941); Olavo
Redig de Campos's Social Centre in Rio
(1942); Firmino Saldanha's Mississippi
(1938) and Mossoró (1940) apartment
buildings in Rio, not to mention the
Ministry of Education and Health itself,
started in 1937 and finished in 1943. All
these are landmarks which have already
endured the test of time.

After the war years the country entered
into a phase of fast industrialization which
helped to raise the level of construction,
also of tremendous real estate speculation,
which of course resulted in a number of
second-rate jobs. However, the initial impulse persisted and today a large number
of good buildings may be credited to the
movement. To the architects whose work
has become better known abroad belong
Paulo Antunes Ribeiro, João Vilanova Artigas, Sergio Bernardes, Francisco Bolonha,
Oswaldo Bratke, Icaro Castro Mello, Ary

Affonso Eduardo Reidy. Museum of Modern Art.
Rio de Janeiro, commenced 1954

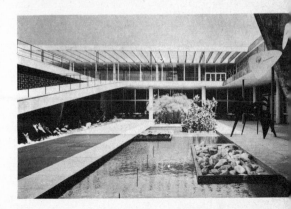

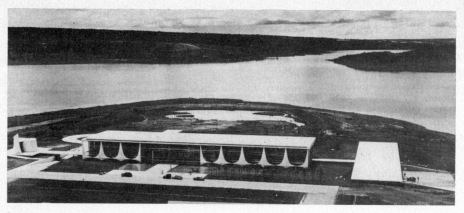

Oscar Niemeyer. President's Palace. Brasilia, completed 1959

probably felt that the brilliance of the sky and of the sunlight, as well as the gorgeous landscape, need no further reinforcement. A great deal of the colour which serves to emphasize the best architectural jobs is due to the surrounding gardens, in connection with which the immense contribution of Roberto Burle Marx must be stressed. The rôle played by Brazilian painters, starting with Candido Portinari's murals and *azulejo* designs for the Ministry of Education must also be noted.

Modern architecture in Brazil has had a paradoxical development, leading it to the summits of creative achievement almost from the start, a result perhaps of the fact that it was handed down and imposed from above by an intellectual *élite* under exceptionally fortunate circumstances. Monumental buildings were put up before any real attempt had been made at solving the urgent problems of providing schools or hospitals or low-cost housing. Until recent times city planning and interior decoration were neglected in favour of more spectacular undertakings. Architects were satisfied with traditional Brazilian furniture or the best that could be brought from Europe, contemporary if possible.

The most striking example of this peculiar development is the dramatic creation by President Juscelino Kubitschek of Brasilia, the new capital for the country, about 1,000 kilometres from the Atlantic coast, in a hitherto virgin territory. Located on gently sloping highlands, half surrounded by a huge artificial lake, this new city, planned for 600,000 inhabitants, was formally inaugurated as the new seat of the Federal Government on 21 April 1960, only three years, one month, and five days after an international jury had selected Lúcio Costa's deceptively simple plan in an open competition among Brazilian architects. In a general outline reminiscent of an aeroplane, the wings are devoted to the super blocks of apartment dwellings; the main axis, along what would correspond to the body of the plane, to the monumental distribution of the Ministries and the Plaza of the Three Powers (Presidential Palace, Supreme Court, and Congress), with the business and entertainment districts round the intersection, which is emphasized by the bus depot, arranged on several levels. Thoroughly planned with deep human concern, yet deliberately aiming at a clear symbolic expression of the city's unique function, Brasilia has carried to the man-in-the-street the concept of planning to an unsurpassed degree, especially through the total elimination of traffic intersections, one of the aspects of planning most easily grasped by the general public.

The unity and integrated character of Brasilia derive not only from Costa's lucid plan but also from Oscar Niemeyer's striking design for most of the buildings carried out to date. There can be no question that the building of Brasilia, in very difficult economic and financial circumstances and involving considerable

sacrifices for the country as a whole, con-
stitutes a magnificently constructive state-
ment of the collective will of the people.
Bibliography: Philip L. Goodwin, *Brazil
Builds*, Museum of Modern Art, New
York 1943; Henry-Russell Hitchcock,
Latin American Architecture since 1945,
New York 1955; Henrique E. Mindlin,
Modern Architecture in Brazil, Colibris,
Amsterdam 1956.

                              HENRIQUE E. MINDLIN

Breuer, Marcel, b. Pecs, Hungary 1902.
In 1920 Breuer moved to Vienna, intending to become a painter and sculptor. After
a brief attendance at the Art Academy he
became disillusioned with its 'tired eclecticism' and looked around for a practical
apprenticeship in one of the crafts, which
would bring him into direct contact with
tools and materials. Before long, he heard
of Walter *Gropius's *Bauhaus, then
located in Weimar; and, late in 1920, he
left Vienna for Weimar and became one of
the youngest members of the first generation of Bauhaus students. Under the
influence of Breuer and others then at the
Bauhaus, the emphasis of the school began
to shift from 'arts and crafts' to 'art and
technology'—or from romanticism and
impressionism to rationalism and objectivity in design. Breuer's principal interest,
from the start, was in the area of furniture
design, and by 1924, at the age of twenty-
two, he took over the direction of the
Bauhaus's furniture department. Before
long his preoccupation with standardized,
modular unit furniture led him to interior
design and standardized, modular unit
housing—and, thus, to architecture.
Breuer's most notable contribution to contemporary design in the 1920s was in the
field of furniture, for he had invented, as
early as 1925, a series of systems that
employed continuously bent steel tubes
(painted or chromium-plated) to form the
structural frames of stools, chairs, and
tables. Indeed, between 1925 and 1928
Breuer literally designed almost every
single piece of modern, tubular steel furniture in use today all over the world. Among
his finest designs was the S-shaped cantilever chair of 1928, which remains the most
commonly used modern commercial chair
in the world today. Much of this important
experimental work in furniture design was
made possible by the move, in 1925, of the

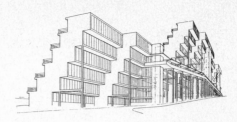

Marcel Breuer. Elberfeld Hospital, 1928. Project

Marcel Breuer, Alfred and Emil Roth. Doldertal
apartments. Zurich, 1935–6

Marcel Breuer. Breuer House. New Canaan,
Conn., 1947

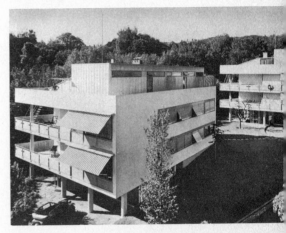

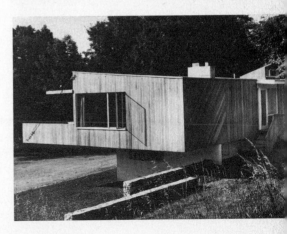

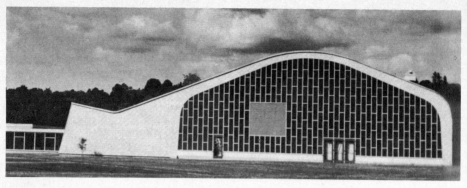

Marcel Breuer. Gymnasium, Litchfield High School. Litchfield, Conn., 1954–6

Bauhaus to Dessau, and the construction of the new Bauhaus by Gropius. Breuer was commissioned to design all the furniture needed in the new buildings, and this commission provided an important stimulus to his work in this field. In later years —especially in Switzerland and in England —Breuer again advanced the art of furniture design by developing some of the first bent and moulded plywood chairs ever manufactured in quantity, as well as some of the first chairs using aluminium as a structural supporting frame.

Meanwhile his interest in architecture had grown, and he left the Bauhaus in 1928 to practise as an architect and interior designer in Berlin. During the next half-dozen years Breuer built several houses and apartments easily as radical as—and often more practical than—the contemporary work of the time by *Le Corbusier and others. Moreover, he entered a number of competitions and otherwise prepared theoretical projects for cities, theatres, factories, etc., that greatly influenced his contemporaries. With the advent of Hitler in 1933, Breuer made preparations to leave Germany and soon entered into partnership with F. R. S. *Yorke in London. The partnership lasted until 1937, when Walter Gropius, who had been appointed Chairman of the Department of Architecture at Harvard, asked Breuer to join him on that faculty. At the same time, Gropius and Breuer formed an architectural partnership in Cambridge, Massachusetts. This partnership lasted until 1941.

While it is difficult, if not impossible, to separate the individual contributions of Gropius and Breuer both to the teaching at Harvard and to the houses designed in their office, it is fair to say that Breuer's contact with individual Harvard students was especially close (he was closer to them in age, and he tended to be extremely practical in his approaches to design problems); and it is fair, also, to say that much of Breuer's attention to detail is evident in the work completed by the Gropius and Breuer partnership. In any event, both Breuer's teaching and Breuer's completed buildings left a profound impression on a new generation of American architects. Among his students, for example, were such men as Philip *Johnson, Paul *Rudolph, John *Johansen, Edward L. Barnes, Landis Gores, and Willo von Moltke—all of them prominent in American architecture and planning today.

In 1946 Breuer moved to New York City, and he has practised there ever since. For the first few years of that practice, Breuer's work was limited largely to houses and smaller, institutional buildings; but in 1952 he was selected to be one of the three architects for the new Headquarters for UNESCO, in Paris. (The other two were the Italian Pier Luigi *Nervi, and the Frenchman Bernard H. *Zehrfuss.) From that moment on, Breuer's work became increasingly important internationally, and larger in scale: his UNESCO Headquarters were completed in 1958; a monastery in Minnesota was under construction at the same time; college buildings all over the

Page 59. Marcel Breuer. St John's Abbey Church. Collegeville, Minnesota, 1953–61

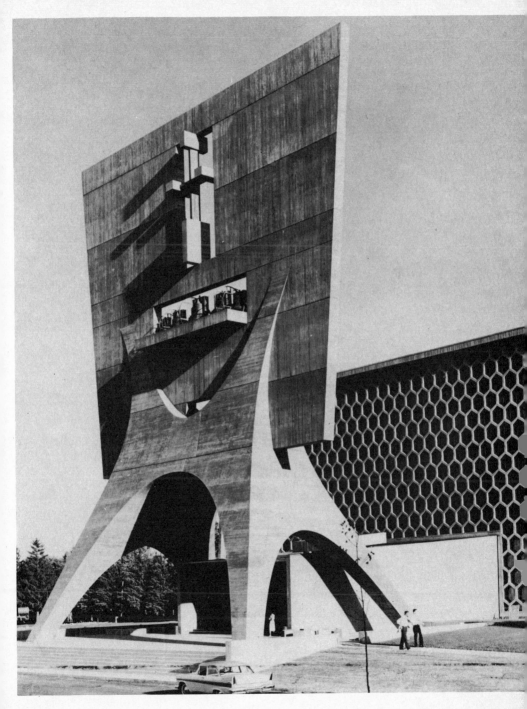

US, large urban projects in South America and in Asia, factories and office buildings in Europe and the US all came his way. At long last he had arrived.

In a sense, Breuer is the last of the true functionalists. In the early 1920s he was greatly influenced by the spirit of the *Constructivist movement, both in Russia and in Western Europe. All his designs were highly articulated: a Breuer chair would express every element separately, both in form and in material; a Breuer house would express different areas of activity in different and separate forms (his H-plans for houses, which separate the day-time areas from the night-time areas, are especially well known); in his construction details, every element of the structure was always clearly defined and separately articulated; and even in his large buildings, such as the UNESCO Headquarters, there was always a clear distinction and separation of functionally different elements—whether different kinds of buildings or different parts of the same building. The resulting clarity in his work has done much to keep modern architecture from becoming eclectic and formalistic. Although some of Breuer's separately articulated elements tended to be poetic rather than purely practical, they always did describe, very literally, what was happening in plan, structure, or building equipment. Still, this clarity of organization has certain drawbacks, for it is often difficult to create a coherent architectural grouping if each part of the group is given separate and equal importance. For this reason, some of the larger projects Breuer undertook in the years after 1952 have consisted of buildings which were individually impressive but failed to add up to truly significant architectural groupings. The UNESCO Headquarters, for example, consists of several separate structures, each of which is highly successful in itself; but as a group these separate structures do not, at present, form a successful architectural unity.

It is too early to evaluate Breuer's work in its entirety, but it is possible to evaluate his influence upon his contemporaries and upon younger generations of architects. Because of the great clarity of his structures and the great clarity of organization of his plans, he has become an enormously successful teacher, for in his work all the fundamentals of modern architecture are clearly distinguishable and presented with imagination and with art.

Bibliography: Peter Blake, *Marcel Breuer, Architect and Designer*, New York 1949; Marcel Breuer, *Sun and Shadow, the Philosophy of an Architect*, New York 1956; *Marcel Breuer, 1921–1962*, Stuttgart 1962; *Marcel Breuer: 1921–1961, Buildings and Projects*, ed. Cranston Jones, London 1962.

                                                    PETER BLAKE

Brinkman, Johannes Andreas, b. Rotterdam 1902, d. 1949. From 1925 in partnership with L. C. van der *Vlugt. The Van Nelle tobacco factory in Rotterdam (1928–30), to whose design Mart Stam also contributed, is, with its transparent structure, one of the most important industrial buildings of the twenties. The slab-shaped Bergpolder point block in Rotterdam was built in 1933–4 (Brinkman, van der Vlugt and W. van Tijen), an early prototype of buildings on stilts. Partnership with J. H. van den *Broek (1937).

Broek, J. H. van den, b. Rotterdam 1898. The names of J. H. van den Broek and Jacob B. *Bakema are inseparably connected with post-war building in the Netherlands, and the reconstruction of Rotterdam in particular. Van den Broek is a professor at Delft Technical College, where he himself graduated in 1924. He started his own practice in 1927 at Rotterdam, entering into partnership with J. A. *Brinkman in 1937 and J. B. Bakema in 1948.

Architecture and social outlook are closely linked in the work of van den Broek and Bakema. The Lijnbaan shopping centre in Rotterdam (1953), a systematically laid-out pedestrian street with low-built shops, was a distinctive contribution to current town-planning practice. The civic centre at Marl (under construction) gives a modern interpretation to the old idea of a citadel, while providing a comprehensive centre for a rising industrial town. A considerable proportion of the two architects' practice is taken up with housing and schools (school buildings at Brielle, 1948–57; Montessori Lyceum, Rotterdam, 1958). Van den Broek and Bakema have carried out other projects also, in which Bakema's description of architecture as the three-dimensional expression of human activity has been realized. These include exhibition buildings (Dutch pavilions at the International Expositions at Paris, 1937, and Brussels, 1958), offices (Van Ommeren, Antwerp, 1939; N. B. ten Cate, Almelo, 1954), department stores (Wassen van Vorst, 1951; Galeries Modernes, 1956, both in Rotterdam), and industrial layouts, laboratories, and research buildings for the Technical High School at Delft. The two churches at Schiedam (1957) and Nagele, in the Nordostpolder (1959) are severely rectilinear buildings which achieve their effects through the interplay of large glazed areas and plane surfaces.

Bibliography: J. H. van den Broek, *Creative krachten in de architectonische conceptie*, Delft 1948; Jürgen Joedicke, *Architektur und Städtebau, Das Werk der Architekten van den Broek und Bakema*, Stuttgart, in preparation.

J. J. VRIEND

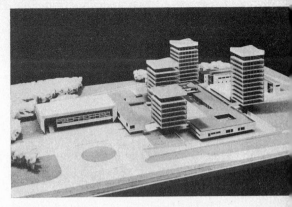

J. H. van den Broek and Jacob B. Bakema. Town Hall Complex. Marl, under construction. Model

Brutalism. Brutalism gave conscious form to a mood that was widespread among younger architects in the 1950s, but in spite of the fact that it expressed a sentiment that was felt in most parts of the Westernized world its origins can be pinpointed in space and time with some precision. Although Giedion is wrong in his etymology ('Brute + Alison') he is right in identifying the Smithson family as the source of the word—either Alison *Smithson or the Smithson's family friend Guy Oddie (who used to call Peter Smithson 'Brutus') was the first person to utter the phrase *The New Brutalism*, some time in the early summer of 1954.

This much being established, what was the intended content of the phrase? The basis was a mood of frustration brought on partly by the difficulties of building in Britain after the Second World War, and partly by disgust at the smugness of the compromising elders who were still able to build because they were well placed with the 'Establishment'. The stylistic preferences of these elders were known as 'The New Humanism' by the political Left, 'The New Empiricism' by the political Right. 'The New Brutalism' as a phrase was intended as a mockery of both, but it also drew attention to certain real qualities in the architecture that was being admired or

designed by the Smithsons and their generation.

They set as their standard the uncompromising ruthlessness of *Mies van der Rohe and *Le Corbusier, their intellectual clarity, their honest presentation of structure and materials. At the same time, they sensed in the work of these masters a continuing tradition, an architecture that lay above and beyond styles and fashions —among the work of the past they admired the clarity and formality of Palladio, the heroic scale of the Anglo-Baroque architects Vanbrugh and Hawksmoor, and the clear-cut and massive forms of early 19th-century engineering structures.

J. H. van den Broek and Jacob B. Bakema. Church of the Resurrection. Schiedam, 1957

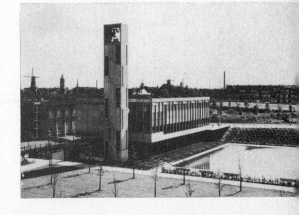

But the architecture that emerged from these admirations was, in the beginning, purely Miesian. No doubt a streak of English puritanism accounts for this initial selection of a simple, elegant structural system, for it was allied to an absolute horror of any pretence or concealment; not only were structure and materials honestly expressed, but services as well. In the school at Hunstanton, England, the first true Brutalist building, not only are steel and brick expressed with an honesty that goes even beyond the acceptable subterfuges of Mies, but pipe runs, electrical conduits, and other services are exposed to view. The austerity of this design was so remarkable that it attracted world-wide attention, and international comparisons were sought. Of these, Louis *Kahn's Art Centre at Yale University was in some ways more convincing than Mies's own work, because Kahn seemed equally preoccupied with the raw nature of the materials and concerned with the expression of the services.

By the time that this was happening, however, the original puritanical extremism of

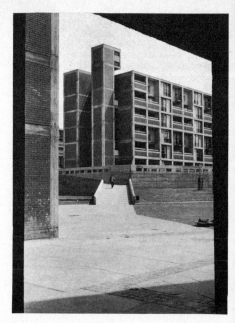

Jack Lynn and Ivor Smith. Park Hill Housing Estate. Sheffield, 1955–61

Le Corbusier. Unité d'Habitation. Marseilles, 1947–52. Detail of piers at ground floor level

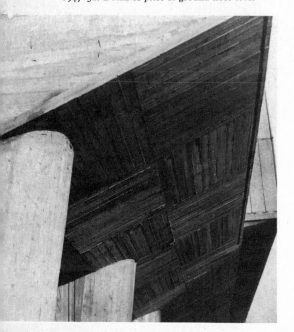

the English Brutalists was beginning to merge with an international movement of different origins and only remotely comparable aims. This movement could be characterized by developments as diverse as the a-formal painting of Jackson Pollock and the a-formal planning of the Chapel at Ronchamp, the *art brut* of Dubuffet and the *béton brut* of the *Unité* at Marseilles. The Brutalism of the uncompromising exhibition of materials became allied to a Brutalism of form; the expressed symmetry of the Hunstanton School and the concealed symmetry of the Yale Art Centre were abandoned in favour of a ruthless honesty in expressing the functional spaces and their inter-relationships. Even that adaptable rectangular geometry, derived from abstract painting, that the older functionalists had been able to accept, was now cast aside, in favour of modes of composition based on the topography of the site and the topology of internal circulation—as may be seen very clearly in the siting and planning of Park Hill, Sheffield, designed in the city architect's office by the newly graduated Jack Lynn and Ivor Smith.

Once the Brutalism of a building such as Park Hill is understood it becomes clear that the application of the term to such fashionably sentimental architecture as that of Leonardo Ricci is improper, as is any attempt to make 'Brutalists' out of—say—Juan *O'Gorman or Paolo *Soleri. Brutalism implies some sort of attempt to make manifest the moral imperatives that were built into the tradition of modern architecture by the pioneers of the 19th century, and the use of shutter-patterned concrete or exposed steel-work is only a symptom of this intention—as Peter Smithson has said, 'We also admire the nature of gold paint, where it is necessary.' The fundamental aim of Brutalism at all times has been to find a structural, spatial, organizational and material concept that is 'necessary' in this metaphysical sense to some particular building, and then express it with complete honesty in a form that will be a unique and memorable image. In the creation of this definitive image the other plastic arts provide, not an aesthetic, but an exemplar of method or a standard of comparison—thus, the admirations of the Brutalists have covered subjects as diverse as US car-styling and the Ise shrines in Japan. Neither have had any visible influence on Brutalist architecture, but both are examples of images created out of the kind of necessary conditions the Brutalists believe to be fundamental, also, to the conception of buildings today. It is this insistence on the primacy of the given and necessary factors in the conception of a building that has caused Sir John Summerson to compare the beliefs of the Brutalists to the Rigorism of Lodoli and other radical theorists of late 18th-century Italian Illuminism.

On this ground, the only Brutalist building in Italy is the Istituto Marchiondi by Vittoriano Viganò, even though at first sight its departures from the common practices of the modern movement appear less extreme than those of the neo-Libertarian sentimentalists. Stylistically, the

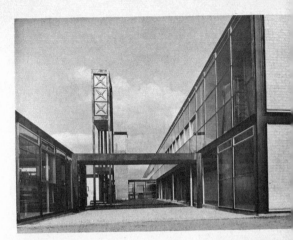

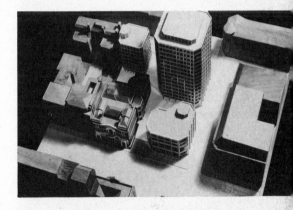

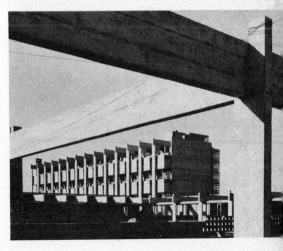

Alison and Peter Smithson. Hunstanton School. Norfolk, 1954

Alison and Peter Smithson. Economist Building. London, under construction. Model

Vittoriano Viganò. Istituto Marchiondi. Milan, 1957

Istituto Marchiondi consciously echoes the ideas, if not the work, of Giuseppe *Terragni and the period of *l'architettura razionalista*, which provide an image that is entirely expressive of the stern, reformative necessities that underlie the conception of this building.

Nevertheless the Istituto Marchiondi draws attention to the relationship of Brutalism to the traditions of architecture. For all its aggressive tone and uncompromising attitudes, Brutalism does not represent a radical departure from the traditional conception of architecture—it is in no way comparable to the technological extremism of Buckminster *Fuller, nor even to the methods of radical functional analysis developed in England by the Nuffield Trust. The most instructive comparisons to be made on this subject are with action-painting and *musique-concrète*. Action-painting abandoned the last vestiges of formal composition but still accepted such 'outworn' traditions as paint, canvas, and a rectangular format for the picture, all of which had been previously rejected at various times by modern painters; *musique-concrète* abandoned the polite fictions of the sounds made by artificial musical instruments in favour of recordings of 'real noises', but it abandoned very little else of what had been left of the traditions of music by earlier modernist composers. Similarly the Brutalists, while abandoning fictitious surface for the 'reality' of steel and concrete and the concept of formal composition as necessary to the art of architecture, have still practised and theorized within the basic traditions of architecture.

To make another comparison between the Brutalists and one of the architects whom they admire, without now imitating his forms: the Smithsons's project for the Economist Building in London has the three component buildings informally grouped around an irregular piazza, whereas the Seagram Building in New York is a single classicist slab, axially sited behind a formal forecourt. The irregular Economist piazza gives a truer image of the organizational and topological necessities of that particular functional programme than an imitation of the Seagram composition would have done, and yet this project accepts the siting of the main built volumes on a pedestrian platform from which

vehicles are banished, as does the Seagram, rather than providing some radical solution of the relationship between building, pedestrians and wheeled traffic.

Brutalism, then, is a tough-minded reforming movement within the framework of modern architectural thought, not a revolutionary attempt to overthrow it. On the other hand, the implicit intention of the Brutalists to return to fundamental functionalist principles in order to make them fulfil their apparent promise may involve the refusal of so many marginal compromises that an effective revolution may unintentionally result.

REYNER BANHAM

Bryggman, Erik William, b. Turku 1891, d. Turku 1955. Bryggman studied at the Design School of the Turku Art Society from 1906 to 1909, and later at Helsinki Polytechnic, where he graduated in architecture in 1916. Directly afterwards he began his professional career with a series of important works in collaboration: the Helsinki War Memorial, with the sculptor Ilkka; the Monument to Liberty at Oulu, with the sculptor Sakselin; and the restoration of the medieval Cathedral at Turku, carried out from 1921 to 1923. In the same year Bryggman opened his own office in the old capital, where he always lived, and where he was joined a few years later by Aino and Alvar *Aalto. The Aaltos's propinquity and collaboration with Bryggman did not last long, however, as the former afterwards moved on to Helsinki, but it came during the most critical period in the development of their architectural thought and resulted in a unique work of collaboration, of great importance in the history of Finnish architecture: the Seven Hundredth Anniversary Exhibition of the City of Turku, which took place in 1929 and is considered to be the first example of modern architecture in Scandinavia.

Bryggman, who was seven years older than Aalto, had carried out a good many works before the Turku Exhibition; they mark the most important stages in that process leading to *Functionalism which was silently developing in the architecture of the young nation. Amongst them may be noted a block of flats for employees of the Finnish Sugar Company at Turku (1923–4), some houses in Turku and elsewhere, and two hotels in Turku: the Seurahuone, with very sophisticated décor (1928), and the Hospitz Hotel (1927–9). His finest work was carried out, however, between 1930 and 1940, starting with Parainen Cemetery Chapel, the Kinopalatsi Cinema at Turku, and the Finnish Pavilion at the Antwerp International Exhibition, all dating from 1930. Next came a series of delightful white country houses, set like crystals amid the virgin nature of the islands in the archipelago: those at Ruissalo and Hirvenssalo (1933); the Villa Kaino at Kaskerta (1935); the Villa Jaatinen (1939); and Vierumäki Sports Club, another work in a purely rationalist style (1930–6). Finally, in this period, we may mention the Library of Turku Academy (1935), and the cemetery chapel in the same city, built between 1938 and 1941. The book tower of the Academy rises in a district of the old city, over which the dark mass of the Cathedral looms in the distance. It is remarkable for the balance of its voids in the large white walls, and for the perfect way it fits in with its surroundings, via a subtle handling of proportions and a complete understanding of the *genius loci*. Turku Cemetery Chapel is Bryggman's best known work, and it is undoubtedly a very fine one, especially in the magical lightness of its internal space, but taken as a whole it is certainly less great, already revealing in certain points the germ of that progressive decline that ultimately affected his performance. The chapel was built to replace one originally erected in 1877 to the designs of F. A. Sjöstrom. Construction commenced in 1938, and was finished with much labour in 1941, despite the war and the great difficulties of supply. In this project more than any other of Bryggman's designs, one feels that the architect has reached deeply into himself and brought to the surface all his most intimate and painful sensibility, but that in doing so he has passed the inexorable limit beyond which it becomes a weakness not to control one's own powers of suggestion. Nevertheless, Turku Chapel is the work in which the architect's personality is expressed most fully, through the medium of a serene rationalism, rarefied and infused by the subtle *frisson* of a pervading romanticism, in a placid and almost still atmosphere, where the dominating whiteness finds its essential complement in the light, which, as it varies, alters the

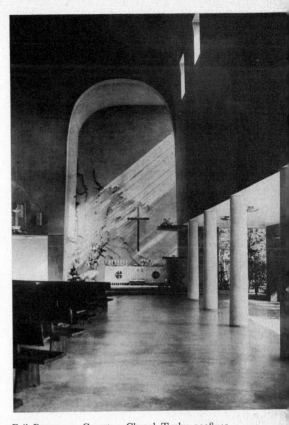

Erik Bryggman. Cemetery Chapel. Turku, 1938–41

weight and the consistency of the architectural elements.

Bryggman's post-war works, in the decade from 1945 to 1955, the year of his untimely death, confirm that Turku Chapel marked the end of his rationalist period in the thirties, just as the 1929 Exhibition proved the turning point between his previous classicism and the functionalism which followed. The buildings of this final period, which we may call one of romantic decline, are numerous, and often very good: they include an estate of timber houses at Pansio, near Turku (1946), the Students' Union and the chemistry laboratory of Turku Academy (1948–50), the Villa Nuuttila on the island of Kuusisto, finely tailored to the site (1947–51) and Riihimäki Water Tower (1951–2).

The last designs which bear Bryggman's

name are probably, in part at least, the work of his office, over which the architect, by now a sick man, gradually lost control. They show a decline towards more complex forms, at times tending to *organic practice, with the careful siting of buildings in the landscape, at others showing a more strictly 'national' inspiration in the handling of volumes, materials and colours, as in his last cemetery chapels. Then his life drew to a premature close, leaving us as a consolation for his loss those authentic works of art, reflecting in their essential forms of line and volume the clear simplicity of his own life and spirit, which have made Turku, already famous for its ancient architectural traditions, Erik Bryggman's city.
Bibliography: Leonardo Mosso, 'L'opera di Erik Bryggman nella storia dell' architetture finlandese', in *Atti SJA*, Turin December 1958.

LEONARDO MOSSO

Bunshaft, Gordon, b. Buffalo, New York 1909. Studied at the Massachusetts Institute of Technology, Cambridge, Mass. In 1937 he joined the architectural firm

Félix Candela. Church of the Miraculous Virgin. Mexico, 1954

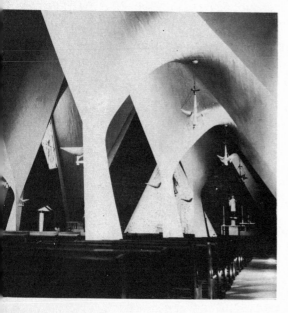

of *Skidmore, Owings and Merrill; since 1946 partner. Bunshaft was responsible for the design, among others, of the Lever Building (New York, 1952), one of the most influential buildings of the last two decades, and the Connecticut General Life Insurance Building (Bloomfield, Conn., 1957).

Burnham, Daniel Hudson, b. Henderson, New York 1846, d. Heidelberg 1912; 1873–91 in partnership with John W. *Root. Burnham and Root designed the Reliance Building at Chicago (1890–4), a classical example of early American steel-frame construction, and the Monadnock Building (1889–91), a skyscraper with load-bearing outer walls of gently modulated profile. After Root's death in 1891, the firm, which had been entrusted with the preparation of the World's Columbian Exposition at Chicago in 1893, veered towards an academic eclecticism. Planning of city centres with axial layouts (Washington, Cleveland, San Francisco, Chicago).

Candela, Félix, b. Madrid 1910. Studied at the Escuela Superior de Arquitectura, Madrid. Towards the end of his studies, Candela had the opportunity of watching one of the best known structures by *Torroja, the Frontón Recoletos, being built. This double barrel-vault spanning 197 feet by 118 feet, or other works by Torroja, probably awakened Candela's interest in *shell vaulting. At all events, he was determined to visit the German shell vaulting specialists Dischinger and Finsterwalder, when the outbreak of the Spanish Civil War in July 1936 prevented his trip. It is anybody's guess if Candela and the exponents of the highly developed German methods of calculation would have seen eye to eye. After Candela had fought in the Civil War on the Republican side, he came to *Mexico in the summer of 1939 via the refugee camps at Perpignan. After twelve years in his adopted country, during which time he, and later his brother Antonio, picked up a living as architects and builders, he began advocating the use of shell vaulting, at first in articles and lectures. The building of the University City gave him an opportunity to construct the first hyperbolic paraboloids, which enabled him to reduce the roof of the Cosmic Ray Building to a thickness of $\frac{5}{8}$ inch. A special advantage of this shape as compared with the sphere or other types of vault, is that the shuttering for hyperbolic paraboloids can be made from straight boards. Due to the relative simplicity of this process, and the great saving in material, Candela's constructions are more economical than other rigid roofs, and this fact alone won his firm numerous industrial commissions. Candela increased his spans with every project and became increasingly bolder in the exploitation of shell vaulting. When he maintains that he is guided less by exact calculation than by an intuitive feeling 'in the manner of the old master builders of cathedrals' we must recall that his intuition has a very firm foundation in his knowledge of materials and stresses, which grows with each new building. As an architect and designer, Candela has distinguished himself with his Church of the Miraculous Virgin in Mexico City (1954) which shows the unmistakable influence of *Gaudí, even though Candela departs widely from the building methods of the lonely Catalan. Later buildings of a non-industrial nature such as the Stock Exchange, several churches and pavilions in Mexico and Cuernavaca and a restaurant in Xochimilco were executed in collaboration with different architects, who were glad to avail themselves of the free outlines of his structures in their search for organic or baroque shapes.

Candela is not lacking in official recognition these days. In 1961 he was awarded the gold medal of the Institute of Structural Engineers in London and almost simultaneously the Auguste Perret Prize of the Union Internationale des Architectes. Shortly afterwards, Harvard appointed him Norton Professor of Poetry.

Bibliography: Max Cetto, *Modern Architecture in Mexico*, Stuttgart and New York 1960; Colin Faber, *Candela, the architect of shell construction*, New York and Munich, in preparation.

MAX CETTO

Candilis, Georges, b. Baku, Russia 1913. Studied in Greece where he met *Le Corbusier in 1933 at the *CIAM Congress in Athens. A scholarship made a stay in Paris possible (1945), and after that (until 1950) he worked for Le Corbusier. Residential buildings in Morocco (with Dony, Josic, and Woods). Planning for Le Mirail near Toulouse. The new town of Bagnols-

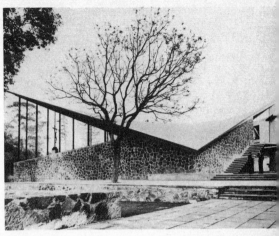

Félix Candela and Enrique de la Mora. Chapel of the Missionaries of the Holy Ghost. Coyoacán, 1956

sur-Cèze in the Rhône valley (started in 1956, with Bodiansky, Woods and Piot), adjoining an old urban centre with which it shares a cultural and sports precinct.

Casson, Sir Hugh Maxwell, b. Southampton 1913. Studied at Cambridge; Craven Scholar, British School at Athens. In private practice from 1937 with the late C. Nicholson; resumed 1946, after war service, latterly with Neville Conder. Professor of Interior Design, Royal College of Art, since 1953. His directorship of architecture at the *Festival of Britain, 1948–51, ensured its remarkable triumph as a piece of organized *townscape; the same powers of urbanistic control are evident in his schemes for Cambridge University (with N. Conder). His Youth Hostel at Holland Park, London, blends sympathetically with the remains of Holland House (17th century), while making no concessions to historicism.

HAROLD MEEK

Castiglioni, Enrico, b. Busto Arsizio near Milan 1914. Designs for complex sculpturally modelled shell constructions, which vault wide areas and mould spaces with the help of light. (Project for the main station in Naples, 1954; for the pilgrimage Church of the Madonna delle Lacrime at Syracuse, 1957.)

Chamberlin, Powell and Bon: Peter Chamberlin, Geoffrey Powell, and Christof Bon. First attracted attention in 1952 with their prize-winning scheme for high-density housing at Golden Lane, London (1953–7), a controversial layout with interesting treatment of multiple ground levels, a preoccupation later (1957) developed in their plan for the Barbican district of London, with separate routes for traffic and pedestrians. Their Bousfield Primary School with its *Miesian exteriors, was awarded the London Bronze Medal for Architecture in 1956; Newington Secondary School, also in London, features a complex folded roof over the assembly hall. Among their other schemes mention may be made of the Sports Centre for Birmingham University, with sculpturesque buildings atop a large podium, and the development plan for Leeds University, which closely integrates the academic layout with the city centre.
Bibliography: 'Detailed Proposals for the Barbican Redevelopment', in *Architects' Journal* (London), 4.6.1959. HAROLD MEEK

Chiattone, Mario, b. Lugano 1891. Studied architecture and painting at the Brera, Milan. Became a member of the *Futurist movement and together with his fellow-student *Sant'Elia exhibited a collection of drawings at Milan in 1914 under the heading 'Structures for a modern Metropolis'.

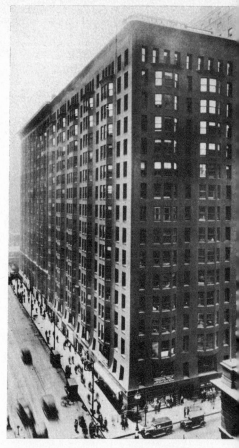

Daniel Hudson Burnham and John Wellborn Root. Monadnock Building. Chicago, 1889–91

Chicago School. This is a term conventionally applied to the characteristic commercial architecture of the American mid-west, especially Chicago, in the last quarter of the 19th century. It has also occasionally been used, but inappropriately, to cover the domestic Prairie style of 1900 that was evolved by Frank Lloyd *Wright and his followers in the same region. The Chicago style of commercial architecture is dominated by two features: the metal frame, as the basic structural system, together with its clear expression

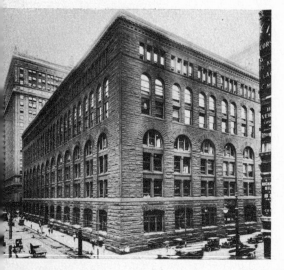

Henry Hobson Richardson. Marshall Field Warehouse. Chicago, 1885–7

on the building's exterior in a simple, often non-historical vocabulary. The Chicago fire of 1871 demonstrated the importance of fire-proof construction and the inability of exposed cast-iron structures to withstand the heat, but the definitive solution to this problem, the protective combination of a metal frame sheathed by brick or masonry, was not arrived at until the construction of the Home Insurance Building, 1883–5, by William Le Baron *Jenney, a ten-storey structure which was subsequently extended. However, this building's structural system was only tentatively expressed in the somewhat conventional detailing and awkward articulation of the exterior, which has none of the suavity of subsequent skyscrapers of the 1890s by *Adler and *Sullivan, *Burnham and *Root, or *Holabird and *Roche. Indeed, the outward appearance of Jenney's pioneer structure does not break with the eclectic Victorian and Second Empire vernacular modes that had been employed previously in Chicago by H. H. *Richardson in the American Express Building, 1872, and by Dankmar Adler in the Central Music Hall, 1879, both typical examples of Chicago architecture before the advent of the skyscraper. Furthermore, a significant stylistic predecessor (though not a specific inspiration) for the Home Insurance Building is the ten-storey mansarded Tribune Tower, New York, 1872–5, by Richard Morris Hunt (1827–95). While this earlier instance of eastern commercial architecture did not employ the metal frame, its pronounced vertical conception certainly is as deserving of the label 'skyscraper' as are the later, more structurally sophisticated towers in Chicago.

If Jenney's structure helped to provide the freedom from height restrictions that were imposed by load-bearing masonry construction, the 'style' of the Chicago School was reoriented by the simple monumentality of Richardson's rusticated, round-arched, but only nominally revivalistic Marshall Field Warehouse, 1885–7, a building which depended for its effect upon an epic expression of its surface material. At first its forms were imitated, as in Adler and Sullivan's Auditorium Building, 1886–9, or in Burnham and Root's Rookery, 1885–7. These derivative structures were rather more elaborate and historically detailed versions of the

Richardsonian paradigm, and the external walls of both were of conventional masonry construction. Subsequently the letter of Richardson's style was dropped, but his direct, expressive compositional principle was transformed into a mode fit for the metal frame and the large glazed openings which now became possible. Jenney's second Leiter Building (now Sears, Roebuck & Co.), 1889–90, is a bold, regular eight-storey volume in which the lines of the structure and the regular window rhythms dominate the almost invisible touches of classicizing detail. Similar qualities are to be observed in the pronounced verticality of the Reliance Building, 1890–4, by Daniel H. Burnham and

Daniel Hudson Burnham and John Wellborn Root. Reliance Building. Chicago, 1890–4

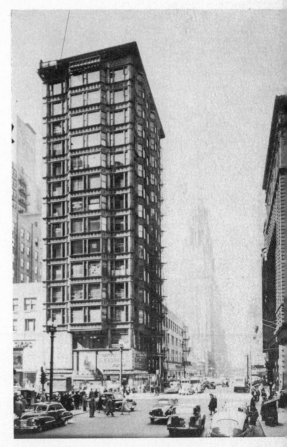

John W. Root, one of the most startling anticipations of the metal and glass style of the mid-20th century. The lower floors of the Reliance Building were built at the same time as Burnham and Root were completing the last masonry skyscraper, the sixteen-storey Monadnock Building, 1889–91, whose simple, rugged elevation contrasts with its light if somewhat inelegant contemporary. Two of Sullivan's finest Chicago School metal-frame skyscrapers of this period were built in St Louis (Wainwright Building, 1890–1) and Buffalo (Guarantee Building, 1894–5), but his most characteristic efforts of the late 1890s are in Chicago: the Carson, Pirie and Scott Store, 1899, and his portion of the façade of the tripartite Gage Building, 1898–9. The Gage Building was the work of William Holabird and Martin Roche (who had made a skeleton framed addition to Burnham and Root's massive Monadnock Building in 1893), and Sullivan was employed to design the façade of the larger right third of the building, accommodating himself to the established structural grid. A comparison of the differing parts of this façade points up the multiple virtues of the Chicago School: the directness and simplicity of the Holabird and Roche portions is in contrast to the more refined, complicated, yet beautifully integrated Sullivan design.

The expressive originality of the Chicago School did not outlast the beginning of the 20th century. The admiration for the academic modes of design, popularized by the Columbian Exposition of 1893 (originally projected in a romantic, almost Richardsonian mode by Root in 1891, but finally executed in a frigid *beaux-arts* manner), did not take hold immediately, but by 1900 the great period of Chicago commercial architecture was over. It did, however, produce a notable, if somewhat isolated, aftermath in such works as Richard E. Schmidt's (b. 1865) Nepeenauk Building, 1901–2, and Montgomery Ward Warehouse (actually by the firm Schmidt, Garden and Martin), 1906–8, in Dwight Perkins's Carl Schurz High School, 1910, and, most provocatively, in Frank Lloyd Wright's Larkin Building, Buffalo, 1904.

Bibliography: Early Modern Architecture: Chicago 1870–1910, New York 1940; Thomas S. Tallmadge, *Architecture in Old Chicago,* Chicago 1941; F. Randall, *History of the Development of Building Construction in Chicago,* Urbana, Illinois 1949; G. Condit, *The Rise of the Skyscraper,* Chicago 1952.

JOHN M. JACOBUS, JR

CIAM (Congrès Internationaux d'Architecture Moderne). The foundation of CIAM in 1928 has been called the beginning of the 'academic' phase of modern architecture: the time certainly appeared propitious for the introduction of some kind of international order into the scattered and independent essays towards a new architecture whose international unity of intention and style had been demonstrated at the Weissenhof exhibition of the previous year.

The effective impetus towards the foundation of CIAM came from Hélène de Mandrot, a sincere and intelligent woman who had aspirations towards being a patroness of the arts. She proposed in the first place a reunion of creative spirits at her château at La Sarraz, Switzerland, but this romantic project was turned to something more purposeful after consultation with Sigfried Giedion and *Le Corbusier. The preparatory document, issued to intending delegates, stated: 'This first congress is convened with the aim of establishing a programme of action to drag architecture from the academic impasse' (it was, in fact, to drag it into another) 'and to place it in its proper social and economic milieu. This congress should . . . determine the limits of the studies and discussions shortly to be undertaken by further congresses.' Although a distinction was thus made between the preparatory congress and later meetings, the date of 26, 27, and 28 June 1928 at La Sarraz is remembered and recorded as CIAM I, in spite of the fact that the properly constituted series of *Congrès Internationaux d'Architecture Moderne* did not begin until after the declaration of 28 June. The contents of the declaration embodied most of the best aspirations as well as the most fashionable fetishes of the architecture of the time. Sample statements read: 'It is only from the present that our architectural work should be derived', and 'The intention that brings us together is that of attaining a harmony of existing elements—a harmony indispensable to the present—BY PUTTING ARCHITECTURE BACK ON ITS REAL PLANE, THE

ECONOMIC AND SOCIAL PLANE; therefore architecture should be freed of the sterile influence of the Academies and of antiquated formulas', and again, 'The most efficacious production is derived from rationalization and standardization.'

The historical irony of these repeated invectives against the Academies is underlined by the dry, formalistic statement of aims that appears as the preamble to the statutes drawn up at Frankfurt-am-Main in 1929 (CIAM II). The aims are given as: (*a*) to state the contemporary architectural problem; (*b*) to restate the idea of modern architecture; (*c*) to disseminate this idea throughout the technical, economic and social strata of contemporary life; (*d*) to remain alert to the problems of architecture.

The Frankfurt Statutes also gave CIAM three operative organs: (1) the *Congrès* or general assembly of the members; (2) CIRPAC (Comité Internationale pour la Résolution des Problèmes de l'Architecture Contemporaine) to be elected by the *Congrès*; and (3) working groups, to apply themselves to specific subjects in collaboration with non-architectural specialists. At the same time the hierarchy of membership was stabilized in the form of national member-groups, to which individuals belonged.

It must be stated that this academic flavour (doubtless given by the 'clerics' such as Giedion, rather than the practising architects) was in no way representative of the work actually being undertaken in these years. The Frankfurt Congress had been called under the auspices of Ernst *May, the city architect and Europe's greatest expert on low-cost housing, and its outcome was a serious report, *Die Wohnung für das Existenzminimum*. CIAM III was held in Brussels in 1930, through the good offices of Victor *Bourgeois, and applied itself to basic problems of land-organization for housing, publishing an equally important report, *Rationelle Bebauungsweisen*. Both reports were at once dogmatic and realistic, somewhat in the manner of the town-planning studies being pursued at the Bauhaus under Hannes *Meyer, and these documents close the 1920s with the last genuine group-efforts of the architects who had met together to build Weissenhof. The next three years were to see fundamental changes.

Already in 1930 it was becoming apparent that CIAM was neither intellectually nor organizationally prepared for the problem to which the logic of its discussions had driven it—town planning. In order to deal with this situation CIAM set to work to standardize the graphic techniques, scales, and methods of presentation used by its members (an enterprise that was not really completed until the adoption of the *Grille-CIAM* after 1949). The Dutch national group, under Cor van *Eesteren, became the working group entrusted with the evolution of an effective symbol language for town planning. These labours, conducted against a background of growing political tensions and disintegrating international relations, proved to be protracted, and CIRPAC met three times (Berlin, 1931, Barcelona, 1932, and Paris, 1933) before it was felt that work was sufficiently advanced for another plenary *Congrès* to be called. This delay of almost three years proved crucial to the whole future of the movement; CIAM underwent a subtle and irrevocable change and took on the character which it was to preserve until its collapse more than twenty years later.

CIAM IV—theme 'The Functional City' —took place in July and August 1933 aboard the S.S. *Patris*, in Athens, and in Marseilles at the end of the voyage. It was the first of the 'romantic' congresses, set against a background of scenic splendour, not the reality of industrial Europe, and it was the first *Congrès* to be dominated by Le Corbusier and the French, rather than the tough German realists. The Mediterranean cruise was clearly a welcome relief from the worsening situation of Europe, and in this brief respite from reality the delegates produced the most Olympian, rhetorical, and ultimately destructive document to come out of CIAM: the *Athens Charter. The hundred and eleven propositions that comprise the Charter consist in part of statements about the conditions of towns, and in part of proposals for the rectification of those conditions, grouped under five main headings: Dwellings, Recreation, Work, Transportation, and Historic Buildings.

The tone remains dogmatic, but is also generalized and less specifically related to immediate practical problems than were the Frankfurt and Brussels reports. The generalization had its virtues, where it brought with it a greater breadth of vision and insisted that cities could be considered only in relation to their surrounding regions, but this persuasive generality which gives the Athens Charter its air of universal applicability conceals a very narrow conception of both architecture and town planning and committed CIAM unequivocally to: (*a*) rigid functional zoning of city plans, with green belts between the areas reserved to the different functions, and (*b*) a single type of urban housing, expressed in the words of the Charter as 'high, widely-spaced apartment blocks wherever the necessity of housing high densities of population exists'. At a distance of thirty years we recognize this as merely the expression of an aesthetic preference, but at the time it had the power of a Mosaic commandment and effectively paralysed research into other forms of housing. The Paris *Congrès* of 1937 (CIAM V) which was to be the last before the war, did little more than make marginal annotations to the Charter.

By the time the war was over, twelve years had passed since the Charter was drawn up, and its proposals had become the established dogma of progressive town planning. In the first years of peace there could be seen attempts to apply the Charter as a universal blueprint all over the world. But even while the *Système-CIAM* was being enforced in the schools and in planning offices its fatal weakness had been recognized, as is made clear by the insertion of a section in *Can Our Cities Survive?* that had no warrant in the Charter: the Civic Centre. At first this appears to be little more than a place where the citizen can go to escape from the Cartesian prison of Dwelling / Work / Recreation / Transportation, but as the study of centres proceeded it became apparent that CIAM's Functional City had been conceived in ignorance of the city's specific functions. Thus the Charter defines Dwelling as the first urban function; but it is also the first rural function; Work and Transportation are functions even of the nomadic life of the desert; Recreation is not specific to cities. The attempt to isolate the specifically urban functions of the city was to be the prime task of CIAM after the war, and since it led to the overthrow of the categories and categorical imperatives of the Athens Charter it was to lead to the

destruction of CIAM, to which the Charter had become more central than either the preparatory document of 1928 or the Statutes of 1929. At first there was no sign of trouble. CIAM VI met in 1947 at Bridgwater, England, a joyous reunion of the heroes of Weissenhof and the followers they had collected in the 1930s; its outcome, a review of buildings erected since CIAM V by the members, edited by Giedion and published under the title of *A Decade of New Architecture*. But at CIAM VII, held at Bergamo in 1949, a new pattern was beginning to emerge, with the growing importance of the Italian delegation and the gathering of numbers of war-toughened students on the fringes of the *Congrès* in order to sit at the feet of the men who were, to them, legendary figures, the makers of modern architecture.

At CIAM VIII, held at Hoddesdon in England, in honour of the Festival of Britain, 1951, the new pattern of CIAM was becoming plain—increasing numbers of students, and official recognition of the inadequacy of the Charter, since the theme was 'The Urban Core'. For this theme the delegates were as unprepared intellectually as they had been for town planning in 1930, and the Congress report, edited by Jacqueline Tyrwhitt, José Luis *Sert, and Ernesto *Rogers, is little more than a compendium of fashionable clichés, such as the need to integrate painting and sculpture into architecture, while at the heart of these so-called studies appears an intellectual and urbanistic vacuum: the centre of the city is considered simply as yet another functionally designated area, an open space, to which the citizens were to be attracted by some mysterious quality of 'spontaneity'.

It was not long before the failure of CIAM VIII was recognized, but in the meantime CIAM IX at Aix-en-Provence had taken place; its theme was officially 'Habitat', but the *Congrès* will be chiefly remembered as a mass rally of Le Corbusier's student fan-club and the proceedings, culminating in an impromptu striptease performance on the roof of the Unité at Marseilles, were marked by adolescent *bonhomie* rather than mature cerebration. Yet it was to be the young who undertook to deliver CIAM from the new 'academic impasse' into which it had lapsed. The group who were entrusted with the preparation of CIAM X (who were therefore known as Team-X) took up a position that, though it drew to some extent on the programme documents for CIAM IX, nevertheless represented a clean break with both the mood and the content of the Athens Charter. Against the large-scale diagrammatic generalizations of the Athenian tradition, Team-X set up the personal, the particular, and the precise: 'Each architect is asked to appear with his project under his arm, ready to commit himself. Today we recognize the existence of a new spirit. It is manifest in our revolt from mechanical concepts of order . . . CIAM X must make it clear that we, as architects, accept the responsibility for the creation of order through form . . . the responsibility for each act of creation, however small.' Though the theme of CIAM X was still nominally 'Habitat', the real business of the *Congrès*, which took place in Dubrovnik in 1956, was the direct challenge presented to the established members by the young radicals of Team-X, *Bakema, *Candilis, Gutmann, the *Smithsons, Howell, van *Eijck, and Voelcker. By the end of the congress, CIAM was in ruins and Team-X stood upon the wreckage of something that they had joined with enthusiasm, and—with equal enthusiasm—destroyed. The sense of the end of an epoch was so strong that the *Congrès* accepted the fact of death with comparative calm; the national groups were instructed to wind up their affairs, and the project of a memorial volume covering twenty-five years of work was seriously discussed. But there were national groups, notably the Italian, who felt that CIAM could still be of service. In addition, Team-X were not averse to international meetings as such, and the combination of these two parties produced, in 1959, a further congress in Otterlo, Holland. In content this was to be similar to what Team-X had intended for CIAM X, and particular projects were indeed discussed, individual responsibility was accepted, and the results, edited by Oscar Newman, were published as *CIAM 59 in Otterlo*. These published documents reveal that close discussion of the particular could often be as trivial as broad discussion of generalities, while the title of the report conceals a bitter dispute among the delegates who, in fact, voted to dissociate their activities from the word 'CIAM'. But the

vote was disputed by some of the delegates who left before the final meeting, and as a result accusations of bad faith were launched against Team-X by founder-members Giedion, Sert, *Gropius, and Le Corbusier (none of whom had been in any way involved with the congress).

This was neither a productive nor a dignified outcome to thirty years of international activity, and the blame for the final collapse of CIAM must be laid chiefly on the inability of the founder-members to resist the temptation to *faire école*. They failed to guard against the academic tendencies in their midst, and became the victims of what Cor van Eesteren termed 'a too formal structure' to which work-programmes had to be subordinated. Nevertheless, in two vital periods—1930–4 and 1950–5—CIAM was the major instrument through which the ideas of modern architecture and town planning were made known to the world, while it performed an equally vital function during the war years in maintaining the nucleus of an international network of communications between progressive-minded architects. It is quite possible that these achievements may ultimately prove to be of greater historical importance than any of the documents that CIAM produced, even the Athens Charter. *Bibliography: Die Wohnung für das Existenzminimum*, Stuttgart 1930; *Rationelle Bebauungsweisen*, Stuttgart 1931; *Logis et loisirs*, Paris 1938; (Le Corbusier) *La Charte d'Athènes*, Paris 1941; J. L. Sert and CIAM, *Can Our Cities Survive?*, Cambridge, Massachnsetts 1942; S. Giedion, *A Decade of New Architecture*, Zurich 1951; Oscar Newman (ed.), *CIAM 59 in Otterlo*, Stuttgart 1961.

REYNER BANHAM

CLASP. Acronym for Consortium of Local Authorities Special Programme. In 1957, a group of local education authorities in England banded together to exploit a system of *prefabricating schools, originally devised in Nottingham under Donald *Gibson to counteract subsidence in mining areas and later extended, as in C. H. *Aslin's Hertfordshire schools, to allow buildings to be erected rapidly from mass-produced prefabricated units at low cost and with a small labour force. Consortium components amount to about half the cost of CLASP schools; £10·6 million worth of

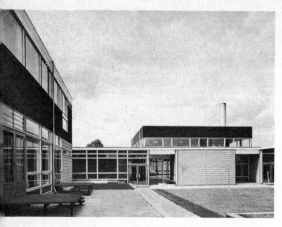

CLASP school. West Bridgford, Nottinghamshire, 1962

work was built in 1964–5, and a second Consortium has been formed of other authorities (SCOLA). The cost of developing the CLASP system since 1957 has been £100,000, but more than £45 million worth of CLASP buildings are either in use or under construction.

A 3 foot 4 inch planning grid is used, with external walls that can change direction at 6 foot 8 inch and 10 foot intervals. An organic grouping of elements with carefully controlled relationships between the spaces creates a deceptive, though usually successful feeling of informality. The same informality, however, when evoked in the choice of external cladding components often appears arbitrary and visually confused, lessening the effect of the carefully related spaces.

A CLASP school was exhibited at the 1960 Milan Triennale, arousing great interest.

Bibliography: Ministry of Education (Building Bulletin No. 19): *The Story of CLASP*, London 1960; 'CLASP in Italy', in *Architectural Review*, May 1963.

HAROLD MEEK

Concrete. *Reinforced concrete.

Constructivism. The movement known as Constructivism originated in Moscow just after the First World War in the work and theories of the two sculptor brothers Naum Gabo and Antoine Pevsner, who issued a Realistic Manifesto in 1920 which indicated the aims of the movement. Other Russian artists associated with the move-

ment in those early years were Vladimir *Tatlin, painter, sculptor, and architect; Kasimir *Malevich, painter and sculptor and founder of the Suprematist movement; and El *Lissitzky, painter and architect. The purpose of the group has perhaps been most succinctly indicated by Naum Gabo, writing in *Abstraction-Création* in 1932, when he said that constructivists no longer paint pictures or carve sculptures but make constructions in space. The distinction between painting and sculpture is thus eliminated and both enter the domain of architecture. Thus Constructivism is a movement that affects all the visual arts, but it emanates in the first place from sculpture. This sculpture being constructions of various elements is essentially the same aesthetically as the constructions in architecture.

Constructivist sculpture consists of constructions in various materials—metals, glass, plastic, and nylon—and one work may be composed of many materials. It was the purpose in making such sculpture to express in symbolic forms the conceptions of life and the universe prompted by modern science. Materials provided by modern industry were logically the most appropriate for this purpose, and thus the constructions of Gabo and Pevsner are expressions mainly in abstract or associative forms that stem from modern science. Constructivism has, by some, been closely associated with Cubism. It was regarded as exhibiting the simple relations of geometric forms to which all natural forms can be reduced according to the dictum of Cézanne that 'Everything in Nature is shaped according to the sphere, cone, and cylinder.' Geometric forms were thus, to some Constructivists, the essential structural forms and Cubist painting was, therefore, either symbolical of Constructivism or actual Constructivist painting. In architecture Constructivism can be regarded as part of the broader movement of *Functionalism, with an accent on constructional expression. Construction in all its aspects was emphasized to the full and in that emphasis all the traditional accessories of a building, such as ornament and style, were discarded so that the aesthetic effect depended on the formal relations of mass and space emanating from the most efficient construction. Any object that was efficiently made for its purpose was regarded as a model to follow; thus the most modern methods of construction, involving the use of new materials made available by industry, whereby structural efficiency could be secured superior to traditional methods, were encouraged, while the efficient machine was cited as a standard of excellence. In this theory there was a good deal of kinship with the early theories of *Le Corbusier, who in his book *Vers une Architecture* cited modern machines, such as the motor-car and aeroplane, as examples of efficient constructions, involving the logical relations of parts to the whole.

In 1921 El Lissitzky, one of the Russian members of the Constructivist movement, came to Berlin and in the following year a Constructivist International was founded with which, in addition to El Lissitzky, the well-known Dutch artist and architect, Theo van *Doesburg, was associated. The manifesto accompanying the foundation, published in *De *Stijl*, affirms the importance of the machine in modern life, and declares that, being designed strictly for its purpose without irrelevancies, it should form a model for building. The principle of Elementarism is also introduced, a kind of philosophy of the elements that form the structure of a building. The manifesto was not a very profound state-

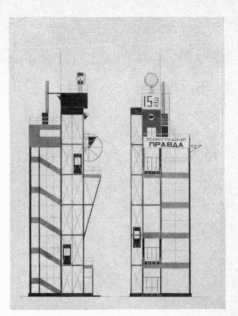

Alexander and Vladimir Vesnin. Pravda Building. Leningrad, 1923. Project

ment of aims and hardly survives critical examination. For example, in the cult of the machine there is a suggested independence of nature and belief in a 'mechanical aesthetic'. Further thought would have made it clear that all machines originate in natural organisms and their functions, while the manifesto is in part a contradiction of the evolution of Cubism based on the principle that geometric forms are, basically, essentially natural forms.

Other members of the Dutch De Stijl group who were associated with the Constructivist movement were Cor van *Eesteren, Gerrit T. *Rietveld, Mart Stam, the painter Piet Mondrian, and the Belgian artist Georges Vantongerloo. In 1923 a further manifesto was issued under the title of *Vers une Construction Collective*, by Theo van Doesburg, Cor van Eesteren, and G. T. Rietveld. In this manifesto it is asserted that the laws of space and colour have been studied and that it was found that their variations and relationships can be resolved into a definite unity, while the

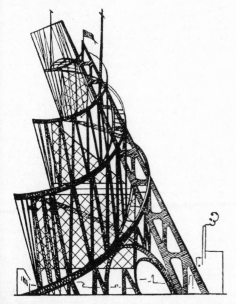

Vladimir Tatlin. Monument to the Third International in Moscow, 1920. Project.

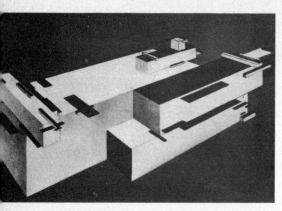

Kasimir Malevich. Suprematist architectural model. 1920–2

El Lissitzky and Mart Stam. 'Cloud Props'. Project. 1924

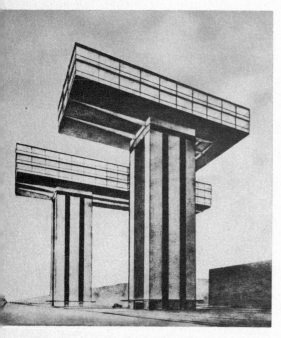

result of the study of the relation of space and time is that the two through colour give a new dimension, and that means have been secured whereby the duality of the interior and exterior of a building can be eliminated. The main point here is, of course, that all the diverse elements which make a construction in the arts can be composed into a unity satisfying to the human spirit, which was repeating in different words what had been said many times before.

Works that might be cited as examples of Constructivism are many and varied. A significant early example is Vladimir Tatlin's design for a monument to the Third International made in 1920, a design of a spiral character in which the bare bones of steel construction are manifest and which could be regarded as either sculpture or architecture. Very much in the same spirit is a much later work, the immense Construction in Space completed by Naum Gabo in 1957 and placed near the Bijenkorf building in Rotterdam. Many of the most interesting Constructivist architectural works are projects, and include a design for the Leningrad *Pravda* offices by the Vesnin brothers made in 1923; a scheme by El Lissitzky and Mart Stam in 1924 for office blocks erected on huge supports bestriding a city thoroughfare, known as the 'Cloud Props' project; Marcel *Breuer's scheme for a theatre in Kharkov made in 1930; and the many industrial fantasies in Jacob Tchernykhov's *Architectural Fictions*, published in Leningrad in 1933. There is one scheme in this book (No. 74) in which buildings at various points are perched on vast cantilevered structures, suggesting construction for construction's sake.

The influence of Constructivism on modern European architecture is difficult to assess. Certain it is that there has been a marked impulse to stress constructional elements in creating architectural effects. Among these is the emphasis given to the structural supporting members of a building, often by leaving the ground floor wholly or partially open, which play a decided part in the architectural ensemble. Such designing has been chiefly associated with Le Corbusier, and it is possible he was influenced by Constructivist theories, although it is equally possible that his theories, resolved independently, gave

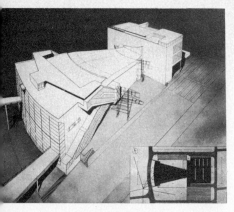

Marcel Breuer. Theatre at Kharkov, 1930. Project

strength to the early Constructivists. The display of structural members in a building, especially large supporting elements, is becoming a more prominent feature of much modern architecture, and formal decorative effects are increasingly dependent on the emphasis on structure. Indeed, in some designs the simulation of structure is actually introduced as a decorative motif and this may be in part due to the movement.

Perhaps the tenet of the Constructivists that has most strongly survived in architectural thought is the identity of efficient construction with beauty, which is a variant of the theory that true and economical fitness for purpose results in beauty. It is a theory held by many noted architects and engineers. For example, the Italian structural engineer, Pier Luigi *Nervi, who has been responsible for some of the most beautiful constructions in concrete, believes that the best chance of a building being beautiful is for it to be structurally right.

Bibliography: El Lissitzky, *Russland, Die Rekonstruktion der Architektur in der Sowjetunion*, Vienna 1930; Jacob Tchernykhov, *Architectural Fictions*, Leningrad 1933; Naum Gabo, *The Constructive Idea in Art*, London 1937; Rex Martienssen, 'Constructivism and Architecture. A new chapter in the history of formal building', *South African Architectural Record*, vol. 26, 1941.

ARNOLD WHITTICK

Costa, Lúcio, b. Toulon 1902. The acknowledged dean of modern architecture in *Brazil as well as its most articulate thinker, Lúcio Costa epitomizes, both in his work and in his writings, all that is more deeply typical of this movement, i.e. the continuing emotional relationship with the colonial past and the lyrical and humanistic approach to the problems of our time.

After graduating in 1924 from the Escola Nacional de Belas Artes in Rio de Janeiro, Costa entered into an early partnership with Gregori *Warchavchik, a Russian architect who had studied in Rome and settled in Brazil and who was responsible for the first modern, cube-like houses built in the country. In 1931, in the wake of the drastic changes brought about by the successful Vargas Revolution of 1930, Lúcio Costa was appointed to the directorship of the School of Fine Arts, which included the School of Architecture, and attempted a renewal of teaching methods, thus bringing to life a whole new generation of young architects oriented in a contemporary direction. Subsequently, in several projects which figure among the most significant milestones of the movement in Brazil, Lúcio Costa was able to express his discriminating good taste and his synthetic vision of the traditional past and the dynamic present of the country. The Ministry of Education and Health, (1937) for which *Le Corbusier was consulting architect and Lúcio Costa for a time the leader of the team of architects, the Brazilian Pavilion at the New York World's Fair, with Oscar *Niemeyer (1939), the Parque Guinle apartment buildings in Rio (1948–50–54), inspire young Brazilian architects to this day.

When in 1937 the DPAHN (National Historical and Artistic Patrimony Department) was formed Lúcio Costa joined it from the start and has never interrupted his devoted study of the history of Brazilian architecture or his work for the restoration and preservation of artistic monuments. Throughout his career, Lúcio Costa has always selflessly supported the work of Oscar Niemeyer, whose extraordinary talent was singled out by him in the early days when the Ministry of Education and Health was being designed, and who thus rose to his decisive role in the development of modern architecture in Brazil.

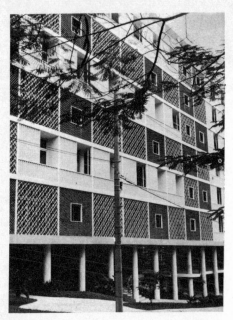

Lúcio Costa. Parque Guinle apartment buildings.
Rio de Janeiro, 1948–54

Recently Lúcio Costa has become more
and more involved in city planning. His
master-plan for Brasilia, which was selected
by an international jury in an open competition in 1956, and which provides a
superb framework for Niemeyer's monumental buildings as well as a beautiful and
rational setting for a better organized
community life in a dignified capital city,
is justly famous.

Bibliography: Except for an article on 'The
Architect and Contemporary Society' published by UNESCO, and one on 'The New
Scientific and Technological Humanism'
published by the Massachusetts Institute
of Technology, Lúcio Costa has to be read
in Portuguese, but the result will be worth
the trouble, especially in the case of the
articles 'A Necessary Documentation',
'Portuguese-Brazilian Furniture', 'Jesuitic
Architecture in Brazil', published in the
*Revista do Serviço do Patrimônio Historico
Artistico*, nos. 1, 3, 5, and of the publications of the Ministry of Education and
Culture of his 'Thoughts on Contemporary Art' and 'A great deal of Building,
a bit of Architecture, and a Miracle'.

HENRIQUE E. MINDLIN

Cuijpers, Petrus Josephus Hubertus, b.
Roermond 1827, d. Roermond 1921.
Studied at Antwerp Academy, follower of
*Viollet-le-Duc. Cuijpers stood at the
watershed between historicism and the
modern movement in the *Netherlands.
Numerous Catholic churches in a freely
adapted Gothic manner. Rijksmuseum
(1885) and main station at Amsterdam
(1889).

Curtain wall. In the evolution of structural
systems two basic types can be distinguished, deriving at various times from
the particular contingencies of place and
civilization: massive structures and skeleton
ones.
In buildings of the first type (Palazzo
Strozzi, Florence, 1489–1507; Notre-Dame
du Haut, Ronchamp, by *Le Corbusier,
1954) every part of the walls performs, without differentiation, the functions both of
loadbearing and of separation; in the second
type (Chartres Cathedral, 1194–1220; Promontory Apartments, Chicago, by *Mies
van der Rohe, 1949) on the other hand, a
system of high strength units, which may
be connected together in various ways,
performs the special functions of a load-
bearing framework, while the other parts
of the wall are devoted exclusively to the
tasks of closing off and separation. All non-
loadbearing walls, adopted at any time by
whatever structural tradition, could in a
certain sense be called curtain walls; in fact
they possess in some respects both the
qualities of a wall (which is immovable,
heavy, and definitive) and those of a curtain
(which is movable, light, and temporary).
In this broad sense the Gothic cathedrals
with their large windows between piers,
the frame buildings of Japan which close
off space with panels of wood and paper,
and those of Central and Northern Europe
which employ brick walls, sometimes
plastered, for partitioning, may be considered authoritative examples of curtain
wall architecture.
However, the feature called by the modern
name of curtain wall (the English term has
universal currency) signifies a particular
kind of external, non-loadbearing wall,
composed of repeating modular elements,
shop-manufactured and erected on site,
which performs all the functions (and only
these) of separation between indoors and
out, and in particular those of defence

against external agencies (atmospheric and otherwise), thermal and acoustical insulation, and regulation of view, light and air. This definition, however, is not always strictly adhered to, either because curtain walling is of recent invention, and has thus not yet been the subject of any deep critical examination, or because its typology is being constantly enriched, thanks to the continual efforts of designers and manufacturers to find better methods of production and application.

The curtain wall is the end-product of a process of development that has involved a number of interrelated considerations connected with technical progress, social and cultural factors, and the emergence of the modern style in architecture. The introduction and perfecting of new structural techniques making use of *steel at the beginning of the 19th century and *reinforced concrete in its second half, gave the impulse to a spreading use of framed structures (Chocolate factory at Noisiel-sur-Marne, by Saulnier, 1871-2; second Leiter Building, Chicago, by Le Baron *Jenney, 1889-90; house in the Rue Franklin, Paris, by *Perret, 1903). The increased employment of this type of walling showed the importance of aiming at two characteristics in particular: slenderness, to keep the maximum floor area available for use, and lightness, so that by reducing the load on the steel frame, the latter might be designed with correspondingly smaller members.

The small dimensions of the steel frames and the progress made by the glass industry permitted an increase in window sizes, a development that was also stimulated by the demand for as much natural light as possible in industrial and commercial buildings. Between 1850 and the early years of the 20th century the window gradually turned into the window wall (Chatham Dockyard Museum, 1867; Reliance Building, Chicago, by *Burnham and *Root, 1890-4; Samaritaine department store, Paris, by Jourdain, 1905), sometimes taking over the whole basic area defined by the façade (Maison du Peuple, Brussels, by *Horta, 1896-9; AEG works, Berlin, by *Behrens, 1908-9). The use of large areas of glass had meanwhile become widespread in greenhouses and winter gardens, pedestrian galleries, railway station roofs and large exhibition pavilions (Crystal Palace,

London, by *Paxton, 1851; Machinery Hall, Paris, by Dutert and Contamin, 1889).

The transformation of the window into the window wall and the employment of large glazed areas drew attention to a number of problems and evoked the first solutions to them; they included such questions as that of insulation, eliminating condensation, developing the secondary glazing framework (Hallidie Building, San Francisco, by *Polk, 1918) and countering the effects of expansion by the careful design of joints and fixing systems. Large industrial buildings and tall office blocks, conceived as endless repetitions of identical cell units, led to the use of a uniform grid for the structural frames. Between the eve of the First World War and the beginning of the Second, the architects of the modern movement carried out a series of experiments, each of which may be considered as perfecting some particular aspect of curtain walling by the use of modern methods of industrial production (Fagus factory, Alfeld, 1911; model factory at the Werkbund Exhibition, Cologne, 1914; Bauhaus, Dessau, 1925-6, all by *Gropius; Bijenkorf department store, Rotterdam, by *Dudok, 1929-30; Maison Suisse, University City, Paris, 1930-2; Salvation Army Hostel, Paris, 1932; Maison Clarté, Geneva, 1932, all by Le Corbusier).

At the same time the theoretical principles of this new means of architectural

Jules Saulnier. Chocolate factory. Noisiel-sur-Marne, 1871-2

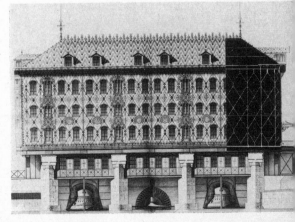

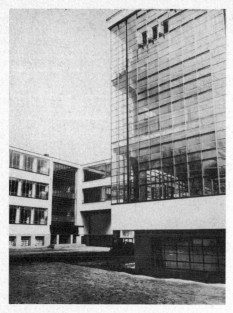

Walter Gropius. Bauhaus. Dessau, 1925–6

Gian Antonio Bernasconi, Annibale Fiocchi and
Marcello Nizzoli. Palazzo Olivetti. Milan, 1954.

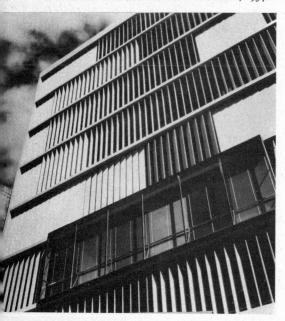

expression were being formulated via educational experiments (*Bauhaus), writings (Le Corbusier) and projects (various schemes of Mies van der Rohe between 1919 and 1922; Gropius and Meyer's design for the Chicago Tribune competition, 1922). It was only after the Second World War, however, that the first experiments began in the real industrialization of the building trade on a vast scale. It was this period that saw the development and spread of the curtain wall in the United States (UN Secretariat Building, New York by *Harrison and others, 1947–50; Lake Shore Drive Apartments, Chicago, 1951 and Seagram Building, New York, 1956, by Mies van der Rohe) and Europe. Architects experimented with its application to different types of building, and discovered new possibilities of expression, with the close collaboration of manufacturers on the alert for new materials and methods.

The classification of curtain wall types is still in its early stages, though certain criteria based on technical and structural considerations seem to provide a valid instrument for critical inquiry:

1. Presence or otherwise of spatial modelling of the façade, obtained with strongly projecting or recessed units. Some types feature three-dimensional treatment: main elevation of the Palazzo Olivetti, Milan, 1954, by Bernasconi, *Fiocchi and *Nizzoli; others employ a flat or two-dimensional treatment: Phoenix-Rheinrohr Building, Düsseldorf, 1960, by Hentrich and Petschnigg.

2. Relationship to the structure's loadbearing frame. Some types do not bring out the framework at all, but cover it like a sheath: Lever House, New York, 1952 by *Skidmore, Owings and Merrill; some pick out only the verticals: Inland Steel Company Building, Chicago, 1954 by Skidmore, Owings and Merrill; or only the horizontals: headquarters of the Fédération Nationale du Bâtiment, Paris, 1950, by Gravereaux and Lopez. Yet others feature both verticals and horizontals: Equitable Savings Building, Portland, Oreg., 1948 by *Belluschi.

3. Differentiation between the wall unit and its frame. Some types are in the form of panels set in a secondary frame, which in its turn is fixed to the loadbearing structure: Crown Hall of the IIT, Chicago, 1955 by Mies van der Rohe. Others use panels of an appropriately rigid section, which is

anchored direct to the main structure: Alcoa Building, Pittsburgh, 1953 by *Harrison and *Abramovitz.

4. Structural make-up of the secondary frame, where it exists. Some types feature vertical elements, others horizontal ones, others again use a grid of both.

5. Method of assembly of individual elements. Some come in single units, others have to be put together from various parts.

6. Method of connecting adjacent units. Some types have edge sections which interlock with the next unit, others use an intermediate feature.

7. Method of packing joints. Some types have rigid joints (welded), others use non-rigid packing (mastic, plastic, etc.).

Bibliography: Curtain Walls, Milan 1956; *Construire en acier*, Zurich 1956; Ian McCallum (editor), 'Machine-Made America' in *The Architectural Review*, London, May 1957, No. 724; W. Dudley Hunt, *The Contemporary Curtain Wall*, New York 1958; R. Schaal, *Vorhangwände —Curtain Walls*, Munich 1961; R. McGrath and A. C. Frost, *Glass in Architecture and Decoration*, London 1961; *Industrial Architecture* (London) 6/1963.

GIUSEPPE GIORDANINO, GIUSEPPE VARALDO, AND GIAN PIO ZUCCOTTI

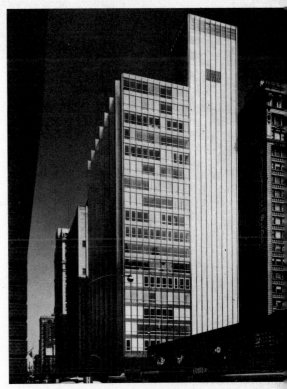

Skidmore, Owings and Merrill. Inland Steel Company Building. Chicago, Ill., 1954

Left. Pietro Belluschi. Equitable Savings Building. Portland, Oreg., 1948

Wallace K. Harrison and Max Abramovitz. Alcoa Building. Pittsburgh, 1953. Erection of a prefabricated unit

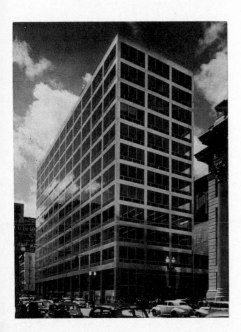

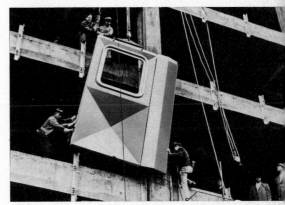

Deilmann, Harald, b. Gladbeck 1920.
Studied and worked as assistant at Stutt-
gart Technical College. Architect of the
Municipal Theatre, Münster, together
with Hausen, Rave, and Ruhnau (1954–6).
Nordwest-Lotto offices, Münster (1960).
Hospitals, cultural buildings.

Deitrick, William H., b. Danville, Va.
1905. Together with *Nowicki and Severud
architect of the arena at Raleigh, N.C.
(1952–3). The roof of the arena is carried
by steel ropes which are suspended from
two sloping parabolic arcs.

Denmark. Danish people have always
drawn inspiration from the major centres
of world culture, but have shown a capacity
to adapt new ideas to Danish landscape and
climate, customs and building practices,
adopting what is new with caution and
criticism. Thus the process whereby
Danish architecture acquired its own
character was markedly evolutionary. Securely anchored in their own tradition of
craftsmanship, the Danes developed a
sense for simple order, natural proportions,
and rhythm, first through half-timbered
work and afterwards through the *modular
brick buildings of the Empire period.
Emotionalism in architecture was always
distrusted and the worst excesses of
eclecticism were avoided. On the other
hand the genuine progressive movement
was slow to make itself felt.
A functional tradition runs through Danish
architecture, from the simple brick buildings of the Empire period, via Gottlieb
Bindesbøll onward to neoclassicism, to
Ivar Bentsen and Kay *Fisker. Bindesbøll's
Medical Association houses and Oringe
Hospital (built in the fifties) are simple
buildings of yellow brick serving a clear
functional purpose. Daniel Herholdt's
work of the 1860s has a clearer sense of
style, but shows the same respect for simple
structures and honest materials. Herholdt
was also the first to use cast-iron in a major
building—Copenhagen University library
(1861). The master builder of Copenhagen
town hall, Martin Nyrop, carried the use
of this material's special properties further,
while Jensen *Klint, securely rooted in the
brick-building tradition, thought he had
arrived at a new and timeless architecture
with Grundtvig's Church (1920–40), a
gigantic paraphrase of the Danish country

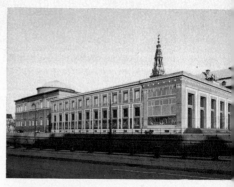

Gottlieb Bindesbøll. Thorwaldsen Museum.
Copenhagen, 1839–48

church. The neoclassicism of 1910–15 was
eclecticism's last outburst. Its two chief
works were Carl Petersen's Fåborg Museum (1912); and the Police Station (1918–
22, by Hack, Kampmann and his two sons,
and Åge Rafn. The chief significance of the
period for the future lay in a severer artistic
discipline and a sharpened sense for the
qualities of craftsmanship and material.
Ivar Bentsen carried on the tradition of
brick building with small unpretentious
houses and good blocks of flats, and since
the twenties Kay Fisker has been the leading exponent of traditionalism, playing a
leading part in the effort to improve the
quality of ordinary housing. The most
important product of Functionalism has
been Århus University (begun 1931), the
first part of which was designed by Fisker
in collaboration with C. F. Møller and Povl
Stegmann. Its many separate buildings
stand skilfully related to one another in a
rolling park-like campus. The laconic and
precise style of the first yellow brick buildings has been continued by C. F. Møller
alone during the past twenty years, without losing the originally projected unity of
design. Fisker's strong personality shows
to advantage in Copenhagen's Voldparken
School and the Maternity Care Building
of the mid-fifties. Kåre Klint carried on
his father Jensen Klint's ideas in Bethle-
hem Church (1937) and also became the
leading figure of furniture design, with
semi-traditional furniture of the highest
craftsmanship. In the post-war years an
agreeable personal atmosphere has been
given to housing developments like Sønder-

gårdsparken (architects **P. E. Hoff** and **Bennet Windinge**) by the location of the buildings and their relation to terrain and landscape gardening. There has been especial emphasis on school building in the past decade, with low single- and double-storeyed buildings which create admirable conditions of intimacy for the pupils. One of the finest of these is F. C. Lund and Hans Christian Hansen's Hansted School in Copenhagen.

The *Art Nouveau movement left little of note in Denmark (see, however, the work of Anton Rosen and Thomas Bindesbøll). International *Functionalism first made itself seriously felt after the Stockholm Exhibition of 1930, which was a revelation for young Danish architects. Vilhelm Lauritzen became an outstanding exponent of Functionalism, coping with contemporary problems such as Copenhagen Airport and Broadcasting House. Mogens Lassen built the first *Le Corbusier-inspired villas and Fritz Schleget became the Danish exponent of a freedom from aesthetic preconceptions established by *Perret with his reinforced concrete work (Mariebjaerg crematorium). The young Arne *Jacobsen also belonged to the revolutionary group, with the charming

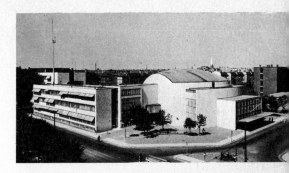

Vilhelm Lauritzen. Broadcasting House. Copenhagen, 1938–45

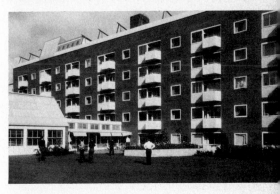

Povl Ernst Hoff and Bennet Windinge. Høje Søborg apartment block. Copenhagen, 1949–51

Left. Peter Vilhelm Jensen Klint. Grundtvig Church. Copenhagen, 1920–40

Kay Fisker, C. F. Møller, and Povl Stegmann. Århus University. Commenced 1931

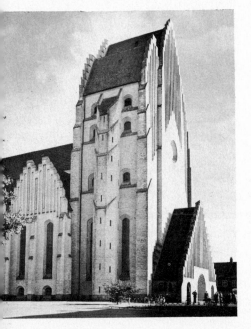

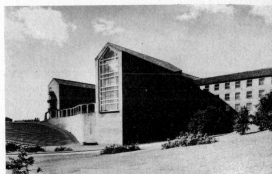

development at Bellevue and later (in collaboration with Møller and Lassen) with the Århus and Søllerod town halls. These edifices were the climax of progressive building in the thirties, before the material shortages of the war and subsequent years brought a return to the cultivation of traditional qualities.

The post-war years have been marked especially by inspiration from the USA, first by *Wright's houses and their adaptation to the landscape, later by *Mies van der Rohe's simplicity. Again Jacobsen was the leading figure, with large administrative buildings and hotels, like Rødovre town hall (1955) and the SAS building in Copenhagen (1959). In his schools and housing Jacobsen convincingly combined foreign inspiration with Danish tradition. Among the younger generation Halldor Gunnløgsson is a fine exponent of a severe classical architecture. Drawing inspiration both from Japanese architecture and from Mies van der Rohe, he has built single houses and (in co-operation with Jørn Nielsen) Kastrup town hall. Jørn *Utzon is the vital, imaginative and original talent whose prize design for Sydney Opera House is now under construction. In Denmark he has so far only completed a number of interesting houses and housing blocks. Utzon is Denmark's most important representative of a dynamic, organic architectural sense. Vilhelm Wohlert and Jørgen Bo have created a delightful background for contemporary art in Louisiana Museum, combining sensitivity with caution towards external effects.

Otherwise it is not so much by individual achievements that Denmark has acquired a certain international recognition as by the conscientious and workmanlike character of her architecture and craftsmanship.

Bibliography: Kay Fisker and Knud Millech, *Danske Arkitekturstrømninger 1850–1950*, Copenhagen 1951; Harald Langberg, *Dansk Byggeskik*, 1955; Monies, Hjort, Røgind, *Contemporary Danish Architecture*, Copenhagen 1956; (Symposium): *The Architecture of Denmark*, London 1949; Esbjørn Hjort, *Housing in Denmark since 1930*, London 1952.

TOBIAS FABER

Deutscher Werkbund. The genesis of the Deutscher Werkbund, which was founded on 6 October 1907 by the German architect Hermann *Muthesius, can be traced back, in part, to the movement in England led by William *Morris and his associates in the middle of the 19th century to revive the standards of craftsmanship in the arts of everyday life that had obtained in the Middle Ages. This movement was associated with the moral requirement that the craftsman should find pride and joy in his labour, and it led to an antagonism to machinery and its crude productions in contemporary industrial art, although it should be emphasized that the antagonism was less to machinery itself than to its bad use by the continual stamping out of crude imitations of historical styles. It must be acknowledged, however, that Morris never really came to terms with machinery, which he felt was responsible for so many of the social and aesthetic evils of the 19th century. Yet the movement led by William Morris revived much of the excellent medieval craftsmanship, with the emphasis on quality of design, of material, and of individual skill. The movement also contributed to the revival of a high standard of domestic architecture which began with the Red House designed by William Morris's architect Philip *Webb in 1859. This was the first of a series of excellent houses designed by Webb, which together with those by C. F. A. *Voysey and Norman *Shaw showed at that time (that is, the last forty years of the century) a new spirit in domestic architecture. Instead of

Jørgen Bo and Vilhelm Wohlert. Louisiana Museum. Humlebaek near Copenhagen, 1958

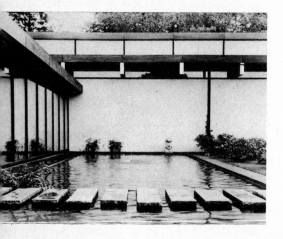

formal symmetrical elevations with planning to match as in Late Renaissance buildings, houses were designed more in accordance with the best fulfilment of their purpose, with rooms in convenient relation to each other, and orientation in accordance with sunlight. This meant design more on medieval lines with often irregular plans, while it was accompanied with an expressive use of the best materials.

From 1896 to 1903 Hermann Muthesius was attached to the German Embassy in London, and during his sojourn he made a thorough study of English contemporary architecture and of industrial art. He returned to Germany with enthusiastic admiration for English domestic architecture and applied art in the Morris tradition and wrote several books on these subjects. He deplored the poor condition of industrial art in Germany, its constant repetition of dead historical styles, and as head of the Prussian Board of Trade for Schools of Arts and Crafts in 1907 he took steps to effect improvements and to infuse new life into industrial art by forming the Deutscher Werkbund. His criticisms of contemporary German art met with a good deal of opposition, both in art circles and from industrialists, but he was able to exercise some influence on the latter by emphasizing the economic aspect of good design and craftsmanship in industrial production, because without these there was a risk that Germany would lose ground in world markets. Several industrialists seemed to realize this and it is not without significance that they appointed well-known architects and designers as design consultants about the same time as the foundation of the Deutscher Werkbund, the most notable being Peter *Behrens, appointed in this capacity to the AEG.

The avowed objects of the Deutscher Werkbund were to select the best representatives of the arts and crafts, industry and trades, to make all necessary efforts to secure high quality in industrial art, and to form a centre for all who aimed at this high quality in their work. Among those who were associated with the venture in its early years, in addition to Muthesius, were Karl Schmidt, Theodor *Fischer, Richard *Riemerschmid, Hans *Poelzig, Heinrich Tessenow, Josef *Hoffmann, and Henri van de *Velde. There was a great insistence on quality of craftsmanship and

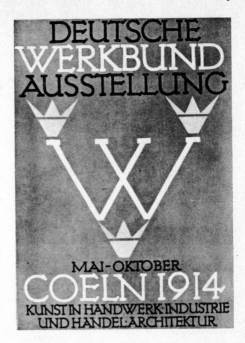

Fritz Hellmut Ehmcke. Poster for the Werkbund Exhibition. Cologne, 1914

material, and it is a question whether aesthetic aspects were sufficiently considered, but this was rectified later when the whole question of aims was considered at the Convention in 1911. The attitude of the members to the use of machinery in production was very different from that of William Morris. They not only came to terms with it, but they welcomed it as a valuable means of large-scale output of quality goods. They viewed machinery as a development of the hand tool, but, like the hand tool, something to be fully controlled and wholly subservient to the artist-craftsman. Another factor that probably influenced the acceptance of the machine by the Deutscher Werkbund was the gradual realization that many machines are beautiful things in themselves, and that such objects as the modern locomotive, motor-car, aeroplane, and modern liner can compare in beauty with the finest of modern buildings.

At the congress held in 1911 Muthesius reasserted the aims of the Deutcher Werkbund, but in addition he placed emphasis on aesthetic qualities and spiritual values which he associated with ideas of form, and he advocated turning for inspiration to that architecture of the past where the realization of form had been of the highest excellence, in the Greek temple, the Roman baths and the Gothic cathedral. This perfection of form was associated, to some extent, in the mind of Muthesius with mathematical calculation, which, together with the acceptance of machine production, led to a belief and advocacy of standardization that he expressed at the annual meeting of the Werkbund in 1914. This point of view, however, met with opposition from Henri van de Velde, a prominent member of the Werkbund, who could not reconcile standardization and the acceptance of canons with the individual creative work of artists. An artist, he contended, was always an individualist, who would never submit to rules and standards. These two lines of thought existed in the ranks of the Werkbund, as indeed they have always existed in discussions of art and architecture.

In this same year, 1914, the Deutscher Werkbund held a very important exhibition of industrial art at Cologne, which some have regarded in retrospect as the most important of the century. Several of the buildings for this exhibition were designed by pioneer modern architects, including Henri van de Velde, Walter *Gropius, Peter Behrens, Josef Hoffmann, and Bruno *Taut, and include some of the most significant early examples of modern architecture in steel, concrete and glass.

Weissenhof Housing Exhibition. Stuttgart, 1927

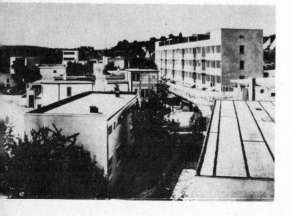

Van de Velde's contribution was a theatre which contained several innovations. Perhaps the most notable building of the exhibition and that which marked the greatest advance was the model factory administrative block and garage designed by Walter Gropius in collaboration with Adolf *Meyer. The contribution of Bruno Taut was a pavilion for the German glass industry which consisted of a twelve-sided glass drum with a pointed glass dome. The First World War arrested the work of the Deutscher Werkbund, but it had already exerted considerable influence throughout Europe and many institutions were formed in other countries to follow its example. An Austrian Werkbund was formed in 1910 and a Swiss in 1913. The Swedish Slöjdsforening was reorganized about the same time to conform with the Werkbund, while in England in 1915 the Design and Industries Association was established which was frankly modelled on the Deutscher Werkbund.

The next really great event in the history of the Werkbund was the exhibition of 1927 which included a housing exhibition on a hill in Weissenhof, a suburb of Stuttgart. It was superintended by Ludwig *Mies van der Rohe, then a vice-president of the Deutscher Werkbund, who invited several European architects to submit designs. Those who accepted invitations were the German architects: Peter Behrens, Walter Gropius, Hans Poelzig, Bruno Taut, Hans *Scharoun, Adolf G. Schneck, Ludwig *Hilberseimer, R. Döcker, Adolf Rading, and Max *Taut; the Austrian architect, Josef Frank; the French architect, *Le Corbusier; and the Dutch architects, J. J. P. *Oud and Mart Stam, while Mies van der Rohe himself designed a block of flats for the scheme. He gave the architects complete freedom in their designs with the one proviso that all the houses should have flat roofs. This housing exhibition proved to be one of the most important events in domestic architecture in the period between the two wars. Its historical value is that it demonstrates, in a concentrated form, the stages reached in the evolution of house design and construction in 1927 by the most progressive architectural thought in Europe. In some of the houses a degree of standardization is employed which would make it possible to build them economically on a large scale.

For example, in the two houses designed by Walter Gropius a steel-framed construction is employed on a grid of about one metre, with asbestos cement sheets as external facing on slabs of cork with suitable internal facing, a method which lends itself not only to mass production but to dry assembly. This is also the case with the block of flats designed by Mies van der Rohe constructed of a light steel frame with standardized wall sections and windows. Similarly the house designed by Hans Poelzig consists of timber sheets fixed to a framed structure. Several of the houses are built of reinforced concrete, including those designed by Le Corbusier in which the essential structure consists of reinforced concrete and steel posts or columns placed at intervals on which the houses are suspended. Flexibility in the design and use of the houses was one of the principal motifs in the designs.

The housing exhibition of the Deutscher Werkbund at Stuttgart was in many ways an exemplification of the principles of modern building advocated by the Werkbund's founder, Muthesius, in 1911. It took place in the year of his death, and its success—for it attracted attention among architectural circles throughout the world—was a reward for his early pioneer efforts. A further triumph for the Deutscher Werkbund was its very successful participation in the Paris exhibition of 1930. The German Government entrusted the task to the Deutscher Werkbund, which appointed Walter Gropius to organize the German section. He was assisted by three of his former colleagues at the Bauhaus, L. Moholy-Nagy, Marcel *Breuer, and Herbert Bayer. The exhibition was dedicated to building and the industrial arts and had two main themes, which were a continuation of those of the Stuttgart housing exhibition: standardization in all fields of building and the mass production of well-designed housing units.

With National Socialism the Deutscher Werkbund was disbanded. It was revived after the end of the Second World War.

Bibliography: Die Form, Berlin, especially IX—1927, and VII—1932; Nikolaus Pevsner, *Pioneers of the Modern Movement*, especially chapter 1, London 1936; Reyner Banham, *Theory and Design in the First Machine Age*, 1–5, London 1960.

ARNOLD WHITTICK

Doesburg, Theo van, b. Utrecht 1883, d. Davos 1931. Van Doesburg, whose real name was Chr. E. M. Küpper, began his career as a painter; his pictures were shown for the first time at an exhibition in The Hague in 1912. In collaboration with the architects *Oud and Wils, van Doesburg endeavoured to transfer his painting of the two-dimensional into something spatial and connect it organically with architecture. In 1916 he founded the *Sphinx* group in Leiden together with Oud, but it did not last long. A year later, he joined a group of artists and architects in De *Stijl, a movement set up to achieve a 'radical renewal of art'. Van Doesburg became the spokesman of the group, whose ideology he helped to formulate.

In 1917, together with Oud, he designed the hall of the latter's house at Noordwijkerhout, near Leiden, in which he sought to reinforce and stress the architecture by means of painting. His use of primary colours, tiled flooring and geometrical leading on the windows is in line with De Stijl methods. In the years that followed, van Doesburg was invited to lecture on the movement's activities at the *Bauhaus in Dessau, and in Berlin. The Bauhaus also took over his book on the basic principles of art, originally published in Dutch (Amsterdam 1919), as the sixth publication in the Bauhaus Books series (*Grundbegriffe der bildenden Kunst*, Munich 1924).

When the Aubette, a dance hall and amusement centre in Strasbourg was reconstructed in 1926–7, van Doesburg was able to realize his ideas on space and colour on a larger scale, in collaboration with Hans Arp. Moving to Paris, he built a studio for himself at Meudon-Val-Fleury (1930–1), which soon became the focus of the Stijl movement. He worked once more in collaboration with Cor van *Eesteren, as he had done already in the early twenties, and turned his attention to applying the principles of De Stijl to town planning. Van Doesburg's death in 1931 meant the end of the Stijl group, but its concepts of space, which he helped to define, have remained a living issue to the present time.

Bibliography: Theo van Doesburg, *De Nieuwe Beweging in de Schilderkunst*, Delft 1917; Theo van Doesburg, *Drie voordrachten over de nieuwe beeldende*

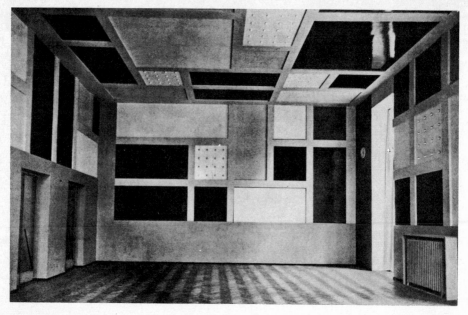

Theo van Doesburg. Aubette. Strasbourg, 1926-7

Kunst, Amsterdam 1919; Theo van Doesburg, *Klassiek, barok, modern*, The Hague 1920; Theo van Doesburg, *L'Architecture vivante*, Paris 1925.

J. J. VRIEND

Drew, Jane Beverly, b. 1911. Studied at the Architectural Association School of Architecture, London. In partnership with J. T. Allison, 1934–9. Independent practice, 1939–45. In partnership with Maxwell *Fry (whom she married in 1942) since 1945. Early work in Kenya led to specialization in tropical architecture. Assistant Town Planning Adviser, West Africa, 1944–5. Schools, housing and colleges in Ghana. Joint work with Maxwell Fry on the University of Ibadan, Nigeria. Projects in Kuwait (1,000-bed hospital); India (hospitals, housing, and a large high school; senior architect at Chandigarh in collaboration with *Le Corbusier); Singapore; Ceylon; South Persia (housing, town planning, hospital extensions, cinemas); and Mauritius (hospitals and housing). Jane Drew served as Bemis Professor at the Massachusetts Institute of Technology in 1961, and has lectured widely elsewhere.

Dudok, Willem Marinus, b. Amsterdam 1884. Although deriving something from both the School of *Amsterdam and De *Stijl, Dudok evolved an independent position of his own. The contrast of solid and void areas, horizontals and verticals recalls De Stijl, but Dudok's brick buildings nearly always retain a massive weightiness. Numerous buildings at Hilversum, where Dudok became municipal architect in 1915: Vondel School (1928–9), Town Hall (1928–30). Netherlands House at the Paris Cité Universitaire (1927–8), Bijenkorf department store at Rotterdam (1929–30, now replaced by the new building designed by Marcel *Breuer).
Bibliography: W. M. Dudok, Übersicht über sein Werk, Amsterdam 1954.

Duiker, Johannes, b. The Hague 1890, d. Amsterdam 1935. Studied at Delft Technical College. Member of De *Stijl and the group connected with the journal *De 8 en Opbouw*. Zonnestraal Sanatorium at Hilversum (1928, together with B. Bijvoet); open-air school at Amsterdam (1930–2), a five-storey fully glazed structure with terraces for open-air lessons.

Eames, Charles, b. St Louis, Missouri 1907. Broke off his studies at Washington University, St Louis, after eighteen months. Architect and designer. Together with his wife Ray he undertakes almost any sort of design from toys to furniture. His own house at Santa Monica, California (1949), a steel-frame building constructed from prefabricated units, is reminiscent of an old Japanese house in its proportions and light appearance.

Ecole des Beaux-Arts. Most influential School of Art and Architecture in the 19th century. The Parisian École goes back to its foundation by Colbert in 1671. Its teaching system rests on lectures and practical work in artists' studios and architects' offices. The Grand Prix de Rome offered by the École provides several years of study at the French Academy in the Villa Medici in Rome. The institute's basic conceptions of architecture lie in the composition of well-proportioned elements in a well-proportioned whole. In practice, the École, where many eminent architects have been trained, has often opposed modern trends in architecture.

Eesteren, Cor van, b. Ablasserdam 1897. Studied at the Academy in Rotterdam, the Sorbonne, and the *École des Beaux-Arts. Belonged from 1923 to the De *Stijl movement. Collaboration with van *Doesburg, especially on housing projects in 1923. For many years President of the *CIAM. Municipal buildings (Amsterdam Plan, 1936).

Eiermann, Egon, b. Neuendorf, near Berlin 1904. Together with Hans *Scharoun, Egon Eiermann is among the most discussed architects of post-war Germany. The work of these two men denotes the span of modern German architecture. If Scharoun designs with a feeling for the possibilities of sculptural massing, Eiermann lays stress on perceptible articulation, logical expression of the structural frame and precise detailing. His buildings create an impression of extraordinary clarity and taut organization. Architecture means to him 'making order visible, from town planning to the smallest building'. Structure and function can nearly always be read off, and his industrial plants reveal the aesthetic charm of visibly displayed technical apparatus. Eiermann develops his designs from functional analysis, in the widest sense of the word, including an assessment of the cultural and geographical background. Two office blocks, built over the same period, for the Essener Colliery (1960) and the Müller Steel Works at Offenbach (1960) depend in their different conceptions on the character of their surroundings: relatively blank wall areas with smallish window openings and quiet, dark panel cladding in the Ruhr town; brightly coloured façades with shady galleries and variable protection from the sun on the Upper Rhine. The tendency towards dogmatic preference for certain shapes is less pronounced in Eiermann than in other architects who are still under the influence of *Mies van der Rohe's image of a clear-cut rectilinear architecture.

Egon Eiermann. Handkerchief Mill. Blumberg, 1951

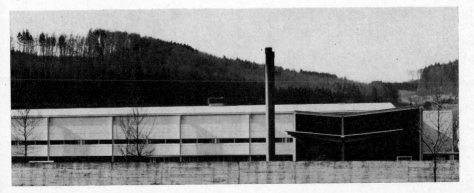

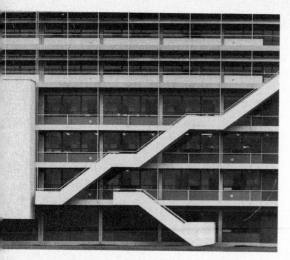

Egon Eiermann. Neckermann Mail Order
Company Building. Frankfurt, 1958–60. Detail
of elevation

Eiermann, who studied under *Poelzig in
Berlin, wrote his thesis on a department
store, and worked at first in the architects'
office of the Karstadt multiple store company. He retained a liking for this type of

Gustave Eiffel. Truyère Bridge. Garabit, 1880–4

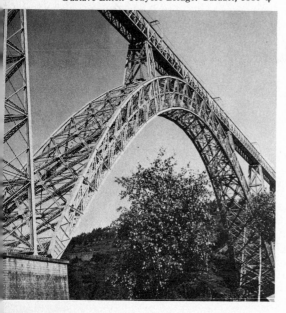

work even after the war (Merkur Department Store at Heilbronn, 1951). The Blumberg Handkerchief Mill (1951) represents
a culminating point in his work, with the
slender tracery of its various viewpoints.
Of Eiermann's church designs, St Matthew's at Pforzheim (1953) and the
Memorial Church in Berlin (1961) have
been built; the war damaged stump of the
latter's tower was preserved and surrounded
by the simple stereometric buildings of the
new church.

For these ecclesiastical buildings Eiermann
used pierced blocks with coloured glazing,
which the light filters through. Similar
textured wall surfaces, which have a purely
decorative purpose, occur at his two depar-
ment stores, the Horten at Heidelberg and
the Merkur at Stuttgart (1961); they are
reminiscent of Edward D. *Stone's work.
But these buildings do not stand comparison with that of the export firm of Neckermann at Frankfurt (1958–60). In contrast
to the patterned surfaces of the two department stores, the Frankfurt building is
vigorously enlivened by external galleries,
fire-escapes, and air conditioning and stair
towers. Eiermann's buildings for the German government display more delicate
outlines and elegant proportions; they include the German pavilion at the Brussels
World Fair (in collaboration with Sep Ruf,
1958) and the German Embassy in Washington, which rises in steps on a sloping
site (work still in progress).
Eiermann, who lectures at Karlsruhe
Technical College, has also made a name
for himself as an industrial designer.

WOLFGANG PEHNT

Eiffel, Gustave, b. Dijon 1832, d. Paris
1923. Gustave Eiffel, a Burgundian by
birth, was intended to be a chemist and
only by chance became a structural
engineer. As consultant to several building
firms and later as an independent consulting engineer, he had the opportunity of
making himself familiar with all the problems occasioned to bridge designers by the
advance of the railways into ever more
difficult territory. He soon realized that
these problems could not be solved if the
metal used was, as hitherto, in the form of
the comparatively heavy and inelastic cast-
iron. New materials, such as rolled iron
and steel had to be used, and these were
now being commercially produced in

sufficient quantities, but new methods and
shapes had also to be invented that did
justice to the better static behaviour of
these materials.

When Eiffel founded his own firm in 1867
he already commanded a sufficiently extensive experience. He also realized the
importance of collaborating with outstanding men such as Nouguier and Koechlin,
and he introduced new methods, whose
precision gave his firm great advantages
over his mostly foreign competitors. Soon
after the end of the Franco-German war,
commissions came in from all over the
world (France, Switzerland, Austria, Hungary, Russia, Portugal, Peru, etc.). Thus
he had ample opportunity of testing the
versatility of the lattice beam he had
developed and which he made the most
important component of a novel structural
system. Apart from numerous bridges,
stations, roof projects, and other structures,
nearly all of which brought technical
advances, his three main designs were: the
Maria Pia Bridge over the Douro near
Oporto (1877–8), the Truyère Bridge near
Garabit in the French Massif Central
(1880–4), and the Eiffel Tower in Paris
(1887–9). These three enormous structures
are all closely related. All three rely
throughout on the application of the
principle on which the lattice beam is based,
viz. the subdivision of beams into three-
dimensional space frames built up from
individually small members and riveted
together from commercially available angle
irons or flats, which afford maximum
rigidity for minimum weight. The Eiffel
Tower is nothing but an extension of the
solution tried out at Oporto and Garabit for
extremely tall bridge supports.

The Tower, in particular, marks an important stage in the development of modern
architecture for the impressive proof it
gives of the fecundity of the engineering
approach: intuitions, substantiated by
calculation, led to entirely new shapes. The
Tower brought the realization of a new
spatial image, made up of joints and fields
of force, to which indeed only graphic
artists like Robert Delaunay and Antoine
Pevsner were receptive, and then hardly
before 1910. Through their intermediation,
and thanks to the interpretations they gave

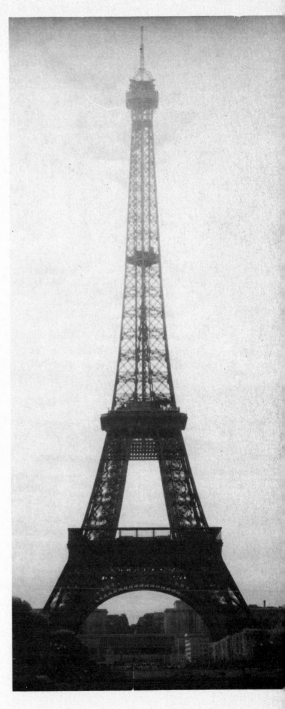

Gustave Eiffel. Eiffel Tower. Paris, 1887–9

of this spatial image, it was beamed back to architecture. The work of *Wachsmann and Le Ricolais on space structures has aroused the interest of architects and for some years now they have been working on Eiffel's multi-centred conception of space.

Eiffel himself pursued the logical direction of his research on the greatest adversary his giant constructions had to contend with: the wind. From 1910 on, he devoted himself to aerodynamic studies, which led to the building of the first wind-tunnel to meet the needs of the aircraft industry (1911), and to the development of the first aeroplane tested in a wind-tunnel (Bréguet LE, 1918).

Bibliography: Gustave Eiffel, *Mémoire présenté à l'appui du projet définitif du Viaduc de Garabit*, Paris 1889; Gustave Eiffel, *La Tour de Trois Cents Mètres*, Paris 1900 (2 folio vols.); Gustave Eiffel, *La Résistance de l'air et l'aviation*, Paris 1913 and 1914; Jean Prévost, *Eiffel*, Paris 1929; Maurice Besset, *Gustave Eiffel*, Milan 1957, Paris 1959.

MAURICE BESSET

Eijck, Aldo van, b. Driebercen 1918. Eijck, who has shown particular interest in problems of education (children's playgrounds at Amsterdam), created 'a house like a small town' when he built the Municipal Orphanage at Amsterdam (1955). This consists of a number of square space units which make up a growing complex of buildings. Municipal work (collaboration in the Nagele Plan).

Ellwood, Craig, b. Clarendon, Texas 1921. Mainly private dwellings of unusually elegant proportions and careful detailing which are reminiscent of *Mies van der Rohe with their slender sections. Carson-Roberts Building, Los Angeles (1961).

Endell, August, b. Berlin 1871, d. Breslau 1925. Self-taught. Designer and architect in the *Art Nouveau style. His most important buildings, the Elvira Photo Studio at Munich (1897–8) and the Bunte Theatre at Berlin (1901), are both distinguished by ingenious surface decoration.

Ervi, Aarne, b. Tammela, Finland 1910. Tapiola Garden City near Helsinki was based on Ervi's 1953 plan, and he himself carried out several of the projects there. Buildings for Turku University (1956–9).

Expressionism. Expressionist architects, like Expressionist painters, had no cultural groupings, with unified programmes and activities, and most architects who came within the ambit of Expressionism did so only for a short period of their development, although this often proved to be the zenith of their artistic careers. In the work of the best of them, various influences must be recognized as existing simultaneously side by side, or at different levels; these may vary from *Art Nouveau to romantic nationalism, from Expressionist art to a kind of late-romantic surrealism, and from rationalism and a search for objectivity to a view of the creative act as an unrepeatable gesture of self- and world-knowledge.

In Germany, during the years immediately prior to 1914, the true artistic avant-garde consisted of architects who owed their allegiance to the *Jugendstil, the course of whose history overlaid that of Expressionism for upwards of ten years. If we look more closely at the anti-classical, anti-internationalist traits that characterize the German version of Art Nouveau, its considerable hang-over from the historical styles and its general tendency to picturesqueness and a taste for organic forms, not projected on to plane surfaces but conceived plastically almost from the start, we shall readily perceive the numerous connecting links with avant-garde German Expressionist movements such as the *Brücke* and the *Blauer Reiter*. In this context one thinks of the work of Eckmann, Pankok, Obrist, *Endell, Joseph Maria *Olbrich, who played a key-rôle at this period with his activities at Darmstadt, and above all of Richard *Riemerschmid with his Hellerau factory (1910) and Henry van de *Velde, for their direct influence on the architects of Expressionism.

A typical feature of the situation in Germany at the time was the way the country was divided up between different cultural centres, each with a strong individual character and relatively independent of all the others, with its own schools of architecture and the applied arts. Efforts were being made to develop a romantic-national style, as a form of escape from eclecticism, that would provide the new German nation with a suitable form of architecture. With Alfred Messel's Wertheim department store (1896) a series of attempts began at simplifying the eclectic Wilhelminian language of the times which implicated all the most distinguished architects currently practising: Theodor *Fischer who taught at Munich (Ulm Garrison Church, 1911), Ludwig Hoffmann, Paul *Bonatz (Main Railway Station, Stuttgart, 1913–27, with F. E. Scholer), and Fritz Schumacher, Professor at Dresden, and later at Hamburg, who had already before 1914 clearly worked out and established an expressive style of his own.

It was Peter *Behrens who achieved the transition to Expressionism with his buildings for the AEG in Berlin (1908–13). We are not concerned here with those elements which clearly anticipate the rationalist style. Behrens's factories are not designed with the kind of utilitarian character associated with the functional tradition, but rather as the representation of a new power, one that directly multiplies nature's goods. In his work may be seen that process of deformation of the national romantic style which is one of the fundamental sources of Expressionist architecture.

Apart from Behrens, there are only two architects before the First World War clearly distinguishable as Expressionists: Hans *Poelzig and Max *Berg. The conventional exterior of Berg's reinforced concrete Centenary Hall in Breslau (1912–13) gives no indication of the exciting three-dimensional treatment inside the enormous dome, 213 feet in diameter. It is impossible to find any reinforced concrete building before this date equally as compelling, and with as little of the schematic about it. Of these three architects, however, it is Hans Poelzig who seems to have adhered most consciously to Expressionism. His large industrial complex at Luban (1911–12) seems even more unprejudiced in design than the best works of Behrens at this period. His volumes are built up of asymmetrical blocks, whose organic unity seems to underline the peculiar individuality of the design. Three years previously, Poelzig had built a large house near Breslau, where the plastic fusion of all the elements towards a volumetric continuity recalls some of van de Velde's villas of the same epoch.

Thanks to the absence of preconceived

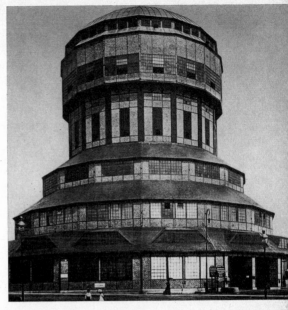

Hans Poelzig. Water tower. Posen, 1911

types, it was industrial architecture that offered the line of least resistance to progressive experiments at the time. This may be seen in the celebrated scheme for a water mill at Weider (1906), and above all in the great structure built by Poelzig at Posen (1911), with a water tower above and an exhibition hall below; brick is used here to clad a steel framework. The bold handling of volumes makes it one of the

Hans Poelzig. Salzburg Festival Theatre, 1920–1. Project

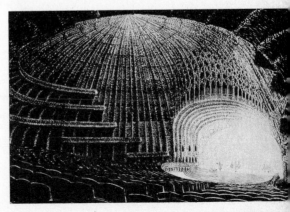

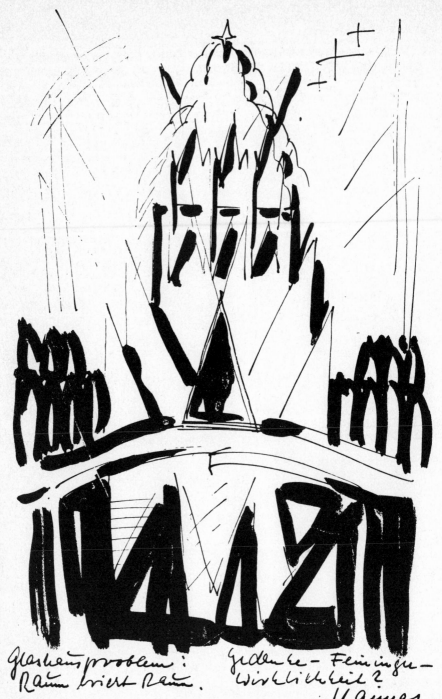

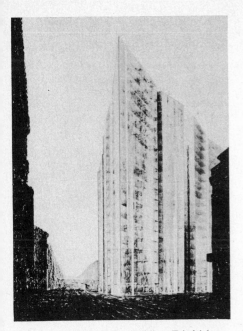

Mies van der Rohe. Office building, Friedrichstrasse, Berlin, 1919. Project (first version)

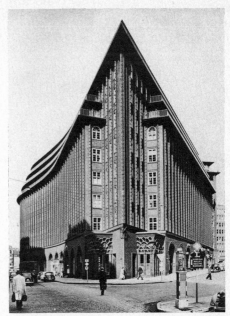

Fritz Höger. Chilehaus. Hamburg, 1922–3

most significant German buildings of its
day—the 'total transposition of a personal
idea into a work' which Kirchner demanded
as the basis for art. A series of sketches
dating from this period are clearly influenced in conception by certain drawings
of Kokoschka, and show a desire to model
a building with an aggressive immediacy
that leaves no part of its surface unmarked
by its author's will.

German culture in the years after the First
World War became progressively more
political in character. The Socialist revolution accompanied Expressionism as a form
of protest for at least ten years, in an
ideologically hybrid identification between
cultural avant-gardism and progressive
politics. Examples of this tendency may
be seen in the Berlin *Arbeitsrat für Kunst*
and *Novembergruppe*. The latter group,
descended from pre-war anarchist papers
such as *Aktion* and *Revolution*, attracted
to it all the foremost representatives of
German artistic life in the years 1918–20;
many architects were members, including

*Gropius and *Mendelsohn. The *Novem-
bergruppe*'s programme attributed particular importance to architecture, regarded
as a direct instrument for raising social
standards. The group was dissolved after
the bloody suppression of the Sparticist
rising, and the ensuing disillusion among
the progressive spirits of the Weimar
Republic contributed decisively to the
emergence of *Neue Sachlichkeit*, which
became the focus of much Expressionist
activity.

The *Bauhaus, too, especially during its
Weimar period, absorbed many features of
Expressionism. The crude pragmatism; the
stark expressive simplicity; a tenacious grip
on reality combined with an ethical sense
of human obligation; all accord well with
the School's methodological programme
as also with a type of design that was a
frequent outcome of Expressionist theory.
It is in this light that some of the works of
the protagonists of rationalism built at this
period may be clearly explained; works
carried out in a style with close affinities
to Expressionism. They include *Mies van
der Rohe's design for a skyscraper (1919)
and his memorial to Rosa Luxemburg and

Page 94. Hans Scharoun. Sketch. 1920

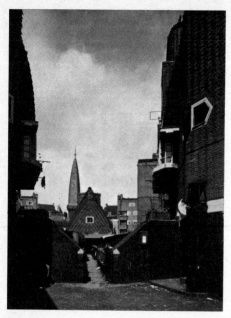

Michael de Klerk. Eigen Haard estate.
Amsterdam, 1921

Paul Bonatz. Head Office, United Steel Works.
Düsseldorf, 1922–4

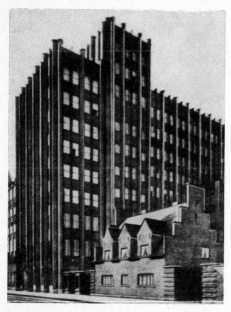

Karl Liebknecht (1926), and Gropius's War Memorial at Weimar (1922) and his theatre at Jena (1923).

Numerous other buildings at this time, however, were built under the direct influence of pre-war Expressionism, thus displaying a cultural lag of about ten years. They may be roughly divided into two distinct groups: one pushing the Expressionist protest in the direction of a progressive intensification of its idiom, either in a lyric vein with Art Nouveau reminiscences, or in a desperate manner leading to the destruction of volume; the other tending towards a national-romantic style. This kind of ambiguity is typical of Expressionism, which proved a fertile source of progressive drives and rationalist activity. Emil Fahrenkamp, for example, built a series of interesting factories in 1923, but later went over to a nationalist style. Wilhelm Kreis, with his Düsseldorf skyscraper, the Wilhelm-Marx-Building (1922–4), and the interior of the planetarium in the same city, produced two works of the highest merit in a near-Expressionist idiom, but later developed a heavy simplified neoclassic manner. *Scharoun, Schneider and the *Luckhardt brothers made use of the figurative manifestations of Expressionism within the orbit of rationalist practice. Rudolf Steiner's Goetheanum at Dornach (1925–8) is linked to Expressionism by its picturesque treatment, but occupies a place apart, as it was designed in accordance with the principles of Anthroposophy.

The School of *Amsterdam, too, whose mouthpiece was the journal *Wendingen, displayed an intensification of the national style; but the situation was somewhat different here from that in Germany, as social contrasts were less extreme. In point of fact, the largest scheme carried out by these architects was the development of low-cost housing estates in South Amsterdam. Hence the Expressionist character of the work is not a manifestation of protest; it derives from a peculiar ability to evolve an endless variety of forms, in a three-dimensional treatment that often achieves almost fairy-tale effects.

The most important Expressionist buildings erected in Germany in the first years after the war comprise: the Chilehaus (Fritz Höger), Ballinhaus (brothers Hans and Oskar Gerson) and Sprinkenhof

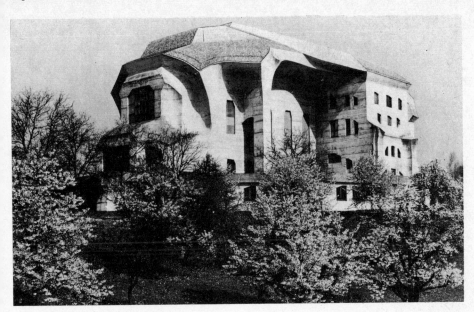

Rudolf Steiner. Goetheanum. Dornach, 1925–8

(Höger and the Gerson brothers), at Hamburg (1922–3), all influenced by Fritz Schumacher; the Einstein Tower by Erich Mendelsohn at Potsdam (1920); and the entrance hall of the Hoechst Dyeworks by Peter Behrens (1920–5). In Behrens's building, the wall surface features continuous punctuation by varying textures and materials, which emphasizes a feeling of unrest and instability that seems to lurk beneath the severe overall design. The brickwork is in shades which range from blue to orange and yellow, a palette which recalls the water-colours of Nolde or Kirchner. Mendelsohn, on the other hand, was influenced by the *Blauer Reiter* movement—he knew Franz Marc and Kandinsky when a student at Munich in 1911—and his Jugendstil reminiscences derive from that source. His sketches, executed between 1914 and 1920, display the same stylistic idioms, and that character of cosmic and stylistic search and lyric effusion as an act of liberation, and at the same time mystical union with the world, that is typical of the *Blauer Reiter's* spiritual posture. His use of sketches to work out his approach to a theme, without reference to structure, is typically Expressionist.

Two other architects deserve special notice: Hugo *Häring and Otto *Bartning. For Häring adherence to the Expressionist aesthetic was tantamount to a recognition of German Gothic as an anti-illuminist culture that shunned the laws of geometry and was hence organic in form (farm buildings, Garkau, 1923). For Bartning, however, architecture is growth and activity, the force of nature itself (Star church project, 1922). Poelzig's development between 1919 and 1930 is in two phases. The rebuilding of the Grosses Schauspielhaus in Berlin, the designs for the Salzburg Festival Theatre and a festival hall at Dresden carry the process of

Erich Mendelsohn. Einstein Tower. Potsdam, 1920. Project

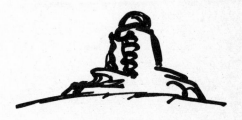

dissolving not only the classic rules of composition but the very constituent elements of the structure itself to extraordinary lengths. A second phase witnesses the reassertion of volumetric values, with a soberer and more monumental style, as exemplified by his designs for the IG-Farben offices at Frankfurt (1928–31) and his broadcasting studios in Berlin.

Under the stress of the menacing political situation in the early thirties, the artistic forces of the time tended to crystallize into groups centring around the democratic opposition or the Nazi party. The sharpening of this crisis betokened the end of Expressionism, which by its intrinsic nature could not tolerate extreme ideological conditions, although it tended to promote and educe them. The 'white architecture of the twenties' became a symbol of the democratic opposition, while Expressionism began to acquire pan-Germanic and nationalist traits, and in its ideological uncertainty was relegated to a position of cultural insignificance.

Bibliography: Walter Müller-Wulckow, *Deutsche Baukunst der Gegenwart*, Leipzig 1929; E. M. Hajos and L. Zahn, *Berliner Architektur der Nachkriegszeit*, Berlin 1928; Vittorio Gregotti, 'L'architettura dell' espressionismo', in *Casabella Continuità*, No. 254, Milan 1961; Arnold Whittick, *European Architecture in the Twentieth Century*, Vol. 1 (up to 1924), Vol. 2 (1924–33), London 1950 and 1953.

VITTORIO GREGOTTI

Festival of Britain, South Bank Exhibition. London, 1951. Aerial view of site

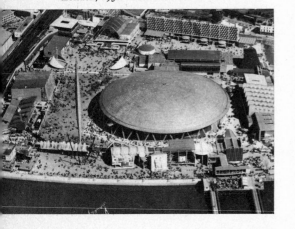

Farmer and Dark. Frank Quentery Farmer, b. 1879, d. 1955 and Bernard Franklin Dark. Practice founded 1934, specializing in industrial buildings, where effects are achieved by essentially simple but carefully developed methods of planning and close attention to details; factories, mills, power stations. In 1957 a 75-inch module system was developed for one- or two-storey timber buildings (Sconce Hills School, Newark, Notts.).

Festival of Britain. A national manifestation organized throughout the United Kingdom in 1951, at the original suggestion of Sir Gerald Barry, to mark the centenary of the Great Exhibition of 1851. Its most important architectural expression was the exhibition laid out on the south bank of the Thames in London (Director of Architecture: Hugh *Casson). This was significant not only for the opportunity it afforded millions of people to see stimulating modern architecture of an almost uniformly high level of design, but because it provided an occasion for displaying the principles of *townscape which had been developing and clarifying themselves over the previous years. Eschewing the formal layouts that had been usual in earlier major exhibitions, recourse was had to a subtly planned disposition of buildings and features, an exploitation of changes of level, progressively evolving views and the dramatic long-distance backdrop of the north bank of the Thames to give an impression of exciting complexity and size that was quite extraordinary for so small a site.

Notable contributions were made by Ralph Tubbs (Dome of Discovery), Arcon (Transport), Maxwell *Fry and Jane *Drew, Edward *Mills (Administration building), R. Y. Goodden and R. D. Russell (Lion and Unicorn), H. T. Cadbury Brown (Land of Britain), Brian O'Rorke and F. H. K. Henrion (The Natural Scene and The Country), *Architects' Co-Partnership (Minerals of the Land), G. Grenfell Baines and H. J. Reifenberg (Power and Production) and Basil *Spence (Sea and Ships).

Bibliography: H. Casson, 'The 1951 Exhibition' in *Journal of the RIBA*, April 1950. See also *Architectural Review* for May 1951.

HAROLD MEEK

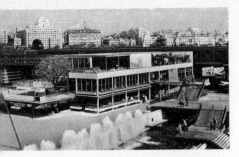

Misha Black, Alexander Gibson, and Design Research Unit. Regatta Restaurant. Festival of Britain, South Bank Exhibition. London, 1951

Figini, Luigi, b. Milan 1903. Graduated there 1926. Founder member of *gruppo 7*. Collaboration with Gino *Pollini. Residential buildings, factories (for Olivetti in Ivrea), exhibition architecture, and interior decoration. The Church of the Madonna dei Poveri erected on a basilica plan (Milan 1952–6) attempts to create an atmosphere of mystical faith with its exposed concrete frame, narrow light slits in the nave and its deliberate impression of a rough, unfinished state.

Finland. The counter-movement to eclecticism began to take shape in Finland in the course of the 1890s. Although preliminary development was gradual, the actual breakthrough in 1900 proved stormy. Following it, virtually no classical shapes emerged again for a long time. The victor was not *Art Nouveau in its true sense, but a Finnish version of it, the so-called National Romantic style, which was inspired by the tradition of primitive Finnish architecture. Axial symmetry was done away with and replaced by the free plan and free massing. Façade architecture gave way to layouts with separate blocks and wings. One of the essential problems of modern architecture had already been encountered: that of the continuity of space. These problems were solved in such an original way in Finland that the best examples have preserved their freshness throughout the past decades. While Art Nouveau often relied on decorative details for its artistic effect, the Finnish National Romantic style depended more on the effect of its materials as such. Timber and granite were favourite media from which strong and expressive effects were derived.

The painter Akseli Gallén-Kallela may be regarded as the spiritual father of the National Romantic movement in Finland, and his studio built in the Wildmark (1894) was the first achievement of the new style. Three architects, Gesellius, Lindgren and Eliel *Saarinen, soon took their place at its head. It was their design for the Finnish pavilion at the Paris International Exhibition of 1900 which precipitated the breakthrough, and their fortress-like log-house building at Hvitträsk near Helsinki (1902) still makes the strongest impression on a spectator to this day. Lars Sonck, the builder of Tampere Cathedral (1902–7) is currently regarded as the most brilliant exponent of the real romantic style. By its side, International Art Nouveau also made its appearance in Finland, assuming the tasks of a rationalist school in comparison with the picturesque romantic style. Its representatives are Selim Lindquist, Onni Tarjanne and Usko Nyström, whose aims were closer to present-day architecture than those of the romantics although they did not always measure up to them as artists.

Lars Sonck and Valter Jung. Bank. Helsinki, 1904

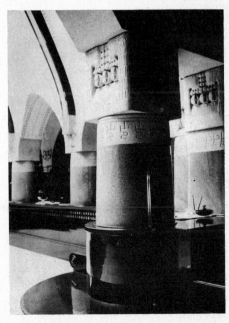

Sigurd Frosterus, a pupil of van de Velde's, and Gustaf Strengell were the leaders of the rationalist opposition and modern architectural ideas emerge in their writings around 1904. Even if they did not manage to defeat the romantics, the rationalists dealt them a decisive blow. The reaction was mainly due to the example set by Eliel Saarinen. He developed his own monumental style, whose fundamental idea is a vertical movement breaking through from the central feature of a horizontal mass; a subject whose pathos greatly appealed to his contemporaries. Saarinen's most important building in Finland is the main station at Helsinki (1904, built 1910–14), but it is less attractive than his general plan for the town—a fully consistent decentralization plan, conceived as early as 1918. After the end of the First World War, it became apparent that belief in the birth of a new art and a new architecture had been vain. Classical motives, albeit freely handled, returned to architecture. Coupled with this tendency now was the influence of Swedish classicism, which prevailed among the young generation. Striving for monumentality during the classicizing intermezzo of the twenties reached its peak in J. S. Sirén's Parliament Building. For many others, such as Erik *Bryggman and Gunnar Taucher, this trend meant a process of simplification, which banished every last moulding from their smooth surfaces. The timeless, functional architecture of the Mediterranean countries was the main exemplar adduced, and in this respect classicism too paved the way for the new architecture. Furthermore, the social thought of the twenties introduced a new element, as shown in the garden suburb of Käpylä at Helsinki (1920–5), planned by Martti Välikangas and others, which is based on old Finnish traditions as much as on the teachings of Ebenezer *Howard.

The new architecture, *Functionalism, only reached Finland in the late twenties. The exhibition at Turku, designed by Alvar *Aalto and Erik Bryggman in 1929, became the manifesto of the movement. The great Stockholm Exhibition of the following year assured the victory of Functionalism in Finland too. Compared with most other countries, the change in Finland was rapid and complete. The first new works by Bryggman, Erkki Huttunen, Yrjö Lindegren, and others showed great maturity, quite apart from Aalto's sanatorium at Paimio (1929–33) and the library at Viipuri (1927–35), which are among the classic masterpieces of modern architecture.

This 'white' Functionalism in Finland does not lack individuality despite its internationalism. A certain stress of solidity is characteristic of most of its products and gives them an expression of real monumentality, which often achieves pathos as in P. E. Blomstedt's work. Bryggman displays an outward lightness which is reminiscent of Continental rationalism but always preserves a romantic colouring.

Although the thirties were so uniform in Finnish architecture, new ideas did develop

Eliel Saarinen. Main railway station, Helsinki. Designed 1904, built 1910–14. Project

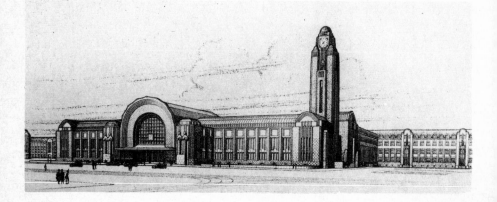

during this period, and more diverse artistic expressions resulted. Aalto above all, whose works from the outset attracted attention outside Finland, demonstrated new powers of design. His cellulose factory at Sunila (1936–9) and the house built along terraces at Kauttua (1938–40) are studies in adapting architecture to landscape. Free shapes and careful use of building materials (in particular of timber) characterize his work from the start (Finnish Pavilion at the New York World's Fair, 1939).

The forties brought a reaction against the severity of Functionalism. The Olympic Village by Hilding Ekelund and Välikangas (Helsinki 1940) marks the retreat of the cube in favour of less demanding functional shapes and the memorial chapel at Turku cemetery (1938–41) by Bryggman appeals to the spectator's emotions. Throughout the war building activity was very limited and the artistic results were modest. The romantic reaction took refuge in eclecticist and decorative motives, so that the fundamental character of the new architecture seemed in some ways to be already as good as lost.

The fifties saw a new upsurge of activity, once more beneath the banners of rationalism and Constructivism. American influences were apparent in the work of Aarne *Ervi and Viljo *Revell. Revell's studio became a kind of headquarters of the rationalist school, from which many of the leading architects of today have emerged. The bright and simple Kudeneule factory at Hanko (1955) may be regarded as Revell's most typical design. He has become widely known as the leader of the team that won the Toronto City Hall competition. Although the fifties were so rationalistic, the trend that started in the thirties still continued. The heavy, vigorous shapes of Finnish architecture are very different from the precise purism of the *International Style; feeling for materials and adaptability to natural surroundings have remained constant. Even in such purist examples as the chapel at Otaniemi (1957) by Kaija and Heikki *Siren, it is for just these reasons that a warmth has been preserved which we generally call 'human'.

These properties are most pronounced in Alvar Aalto's buildings. Although at first he renounced free shapes, his designs preserve a plastic unity despite their

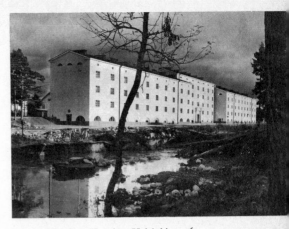

Gunnar Taucher. Housing. Helsinki, 1926

Jorma Järvi. High School. Helsinki, 1955. Assembly Hall

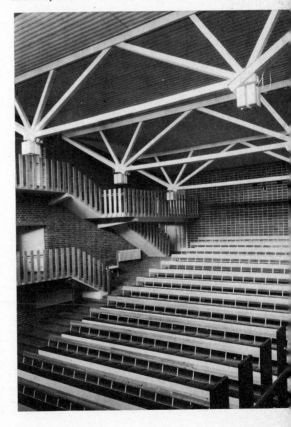

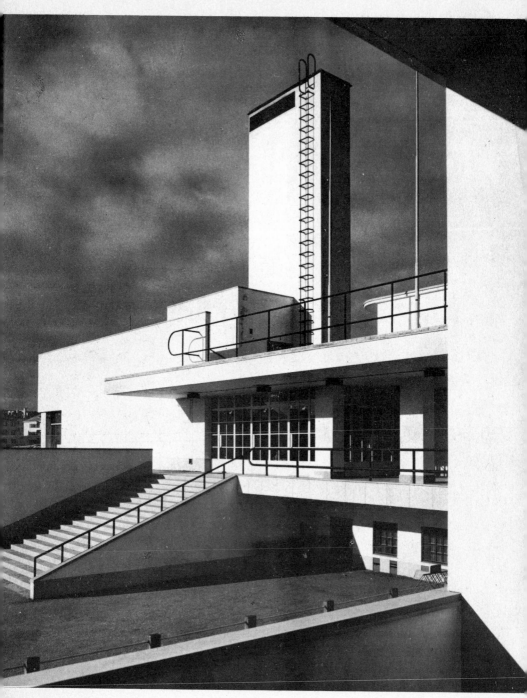

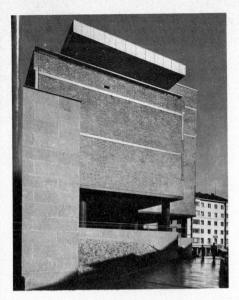

Alvar Aalto. Boarding School. Helsinki, 1952–6

Page 102. Yrjö Lindegren and Toivo Jäntti. Olympic Stadium. Helsinki, 1934–40 and 1952

Kaija and Heikki Siren. Chapel, Otaniemi Technical College, 1957

rectangularity (Town Hall at Säynätsalo, 1950–2; boarding school at Helsinki, 1952–6). Later he returned to free shapes and transferred them from the interiors to the way his buildings were massed (Cultural Institute at Helsinki, 1955–8; church at Vuoksenniska near Imatra, 1956–58). His palette as always is built up from natural materials and has become still richer. Apart from timber he now employs exposed brickwork, copper, ceramics and marble. Aalto has not founded a school of architects but his influence on Finnish architecture is none the less extraordinarily great, thanks to his ability to point out new directions and to serve as a criterion of architectural quality.

Lindegren (extensions to the Olympic Stadium at Helsinki, 1952; 'Snakehouse' residential district at Helsinki, 1951) and Aulis Blomstedt have also gone their own roads. The less numerous and more modest works of Blomstedt achieve their effect by their outstanding sureness of proportion to which he has devoted special research. New trends reached Finland, too, towards the end of the fifties. The free shapes of *shell vaulting have remained more or less at the design stage, however, and this situation is not yet resolved.

Bibliography: Nils Erik Wickberg, *Byggnadskonst i Finland*, Stockholm 1959;

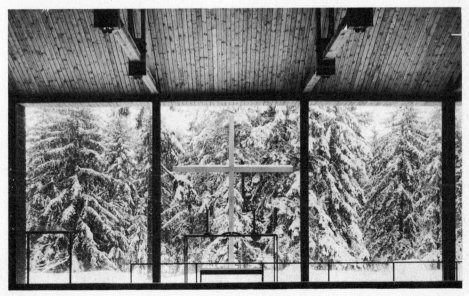

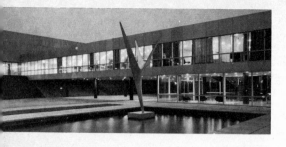

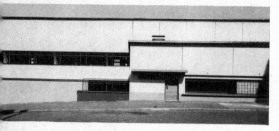

Viljo Revell. Kudeneule Textile Works. Hanko, 1955

Aulis Blomstedt. Extension to a Workers' Club. Helsinki, 1959

Hans J. Becker and Wolfram Schlote, *Neuer Wohnbau in Finnland*, Stuttgart 1958, Milan 1960.

KYÖSTI ÅLANDER

Fiocchi, Annibale, b. Milan 1915. Director of the architectural department of Olivetti's. Housing estates and factories in Ivrea (together with *Nizzoli, *Figini and *Pollini and Mario Oliveri), Palazzo Olivetti, Milan (with Gian Antonio Bernasconi and Nizzoli, 1954).

Fischer, Theodor, b. Schweinfurt 1862, d. Munich 1938. Collaborated with Paul Wallot on the Reichstag Building, Berlin. Taught and built in Stuttgart, Munich, and elsewhere. Evangelical Garrison Church at Ulm (1911), numerous offices, schools, museums.

Fisker, Kay, b. Copenhagen 1893. Studied at the Academy of Fine Arts, Copenhagen. The influence of international Functionalism is evident in Fisker's buildings, but he has not abandoned the tradition of Danish brick architecture. Considerable teaching activity. Architect of Århus University, together with Povl Stegmann and C. F.

Møller (work commenced 1931), school at Husum (1949–51), large housing estates.
Bibliography: Hans Erling Langkilde, *Arkitekten Kay Fisker*, Copenhagen 1960.

Floorscape. The use of patterns and textures in the ground as a design element, either contributing to overall visual appeal, suggesting lines of directivity to the pedestrian, or simply emphasizing space.
Bibliography: Elizabeth Beazley, *Design and detail of the space between buildings*, London 1960; Gordon Cullen, *Townscape*, London 1961.

France. The history of modern architecture in France is characterized by the tenacious resistance to new ideas put up by the reactionary forces and the continuance of a type of thought aiming at reform, which has been asserting itself equally stubbornly for a hundred years. From this polarity a fascinating historical picture emerges and, at the present time, a conflicting situation that can only be surveyed with difficulty. Academic resistance has centred round the Paris *École des Beaux-Arts, with practically all the means of a centralized, official apparatus at its disposal. The attitude of this court of official opinion was not only of importance to France; European and American reaction took its cue for decades from the example of the École des Beaux-Arts. Though the academicians succeeded in keeping commissions away from the younger generation and withholding from them the opportunity for experimentation, they could not prevent men in every generation who had espoused a revolutionary attitude from making their influence felt even far beyond the frontiers of their own country.
The conflict flared up when *Viollet-le-Duc, in his own feud against the Beaux-Arts, professed a doctrine relating form to material and function, which his investigations into Gothic architecture had suggested to him (*Dictionnaire de l'Architecture*, 1854 ff., *Entretiens sur l'Architecture*, 1863–72, American translation 1875–1881). This doctrine has influenced practically all pioneers of modern architecture, from *Richardson, via *Berlage and *Horta, to *Perret, *Le Corbusier and even F. Ll. *Wright. It met with most approval from the engineers, who saw in the return of architecture to structural form an ideal

which they themselves did not dare to proclaim publicly. Their colossal structures (Douro and Garabit bridges by *Eiffel, 1877–84; Eiffel Tower and *Contamin's Machinery Hall, 1889; Arnodin's Ponts Transbordeurs at Nantes and Marseilles, 1900–5) seemed to confirm the doctrine of the essential dependence of form on function, and the new formal and spatial concepts were indeed traced back to a strict adherence to this thesis. The prestige of such works has outlasted the change of generations. No wonder then that Choisy's still influential *Histoire de l'Architecture*, which was published towards the end of that golden age of construction in 1898, tackles the history of form in a purely engineering spirit.

The iron style had just reached its Baroque phase in Art Nouveau (*Guimard's Métro station entrances, 1900, Frantz Jourdain's Samaritaine department store, 1901) when a new generation tried taking the new material of reinforced concrete as the starting point for a new style, based on the same functional principles. A clear, strictly geometrical vocabulary of form, with classical overtones in the case of Perret, takes the place of the spatially complicated iron structures. Until the First World War the architectural use of reinforced concrete was restricted to a few examples (Perret, *Garnier). But these pioneers deserve the credit for having made the new material fit for architecture, while restoring validity again to the principle of truth to structure. The conflict with official architecture now assumed a sharper character than at the time of the iron engineers whose sphere of activities only overlapped with academicism at the edges.

Only after the war did the 'new style' emerge from a combination of architectural form with the new spatial concept that had crystallized between 1907 and 1914 in the graphic arts: Cubism. Since then Le Corbusier's genius towers over the horizon of French architecture. Around him and beside him, however, though seldom quite independent of him, new paths were explored. During the twenties the interchange of ideas with other centres of the movement —Germany and Holland—was particularly active. It was promoted by such journals as *L'Esprit Nouveau* (edited by Le Corbusier and Ozenfant, 1920–6), *Les Cahiers de l'Effort Moderne* (edited by Léonce

Rosenberg, 1925–7) and the *Architecture Vivante* series (edited by Badovici and Morancé from 1923); by exhibitions such as the International Exhibition of Applied Art, Paris, 1925, the unequalled exhibition of the Deutscher Werkbund (with the *Bauhaus as a focal point) in the Salon des Artistes Décorateurs, Paris, 1930, and the participation of French architects at the Werkbund Exhibition in Stuttgart, 1927, and at the International Building Exhibition, Berlin, 1930, etc. Adolf *Loos worked in Paris from 1923 till 1928 (Maison Tzara, 1926) and exerted a deep influence

Hector Guimard. Métro entrance. Paris, 1900

Henri Labrouste. Bibliothèque Ste Geneviève. Paris, 1843–50

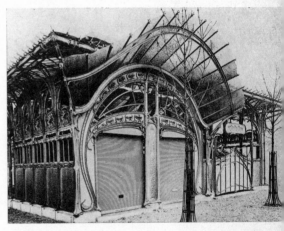

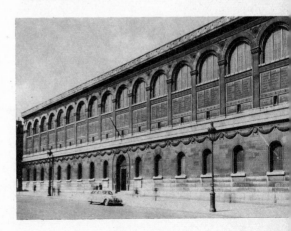

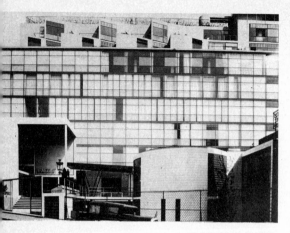

Le Corbusier. Salvation Army Hostel. Paris, 1931–2

on the younger architects. Le Corbusier and Jeanneret, André *Lurçat, Robert *Mallet-Stevens, Gabriel Guevrekian, Jean Badovici, Michel Roux-Spitz built houses and villas for avant-garde patrons, all typical examples of the *International Style; suffice it to mention the steel and glass house built by Pierre Chareau for Dr Dalsace, 1931.

The exponents of the new architecture, however, lacked the powerful support which their colleagues in Germany and Holland enjoyed in the form of major commissions from municipal authorities for the design of housing estates. It was only as late as 1930–5 that opportunities for other work arose on a limited scale. Thus besides a few blocks of flats (preceded twenty years earlier by those of Henri Sauvage in the Rue Vavin which had not received the attention they merited), the Hôtel Latitude 43 was built at St Tropez in 1933 by Pingusson and the school at Villejuif by Lurçat in 1931–3. The housing estates of Eugène *Beaudouin and Marcel *Lods at Drancy (the first point blocks) and Bagneux followed, with their open air school at Suresnes (1932–5) and the Maison du Peuple at Clichy (in collaboration with Jean *Prouvé). A development opened up that might have led to a kind of 'Scandinavian style' if stagnation on the property market, the hostility of the authorities and the deplorable success of the compromise-architecture at the Paris International Exhibition of 1937 had not barred the way.

The years following the Second World War created a completely new situation: a building boom, shifting the emphasis to State-backed housing schemes (annual target: 350,000 dwellings), with the problem extended to dimensions that required the creation of mixed teams of architects, engineers, and sociologists, and the emergence of town- and country-planning projects to a position of major importance. The unique opportunity of this first reconstruction period has been missed in France as thoroughly as elsewhere. Le Corbusier's advanced scheme for St Dié was not carried out; the aged Perret created a grandiose urban abstraction at Le Havre, but his pupils can breathe no life into it. Pison's research into contemporary farm buildings was not followed up. The remainder is mediocrity. It looks above all as if French architecture has succumbed to an empty inhuman geometry, from which it can at best only save itself by recourse to an inadequate, if technically brilliant, formalism in ostensibly purpose-free buildings (French Pavilion at Brussels, 1958).

Eugène Beaudouin and Marcel Lods. Cité de la Muette, Drancy near Paris, 1933

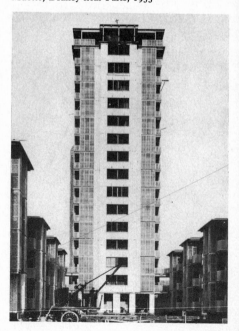

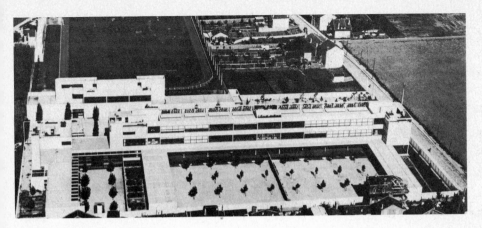

André Lurçat. School. Villejuif, 1931–3

A new generation, whose most outstanding representatives have been trained by Le Corbusier or who at least acknowledge allegiance to him has led to a marked change since about 1955. These younger men show a common tendency, which may be traced back to Le Corbusier, to consider all architectural problems in the light of a 'humanisme total', whether it is a matter of individual buildings or of town planning. In the manipulation of technical resources, apart from the influence of the masters of reinforced concrete such as *Freyssinet, André Coyne and Bernard Lafaille, the work of Jean Prouvé is exerting an increasingly more marked effect. His example makes up for the temptation offered to their followers by the monumentality of Le Corbusier's later works and the abstract transparency of Mies. Hence an original French style is beginning to establish itself, whose principal features can already be recognized in numerous buildings and projects. These include the new town of Bagnols-sur-Cèze and the planning for the Toulouse satellites at Le Mirail (*Candilis team), the blocks of flats at Croix and St Germain (Shape-Village), the Paris Museum of Folk Art (Dubuisson), the Vieille-Église housing estate at Croissy (Chemineau and Mirabaud), tall blocks of flats, shops and district heating plant at Bagneux (Gomis, Bodiansky, Gillet), residential and school buildings, the cathedral at Algiers (Herbé and Le Couteur), the Les Bureaux housing

estate at Sceaux and the Museum at Le Havre (Lagneau team), the experimental plastic house by Schein and Magnant, the studio house at St Rémy, the 'Mex' type adaptable prefabricated houses and the St Antoine University Clinic by A. Wogenscky, who was the architect in charge of building the Unités d'habitation when head of Le Corbusier's office.

Men of the older generation have also contributed to this renaissance, e.g. Lods with his large housing estate, Marly (with Honegger and Beuté), André Sive with several housing schemes, Beaudouin with the Cité Rotterdam at Strasbourg and the point blocks in Berlin (Hansa district) and Pantin (with Lopez), Emile Aillaud with industrial buildings in Lorraine and the ribbon and round tower housing estates at Aubervilliers and Bobigny, Pierre *Vago with the Basilica at Lourdes (with Freyssinet), and Ecochard with town planning and large-scale buildings in North Africa and the Near East. Mention should also be made of the office buildings by Lopez and Gravereaux (Rue Lapérouse and Rue Viala in Paris, with Prouvé) and by Edouard Albert at Paris and Orly, the Technical College (INSA) at Lyons (Jacques Perrin-Fayolle with Prouvé), the Faculty of Philosophy at Poitiers (Ursault), the medical faculty at Marseilles (Egger), the training workshops of the Electricité de France near Soissons (P. and P. Sirvin), Ginsberg's residential blocks in the west of Paris, and several shopping centres and

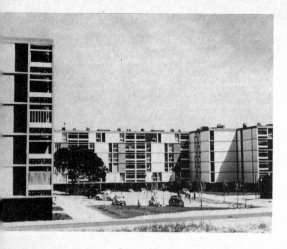

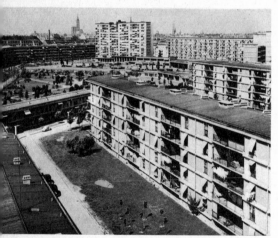

Georges Candilis, Bodiansky, Woods and Piot.
Bagnols-sur-Cèze. Commenced 1956

Eugène Beaudouin. Cité Rotterdam. Strasbourg,
1951–3

industrial and exhibition buildings. The
churches form a group of their own: Rueil
(Sonrel and Duthilleul), Neuilly (Coulon),
Mazamet (Belmont), Baccarat (Kazis),
Fontaine-lès-Grès (Marot), Pontarlier and
Villejuif (Rainer Senn), the Franciscan
Monastery at Orsay (Brothers Arsène-
Henry) and the Dominican Monastery at
Lille. The influence of the Dominican
journal *Art Sacré* played a decisive rôle
here.

Since 1925, Charlotte Perriand has been
in the forefront of the fight for functional
equipment in the home. The feud between
Formes Utiles (André Hermant) and
Esthétique Industrielle (Jacques Viénot) has
led to the solution of many minor problems
in the field of industrial design. The
Architecture Mobile Association is carrying
out basic research, the sculptor H. G.
Adam encourages his pupils to co-operate
with architects, and the Cercles d'Études
Architecturales have become a forum for
modern architecture and an important
centre for international exchange. This
revival of the spirit of experimentation on
which the best French tradition has always
been based can be furthered by the reform
of architectural education, which was at
last taken in hand in 1962 and which
should lead to the suppression of the
de facto monopoly of the Beaux-Arts.
Bibliography: S. Giedion, *Bauen in Frank-
reich, Eisen und Eisenbeton*, Leipzig 1929;
Marie Dormoy, *L'Architecture Française*,
Paris 1938; *25 Années UAM* (*Union des
Artistes Modernes*), Paris 1956; J. Schein,
Paris construit, Paris 1961.

MAURICE BESSET

Guillaume Gillet. Notre Dame de Royan, 1954–9

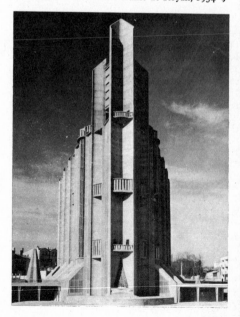

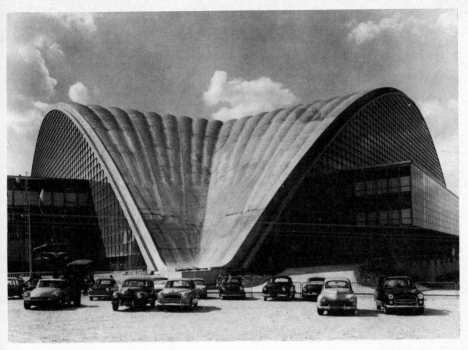

Camelot, De Mailly and Zehrfuss. Centre Nationale des Industries et Techniques. Paris, 1958

Freyssinet, Eugène, b. Objat, France 1879, d. 1962. Freyssinet was a pupil of the reinforced concrete pioneer Charles Rabut. In 1907, when just twenty-eight years old and employed as an engineer by a road-works authority in Central France, he built the bridges of Boutiron and Le Veurdre (destroyed 1940–4), which together with the contemporary early works of the Swiss *Maillart are considered among the boldest and most elegant creations of the early days of *reinforced concrete bridge building. A design for an arched bridge with a span of 607 feet (1913) was not executed due to the outbreak of war, but served as a basis for a number of later bridges by Freyssinet, right up to the Traneberg Bridge in Stockholm (1932, 597 foot span) and the bridges on the Caracas-to-La Guaira motorway (1950–5, average spans 476 feet). The St Pierre-du-Vauvray Bridge was built in 1922, its thin deck slab borne by a daring twin-arch 433 feet in span (destroyed 1940–44). Apart from the road and railway bridge over the Elorn estuary in Brittany, with three piers (1926–9, span 3 by 564 feet, partly destroyed 1944, since then rebuilt), Freyssinet's most popular works were the two airship hangars at Orly (1916–24, each 984 foot long and 205 foot high, destroyed 1944). These giant structures are important in the history of architecture not just because of their tremendous size and their technical innovations, but perhaps even more because of the matter-of-factness with which harmony of forms results from the choice of rational, albeit unusual, structural solutions despite unfamiliar dimensions. St Pierre-du-Vauvray and Orly are examples of pure functional beauty raised to the highest pitch of drama. Exceptionally bold intuitions of form were realized in them without their effect being weakened by any later 'cosmetic' alterations.

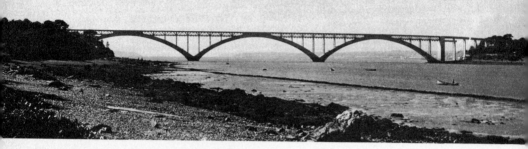

Eugène Freyssinet. Elorn Estuary Bridge. 1926–9

Apart from bridges, Freyssinet designed mainly industrial buildings, warehouses, etc., in his 'industrial period' (he was technical director of the Entreprises Limousin from 1913 to 1928). During this time he produced a series of now famous examples in the field of *shell and vaulted structures. Due to the difficulty of shuttering, the execution of curved shapes in reinforced concrete is troublesome and expensive. Freyssinet therefore attempted, on the one

Eugène Freyssinet. Airship hangar. Orly, 1916–24

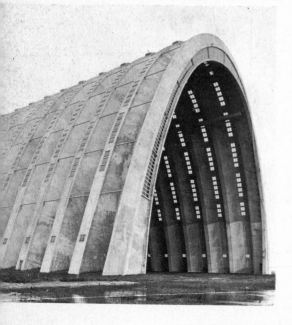

hand, to achieve extensive standardization of these shapes, and on the other hand to improve the static behaviour of reinforced concrete by means other than stiffening deformations. He had the idea of subjecting the reinforcement to tensile stresses. These tensile stresses were intended to compensate for the compressive stresses which are engendered in the finished building by the self-weight of the concrete and the additional live loads. This led to the invention of pre-stressing, as it is now called, in experiments which go back to 1926 (his 'scientific period'). Freyssinet used it from 1933 onwards for the most varying tasks in multi-storey and underground structures (dam building in North Africa and harbour construction at Brest, 1937–9, and in particular Le Havre, 1946–52, runways at Orly, 1946–7, bridges and water tanks of up to 9,000 cubic yards capacity).

The shapes resulting from pre-stressed concrete are considerably flatter, slenderer and more highly stressed than those of normal reinforced concrete. The Marne bridges Freyssinet rebuilt with an average span of 230 feet thus have a stress ratio of 1:45. The strength of the units, which are prefabricated on the bank and assembled like steel beams, depends on the centre-piece of the bridge which is 2 feet thick. This type of construction, which was tried out on bridges, could be taken over for the underground Basilica of Pius X at Lourdes, where a maximum clear width had to be achieved for a minimum overall height. Here, as at Orly, repetition of a single technical shape worked out to the last detail, resulted in a monumental effect of

a truly architectural nature. As in certain designs by Pier Luigi *Nervi, pure structure becomes most impressive architecture.
Bibliography: Maurice Besset, *Eugène Freyssinet*, in *Les Architectes Célèbres*, Vol 2, Paris 1959.

MAURICE BESSET

Fry, Edwin Maxwell, b. 1899. Studied at Liverpool School of Architecture. Partnership with Walter *Gropius, 1934–6; with Jane *Drew, 1945–50. From 1951 to 1958 practised as Fry, Drew, Drake and Lasdun; since 1958, Fry, Drew, Drew and Partners. A pioneer of modern architecture in *Great Britain; his Kensal House housing scheme at Ladbroke Grove, London (1936, in collaboration) was the nearest British prewar approach to a continental *Siedlung*. Schools, hospitals, housing, offices; educational buildings in West Africa, where he worked as a town planner from 1943 to 1945. Senior Architect at Chandigarh, 1951–4, in collaboration with *Le Corbusier.

Fuller, Richard Buckminster, b. Milton, Massachusetts 1895. Not an architect in the usual sense of the word, but instead a unique reflection of those 20th-century concepts related to the machine aesthetic, Fuller has received recognition from the architectural profession for his unique gifts only in the last few years. His formal education was sketchy and did not progress much beyond two years at Harvard, 1913–15. After service as a naval officer during the First World War and after occupying a number of positions in business and industry, he perfected a kind of machine for living in which he called the 'Dymaxion (dynamic plus maximum efficiency) House' in 1927. In contrast to the poetic expressions of the machine age which were so frequently manifested in the buildings of the 1920s in Europe, and especially in Le *Corbusier's lyrical Villa Savoye, 1929, Fuller's product was a machine for living in in a literal rather than in a metaphorical sense. Unlike the contemporary masterpieces of European Purism and related movements, Fuller's Dymaxion House was not in any consequential way an object for aesthetic contemplation, but is more correctly viewed as an assemblage of mechanical services in conjunction with living areas. In 1932–5 Fuller developed a motorized version of this idea in his 'Dymaxion Three Wheeled Auto'.

Since then Fuller has devoted much time and effort to the art of structures, and these studies have led to the perfection of his Geodesic Domes, structures of metal, plastic, or even of cardboard based upon octahedrons or tetrahedrons. He came to use the domical shape not for a traditional, architectural reason—not, for instance, because it was an 'ideal' form—but because of its natural efficiency in providing the greatest space enclosed in relation to the surface area of the enclosing form. In their use of standardized parts, these Geodesic Domes are, in a sense, the most recent descendants of the assembly techniques that were first employed by Sir Joseph *Paxton in the Crystal Palace, London, 1851. The largest of these domes that has been erected was the repair shop for the Union Tank Car Co., Baton Rouge, La., 1958, with a diameter of 384 feet, a span that exceeds those of the mammoth 19th-century exhibition halls, such as the Machinery Hall at the World Exhibition, Paris, 1889 (362 feet). More recently Fuller has produced a new system known as

Richard Buckminster Fuller. Dymaxion House, 1927. Model

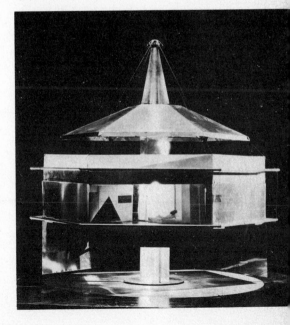

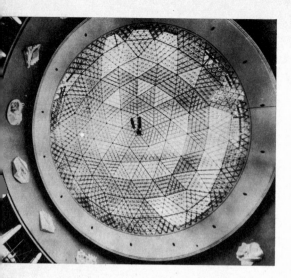

Richard Buckminster Fuller. Ford Motor
Company. Dearborn, Mich., 1953. Dome

Tenegrity Structures (a contraction of
Tensional Integrity), examples of which
were exhibited at the Museum of Modern
Art, New York, in 1960.
Understandably more popular with students
than with the established elements in the
architectural profession, Fuller has enjoyed
notable success as a visiting lecturer in
various architectural schools in the USA,
among them being Cornell, Massachusetts
Institute of Technology, University of
California, University of Pennsylvania,
Princeton University, University of Michigan and Yale University. In 1952 Fuller
received the Award of Merit of the New
York Chapter of the AIA, and in 1959 the
national organization of the same body
recognized his work with the award of an
honorary membership.
Bibliography: Robert W. Marks, *The
Dymaxion World of Buckminster Fuller*,
New York 1960.

JOHN M. JACOBUS, JR

Functionalism. 'Form follows function'
is the catchphrase that spells modern
architecture to most laymen. In the 1920s
it seemed like a strange idea, cold and
forbidding; today, although widely accepted
(and even more widely misunderstood),
'form follows function' continues to evoke
the image of modern as opposed to traditional architecture more readily than any
other slogan. Yet there is no architectural
principle that can claim a more ancient and
distinguished tradition. Form has followed
function from the paleolithic cave-dwellers
to the neolithic lake-dwellers; it followed
function in Roman forts and aqueducts, in
medieval castles and the Great Wall of
China, in 18th-century English warehouses, and in 20th-century Manhattan
office piles. Functionalism, in short, is as
old as building itself.
Critics of functionalism sometimes suggest that functionalism stops where architecture begins. This is unfair both to
functionalism and to architecture. The
functionalist period in the development of
a new architecture is much like the formative childhood period in the life of a man.
As he matures, he may reject many of the
fads and prejudices of his teen-age; none
the less, the basis of his personality was
laid during those earlier years.
The personality of modern architecture
had its genesis in the 1850s, the formative
years of present-day Functionalism. Both
the followers of *Le Corbusier and of
Frank Lloyd *Wright—now apparently
poles apart—derived much of their early
inspiration from the 19th-century doc-
trines of Eugène *Viollet-le-Duc, the
French architect and theoretician, who is
best known for his restorations of medieval
castles. Less well known, but more important, are his attempts to rationalize (or
'functionalize') the art of architecture into
a logical system with simple rules. Le
Corbusier's writings of the early twenties
—for example, his *Vers une architecture*—
read like Viollet-le-Duc brought up to date;
and Wright told his architect-son to read
Viollet-le-Duc, because his writings would
give him all the basic education he needed.
The first rule of Functionalism grew
directly out of the credo that form must
reflect function—or 'express' function, as
architects like to say. This was paraphrased
to mean that all the different elements in a
building should be separately 'expressed':
for example, the structural columns and
beams should be made clearly visible,
inside and out, and separated from non-
structural wall panels and partitions, so
that the structural frame would clearly
'express' its function of holding up the
floors and the roof.

The second rule of Functionalism came about in a more roundabout way. Because the early Functionalists got much of their inspiration from the machine itself, machine forms became greatly admired. The fact that such forms did not always make much sense in buildings did not matter; after all, Louis *Sullivan used plant forms for terra-cotta ornament because natural organisms were something that *he* admired—so why should not machine forms like cylinders, cones, cubes, and other geometric shapes be used by the admirers of machine organisms? None of this need have come as a surprise. As early as 1920, Le Corbusier had written jubilantly: 'Thus we have the American grain elevators and factories . . . the American engineers overwhelm with their calculations our expiring architecture.' However, Le Corbusier was not quite so overwhelmed as he may have seemed. For while he was praising functional buildings put up by practical men, he also announced, in the same breath, that 'architecture is the masterly, correct, and magnificent play of masses brought together in light . . . cubes, cones, spheres, cylinders, or pyramids are the great primary forms which light reveals to advantage . . . these are *beautiful forms, the most beautiful forms* [his italics]'. In other words: Functionalism is wonderful—as long as it produces beautiful forms.

But while these sophisticated Functionalists were busy in the 1920s and 1930s developing a style out of the raw material of engineering, there grew up, on the side-lines, another kind of functionalist. He was the builder, the businessman, the engineer, who really believed all that he had read in the papers about cheaper, more practical, more form-fitting architecture. If 'form follows function', he argued, does not efficient function automatically produce beautiful form? Well, it seemed to—in some instances at least: How about aeroplanes? How about some bridges, ships, tools, factories, dams? And if you can produce beauty by some kind of automatic function-computer, why bother with all the talk about art? The output of these literal functionalists is all around us today, for everyone to see. Every big American city is studded with office and apartment buildings designed—if that is the word—by some sort of automatic 'functional' process: the exterior shape is determined by zoning laws; the exterior surface is papered with *curtain wall patterns picked out of a manufacturer's catalogue; the interior layout is determined by rental experts, the core by the stop-watches of elevator specialists; the roof is designed by the cooling tower fabricators; and the lobby by the newspaper distributors. Result: chaos—in the name of 'functionalism'.

Unfortunately, the 'sophisticated Functionalists' have only themselves to blame. They laid the trap when they began to apologize for the new style by claiming it was less expensive to build and less expensive to maintain. Few, if any, ever came out and said publicly that Functionalism was a coherent system of organization, a completely integrated method of putting a building together, and that it should be judged entirely on its own merits.

The present confusion over Functionalism has not been caused entirely by the innocent or the opportunistic. Functionalism needs to re-examine its own premises to see how many of them still make sense. Is it really justifiable to adhere so rigidly to a machine aesthetic? Does it really make sense to articulate and to express all things —to separate a building's elements only to have to link them together again afterwards? 'Expressing structure' is fine in many kinds of buildings; in many others, however, expressing the structure may turn out to be a big headache. And when you come to expressing mechanical equipment—elevators, or cooling towers—then the question arises, why not express the plumbing, the wiring, and the heating, too? Moreover, as the need increases for flexible space uses (in schools, offices, factories, almost any type of building), the urge to articulate each plan element must be suppressed; for, after all, the plan requirements may change overnight.

Functionalism, however, though in transition, is far from dead. It remains a rigorous and demanding discipline, an excellent textbook for young architects, a fine standard by which to judge many a building put up today.

Bibliography: E. R. de Zurko, *Origins of Functionalist Theory*, New York 1957.

PETER BLAKE

Furness, Frank, b. Philadelphia 1839, d. 1912. In buildings such as the Provident Life and Trust Bank (Philadelphia, 1872)

Furness employed neo-Gothic features to create an architecture of powerful gravity and impressively integrated massing. His decoration is entirely original and employs free geometric or organic shapes derived from nature. Louis *Sullivan worked in his office for a time.

Futurism. The Futurist movement, which began in 1909, ignored architecture until 1914. In that year two young architects, Antonio *Sant'Elia and Mario *Chiattone, presented a revolutionary picture in Milan of the *Città Nuova*, the city of the future, in a series of designs and projects. In the catalogue of the exhibition a powerful harangue by Sant'Elia was published, which pleads the historical and human necessity for a radical renewal of Italian architecture, that had fallen into an academic eclecticism lacking any vital spark. The author was clearly familiar with the writings of Boccioni and Marinetti, although he had not joined the Futurist movement himself, and his proposals to 'harmonize the environment with man', in the light of the extraordinary and decisive developments of science and technology, frequently chime in with the views expressed in Futurist manifestoes on the other arts.

Marinetti, discovering the Futurist elements in Sant'Elia's thought, determined to integrate the movement's programme

Mario Chiattone. Block of flats. 1914. Project

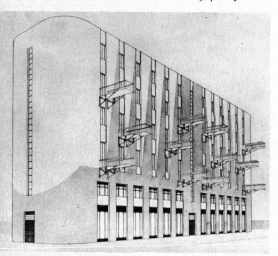

with this fascinating and open-minded piece of writing on architecture. He persuaded Sant'Elia to join the group, introduced some modifications to his text (which made no mention of Futurism in the original version) and published it again in July of the same year, 1914, under the title of *Manifesto dell'Architettura Futurista*. The manifesto proclaimed that 'everything must be revolutionized. Architecture is breaking loose from tradition. It is forcibly starting from scratch again', and a 'preference for what is light, practical, ephemeral and swift' was praised as being Futurist, in accordance with Boccioni's aesthetic theories on 'plastic dynamism'.

This manifesto was the most important objective that Futurism achieved in the field of architecture. It has become famous and has acquired great historical value because in its way it helped to bring *Italy into the mainstream of modern developments in European architecture. In actual fact, it was only a matter of words: no important Futurist work was ever built in Italy. The finest thing that has come down to us from this period of lively controversy is simply the series of splendid drawings by Sant'Elia himself, which portray, in part at least, the architecture of Futurism. To these may be added the designs of Chiattone, most of them unpublished until 1962, and based furthermore on a static system that foreshadows the aesthetics of the *Novecento Italiano*, far removed from the 'plastic dynamism' that is at the basis of Futurism.

Fourteen years had to pass before Futurist architecture was thought of again. In 1928 one of the keenest and most convinced supporters of the idea of Futurism in architecture, the painter and journalist Fillía, organized the 'First Exhibition of Futurist Architecture' (it was also to be the only one) 'under the high patronage of His Excellency Mussolini'. The artists who took part were of various origins and tendencies: Antonio Sant'Elia, Mario Chiattone, Alberto Sartoris and Virgilio Marchi (architecture); Ivo Pannaggi, Giacomo Balla and Fillía (interior decoration); Enrico Prampolini, Fillía and Nicola Diulgheroff (stage designs); Fortunato Depero, Diulgheroff and Prampolini (exhibition architecture); and various other artists with posters and objects of daily use. Most of the schemes illustrated were only

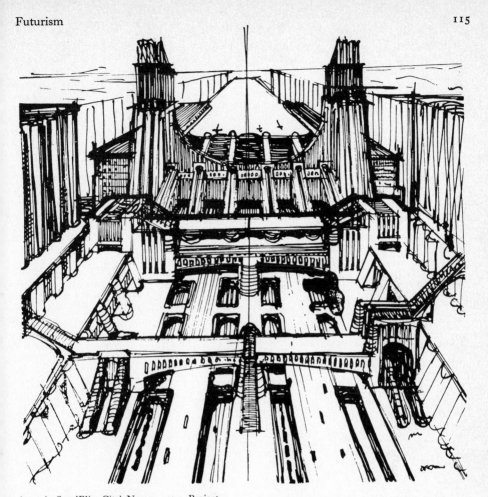

Antonio Sant'Elia. Città Nuova. 1914. Project

projects. The sole works of architecture, apart from exhibition designs, built up to then (by Sartoris) were tied in with the European rationalist movements and ignored 'plastic dynamism'. But Fillía continued to believe in the possibility of Futurist architecture developing as Fascist architecture, and to promote and spread this idea he founded and edited a number of journals (*La città futurista*, *La città nuova*) and wrote articles and books (*Arte Fascista*, 1928; *La nuova architettura*, 1931).

Of works that were actually built a few 'Futurist villas' may be mentioned (at Turin and Albisola), and some exhibition pavilions (by Depero at Monza, 1924; by Fillía at Turin and Florence, 1928). Stage designs were carried out by Enrico Prampolini, Virgilio Marchi and Anton Giulio Bragaglia, amongst others, for the Teatro degli Indipendenti in Rome, which was run by Bragaglia.

The work in which Futurism, with all its poetry, culminated was the 'Exhibition of the Fascist Revolution' held in Rome in 1932. Organized by architects, painters and designers who were mostly drawn from the ranks of Futurism, it was the only manifestation of Fascist art that achieved any historic *rapport* with the rest of Europe, by displaying a kind of *Constructivism which could be compared with that of Russia. While the Futurist requirements of plastic dynamism, simultaneity and speed ('empty words in architecture' Mario Chiattone wrote) were being met by stage design techniques at the Exhibition, the principles of the *Novecento Italiano* were winning acceptance in architecture: 'plastic values' taken from national tradition, and accepted by Fascism as those truly expressive of the times. Sant'Elia had died twenty years before, shortly after *Gropius's Fagus factory was built. Now Marinetti, the leader of Futurism, was appointed by Mussolini to the Accademia d'Italia.

Bibliography: Virgilio Marchi, *Architettura futurista*, Foligno 1924; F. T. Marinetti, Enrico Prampolini and Escodame, *Sant' Elia e l'architettura futurista mondiale*, Milan 1931; Alberto Sartoris, *Sant'Elia e l'architettura futurista*, Rome 1944; Fillía, *La Nuova Architettura*, Turin 1931; Reyner Banham, 'Futurism and Modern Architecture' in *RIBA Journal*, February 1957; Rafael Benet, *Futurismo y Dada*, Barcelona 1949; Drudi Gambillo and Teresa Fiori, *Archivi del Futurismo*, Rome 1958; Reyner Banham, *Theory and Design in the First Machine Age*, London 1959.

GIULIA VERONESI

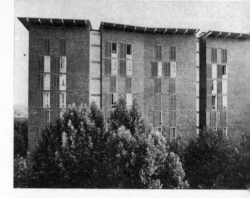

Ignazio Gardella. Block of flats for employees. Alessandria, 1952

Gardella, Ignazio, b. Milan 1905, first winner of the Olivetti National Prize for architecture, is a lecturer at the University Institute of Architecture, Venice. In the current architectural scene in Italy, Gardella is a figure of particular importance. In contrast to the other architects of his generation, he has not had recourse to any social or aesthetic ideologies for the genuine rationalism he has displayed from his first works. This attitude, nevertheless,

Ignazio Gardella. Mensa Olivetti. Ivrea, 1959

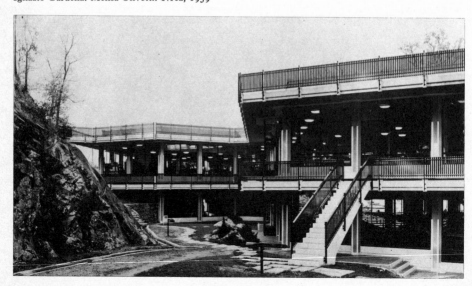

has permitted him to work quite naturally by the side of the most committed of his colleagues. He has collaborated with them fruitfully at the various Triennali, in architectural and town planning competitions and in projects of all kinds. His work is characterized by its elegance and purity of composition, in a lyric vein which he has used to provide magisterially free and simple solutions to the most complex problems.

He began his career with interior decoration and rebuilding schemes. The most noteworthy among the latter are: the renovation of the theatre at Busto Arsizio in 1934, and an extension of the Villa Borletti in Milan (1935), which first brought him to notice. In the following year came his finest work to that date, and one that remains 'an outstanding example of Italian rationalism' (Mazzariol): the Anti-tuberculosis Dispensary at Alessandria (1936–8), in which the most interesting lines of Gardella's architecture are defined: clarity in the handling of plane surfaces and a judicious use of materials as essential instruments of expression. In this connection, the extensive employment of brick to face a reinforced concrete building shows Gardella's tendency to respect local traditions, at least as far as the use of colour goes.

The splendid Dispensary (soon to become dilapidated through neglect on the part of the city authorities) was the first and most significant of Gardella's architectural activities in Alessandria, where he has left a distinctive imprint, building the major part of his own most important works there: the Provincial Laboratory for Hygiene and Prophylaxis (1937–9); a block of flats for employees (1952), in which he tried, by an interesting play of movement on the elevation and the use of deeply projecting eaves, to go beyond a purely 'rationalist' scheme; a building for the Borletti works, in 1951; the Children's Hospital, in 1955; and finally, a Vocational School, currently under construction. During the same period Gardella was building elsewhere too. In 1946, in a block of flats he designed at Castana, particular emphasis was laid on an attempt to reinterpret regional and traditional elements in a modern key. This characteristic has led Gardella little by little a long way from his initial standpoint; his architecture, diverging as it does some-

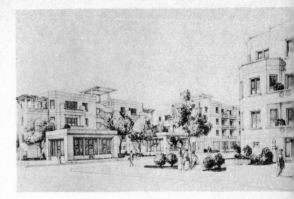

Tony Garnier. Residential district. Cité Industrielle. 1901–4. Project

times from strict rationalism has sparked off a good deal of controversy, though no one disputes his taste or technical skill.

He has built blocks of flats and villas, and a group of terraced houses (1952) in the new suburb of Cesate Milanese, where he also plans to erect a brick-built church with historic overtones and a layout of subtle geometric invention in the contemporary spirit. He returns again to the poetic 'rationalist' manner, albeit exceptionally, with the white annexe he designed for the Museum of Modern Art in Milan (1953). Thereafter he often subordinates the free workings of his own imagination to the promptings of the environment in his schemes, which include a house on the Grand Canal in Venice, and a villa on the Riviera, His most significant design currently under construction, apart from the Vocational School at Alessandria, is the Olivetti Studies Centre at Ivrea.

Gardella was a member of the executive committee of the 1959 Milan Triennale.

Bibliography: G. C. Argan, *Gardella*, Milan 1959; Giuseppe Mazzariol, 'Umanesimo di Gardella' in *Zodiac 2*, Milan 1957.

GIULIA VERONESI

Garnier, Tony, b. Lyons 1869, d. La Bédoule 1948. Tony Garnier is a unique case. His first job, the project for an industrial town designed in 1901–4, when he was a Rome Scholar of barely thirty, contains not only a wealth of fertile, revolutionary ideas but so many concrete suggestions as well for the most diverse architectural

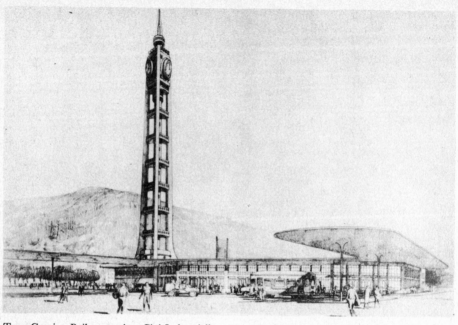

Tony Garnier. Railway station. Cité Industrielle. 1901–4. Project

problems of the modern town that as a mature master later on he had only to dip into it to cope with his manifold commissions: in particular the 'Grands Travaux de la Ville de Lyon', the abattoir of La Mouche (1909–13), the Olympic Stadium (1913–16), the Grange Blanche Hospital (1915–30), the War Memorial (1924), the telephone exchange (1927) and the residential district known as 'Les États Unis' (1928–35). Even the still much-copied town hall of Boulogne-Billancourt (1931–4, in collaboration with Debat-Ponsan) can be traced back to the 'Cité Industrielle'. But this does not mean that the untiring, ever-searching Garnier even considered resting on his early-won laurels.

Even the idea that lies at the basis of Garnier's 'Cité Industrielle' is revolutionary in its novelty. The town planning of his time had not progressed beyond Camillo Sitte's *Stadtbaukunst* (1889) and the English garden city, both of which only cope with certain aspects of the problem. Thanks to his Socialist leanings, Garnier conceived a town organism which—without churches and barracks!—fully serves the human needs of an industrial age. His

choice of material which determines the shape of the individual buildings is no less bold; only a few experimental buildings were erected in reinforced concrete in 1901. In addition, Garnier invented the shapes best suited to reinforced concrete, which have become standard features in modern architecture: continuous strips of glazing, glass walls, *pilotis*, and flat roofs. The 'free plan' derives from his cantilevered structures, which (with the exception of *Perret, 1903) he was the first in Europe to achieve. In addition, there are surprising technical innovations such as electric heating, thermostats, service cores, and a novel system of ducting worked out to the last detail. The shapes are of a baffling modernity. Their ascetic geometry recalls the harmonious cuboid houses of Adolf *Loos (e.g. Garnier's own house at St Rambert, 1911). No less advanced are the designs of the buildings and the general disposition of the town: a residential district without enclosed courtyards but featuring continuous green areas and traffic-free pedestrian precincts; single-storey schools in open layouts; hospitals planned in separate blocks; numerous sports stadia;

a community centre that anticipates contemporary social centres; separation of vehicular and pedestrian traffic; clear distinction between the different functions of a town (living, work, leisure, education, traffic), in a way that has only been theoretically planned by *CIAM since 1928. All the fundamental ideas of modern architecture and town planning have not just been hinted at in Garnier's project but are carefully thought out in detail. Only the outbreak of the First World War prevented their actual realization at Lyons from 1915 to 1920.

Garnier's name was little known outside Lyons up to the time of his death. His influence, however, extended far beyond the circle of faithful pupils who had gathered round him. Long before the publication of *Une Cité Industrielle* and its later shortened version, Garnier's ideas were known in progressive architectural circles; they played a considerable part in *Le Corbusier's ideas on town planning. Only after his death was Garnier's importance fully recognized as one of the key figures of the start of the century.

Bibliography: Tony Garnier, *Une Cité Industrielle*, Paris 1917; Tony Garnier, *Les Grands Travaux de la Ville de Lyon*, Paris 1919; Jean Badovici and Albert Morancé, *L'œuvre de Tony Garnier*, Paris 1938; Giulia Veronesi, *Tony Garnier*, Milan 1948.

MAURICE BESSET

Gaudí, Antoni, b. Reus, Catalonia 1852, d. Barcelona 1926. Gaudí, who came from a family of coppersmiths, began his architectural studies in Barcelona at the age of seventeen and graduated in 1878. At school his radical nonconformity often earned him bad marks in his examinations. He felt little attraction for the official courses, whereas, during his years as a student, he was an assiduous frequenter of the philosophy classes of Llorens y Barba and the lectures on aesthetics by Pau Milà y Fontanals. In his youth Milà y Fontanals had lived in Rome during its romantic period, where he had moved in the circle of the Nazarenes, Overbeck and his fraternity. As a consequence he had developed in a direction parallel to the English Pre-Raphaelites, with a passionate attachment to the Middle Ages, symbols, mystery and a certain esotericism. In Catalonia this kind of mentality had been brought about by the nationalist movement, some seeing in a return to the Middle Ages a return to Catalonia's Golden Age, others displaying a primitivist reaction which sought the fount of life in the realm of folk-lore and in communion with the nature of one's native land.

Gaudí's ideas were decisively influenced by this school of thought, which led him to a veneration for craftwork and the honesty of medieval art; to a mechanistic logic inspired by *Viollet-le Duc's conception of medieval architecture; and to nature as a source of inspiration, not only for decorative details but for structures as well. While he was a student, he worked as an assistant to Villar and Fontseré on the

Antoni Gaudí. Palau Güell. Barcelona, 1885–9

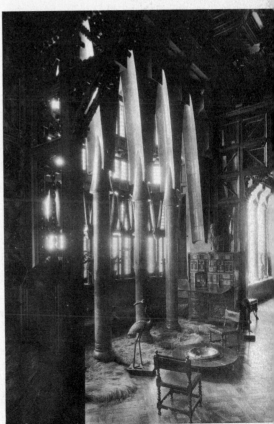

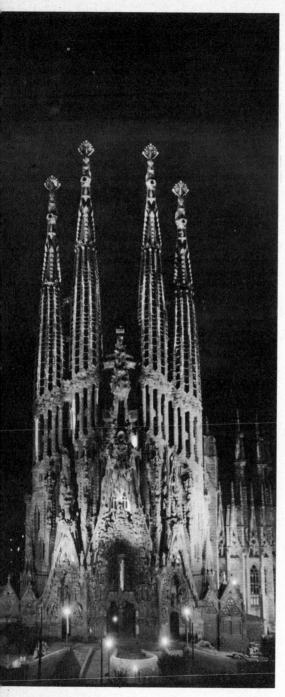

church at Montserrat and on the waterfall in the Ciutadella Park in Barcelona. His contribution consisted of decorative details derived from a stylization of themes from nature in the Japanese manner and from the use of ironwork features with strongly accentuated joints. His workshop experience marked him off from those architects who were merely academic draughtsmen and helped him to grasp three-dimensionally the way things are made, with tangible material.

In 1878, shortly after graduating, he designed the Casa Vicens, in the Carrer de les Carolines at Barcelona, a building suggestive of Islamic prototypes with its stepped prismatic blocks, its alternations of stone and brick, and its brilliant decoration in polychrome tiles. Constructed as it was at a period when revivalism was in full flood, it had the merit of belonging to no known style. This recourse to Islamic details was one of the levers Gaudí used, in conjunction with neomedievalism, to throw off the weight of academic prejudices and try to arrive at his own means of expression, which was characterized by a feeling for the modulation of indirect light in interiors, and something that was to be as much part and parcel of his architecture as it was to be opposed to the colourless art of the academics: his polychrome use of ceramics, mosaics, glazing and painting. Although naturalism was limited at the Casa Vicens to palm leaves featured in the wrought-iron work and the decorative ceramics which displayed ivy and raspberry tendrils, Gaudí took a step further with the street lamps he designed for the Plaça Reial in Barcelona, where he imitated forms derived from the growth of plants. The same period marks the beginning of his interest in structural problems, with the parabolic arches he employed in warehouses built for the Mataró Workers' Cooperative (1878–82), and in social questions with his schemes for workers' housing drawn up for the same co-operative.

In 1883, Gaudí was commissioned to continue the work on the Church of the Sagrada Familia, a building of great size that was progressively to monopolize his activities. A neo-Gothic design by Villar was already in existence, which Gaudí

Antoni Gaudí. Church of the Sagrada Familia. Barcelona, 1883–1926

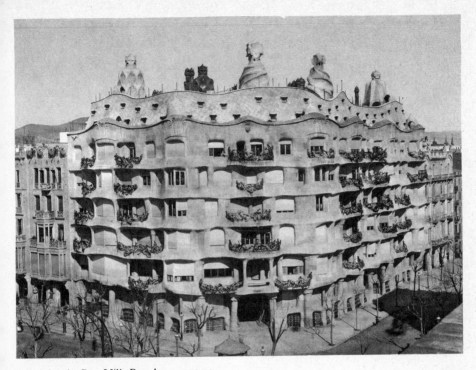

Antoni Gaudí. Casa Milà. Barcelona, 1905–10

abandoned, but the lines of the apse, the first part he built, still contain many Gothic reminiscences, although the mouldings and decorative details are drawn much more closely from nature. It is to this period that the Palau Güell belongs in the Carrer Nou de la Rambla, Barcelona, now the calle Conde del Asalto (1885–9), where Gaudí's structural experiments—the use of parabolic arches is the most evident one —create a personal style, adapted to the exclusive use of stone, timber and wrought-iron. This palace, and his designs for a large building for Catholic missions in Tangiers, with towers that recall the parabolic cupolas of villages in the Chad, formed the basis of his complete liberation from the historic styles, and his approach to a 'biological' style.

Work on the Sagrada Familia continued with the Nativity façade of the east transept. This consists of three open portals between four interpenetrating square-based towers, set diagonally, which rise to

a height of 351 feet and terminate in thin, curved, circular features crowned by a piece of capricious play with intersecting surfaces, covered in mosaic. A complex and lively world, modelled for the most part by Gaudí himself and comprising an immense variety of plants and animals, throngs the great concavities below the gables, which are covered in imitation snow carved out of stone and carry a series of sculptures depicting the childhood of Christ. While in his previous works naturalism was used purely decoratively, in this instance the sculptures of living forms, connected up by a series of continuous curved surfaces, make up a form of cladding that covers the structure completely and models it independently.

Henceforth, as in the Casa Batlló in the Paseo de Gracia, Barcelona (1905–7), natural and organic forms no longer simply comprise a kind of ornament superimposed on the building but go on to constitute essential structural elements, as in the case of the bone-shaped columns, the undulating façade covered with polychrome mosaics like a sheet of sea-water set on end, and the imbricated roof like an armadillo's back. This type of effect is a transitional one between the sculptural plasticity of Gaudí's earlier years (1878–91), and the structural plasticity of his later period.

This structural plasticity has as one of its chief features the system of design Gaudí used for the Colonia Güell Church (1898–1914), which was planned by means of a string model representing the structural ribs of the building, from which were hung weights proportional to the loads which each member would have to carry. The polygons formed by these strings gave the inverted shape of the building's columns. It permitted a type of vaulted structure without buttresses of any kind, since all thrusts are taken up by suitably inclined pillars. This method was later used in designing the naves of the Sagrada Familia.

In the Güell Park (1900–14) Gaudí made systematic use of inclined supports of unwrought stone for retaining walls and bridges, where he raised great masses of stone on flimsy columns in a tense desire to flaunt gravity. An important feature in this park is the abundant employment of ceramic and glass mosaic, which presents an extraordinary ensemble of powerfully expressive abstract compositions, in which Gaudí makes frequent use of broken plates, china dolls, bottles, etc., in a fabulous fantasia, like the elements of a collage.

The Casa Milà (1905–10), called la Pedrera (the quarry) is perhaps Gaudí's most original work. An interesting structural feature is the way the entire weight is carried between the external elevations and the columns which surround the patios. The handling of the internal space is also noteworthy, with its numerous acute and obtuse angles and undulating walls. Plastically speaking it constitutes a great stone sculpture of organic shape, with a rhythm of undulating horizontal edges, comparable to eyebrows or lips, pierced by windows, which preserve the expression of human eyes or mouths, somewhat in the manner of sculptures by Henry Moore or Barbara Hepworth. Gaudí's structural masterpiece was reached in 1909 with his Sagrada Familia schools, walled and roofed by undulating membranes of thin brick.

Towards the end of his career, Gaudí asserted that the straight line belonged to men, the curved one to God. Shortly before his death he invented a system of well-nigh universal application, based on hyperboloids and paraboloids, though his designs were never purely geometrical. They always preserved a close tie with familiar living shapes: bones, muscles, wings and petals, and at other times with caves and even stars and clouds.

Terrifying and idyllic features may be encountered side by side in Gaudí's work, in a way that closely recalls Surrealism. This impression is accentuated by the fortuitous objects in his collages, and gives Gaudí's architecture, despite his profoundly rational approach to structure, a character that is impassioned, savage and poetical to the point of frenzy.

Bibliography: Alexandre Cirici-Pellicer, El arte modernista catalán, Barcelona 1951; J. F. Ràfols, Gaudi 1852–1926, 3rd edition, Barcelona 1952; Joan Bergós, Antoni Gaudí, L'home i l'obra, Barcelona 1954; George R. Collins, Antonio Gaudí, New York 1960; James Johnson Sweeney and Joseph Lluis Sert, Antoni Gaudí, London 1960.

ALEXANDRE CIRICI-PELLICER

Germany. In 1828 the architect Heinrich Hübsch published a brochure with the title In which style should we build? In it he put forward the thesis that it was impossible to create new and beautiful forms in architecture. But the combination of these forms, and the 'arrangement of the parts . . . could reveal much that was individual'. These words sum up the malaise of the 19th century. The romantic period in German architecture after Friedrich Gilly had omitted to develop an exclusive manner in which the whole was subjected to a common rule like its parts. In practice, of course, the combination of adopted antique or Gothic features led to a new kind of style. The German romantic period was already familiar with unlimited repetitions of particular forms, the renunciation of dominating axes, flowing plan forms and the alternating interpenetration of space and buildings, and it already took account of the optical displacements and intersections that ensue when the spectator moves about. It is not by chance that the early *Mies van der Rohe was influenced by the country house projects of *Schinkel.

In the face of the tasks confronting the 19th-century architect this anticipation of the principles of modern architecture seems to lack binding force or significance. Infinite space was one thing, back yards in the Ackerstrasse, Berlin, another. Industrial expansion and increasing population created an inescapable situation in the second half of the 19th century. There were no models for factories, commercial buildings or above all for apartment blocks on a large scale; there was a reluctance at first to accept these tasks as worthy of architecture. The readiness for technical experimentation which led to revolutionary solutions in building with iron and *steel in *Great Britain, *France and the *United States, was less pronounced in Germany. Internationally important innovations in building technique only appeared in the 20th century with the glass architecture of the years around 1910, Max *Berg's reinforced concrete dome (Centenary Hall, Breslau 1912–13), the *shell structures of the twenties and the scientific study of building as developed by the *Bauhaus.

*Art Nouveau, which marked the beginning of extensive reform movements, began with private houses. *Muthesius studied English country house styles while serving as an attaché at the German Embassy in London, *Riemerschmid and *Behrens started their architectural careers by building their own houses. This limitation was not meant as a renunciation, for the new style was not going to be determined by popular taste but, as Henry van de *Velde expressed it, by the 'ethos of the most intimate of man's possessions', the ethos of his own home. The Darmstadt Exhibition on the Mathildenhöhe (1901) which mainly featured such individual homes was thus not a private but a public event of considerable significance.

German Jugendstil had a higher moral content than Art Nouveau in France or Belgium. Appreciation for what was good and solid, honesty in the expression of materials and functions and the craft mentality were able to continue in force even when these new art forms had ceased to bloom. Enterprises such as the Vereinigte Werkstätten at Munich, the Werkstätte für Handwerkskunst at Dresden and above all the *Deutscher Werkbund founded in 1907, to which the most significant practitioners of Art Nouveau belonged, carried on the

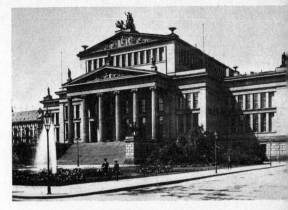

Karl Friedrich Schinkel. Playhouse. Berlin, 1818–31

message. Parting from Art Nouveau proved the easier since no German architect had fulfilled the intentions of the new style as had Victor *Horta in Brussels, *Mackintosh in Glasgow, *Gaudí in Barcelona or even *Guimard in Paris. August *Endell's buildings, the wittiest creations of German Art Nouveau in architecture, remained examples of decorative art, two-dimensional surfaces attached to three-dimensional buildings. The Belgian Henry van de Velde built too late in Germany to exert a significant influence on architectural developments there.

August Endell. Buntes Theater. Berlin, 1901

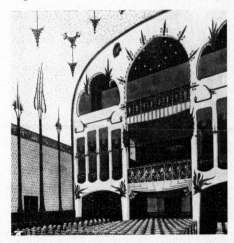

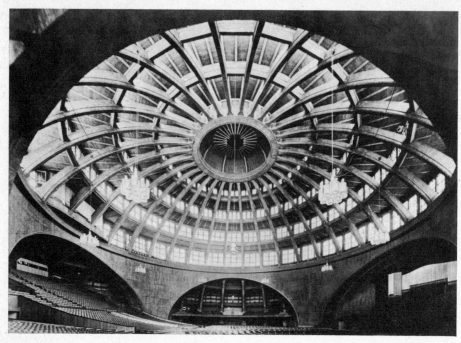

Max Berg. Centenary Hall. Breslau, 1912–13

The Werkbund Exhibition at Cologne in 1914, where van de Velde erected a theatre in the generous flowing lines of the latest Art Nouveau, featured two buildings that anticipated the future: Bruno *Taut's pavilion for the German glass industry and the model factory by Walter *Gropius. A new building material, *glass, and a new building assignment, the factory, had led to a new aesthetic. Both buildings exhibit the close connection between function and expressive form which lasted until well into the twenties. Peter Behrens's turbine factory in Berlin (1908–9) with its heavy roof and Hans *Poelzig's chemical factory in Luban (1911–12) with its decorative masonry and carefully proportioned fenestration are not the monuments of a purely objective architecture which they have been made out to be. Nearly all important architects who played a significant rôle in the twenties have gone through an Expressionist phase: *Mendelsohn, Poelzig, the brothers *Taut and *Luckhardt, *Scharoun, Mies van der Rohe with his glass-tower visions and the memorial to Karl

Liebknecht and Rosa Luxemburg (1926) and Gropius with the sharply thrusting architectural sculpture of his War Memorial (Weimar, 1922).

The Bauhaus at Weimar and later at Dessau became the high school of 'Neues Bauen' (a name coined by Hugo *Häring). If the educational foundations were laid here, and the Dessau school buildings themselves were examples of the most avant-garde type of architecture, the real testing of the new architecture took place in the big cities. Berlin was the centre. Ever since Martin Mächler's new zonal plan of 1920, a kind of creative activity prevailed here, which did not confine itself to individual buildings but pursued a town planning concept. The 'white towns', Berlin's urban estates amid green settings, bear witness to this even today. The Weissenhof estate at Stuttgart, 1927, was largely built by Berlin architects, who moreover—despite stylistic differences—had joined together in an association, the *Ring. The new ideas radiated from Berlin. Bruno Taut, who was city architect in Magdeburg for a time, Ernst *May, who built excellent housing estates at Frankfurt, Richard Döcker in Stuttgart, Otto Haesler in Celle and Kassel were in the forefront. Contacts with Holland and France strengthened the avant-garde. Mies van der Rohe's German pavilion at the Barcelona International Exhibition of 1929, a subtle composition of space-creating planes, proved that this type of architecture was recognized by the government too as representative of the new republic. Northern Germany, where Fritz Schumacher in Hamburg laid the foundations for a type of country planning that reached beyond the limits of civic design, was the home of an architecture which rested on the local tradition of building in brick and kept its expressive character somewhat longer.

The advent of National Socialism called a sudden halt to the 'New Architecture'. The Bauhaus was dissolved and architects such as Gropius, *Hilberseimer, *Breuer, *Wagner, Mies, Mendelsohn, May and Hannes *Meyer emigrated. In contrast to Fascism, National Socialism tolerated no modern architecture within the State. The official style was a monumental, sterile, *neoclassicism. For residential buildings, a Biedermeier-like native style supervened, which had already gained ground shortly after the turn of the century and had put up a considerable proportion of all buildings even during the heroic period of the modern movement. Only industrial buildings continued to permit functionally justified and aesthetically pleasing designs to be carried out; it amounted to a kind of internal emigration.

The tabula rasa after 1945 was complete. The character of German architecture in the twenties had been largely formed by the pioneer work carried out before the First World War; that after the Second World War stood alone. The task was immense. The demand for homes in the Federal Republic was estimated at 6.5 millions in 1948. Even at the end of 1960 the deficit was still estimated at 1.3 millions, to which another 1.5 millions must be added, to replace condemned property. Of the present 14 million living units less than half include a bath!

550,000 new homes a year is an achievement. But it has not brought with it a new way of living. There is nothing equivalent to the English New Town movement or

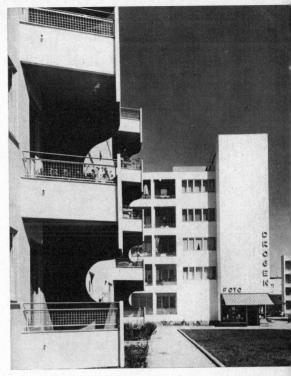

Hans Scharoun. Siemensstadt housing estate. Berlin, 1930

Mies van der Rohe. German pavilion at the International Exhibition. Barcelona, 1929

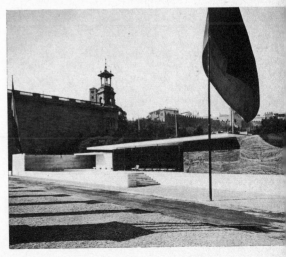

*Le Corbusier's *Unités d'Habitation*. German architects had to build before they had time to think. The costly relief measures that have been devised for nearly all the larger cities nowadays to prevent their centres from becoming completely choked are more concerned with traffic restrictions than town planning. Only in individual cases such as Hanover have planning measures proved more far-sighted. Hamburg is considering building a second centre. New satellites like Sennestadt near Bielefeld by Bernhard Reichow (where there are no traffic crossings), the Neue Vahr near Bremen or the planned Nordweststadt near Frankfurt offer more pleasing prospects. In the Hansa district of Berlin, a central area in a parkland setting, major international architects have left their mark. But this enterprise which was opened in 1957 as the Interbau-Exhibition has remained a

Helmut Hentrich and Herbert Petschnigg. Phoenix-Rheinrohr skyscraper. Düsseldorf, 1957–60

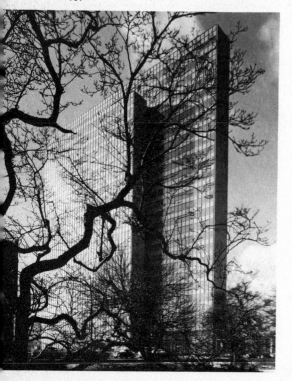

medley of remarkable individual buildings; no town planning principle can be deduced from the layout, rudely bisected as it is by a traffic artery. Even the much publicized *Hauptstadt Berlin* competition has remained without visible effect.

If any force towards integration in urban or country settings has hitherto been lacking, the isolated achievements of individual architects are admirable. Individual projects rate differently. High points are the prestige buildings of industry or communities: administrative buildings like the three-slab point block of the Phoenix-Rheinrohr at Düsseldorf by Hentrich and Petschnigg (1957–60) whose elevational treatment does not come up to the standard of the splendidly articulated massing; cultural buildings such as the municipal theatre at Münster (1954–6) whose team of architects have intelligently incorporated a neoclassic ruin into the building complex; or the municipal theatre at Gelsenkirchen (1958–9) with its transparent theatre mechanism. Extensive re-thinking on the subject of concert halls has gone into the Stuttgart Liederhalle (by Abel and Gutbrod, 1955–6) with its somewhat overlavish décor, and especially into Scharoun's Berlin Philharmonic, with the audience orientated towards the centrally placed orchestra (under construction). Church buildings are on a high level with designs by Dominikus *Böhm, *Bartning, Baumgarten, Lehmbrock and Oesterlen; the churches of the archdiocese of Cologne stand out by their special quality. This is where Rudolf *Schwarz built many of his churches, three-dimensional images of an incontestably timeless quality.

Modern German architecture has no claim on any of its great masters any more. Gropius has built one private house and a block of flats for the Interbau in Berlin since the last war. Mies did not get his first German commission until 1960, an office block for Krupp's of Essen. But his influence above all can be felt in Germany either directly or indirectly in the way that his ideas have been treated by American architects such as *Skidmore, Owings and Merrill. The rectangular cube, the dissolution into glass, the narrow profile and the separation into load-bearing members and infill areas are features which are met with in many of the buildings by Friedrich Wilhelm *Kraemer, Johannes Krahn,

Gerhard Weber and Otto Apel. In this middle generation, which was young in the twenties and today occupies chairs at the colleges and academies, Egon *Eiermann and Hans Scharoun represent extreme positions: Eiermann who is concerned with the lucidity and perspicuous arrangement of the formal image and with elegance of design; Scharoun who works on each assignment as though the planning problem it exemplifies had never occurred before.

In the youngest generation freedom of conception, psychological command and originality of design are manifestly gaining ground. Wolske with his Beethovenhalle in Bonn (1959) has built a vast festival hall in the spirit of Scharoun. The Berlin Academy by Düttmann (1959–60) is a lively organism free from chilly reserve. Blocks of flats and houses by Oswald Mathias Ungers or houses by Reinhard Gieselmann seem to provide a parallel to international *neoplasticism or *Brutalism, but in actual fact they should be regarded rather as playing with plastic forms in the course of fulfilling the building programme.

Buildings by engineer-architects often determine the aspect of an extensive environment more strongly than architecture, in its narrower sense, is able to. Amongst television towers, the one in Stuttgart by Fritz Leonhardt (1954–6) has remained unequalled in its slender grace. The Nord bridge in Düsseldorf and the Severin bridge in Cologne are bold, suspended structures, the one at Cologne having been suspended asymmetrically from a single pier, out of planning consideration for the nearby Cathedral towers. Despite their international renown, Frei *Otto's tent roofs have not yet assumed the position in Germany that they may one day occupy, since they have been labelled as exhibition architecture. It would not be the first time that structural innovations had left their stamp on a new style.

Bibliography: Hermann Beenken, *Schöpferische Bauideen der deutschen Romantik*, Mainz 1952; Fritz Schumacher, *Strömungen in deutscher Baukunst seit 1800*, Leipzig 1935; G. Hatje, H. Hoffmann, K. Kaspar, *New German Architecture*, London 1956; *Planen und Bauen im neuen Deutschland*, Cologne 1960; U. Conrads and W. Marschall, *Modern Architecture in Germany*, London 1962.

WOLFGANG PEHNT

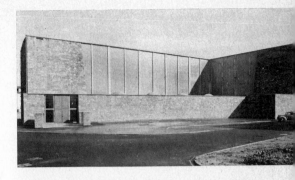

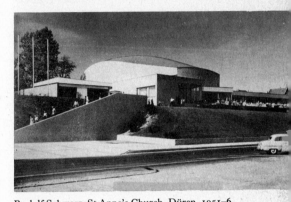

Rudolf Schwarz. St Anne's Church, Düren, 1951–6

Siegfried Wolske. Beethovenhalle. Bonn, 1959

Friedrich Wilhelm Kraemer. Technical and Evening College. Dortmund, 1956–9

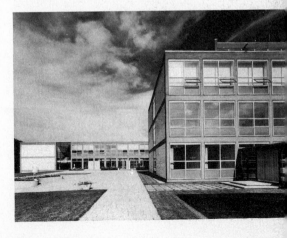

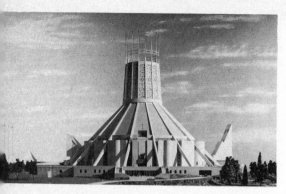

Frederick Gibberd. Metropolitan Cathedral of
Christ the King, Liverpool. Under construction.
Model

Gibberd, Frederick, b. Coventry 1908.
Studied at Birmingham School of Architecture; in private practice since 1930.
Planning consultant to several borough
councils and, since 1947, architect planner
of Harlow New Town. Gibberd has
designed a wide range of buildings, including flats, housing schemes and hospitals: Scunthorpe steelworks and power
house, 1947–9; London Airport, 1955;
National Dock Labour Board Offices,

D. E. E. Gibson. Broadgate House. Coventry, 1953

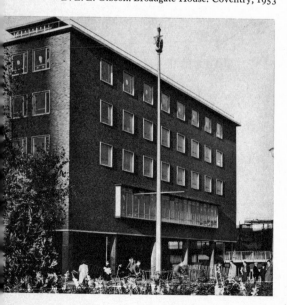

London, 1956; Hinkley Point Atomic
Power Station, Somerset, 1957; Ulster
Hospital, N. Ireland, 1953–62; technical
colleges at Hull, Kidderminster and Stour-
bridge. His prize-winning design for the
Roman Catholic Cathedral at Liverpool
shows the influence of *Niemeyer's Brasilia
Cathedral. Gibberd has written a popular
history of English architecture (1938), and
a definitive work on town design (1953).

HAROLD MEEK

Gibson, Sir Donald Evelyn Edward, b.
Manchester 1908. Studied at Manchester
University School of Architecture. He was
City Architect of Coventry (1939–55) when
it was devastated by German air raids in
the Second World War, and his powerful
feeling for urban form and unswerving
professional integrity succeeded in re-
creating a city centre there in which fewer
opportunities have been missed than in any
other city of *Great Britain, whose reconstruction of blitzed areas has generally
attained a mediocre standard. From 1955
to 1958 he was County Architect of Nottinghamshire where the *CLASP system
of prefabrication for schools was initiated
under his auspices. In 1958 he became
Director-General of Works in the War
Department, where he brought CLASP
construction into use for buildings of
various types, including the Army's Com-
puter Headquarters at Worthy Down.
Since 1962 he has been Director-General
of Research and Development in the
Ministry of Public Building and Works.

HAROLD MEEK

Gill, Irving John, b. Syracuse, New York
1870, d. 1936. First worked in the office of
*Adler and *Sullivan in Chicago; after
1896 in San Diego on his own. His early
buildings are in the 'Schindel' style,
followed since about 1906 by work in
which simple geometric elements assume
importance: 'the straight line, the arc, the
cube and the circle, the mightiest of all
lines' (Wilson Acton Hotel at La Jolla,
1908; Dodge House, Los Angeles, 1916).
His whitewashed, flat-roofed asymmetrically disposed *reinforced concrete buildings, which often display no mouldings of
any kind, were inspired by Spanish mission
stations in California and are markedly
similar to the Cubist architecture of Adolf
*Loos.

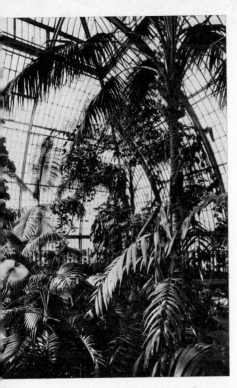

Burton and Turner. Palm House. Kew, 1844

Towards the middle of the 19th century the glass industry entered a period of intensive development; the end of the century saw the introduction of the first mechanized processes, backed by a systematic investigation of the physics and chemistry of glass. Hand manufacture and mouth-blowing are only employed today for special products and *objets d'art*.

The remarkable progress made by the glass and iron industries afforded new techniques for confronting the architectural problems of the early 19th century. The Galérie d'Orléans by Fontaine (Paris, 1829) is the prototype of all large pedestrian galleries, and is probably the first example of a large area with opaque walls covered by a glazed, translucent vault. A number of large greenhouses erected in France and England between 1830 and 1850 (at the Jardin des Plantes, Paris, by Rouhault, 1833; Chatsworth Conservatory by *Paxton, 1838; Palm House at Kew by Burton and Turner, 1844) exhibited a strictly functional character while reaching hitherto unfamiliar dimensions. Such structures became popular and were sometimes transformed into places of public resort (Jardin d'Hiver, on the Champs Elysées). With the Crystal Palace in London (1851) Joseph Paxton, by transferring the structural principles of the great greenhouses to the first exhibition pavilion, demonstrated the high degree of perfection that had been achieved in the manufacture and

Glass. Glass production has its origins in remote antiquity. The Phoenicians and Egyptians already made objects from molten glass; the Romans had a glass industry capable of producing precious objects, and the introduction of glass-blowing is probably due to them. On the fall of Rome, Byzantium took over the leading rôle in the sphere of glass production. With the end of the eastern empire Byzantine artists in glass transferred to Venice, which soon became one of the most important centres of production. The German glass industry developed during the Middle Ages; from the 15th century Bohemian products began to acquire importance. Between the 17th and 18th centuries glass manufacture spread throughout France, Belgium, England, Spain and Russia; by the beginning of the 19th century it had reached North America as well.

Victor Horta. Maison du Peuple. Brussels, 1896–9. Detail of façade

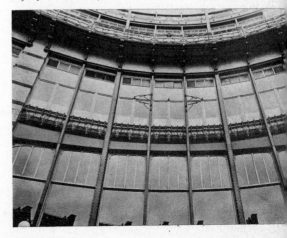

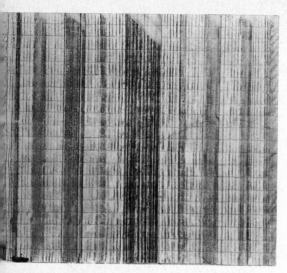

Ludwig Mies van der Rohe. Office block,
Friedrichstrasse, Berlin, 1919. Project (first
version)

Bruno Taut. Glass pavilion at the Werkbund
Exhibition. Cologne, 1914

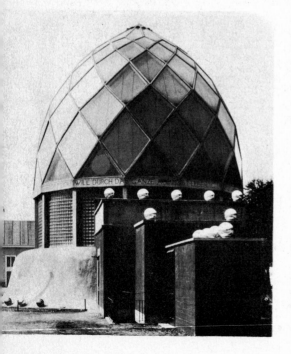

application of glass. The skill with which he
designed in new materials, without harking
back to academic tradition, was the result
of his habit as a greenhouse designer of
pursuing functional ends rather than those
of formal prestige.

The large glazed gallery became a basic
architectural feature of Paris International
Exhibitions in the second half of the
19th century, reaching in Dutert and
Contamin's Machinery Hall (1889) the most
complete expression of synthesis between
a great and original steel structure and its
transparent covering. In 1853, Baltard
built les Halles Centrales at Paris, roofed
partly in glass on an iron framework. After
1850 the use of huge transparent roofs
became common in railway stations
(Paddington Station, London, by Brunel
and Wyatt, 1854; Lime Street Station,
Liverpool, by Turner). In 1876 Boileau and
*Eiffel covered the 'Bon Marché' stores in
Paris with a complete glass roof. Large
glass roofs were adopted by *Berlage for
the Amsterdam Stock Exchange (1898–
1903) and by Otto *Wagner for the Savings
Bank in Vienna (1905) to give top lighting
to areas of major importance or prestige.
In less than a century the large glass roof
had become a definite part of the architect's
structural technique and repertory of
expression.

'The history of architecture shows that
down the centuries an unremitting battle
has been joined on behalf of light against
the obstacles imposed by the laws of
gravity: the history of windows' (*Le
Corbusier). Before the introduction of
modern structural systems the sizes of
vertical load-bearing elements in buildings
(especially multi-storey ones) of the traditional type were necessarily so large as to
confer on elevations more the character of
pierced walls than of surfaces with integrated fenestration.

The process of development whereby the
window ultimately extended its dimensions
to occupy practically the whole façade
began about the middle of the 19th century,
when cast-iron, which had already been in
use for half a century for internal construction, began to take the place of solid
walling on external elevations too (Harper
and Brothers' Building, New York, by

Page 131. Frank Lloyd Wright. Laboratory tower
for S. C. Johnson & Son. Racine, Wis., 1949

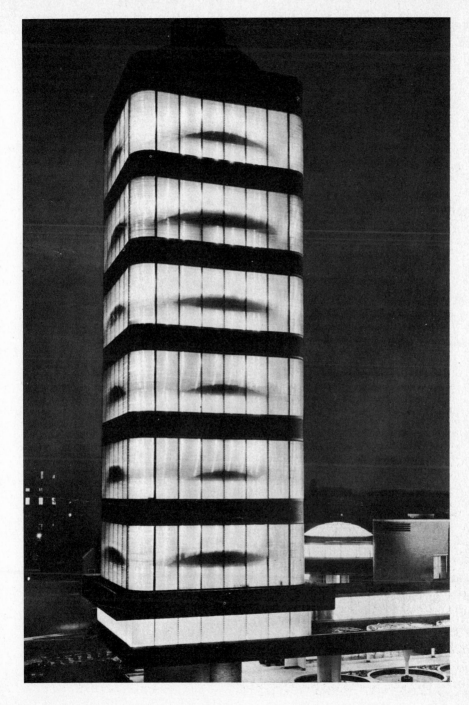

*Bogardus, 1854; riverfront buildings at St Louis, by unknown architects, 1850–80). The tendency to increase the ratio of glass to the total surface area was facilitated by the introduction and perfecting of completely framed buildings, firstly in cast-iron and later in steel, by William Le Baron *Jenney and other architects of the *Chicago School, thus answering the demand for as much natural light as possible for every room in those first large office blocks. With the Reliance Building of *Burnham and *Root (1890–4) and *Sullivan's Carson, Pirie and Scott department store (1899), the façade assumes a modular texture, with continuous rows of closely spaced but ample windows. The so-called 'Chicago window' is rectangular in shape, running horizontally, and features several lights with a large central pane.

*Horta, in his Maison du Peuple, Brussels, 1897, and *Behrens in his AEG works, Berlin, 1909, adopted continuous glass surfaces for almost the whole façade. Le Corbusier in the Pavillon Suisse, University City, Paris, 1930–2, reduced the formal importance of the steelwork, making it

Le Corbusier. Notre-Dame du Haut. Ronchamp, 1950–4. Detail of the south wall from inside

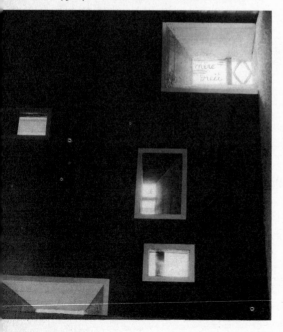

seem in the fully glazed wall simply the basic frame for a single great window.

Thus in addition to its traditional functions of providing daylight and view, glass began to be used for all the requirements of separation and insulation between interior and exterior. The window was extended to become the window wall. In the examples cited this is still contained within a single mesh of the structural grid, but elsewhere the continuity of the window units was developed until a continuous glass screen runs in front of the horizontal members (Fagus factory at Alfeld by *Gropius, 1911; Maison Clarté, Geneva, by Le Corbusier, 1932); or in front of the vertical members (model factory at the Werkbund Exhibition, Cologne, by Gropius, 1914; Salvation Army Hostel, Paris, by Le Corbusier, 1932); or in front of the whole structural grid of the façade (Hallidie Building, San Francisco, by *Polk, 1918; Bauhaus, Dessau, by Gropius, 1926; UN Secretariat, New York, by *Harrison and others, 1947–50).

While the window was becoming a glass façade, *Mies van der Rohe was investigating the theoretical bases for skyscrapers completely clad in glass with his projects for a skyscraper at Friedrichstrasse Station, Berlin, 1919, and a tower of glass and steel, 1921. These came to represent a typical manifestation of modern architecture, as defined in particular by two design features: simple volumes and glass surfaces. Outstanding examples of this type became numerous both in North America and Europe: Lake Shore Drive Apartments, Chicago, 1951 and the Seagram Building, New York, 1956, both by Mies van der Rohe; Lever House, New York, 1952, and Carbide Building, New York, 1960, by *Skidmore, Owings and Merrill; Torre Galfa, Milan, by Bega, 1959; Mannesmann Building, Düsseldorf by Schneider-Esleben, 1960.

Meanwhile developments were taking place in the design of structural frames; sometimes these were co-planar with the enclosing walls, at others they were set back, with the walls cantilevered out. This was the source of further compositional research on windows. Le Corbusier's 'Five points for a new architecture' (c. 1920), Mies van der Rohe's scheme for an office block in reinforced concrete (1922) and other projects led to the introduction and

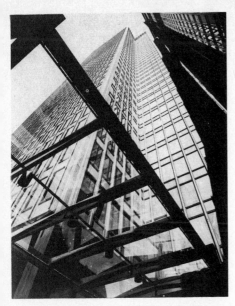

Ludwig Mies van der Rohe. Seagram Building.
New York, 1958

widespread use of strip windows (Kiefhoek Estate, Rotterdam by *Oud, 1925; Van Nelle tobacco factory, Rotterdam, by *Brinkman and van der *Vlugt, 1928–30; Schocken department stores, Chemnitz, by *Mendelsohn, 1928; tobacco factory at Linz, by Behrens and Popp, 1930–5) and windows freely shaped and set in elevations (Lovell House, Los Angeles, by *Neutra, 1927; open-air school, Amsterdam, by *Duiker, 1930–2).

The possibility of obtaining ever greater areas of glass, the adoption of slender modern structures with large spans, the boldness with which traditional materials were being used in a new spirit, and the tendency to emphasize spatial continuity between adjacent rooms and between interior and exterior led to the emergence of completely transparent glazed walls with the structural frame reduced to a minimum (Tugendhat House, Brno, by Mies van der Rohe, 1930; pavilion at the Stockholm exhibition, 1930 by *Asplund; Villa Savoye, Poissy, by Le Corbusier, 1929–30). Commercial buildings with special need for transparency (windows of shops and large stores) and the incidence of particular requirements for spatial continuity (par-

tition between the reading room and stacks in the Bibliothèque Nationale, Paris, by Labrouste, 1858–68) had initiated this process already in the 19th century. Modern architectural theory and the new types of glass available have brought this development to its culmination.

The vocabulary of current architectural expression has also been enriched by the unusual, and sometimes fanciful use that has been made of special products of the glass industry: thick slabs of glass for the treads of top-lit stairs (Brewster Apartments, Chicago, by Turnock, c. 1890; Maison Clarté, Geneva, by Le Corbusier, 1932); glass bricks for walls and roofs; rows of glass tubing making up walls and ceilings (Johnson Wax offices, 1936, and laboratory tower, 1949, Racine, Wis., by *Wright); polarized glass for heat protection (Van Leer works, Amsterdam, by *Breuer, 1957–8); blown glass polyhedra for spatial compositions (Veneto Pavilion at the 'Italia '61' Exhibition, Turin, by Scarpa, 1961).

A new interpretation has similarly arisen of the ancient tradition of decorative glass, whose forms have been adapted to modern structural and architectural requirements (Steel Church, Cologne by *Bartning, 1928; Cathedral of St Michael, Coventry, by *Spence, 1954–62). Cartoons for stained glass windows were designed by outstanding modern artists (Chapel at Vence by Matisse, 1947), and new techniques for treating the glass (Notre-Dame du Haut, Ronchamp, by Le Corbusier, 1954) or binding the component parts of the design together (Church at Audincourt, by Novarina, Léger and Barillet, 1950–1; Church at Athis-Val by Laurence and Rocher, 1954) were explored. Finally, the task of directly expressing the decorative significance of the glass has been transferred to the design of the framework itself (Robie House, Chicago, by Wright, 1909; Church of Notre Dame, Le Raincy, 1923, and Ste Thérèse, Montmagny, 1926, by *Perret; glasswork in the Italian Pavilion at the Brussels International Exhibition, by *Gardella, 1958).

Bibliography: F. Franceschini, *Il vetro*, Milan 1955; R. McGrath and A. C. Frost, *Glass in Architecture and Decoration*, London 1961.

GIUSEPPE VARALDO
GIAN PIO ZUCCOTTI

Goff, Bruce, b. Alton, Kansas 1904. Designer of houses which clearly show their derivation from Frank Lloyd *Wright. Goff drives poetic impulse to formal caprice (circular and spiral buildings with continuous flowing space; house made up of cubic units).
Bibliography: Progressive Architecture, Dec. 1962.

Gollins, Melvin, Ward and Partners. Frank Gollins, James Melvin, Edmund Fisher Ward. Extensive practice distinguished for ability to handle large masses and exploit the results of careful research. Works include Castrol House, London (with *Casson and Conder), Cleveland Technical College, Redcar, and developments at the Western Bank area of Sheffield University, for which they have designed a library to hold a million books.

Sir Owen Williams. Boots' Factory. Beeston, near Nottingham, 1930–2

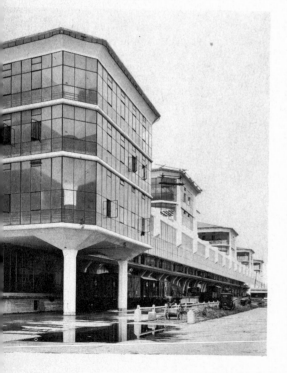

Great Britain. Modern architecture developed in France and Central Europe in the first three decades of the century, but it was late in coming to England. It is true that English domestic architecture seen in the work of Philip *Webb, Norman *Shaw, and C. F. A. *Voysey in the late 19th and early 20th centuries eloquently demonstrated designing that was logically and tastefully in answer to needs, and that this had a great influence in Europe, but the task of further development along such lines over a bigger field of building continued first in Germany, Austria, and to a lesser extent in France. Except for rare, isolated, examples it was not until the thirties that development along vigorous functionalist lines, in the broadest sense, was again manifest in England. Among the few exceptions was the Royal Horticultural Hall in London, designed by J. Murray Easton and Howard Robertson in 1923. This hall is constructed of *reinforced concrete parabolic arches, which hold together a step structure with four tiers of windows. It is a functional and expressive use of reinforced concrete and makes a beautiful and impressive interior.

Among the most important, slightly later, examples of modern architecture in England are the early works of a structural engineer, Sir Owen *Williams, of which the most notable are the large factory for Boots the Chemists at Beeston, near Nottingham, completed in 1932, the Empire Swimming Pool at Wembley (1934), and the Peckham Health Centre (1936). All these works are in reinforced concrete, the structure of which largely determines the appearance of the buildings. The Boots factory shows the influence of the *Bauhaus at Dessau, designed by Walter *Gropius. It is a large building and consists of reinforced concrete mushroom columns supporting concrete floors, the whole enclosed in glass walls, the only break in the glass being the edges of the concrete floors. By this simple mushroom-slab construction and the glass walls this building marked a big step forward in factory design in England and it was increasingly imitated. The Swimming Pool at Wembley was, at the time of its completion, the largest covered bath in the world. It was built on the reinforced concrete frame principle on a horizontal grid and vertical unit, which permitted the extensive employment of standardized parts. The roof is constructed of a series of three hinged arches held by vertical concrete shafts, which project above the plane of the low-pitched roof and perform a similar function to that of buttresses in a Gothic church. The Peckham Health Centre was a pioneer venture of two doctors, and Sir Owen Williams provided them with a modern three-storey structure of reinforced concrete with glass screens for external walls, thus admitting the maximum of light. Design is determined by purpose, and here the newest methods of construction are devised to satisfy that purpose as efficiently as possible. So as to enhance the enjoyment of sunlight and the surroundings the wall on the south-west side becomes in the two upper storeys a series of bay windows. Following similar lines, with extensive use of glass walls, is the Royal Corinthian Yacht Club building at Burnham-on-Crouch designed by Joseph Emberton in 1930. With its long balconies in front of glass walls, giving horizontal emphasis, it harmonizes with its position by the sea.

Some of the most notable contributions to modern architecture in the thirties in England are to be found in individually designed houses, and the torch of Webb, Voysey and Shaw seems to have been recovered by architects like Amyas Connell, Basil Ward and Maxwell *Fry, although the torch burns a somewhat different flame. What they have in common are plans and sequence of rooms, determined by convenience, ignoring any preconceived ideas of balance and symmetry. They are mostly built of reinforced concrete, with irregular plans, large windows towards the sun and flat roofs. The first of these houses was the famous 'High and Over' at Amersham, Buckinghamshire, designed by Amyas Connell in 1929. The house has three storeys, consisting of three arms radiating from a central octagonal hall which extends the whole height of the house. Another house built at Grayswood in 1933 by Connell in association with Basil R. Ward has a very irregular plan rather like an irregular triangle, but a perfect orientation is secured with the three principal ground-floor rooms—living-room, study, and dining-room—and the three bedrooms on the front floor all facing south. The irregular plan is reflected in the general appearance which composes

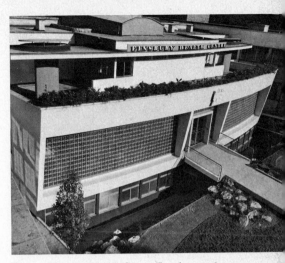

Tecton. Finsbury Health Centre. London, 1938–9

into a very agreeable relation of masses. This was one of the most ingeniously designed modern houses in Europe. It was followed by several other houses by the same architects, and these, and the stimulus given to English architects by the migration of famous German architects to England between 1933 and 1936, including Walter Gropius, Marcel *Breuer, and Erich *Mendelsohn, led several architects to design houses in a similar progressive manner. Among them was Maxwell Fry, who was Gropius's partner for a few years. After Gropius left for America, Fry built several houses on the most modern lines, one of the most effective being a house in Frognal, Hampstead (1938), which has a glass wall on the first floor opening on to a balcony. Fry was also responsible for a working-class housing scheme in Ladbroke Grove, London, which was, from the standpoint of light, good planning and spacing, the most advanced scheme of its kind in London at the time of its erection. Other architects who produced good modern work in which the new methods of construction were employed expressively were the *Tecton Group, who built the Highpoint block of flats at Highgate and the Finsbury Health Centre, both works in the modern idiom, but who became known chiefly for their constructions for the London Zoo: the Gorilla House and the Penguin Pool, where

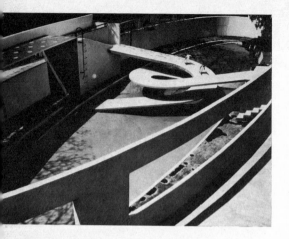

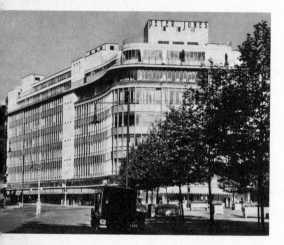

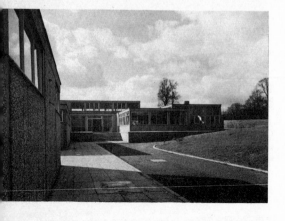

concrete has been used with good effect in a sculptural manner to show off the comic antics of the penguins. Mention should also be made of the Peter Jones Department Store in Sloane Square, London, designed by William Crabtree in association with Slater and Moberley and C. H. Reilly. Here the main supports of the building are set back from screen walls and the whole has a very light appearance.

In the early post-war period a great deal of experiment was conducted with new methods of house construction, but only a few of the many types survived and led to further developments. Probably the most outstanding post-war architecture in which the resources of modern building were used most intelligently was in schools, particularly those built in Hertfordshire. In these early post-war days materials were difficult to obtain in adequate quantities, and there was a shortage of skilled labour. Techniques were therefore adopted that permitted a fair degree of prefabrication and standardization which would contribute to speedy building. By these methods and designing that aimed at good lighting, large windows and cross-ventilation, some excellent school buildings were erected rapidly.

A notable and typical example of the Hertfordshire schools is the Hampden Secondary School for which the County Architect, C. H. *Aslin, was responsible with W. A. Henderson as the architect in charge. It was built in 1949–51 to accommodate 450 children, with a grouping of buildings according to the functions of general teaching, assembly, crafts and science, physical training and administration. The buildings are mainly two-storey, thus representing a departure from the previous post-war one-storey school building; yet the standard steel-frame structure employed in the latter was used in the Hampden School with cladding of concrete blocks. The irregular yet functional grouping and the long horizontal rectangular massing composes well with the landscape. Other

Tecton. Penguin Pool, London Zoo, 1938

William Crabtree, Slater and Moberley and C. H. Reilly. Peter Jones Department Store. London, 1938

C. H. Aslin. Junior School. Croxley Green, Hertfordshire, 1947–9

notable post-war schools in Great Britain
are the secondary school at Hunstanton
in Norfolk, completed to the design of
Alison and Peter *Smithson in 1954,
another functional grouping where the
assembly and administration are on the
ground floor and classrooms on the upper
floor, mostly with glass walls. A notable
example in London of a well-planned
school characterized by lightness and large
glazed areas is the Bousfield Primary
School, Old Brompton Road, designed by
*Chamberlain, Powell and Bon.
In 1951 three notable concert halls were
built: the Royal Festival Hall in London,
the Colston Hall in Bristol, and the Free
Trade Hall in Manchester, the last two
being rebuildings. In all these halls very
special attention was paid to acoustics. In
the Festival Hall designed by Robert
*Matthew, the architect of the London
County Council, a large area of slate is
incorporated in the floor between the
steeply raked auditorium and the orchestra
so as to reflect sound. Vision is extremely
good from every seat, and the whole building is an excellent design for its function,
with a clever use of materials, while the
large glass walls of the landings and rear
corridors afford views over London and
its river.
Some of the best large-scale housing in
Britain is to be seen in certain blocks of
flats in London and the vicinity, and in
some of the two- and three-storey blocks in
the new towns, such as Stevenage, Harlow,
Basildon and Crawley near London, in
Peterlee, Durham and the Scottish new
towns of East Kilbride, Glenrothes and
Cumbernauld.
The LCC Roehampton estate is one of the
largest and most impressive of local authority developments. It accommodates nearly
10,000 persons, and consists of ten-storey
tower blocks, six-storey slab blocks, four-
storey maisonette blocks, and rows of two-
and three-storey dwellings. The estate is
situated in wooded undulating country,
and the diverse buildings group pleasantly
and look well in the landscape. The treatment of the slab blocks with their open
ground floors is influenced by the work of
*Le Corbusier, but they are marred by
gallery access. Other notable housing
estates in London are the Spa Green Flats
in Finsbury by Tecton (1946–50); Churchill
Gardens by *Powell and Moya (1947–53);

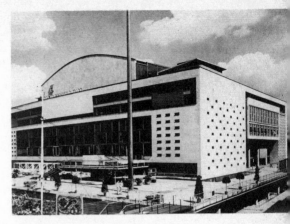

Robert H. Matthew. Royal Festival Hall.
London, 1951

and the Golden Lane estate in the City of
London by Chamberlin, Powell and Bon
(1953–7). The dominating buildings in all
these groups are tall slab blocks, seven to
ten storeys, and they all succeed in being
aesthetically pleasing because of well-
designed patterns made by the windows
and balconies, and by the relation of the
blocks to the spaces between. Although
they are all low-cost housing there is an
agreeable effect of spaciousness between
the blocks, while at the same time an effect
of intimacy is occasionally obtained as in a
group of shops and public house within the
Churchill Gardens development.
Two interesting schemes with very different purposes have a strong architectural
kinship: a tower block with four wings of
small low-cost flats in Bethnal Green (1959)
and a block of luxury flats in St James's
Place, overlooking Green Park (1961), both
by Denys Lasdun & Partners. The architectural idiom is similar in both: large
glazed areas related to plain flat rectangular
shapes of walls and balconies. The effect is
particularly felicitous in the views of the
St James's Place flats from various points
in Green Park.
The best low-cost two- and three-storey
housing during the fifties is undoubtedly
in the new towns; one of the reasons for
this is that many of the new town development corporations have commissioned
well-known architects to design for them.
Examples typical of the best are some parts

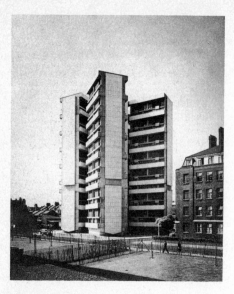

Denys Lasdun and Partners. Cluster Block.
Bethnal Green, London, 1958–60

of Basildon which, in the layout, are
adaptations of the Radburn planning of
residential areas. In these, by rear access
of vehicles to houses, some degree of
segregation of vehicular traffic and pedestrians is secured. Three areas: Barstable
planned by the development corporation
architect Anthony B. Davis; Vange by
Sir Basil *Spence; and Kingswood by
William Crabtree are examples where this
segregation has been achieved with some
varied and attractive housing. In Peterlee
new town some very compact housing
was designed by two development corporation architects, Peter Daniel and
Frank Dixon in collaboration with the
painter Victor Pasmore. Some of the
patterns of the rectangular façades are
reminiscent of Pasmore's abstract pictures.
As a whole industrial architecture of the
fifties shows a decided improvement on
that of the thirties where the custom of
having a symmetrically designed Georgian
office in front of a series of sheds was all
too common. In the fifties there has been a
more marked tendency to integrate the
various parts into a satisfactory architectural ensemble; some of the best examples
can be seen in the spacious industrial areas
of the new towns, four of the most notable

being at Stevenage, Hemel Hempstead and
Crawley round London, and East Kilbride
near Glasgow.
Perhaps the most original industrial architecture of the post-war period is seen in
power stations, in both the conventional
stations using coal or oil and the nuclear
power stations, a type of building of which
Britain has been a pioneer. In the early
thirties most power stations were built
with heavy walls of brick, but this was felt
to be unnecessarily substantial, and the
tendency has been towards a much lighter
cladding of glass, aluminium, asbestos and
other thin, light materials. Some well-
designed power stations have resulted, a
number of which are by *Farmer and Dark.
A good example is the Marchwood Power
Station on the Hampshire coast near
Southampton. This building in which
aluminium *curtain walling is employed
forms a long horizontal mass by the sea
with two tall chimneys. With nuclear
power stations different problems of design are presented because they include
immense reactor buildings which have to
be of very sturdy construction. All the
massive nuclear power stations so far built
—those at Berkeley and Hinkley Point
near the Bristol Channel are examples—
are different in design. The most recent,
that at Sizewell in Suffolk, designed by
Frederick *Gibberd, has something of the
massive character of a medieval fortress or
defensive castle. Instead of the nuclear
power stations spoiling scenic beauty, as
was feared, they have become interesting
features in the landscape.
A main development in British architecture during the fifties can be seen in
office and apartment blocks. Consent is
now given for higher buildings in certain
circumstances, and this has resulted in
many office blocks in London being built
well above the previously permitted 100
feet (generally about nine or ten storeys)
to fifteen, twenty, thirty storeys or even
more. The chief distinguishing architectural feature of office blocks since about
1952 is the curtain wall, and a tower block
of about fifteen or twenty storeys rising
from a lower block of about two or three
storeys. Notable buildings of this kind in
London are Castrol House, designed by
*Gollins, Melvin Ward & Partners; Thorn
House, designed by Sir Basil Spence; and
the Vickers Building, designed by Ronald

Ward & Partners, which is the highest office block built in London, having thirty-four storeys. There is a danger that the pattern of tower and low podium block if not designed with some originality may become monotonous, and thus architects, alive to this, are introducing more varied treatment such as the curved façade of the Vickers tower, and the Y plan of the new multi-storey Hilton Hotel in Park Lane. This plan serves the function of giving a maximum number of bedrooms views over Hyde Park. With parts of the building of various heights combined with a tower block, the architecture of office buildings is becoming a matter of the large-scale relation of masses, while in the treatment of curtain walls and end walls architecture is moving closer to the art of the painter with effects that depend on the abstract pattern of colours and textures.

Bibliography: J. M. Richards, *An Introduction to Modern Architecture*, 1st edition, London 1940, 3rd edition, London 1961; Edward D. Mills, *The New Architecture in Great Britain 1946–1953*, London 1953; John Summerson, *Ten Years of British Architecture*, London 1956; Trevor Dannatt, *Modern Architecture in Britain*, London 1959.

ARNOLD WHITTICK

Greene, Charles Sumner and Henry Mather. Charles Sumner, b. St Louis 1868, d. Carmel 1957. Henry Mather, b. Cincinnati, Oreg. 1870, d. Altadena, Calif. 1954. Studied at Massachusetts Institute of Technology, Cambridge. The Greenes' houses are among the best examples of Californian regionalism at the turn of the century, with their interpenetration of internal and external space, projecting roofs, flat gables and warm materials (timber, shingled walls, coloured windows). Blacker House (1907) and Gamble House (1908–9) at Pasadena, Calif.

Gropius, Walter, b. Berlin 1883. One of the outstanding architects and teachers of the 20th century, Walter Gropius is the son of an architect who occupied an important official position in Berlin. It is not without significance that his great-uncle, Martin Gropius (1824–80) was an architect of some reputation who designed, among other notable buildings, the great hall of the new Gewandhaus at Leipzig, and who

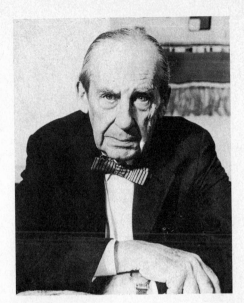

Walter Gropius

was also Principal of the Arts and Crafts School in Berlin and Director of Art Education in Prussia.

Walter Gropius received his training in architecture first at Munich from 1903 to 1905 and then in Berlin to 1907, when he entered the office of Peter *Behrens where so many young architects later to become famous had also worked, among them *Mies van der Rohe and *Le Corbusier, who, however, stayed only for a short time. In 1910, after three years in Behrens's office, Gropius started on his own as an industrial designer and architect. His designing covered a wide range and included interior decoration schemes, wall fabrics, models for mass-produced furniture, motor-car bodies, and a diesel locomotive. His first important building was the Fagus shoelace factory at Alfeld-an-der-Leine, built in 1911 in collaboration with Adolf *Meyer. This building marked a step forward in steel and glass construction. It is three-storeyed, the steel frame supports the floors, and the walls have become glass screens, the non-structural character of which is emphasized by the absence of vertical supports at the corners. At the famous *Deutsche Werkbund Exhibition at Cologne in 1914 Gropius and

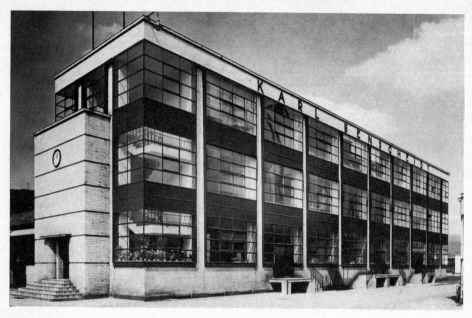

Walter Gropius and Adolf Meyer. Fagus factory. Alfeld-an-der-Leine, 1911

Meyer designed the Administrative Office Building which proved to be a very notable contribution to modern architecture. The building is symmetrical, the central portion of the front façade is faced with brick, and at the ends are spiral staircases enclosed for two storeys by glass towers. The glass screen held by a very light steel framework continues on the first floor along the narrow sides and for the whole length of the rear of the block, thus imparting the character of unusual lightness. The circular glass towers enclosing the staircases represent the first use of an architectural motif that was to become an important feature in many modern buildings, especially departmental stores. It was often used by Erich *Mendelsohn with fine effect. Gropius and Meyer also designed the hall of machinery and open garages at

Walter Gropius and Adolf Meyer. Model factory at the Werkbund Exhibition. Cologne, 1914

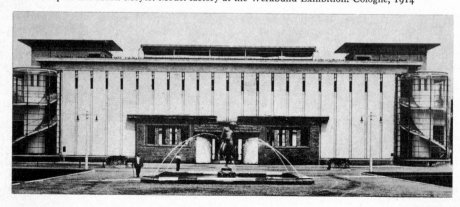

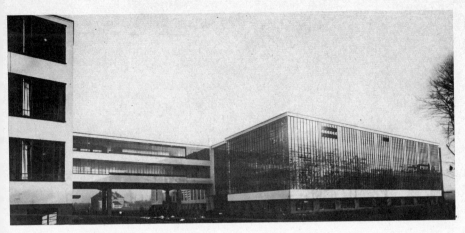

Walter Gropius. Bauhaus. Dessau, 1925–6

the back of the office block. The former had a slightly pitched roof with steel stanchions curving from the walls.

From 1914 to 1918 came the break of the First World War when Gropius served in the German Army. In 1915 he was given the position by the Grand Duke of Saxe-Weimar of Director of the Grossherzog-liche-Sächsische Kunstgewerbeschule and the Grossherzogliche-Sächsische Hoch-schule für Bildende Kunst at Weimar, and after the cessation of hostilities in 1919 he combined the two under the name of Das Staatliche *Bauhaus, Weimar, because Gropius believed in the unity of design and craft, of art and technics. He was Director first at Weimar from 1919 to 1925 and then at Dessau from 1925 to 1928 when he resigned because he wished to devote his energies more wholeheartedly to archi-tecture untrammelled by official duties.

While at the Bauhaus, however, he was the architect of several buildings and the designer of several projects, his most important building during this period being the world-famous group of buildings for the Bauhaus at Dessau, which was completed towards the end of 1926. Among other works was the rebuilding of the Municipal Theatre at Jena in 1923, designed in collaboration with Meyer, and two very interesting projects, one a build-ing for an international academy of philo-sophical studies and the other a 'Total Theatre'. The former, designed for a site near the University of Erlangen, belongs

to 1924 and shows the tendencies in his planning that two years later resulted in the Bauhaus building. The 'Total Theatre' design was made in 1927 in collaboration with Erwin Piscator, the Berlin theatrical producer. The purpose was to design a theatre that could be changed to accord with the type of play, changed, that is, from the Greek theatre with the semicircular orchestra, to the circus with the central arena and to the modern picture-frame stage. The theatre was so designed that the tiers of seats could be revolved in sections to enable the change from one form to another to be effected quickly. A model

Walter Gropius. Siemensstadt housing estate. Berlin, 1929

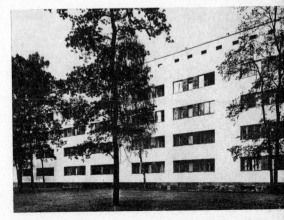

was exhibited at the 1930 Paris Exhibition, but it was never built. The movement towards building theatres of flexible construction, however, has grown considerably during the century, and Gropius's project has been a significant contribution towards the feasibility of the idea.

Gropius was not only an architect and industrial designer, but a sociologist who wanted to build on the basis of a rational interpretation of the needs of people. During the latter part of his directorship at the Bauhaus he studied the problem of obtaining the best living conditions in cities while preserving their urban character. He aimed to produce city dwellings in which the inhabitants obtained as much sunlight, space, and air and trees and lawns as possible at very much the same density as then existed. To achieve this he evolved the tall slab-like apartment block of about ten storeys, arranged, not parallel with the street but transversely with it, orientated according to the sun, with cross-ventilation and with broad stretches of garden between the blocks and open at both ends. He showed that with higher blocks housing people at the same density there is far more space and the angle of light is less.

Gropius was able partially to realize his ideas in the Dammerstock housing scheme near Karlsruhe in 1927–8, where he not only designed some of the five-storey blocks but acted as a co-ordinator for eight other architects. In this scheme several blocks are arranged in parallel lanes transversely with the streets. A more ambitious realization was in the large Siemensstadt estate near Berlin, in which Gropius was the supervising architect with several others collaborating, while he was himself responsible for two of the blocks. The general layout consists of long five-storey blocks, orientated north–south so as to get the maximum sunlight, widely spaced with stretches of grass and tall trees with light, delicate foliage between. The blocks have pale plain walls with large windows, and they are planned with two flats per landing. These Siemensstadt flats have exerted a wide influence and have been much imitated.

With the accession to power of the National Socialists in 1933 conditions became difficult for liberal and modern minded architects, so in 1934 Gropius left Germany for England. He settled in London and entered into partnership with E. Maxwell *Fry, one of the most successful of the younger British architects. Together they designed several interesting schemes, the work actually completed including the film laboratories for London Film Production at Denham (1936); two houses, one in Sussex (1936) and one in Old Church Street, Chelsea (1935); and Impington Village College, Cambridgeshire (1936), one of four village colleges erected by the County Council. This was Gropius's most important contribution to architecture in England. It is a one-storey building with single depth classrooms, fan-shaped hall, and club amenities, all very happily sited amongst lawns and trees to serve the dual purpose of a secondary school and community centre for adults.

Early in 1937 Gropius accepted an invitation to become Senior Professor of Architecture at Harvard University, USA, and the following year he became Chairman of the Department of Architecture. He very quickly demonstrated his practical ability as an architect by building his own house, which was completed in the year of his arrival. It has much of the classic restraint of the houses that he had designed for himself and the Bauhaus leaders in 1926. This was followed by a large number of private residences that he designed in collaboration with other architects in America. In the year of his arrival he entered into partnership with the Hungarian architect, Marcel *Breuer, who had been a student and master at the Bauhaus. In the years of their partnership in addition to several houses, including one for Breuer himself, they designed the Pennsylvania Pavilion, New York World's Fair in 1939, and an interesting housing scheme at New Kensington near Pittsburgh in 1941, in which year the partnership with Breuer terminated. The New Kensington housing was for the workers in an aluminium factory, and the houses were built on the slopes of the hills above the factory. They were irregularly sited and in accordance with the best orientation, following the contours of the hills; they were reached by winding paths.

Page 143. The Architects Collaborative. Harvard Graduate Center. Cambridge, Mass., 1949–50

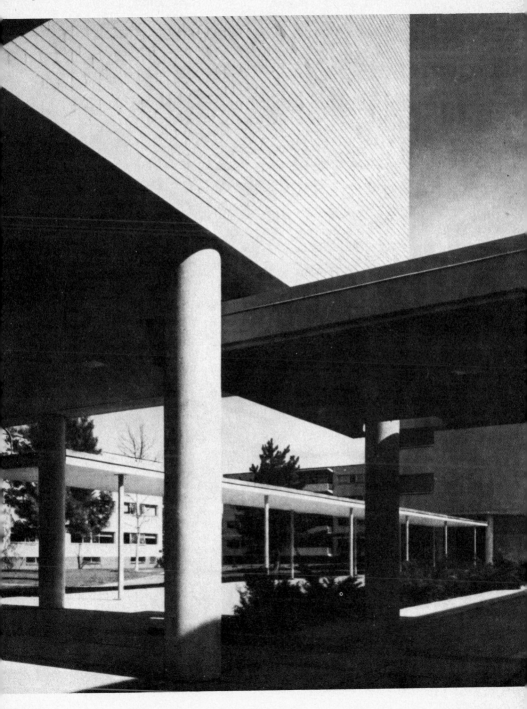

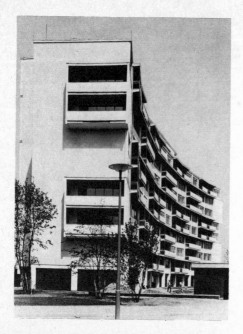

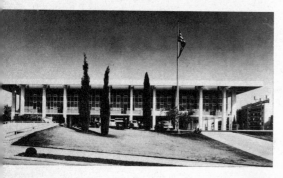

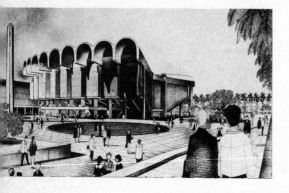

When in Germany, in 1932, Gropius had begun experiments with standardized building elements for mass-produced housing, and he resumed these experiments during the war years 1943–5. The earlier ideas were concerned with copper-sheet houses, but these later developments were with timber panels based on a module both horizontally and vertically of 40 inches. After experiments made in collaboration with Konrad *Wachsmann in Long Island, these houses were erected on a considerable scale in California.

In 1945 Gropius went into partnership with several architects of the younger generation forming a team of eight under the name of 'The Architects Collaborative' (*TAC). In this enterprise Gropius was the guide and leading spirit. That he was able to enter with enthusiasm into so large a group demonstrates his great belief in the value of team-work which he had always felt to be necessary in modern building. The team was responsible for much interesting work which made a noteworthy contribution to mid-20th-century American architecture. It includes several private residences, all of which are worthy of study for their planning and siting; the Junior High School, Attleboro, Mass. (1948); the Harvard University Graduate Center, Cambridge, Mass. (1949–50), which consisted of a group of seven dormitory blocks in relation to the social centre; and the Harkness Commons, a grouping in which the open spaces between the buildings were very carefully related to function. In 1953 the team built the McCormick Office Building. In 1961 Gropius was invited to London to design a building for the Monico site in Piccadilly Circus, the former scheme for which had been rejected by the authorities as not being of sufficient architectural merit for this important site.

Gropius's buildings are distinguished by an adventurous use of the modern materials of steel, concrete and glass, while he may be regarded as perhaps the principal innovator in the utilization of the complete

Walter Gropius and Wils Ebert. Block of flats. Interbau Exhibition. Berlin, 1957

The Architects Collaborative. US Embassy. Athens, 1961

The Architects Collaborative. Bagdad University, 1960. Project glass screen in forming the outer shell of a building, thus admitting the maximum of light. Architecturally his work is always distinguished by a classic restraint and excellence of proportion of which the houses for the staff at the Bauhaus at Dessau are an example. But important as Gropius is as an architect, he is possibly even more important as a teacher and an influence. He was a great believer in the intelligent application of standardization and prefabrication, but above all he wanted a building to be the product of team-work in which each member of the team appreciated fully the relation of his contribution to the whole design. Gropius regarded this as a symbol of community living and the intelligent integration of society.

Bibliography: Sigfried Giedion, *Walter Gropius*, Paris 1931; Sigfried Giedion, *Walter Gropius: Work and Teamwork*, Stuttgart, Paris, New York and London 1954; J. M. Fitch, *Walter Gropius*, New York 1960. See also Bauhaus.

ARNOLD WHITTICK

Gruen, Victor, b. Vienna 1903. Studied under Peter *Behrens. Emigrated to the United States in 1938. Mainly town and country planning (e.g. Fort Worth, Texas). His conception of 'shopping centres' was epoch-making, sited out of town and catering for the needs of modern street traffic (Northland Shopping Centre, Detroit, 1952).

gruppo 7. Architectural co-operative of seven (predominantly Milanese) architects, Luigi *Figini, Guido Frette, Sebastiano Larco, Adalberto Libera, Gino *Pollini, Carlo Enrico Rava and Giuseppe *Terragni. The group, founded in 1926, appeared publicly in 1927 with an exhibition at the Biennale in Monza and was invited in the same year to the Werkbund Exhibition at Stuttgart. It stood for an architecture founded on the regional analysis of building functions and attempted to create an Italian tradition in modern building. 'The desire for sincerity, order, logic and clarity above all, these are the true qualities of the new way of thinking.' (Series of articles in *La Rassegna Italiana*, December 1926 to May 1927.)

Guimard, Hector, b. Paris 1867, d. New York 1942. Studied at the École des Arts Décoratifs and at the École des Beaux-Arts in Paris, where he later taught. Guimard was influenced by Victor *Horta, the most gifted and eminent architect of the French *Art Nouveau. His main work consists of the Castel Béranger, Paris (1897–8), the imaginative entrances to the Paris Métro, reminiscent of the organic forms of nature (1900), and the Humbert de Romans Building, Paris (1902), a large auditorium with a steel frame.

Hankar, Paul, b. Frameries 1859, d. Brussels 1901. The architect Paul Hankar was one of the moving figures in Belgian *Art Nouveau, together with Victor *Horta and Henry van de *Velde. He learnt his profession in the office and on the building sites of the architect Henri Beyaert from 1879 to 1894, when Beyaert died. During this period Hankar was personally responsible for the restoration and interior

Paul Hankar. Maison Kleyer. Brussels, 1898

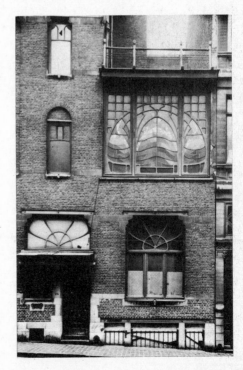

decoration of the Church at Everberg in Brabant.

Hankar took over from his master certain elements of his style, such as the harmonious blending of white stone, blue stone and brick, but introduced modernist details into this traditional type of structure: wrought-iron grilles, consoles, handrails and balconies, and sgraffito murals. A number of medieval and oriental reminiscences are incorporated in his work, too: openings set asymmetrically, stilted arches, battlements, penthouses, broad cornices and heavy modillions, which conspire to produce a picturesque effect. He conceived of architecture as a synthesis of the plastic arts and designed the interior decoration and furniture for most of the private houses he built. He originated an Art Nouveau type of shop-front and fittings which gained rapid acceptance in Europe. He died before being able to carry out a major project, the *Cité des Artistes*, for which he had drawn up the plans.

Bibliography: Charles de Maeyer, *Paul Hankar*, Brussels 1962.

ROBERT L. DELEVOY

Häring, Hugo, b. Biberach 1882, d. Biberach 1958. Häring advocated in his writings and buildings a theory of organic building which differs from the *organic architecture of Frank Lloyd *Wright.

Häring studied at Stuttgart Technical College (under Theodor *Fischer) and at Dresden. In 1912 he established his own architectural practice in Berlin. In 1924 the *Zehnerring* was founded to fight the tendencies propagated by the then city architect Ludwig Hoffmann, and this group was later enlarged to become *Der *Ring*. The *élite* of the modern architects of Germany belonged to it, and Häring, as its secretary, was the leader of the association. In 1933 the *Ring* was dissolved by the Nazis. Though *Gropius and *Mies van der Rohe emigrated, Häring remained in Germany; he was the head of a private art school. In 1943 he returned to his native town of Biberach, where he died in 1958 after a long, painful illness.

Häring was responsible for a number of important works, of which the Garkau farm buildings (1923) have become particularly famous; his real importance, however, lies in the theoretical field. He expounded his views on organic building

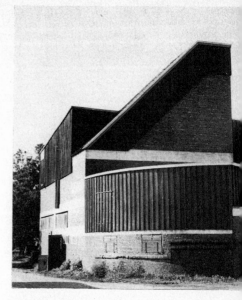

Hugo Häring. Farm buildings at Garkau, near Lübeck, 1923

in numerous articles and lectures. He maintained that the work of rejuvenating architecture had to proceed in two stages. The first is concerned with research into changing needs, and aims at fitness for purpose and the 'organism'; the second, on the other hand, deals with 'design'. While other contemporary trends in the twenties (*Le Corbusier, for example) determined what shape fitness for purpose would take by using geometric forms accepted as *a priori* beautiful, Häring attempted to develop the design from its fitness for purpose without preconceived ideas of shape. 'We want to search for things and let them unfold their own design. It goes against the grain . . . to determine their shape from the outside, to subject them to a set of derived laws' ('Wege zur Form'). Häring emphasized that organic building did not mean copying the forms of nature but that—as in nature—shape arose from function.

The thesis sometimes propagated by his followers, that organic building demanded curved shapes, not based on orthogonal principles, was rejected by Häring. 'The identity of an object must determine the type of form appropriate to the individual building' ('Geometrie und Organik'). The decisive criterion in organic building is the determination of form from an object's identity. A building derives its shape from the function which it has to discharge as the tool (or 'organ' as Häring called it) of man. The house as the tool of its inhabitants is the starting point of his thinking.

Häring's ideas, which in the twenties were limited to a small circle, became increasingly important with the new phase of modern architecture that started about 1930. Today, architects as distinct as Alvar *Aalto, Louis *Kahn and Hans *Scharoun hold similar views.

Bibliography: Hugo Häring, 'Wege zur Form', in *Die Form*, No. 1, 1925; Hugo Häring, 'Geometrie und Organik', in *Baukunst und Werkform*, No. 9, 1951; Heinrich Lauterbach and Jürgen Joedicke (editors), *Organhaftes Bauen* (= Dokumente der Modernen Architektur 4), Zurich and Stuttgart in preparation.

JÜRGEN JOEDICKE

Harrison, Wallace Kirkman, b. Worcester, Mass. 1895. Studied at the École des Beaux-Arts, Paris. Worked on the Rockefeller Centre (1931–47). Partnership first with *Hood then with Fouilhoux and Max *Abramovitz. Harrison and Abramovitz are among the greatest American architectural firms and have specialized in office buildings. Storey-high units of aluminium or steel were used for the *curtain walls of such buildings as the Alcoa Building in Pittsburgh (1953) and the Socony Mobil Building in New York (1956). Harrison, who possesses excellent organizational ability, was principal architect for the United Nations Buildings, New York (1947–50, esquisse by Le Corbusier). As coordinator he is directing the construction of the Lincoln Center, a cultural project in New York (building in progress).

Haussmann, Georges-Eugène, b. Paris 1809, d. Paris 1891. As prefect of the Seine department under Napoleon III, Haussmann carried out a series of town-planning schemes in Paris that determined the present face of the city: construction of bridges and prestige buildings, opening up of streets and boulevards to meet military, ceremonial, hygienic and traffic requirements.

Havlíček, Josef, b. Prague 1899, d. 1962. Studied at the College of Technology and the Academy of Fine Arts at Prague (1916–26). Housing, offices, hospitals, large-scale urban works. His 1930 buildings, white blocks with continuous horizontal strips of windows, are amongst the most disciplined examples of the *International Style.

Hilberseimer, Ludwig, b. Karlsruhe 1885. Worked in Berlin till 1928, then at the *Bauhaus in Dessau; since 1938 at the Illinois Institute of Technology in Chicago. Town-planning work of fundamental significance.

Bibliography: Ludwig Hilberseimer, *Grossstadt-Architektur*, Stuttgart 1927.

Hoffmann, Josef, b. Pirnitz, Moravia 1870, d. Vienna 1956. Hoffmann studied architecture in Vienna under Otto *Wagner, whose most faithful and convinced disciple he became. The rationalistic theories that underlay Wagner's teaching had a decisive influence on the course steered by Hoffmann, but the latter's famous elegance and refinement of taste was far removed from the severity of *Loos. He did not, in fact, despise ornament and this led him to show particular interest in the production of craft objects. He taught at the School of Applied Arts from 1899 onwards, and together with Koloman Moser set up a group of studios and workshops, which under the name of *Wiener Werkstätte* enjoyed widespread success and fame for thirty years.

In 1897 he joined with other young artists, including Joseph *Olbrich in founding the Wiener Sezession. Under the influence of the Glasgow School and of Belgian and French *Art Nouveau, its aims were more radically modernist than those of Wagner's school. Ten years later, he moved towards a new cultural avant-garde that centred round the painter Gustav Klimt, with whom Hoffmann founded the *Kunstschau* called 'the Secession from the Secession'. Meanwhile Hoffmann's first works of architecture gave him a European celebrity, which was confirmed by the commission he received to build a large house in Brussels for the Stoclet family. In the opening years of the century he had designed exhibition pavilions, schemes for internal decoration and four houses (Moser, Moll, Henneberg and Spitzer). With the Purkersdorf Sanatorium (1903) he became one of

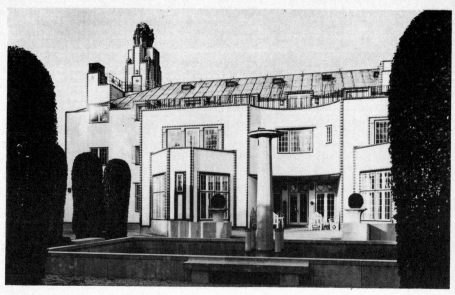

Josef Hoffmann. Palais Stoclet. Brussels, 1905

the foremost exponents of the new style in architecture. His Palais Stoclet (1905) is an architectural masterpiece that evokes the exquisite poetry of Post-Impressionism and Symbolism. Although completely based on rationalist theories it is rich and refined to the point of decadence, a monument of the last bourgeois age which represents a milestone in Hoffmann's own career, and in the history of European architecture, at the moment when it was turning towards the new century.

In the years that followed, up to the eve of the First World War, Hoffmann built dozens of villas in Vienna with only a few basic variations. At the 1914 *Deutscher Werkbund Exhibition in Cologne, for which he designed the Austrian Pavilion in an elegant style of vaguely neoclassic derivation, he encountered in the work of *Gropius a new and more vigorous form of architectural modernity: one which was to mark, inevitably, the decline of his own, with its exquisite refinements of 'taste'.

In 1912 he began the construction of a villa colony at Vienna-Kaasgraben, which was interrupted by the war; his architectural work was only resumed in 1920, though the activity of the *Wiener Werkstätte* had continued. In 1920, too, he was

appointed city architect of Vienna. But with the rise in Europe of De *Stijl, the *Bauhaus and *Le Corbusier's *Esprit Nouveau,* something a little anachronistic in Hoffmann's work was to leave it henceforth slightly on the margin of modern architecture, whose social content was also radically new. Hoffmann himself was aware of this. The housing schemes he carried out in 1924 and 1925 for the City of Vienna, and his terrace houses in particular for the 'Internationale Werkbundsiedlung' of 1932, are built in a style of extreme architectural purity that recalls the houses of *Neutra, Loos, *Rietveld and *Lurçat. They are the last proofs of Hoffmann's conscious and

Josef Hoffmann. Design for an auditorium. 1922

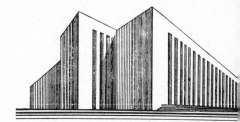

deliberate 'presence' in the process of total revolution through which architecture was passing in those years of unmitigated controversy. The next year, 1933, he decided to close down the famous *Wiener Werkstätte* for good. He designed the Austrian Pavilion for the 1934 Venice Biennale, and, after the last war, some blocks of workers' housing. He died in Vienna in 1956, while a large exhibition devoted to his work was on show in Brussels.

Bibliography: Ludwig Hevesi, *Acht Jahre Sezession*, Vienna 1907; Leopold Kleiner, *Josef Hoffmann*, Berlin, Leipzig and Vienna 1927; Armand Weiser, *Josef Hoffmann*, Geneva 1930; L. W. Rochowanski, *Josef Hoffmann*, Vienna 1950; Giulia Veronesi, *Josef Hoffmann*, Milan 1956.

GIULIA VERONESI

Holabird, William, b. Amenia Union, N.Y. 1854, d. Evanston, Ill. 1923. Trained in the office of William Le Baron *Jenney, later in partnership with Martin Roche. The Tacoma Building (Chicago, 1889) by Holabird and Roche is the aesthetic consequence of the introduction of steel frames for tall buildings; an extensive dissolution of the façade into glass, punctuated by projecting bays, and the abandonment of historical ornamentation.

Holford, Lord, b. S. Africa 1907. Studied at Liverpool University School of Architecture. Rome Scholar, 1930. Professor of Civic Design at Liverpool, 1937; Professor of Town Planning, University College, London, 1948. Houses, factories, public buildings. Planning proposals for the County of Cambridge, 1950. Report on St Paul's precinct, 1956; three-level plan for Piccadilly. His fourteen-storey block of flats at Kensal (1958) has been called the first large-scale *modular building. President RIBA, 1960–2. Life Peer (Baron), 1965.

Holzmeister, Clemens, b. Tirol 1886. Churches, residential and public buildings. Worked in Turkey (Ministry of War, Summer Palace for Kemal Pasha). New Salzburg Festival Theatre (1960).

Hood, Raymond M., b. Pawtucket, R.I. 1881, d. Stamford, Conn. 1934. Gained first prize in the competition for the Chicago Tribune Building (1923–5, a neo-Gothic design); c. 1930 in collaboration

with a partner he built the McGraw-Hill Building, New York, no longer revivalist in style, and the Daily News Building (1930) which anticipates the marked vertical stress of the Rockefeller Center.

Horta, Victor, b. Ghent 1861, d. Brussels 1947. A keen disciple of *Viollet-le-Duc, Horta was a leading figure of continental *Art Nouveau and the creator of an original vocabulary of ornament. He helped to open up new paths to 20th-century architecture by doing away with the traditional plan of the private house and providing an architectural expression for the new building programmes set in train by the social and cultural developments of his time. He was also instrumental in devising a number of subtle structural forms that drew on the resources of iron and glass.

Horta began his architectural studies at Ghent Academy (1876) and continued them at the Académie des Beaux-Arts at Brussels. After spending some time in the office of Balat, a neoclassic architect of repute, he built a group of three little houses in the Rue des Douze Chambres at Ghent (1886), where his great architectural ability is already obvious despite the modest scale

Victor Horta. Hôtel Tassel. Brussels, 1892–3

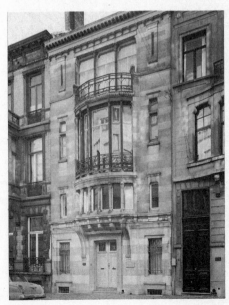

of the project. This first design of his, honest, straightforward and economical, gave little indication of a work that was to appear six years later, whose astonishing architectural and decorative richness revealed its author as someone of great creative maturity, albeit still young (thirty-one): the Hôtel Tassel, built between 1892 and 1893 at 6 Rue P. E. Janson, Brussels. This house, a veritable manifesto of Art Nouveau, is revolutionary in form and structure and is regarded today as one of the classic monuments in the history of architecture. It is the product of an expanding bourgeois economy, strong craft traditions and a country that has achieved a high degree of industrialization; but above all, the Hôtel Tassel is remarkable for the novelty of its plan: instead of the corridor usual in Belgium, Horta substituted an octagonal hall, from which a broad staircase leads off, giving access to the various rooms at different levels. This arrangement breaks with the practice of uniform layout floor by floor, foreshadowing the 'plan of volumes' conceived by *Loos in 1910 and *Le Corbusier's two-storey system of 1930.

Victor Horta. Hôtel Solvay. Brussels, 1895–1900

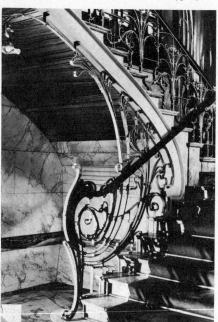

The Hôtel Tassel is also remarkable as being the first private house to make use of iron, both as a structural material (a huge winter garden on the ground floor is carried on an exposed iron frame, while an elegant iron column supports the staircase) and to supply decorative elements in a flexible linear style, exemplified by the wrought-iron handrails of the staircase and balconies. It is in this building, too, that an impressive repertoire of two-dimensional forms was initiated, based on a close study of plants and flowers: the 'whiplash line' or 'Horta line' literally covers the floors, walls and ceilings; it lashes out everywhere, coiling, interlacing, flying loose, climbing across glazing bars, encircling the feet of furniture, branching out in chandeliers and outstripping, often to excess, every structural requirement.

In the Hôtel Solvay (224 Avenue Louise, Brussels), built between 1895 and 1900, Art Nouveau can be seen in its maturity: it is an astonishing symbiosis, of Baroque and classical, sentiment and reason, craftsmanship and industry, colour and form, with aesthetics dominating technology. This building, wholly fitted out and furnished by Horta, is undoubtedly the most significant and complete example of its period. Horta built numerous houses in Brussels before the First World War in the same style (Autrique, 1893; Winssinger, 1895–6; Van Eetvelde, 1897–1900; Aubecq, 1900). The Maison du Peuple he designed for the Brussels branch of the Workers' Party (1896–9), and the department stores 'A l'Innovation' (Brussels, 1901) and 'Grand Bazar' (Frankfurt, 1903) all employ the structural resources of iron in the service of a new programme. The large glazed façades of these three buildings prefigure the light transparent envelopes that have led to the disappearance of the load-bearing wall.

In 1912 Horta was appointed a professor at the Académie des Beaux-Arts, whose head he eventually became (1927–31). After a stay in the United States (1916–19), his architecture assumed an austere, classical direction; the picturesque and calligraphic tendencies of Art Nouveau were conclusively superseded by the straight line. The Palais des Beaux-Arts in Brussels (1922–8) is the principal work of this period; well laid-out and designed in concrete, it was the first cultural centre of

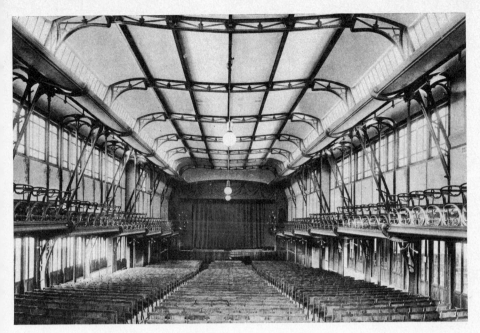

Victor Horta. Maison du Peuple. Brussels, 1896–9

a type that was to gain wider diffusion after the Second World War.

Bibliography: Robert L. Delevoy, *Victor Horta*, Brussels 1958.

ROBERT L. DELEVOY

Howard, Ebenezer, b. London 1850, d. Welwyn Garden City 1928. In his book *Tomorrow: A peaceful path to reform* (London 1898) Howard advocates garden cities to counter flight from the land and the overpopulation of towns. His idea of an economically independent garden city surrounded by an agricultural belt and numbering approximately 30,000 inhabitants led to the foundation of the Garden Cities Association. First garden city: Letchworth near London (1903).

Howe, George, b. Worcester, Mass. 1886, d. Cambridge, Mass. 1955. Studied at the École des Beaux-Arts in Paris. Partner in the firm of Mellor, Meigs and Howe (residential buildings). Architect of the Philadelphia Savings Fund Society Building (1932), together with William *Lescaze.

Howell, Killick, Partridge and Amis. William Gough Howell, John Alexander Wentzel Killick, John Albert Partridge, Stanley Frederick Amis. Practice with a style characterized by a powerful striving after plastic originality. Their project for the Department of Commerce and Social Science at Birmingham University features *Gaudí-like façades of precast concrete balcony units; a redevelopment plan for St Anne's College, Oxford, consists of a series of curved blocks with highly modelled surface treatment, set in a wide oval round the college garden.

International Style. The term International Style, although recurrently under attack since it was first introduced a generation ago in the book of that name (New York 1932), has become—in considerable part by default—perhaps the most useful name for the dominant architectural current of the second quarter of the 20th century. Within the broad historical range of modern architecture, from the European and American modes of such men as *Voysey, *Horta and *Sullivan in the 1890s to the present 1960s, it defines a type of architectural design which came into existence in the early 1920s, developed at the hands of a few leaders to classic expression by 1930, and from that time on found wider and wider acceptance throughout the world.

Foreshadowed by the domestic building of Adolf *Loos, the early industrial constructions of *Perret, *Behrens and *Gropius, much work by engineers, European and American, and even the Futurist visions of *Sant'Elia, the new architecture of the pioneers among the second generation of modern architects, particularly the French-Swiss *Le Corbusier, the German Gropius and *Mies van der Rohe, and the Dutch *Oud and *Rietveld, representing a convergence of social and aesthetic aspirations characteristic of the second decade of the century, found early expression, mostly in projects, in the years 1919–23 immediately after the First World War. The large-scale projects of Mies (his glazed towers of 1919 and 1921), the Chicago Tribune Tower design of Gropius and Meyer (1922), and the spaced cruciform skyscrapers of Le Corbusier's 'City of Three Million', also projected in 1922, indicated a generic debt to American achievement in building, and by the mid century the International Style would even come to seem to many a characteristically American style. But for all the debt of

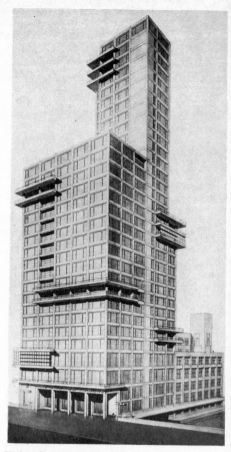

Walter Gropius and Adolf Meyer. Chicago Tribune Tower. 1922. Project

Le Corbusier. Second Citrohan House. 1922. Model

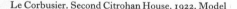

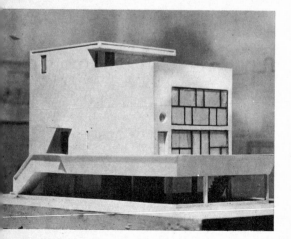

younger architects outside America to *Wright, especially in Holland and Germany in the fifteen years following 1910, the initiation of the new style—if style it be—was Western European, even specifically French, Dutch, and German; and it did not even begin to be accepted in other European countries—England, Sweden, Denmark, Finland, Russia and Italy—or in the New World until the late 1920s. As it spread internationally in the 1930s, however, political reaction and economic stagnation interrupted further development in several countries of Europe, notably Germany, Russia and France. On the other hand, by the late thirties, notable work was under way from Helsinki to

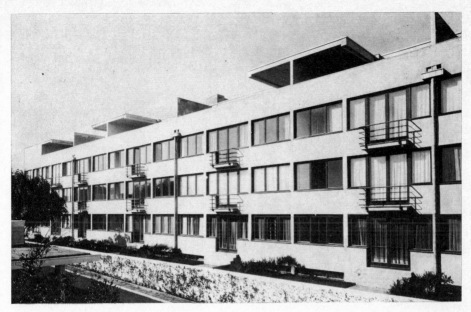

Ludwig Mies van der Rohe. Block of flats on the Weissenhof Estate. Stuttgart, 1927

Rio de Janeiro; and when building revived in the late 1940s after the Second World War the International Style had come to be almost universally accepted throughout the whole non-Communist world wherever modern technological advances were already an accomplished fact or even a relatively new importation.

As late as 1952 it was possible to claim (see the article 'The International Style Twenty Years After' in the *Architectural Record*) that, despite all the modulations, reactions and divagations up to that time, the International Style was still the essential core of international architectural practice. A decade later, now that the stylistic divergences of the last thirty years have become more strikingly apparent, the International Style probably still remains the basis of further architectural development since it was, very definitely, the discipline under which almost all architects under sixty were formed. To offer historical parallels not too pretentiously disparate in their chronological range, the divergent aspirations and achievements of the later 1930s, 40s, and 50s bear somewhat the same relation to the classic stage of the International Styles of the 1920s as the modu-

lations that followed the High Gothic in the mid and late 13th century or those that followed the High Renaissance in the mid and late 16th century. On these analogies the International Style, as the 'high' phase of modern architecture, may indeed continue to provide the basis of architectural developments for several generations—and even centuries—to come.

Returning to the book of 1932 which attempted at the end of the classic phase to formulate the International Style which had come into being through the preceding decade since 1922, certain quotations may still be relevant: 'The unconscious and halting developments of the 19th century, the confused and contradictory experimentation of the beginning of the 20th have been succeeded by a diverted evolution. There is now a single body of discipline, fixed enough to integrate contemporary style as a reality and yet elastic enough to permit individual interpretation and to encourage general growth. . . . The idea of style as the frame of potential growth, rather than a crushing mould, has developed with the recognition of principles such as archaeologists discern in the great styles of the past: . . . There is, first,

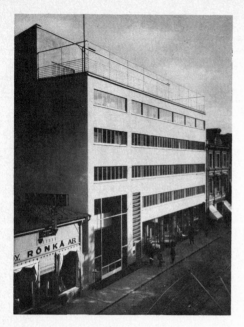

Alvar Aalto. Building for the newspaper Turun Sanomat. Turku, 1928–30

Eero Saarinen. General Motors Technical Center. Warren, Mich., completed 1955

a new conception of architecture as volume rather than as mass. Secondly, regularity rather than axial symmetry serves as the chief means of ordering design. These two principles, with a third proscribing arbitrary applied decoration, mark the productions of the International Style. This new style is not international in the sense that the production of one country is just like that of another. Nor is it so rigid that the work of various leaders is not clearly distinguishable. . . . In stating the general principles of the contemporary style, in analysing their derivation from structure and their modification by function, the appearance of a certain dogmatism can hardly be avoided. (But) the international style already exists in the present; it is not merely something the future may hold in store. Architecture is always "a set of actual monuments, not a vague *corpus* of theory".'

Some of those actual monuments may well be named, in addition to the skyscraper projects mentioned earlier. These, however, it should be noted, have proved especially premonitory of what may be considered the 'American' phase of the International Style of the 1950s, which could now be illustrated with monuments as far apart geographically as the Edifico Polar in Caracas, Venezuela, by Vegas and Galia and the SAS building in Copenhagen, Denmark, by Arne *Jacobsen, not to speak of prominent examples in countries such as England, Germany, Italy, Belgium and South Africa.

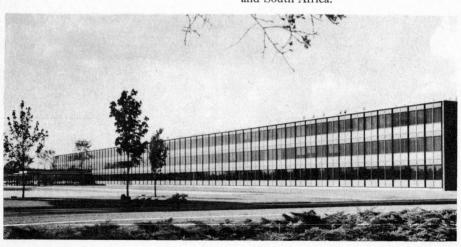

Perhaps the first modest realization of the ideals of the still unformulated International Style was a jewellery shop of 1921 in the Kalverstraat in Amsterdam by G. T. Rietveld inspired by the Dutch *neoplasticism. Parallel with this came the unrealized projects of Le Corbusier for 'Citrohan' houses (1919–21) and those by Mies van der Rohe for a brick country house and for a concrete office building (1922). Major works of the mature International Style followed, with Gropius's *Bauhaus at Dessau (1925–6), Le Corbusier's Cook and Stein houses (1926 and 1927), Oud's low-cost housing at the Hook of Holland (1926–7), Gropius's housing at Törten, Siemensstadt and Dammerstock (1928 and 1929), not to speak of his Dessau Employment Office (1928), perhaps his most perfect work; and finally Mies's German Pavilion at the Barcelona Exposition (1929) and his Tugendhat house in Brno, Czechoslovakia, and the Savoye house at Poissy outside Paris by Le Corbusier (both 1930). Immediately after 1930 definite modulations began to appear away from some of the austerities of the classic phase, particularly in Le Corbusier's Swiss Hostel (1931–3) at the Cité Universitaire in Paris with its rubble rear wall of irregular curvature and its somewhat sculptural *pilotis* of rough concrete. Thus in the very years of the early 1930s, when the new style was spreading most rapidly throughout the world on the way to its almost universal acceptance after the Second World War, one at least of the founders was still in the lead in moving away from the rigid machinolatry implicit in the most advanced aspirations of the 1920s. But this should not be overemphasized. In the very years of the early 1950s, when Le Corbusier in his Church of Notre-Dame du Haut at Ronchamp in France and his High Courts of Justice at Chandigarh in India was reaching the extreme point of his reaction against the International Style, Mies van der Rohe in his Lake Shore Drive apartments was providing a new model of the tall building, based on his projects of the 1920s, destined to be enormously influential internationally; while Eero *Saarinen, whose early death in 1961 deprived the post-war world of one of its most typically versatile and divergent designers, was still faithful to the Miesian version of the International Style in his first major work, the General Motors Technical Center at Warren, Mich.

It still seems just, therefore, to return to the initial paragraph of this article and to state once more that the International Style was the dominant architectural development of the second quarter of this century, and that its core of tradition, at least, as well as its continued employment in vulgarized modes—to which the term is by some derogatorily restricted—is still the basis of the world's architecture even in the 1960s and may well remain so for many decades.

HENRY-RUSSELL HITCHCOCK

Iron. *Steel.

Italy. 'Since the 18th century there has been no architecture': it is with these words that *Sant'Elia opened his Manifesto of 1914. It would have been truer to say that since the 18th century Italy had produced no great architect, no new directions in architecture and no great school. Nevertheless, there has not been any substantial change from 1914 to the present day, despite Sant'Elia and despite *Nervi: for two centuries now, Italian architects, when they have not built like the ancient Romans, have trodden in the steps of foreigners; only *Terragni has dared to strive for independence. The few interesting architects of the *Stile Liberty* (the Italian *Art Nouveau), *Basile, D'*Aronco and *Sommaruga looked to the Belgians and French; while Vienna provided the models for Sant'Elia himself (influenced by the school of Otto *Wagner) and the Lombard rationalists prior to 1927, who were followers of *Loos and *Hoffmann. After 1927 the young 'Europeanists' of the modern movement reorientated themselves to *Le Corbusier, *Mies van der Rohe or *Gropius. This generation, which is now fifty or sixty years old, still represents the best in Italian architecture today.

Naturally, in the work of each of them, from Basile to *Albini, and from Sant'Elia to Nervi, the personal imprint is stronger than the foreign one; but it has not been as determinative either of the essential content or the original form as the foreign sources have; it is the latter, revived and worked over again, that one sees reflected there. One original element, in the years between the wars however, intervened amid the various foreign influences, as a dangerously suggestive constant: the *Novecento Italiano*, the only cultural movement that was typically Fascist (hence the 'Italiano'), recruited from the 'reactionaries of the modern revolution' (as one of its founders wrote), or rather from the 'revolutionaries of the Fascist reaction' as its critics saw it. But unlike the revolutionary architects of *Germany and the *Netherlands, the protagonists of the *Novecento Italiano* did not start from scratch. They carried out a modernist reform based on the principles of neoclassical architecture and the aesthetics of *valori plastici*, modified in the light of Cubism, or its Italian derivative, *Futurism. Giuseppe Terragni revivified this

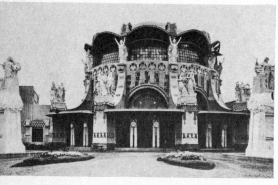

Raimondo d'Aronco. Main Building at the Applied Art Exhibition. Turin, 1902

Matté Trucco. Fiat Works. Turin, 1927. Car ramp

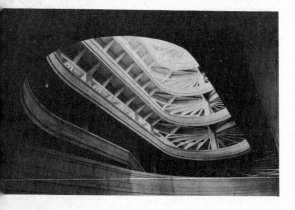

movement by the support of his artistic genius; he was its most important architect, not only by reason of the absolute value of his works, and of the Casa del Fascio (Como, 1936) in particular, but above all because of the complexity of the problems he set himself in attempting to break down the 'national' barriers to his lively historical feeling for architecture; and by historical we mean European. Luciano *Baldessari worked with similar aims, building the fine Press Pavilion at the Vth Milan Triennale (1933).

The ferment of new ideas came to the boil in 1927, in particular with the work of the seven young architects united under the banner of *gruppo 7, who formulated their ideas in a number of publications and helped to promote the foundation of the *Movimento Italiano per l'Architettura Razionale*. But as architecture, more than any other art, was tied up with politics, the ambiguous attitude of the *Novecento Italiano* was passed on to the new movement. The subsequent confusion was great, since both opposing trends, the 'modern' and the 'ancient Roman' (whose leader was Piacentini) declared for Fascism. In reality the interests and claims of both sides were equally demagogic, and periods of inauspicious alliance were not lacking either. The journal *Quadrante*, edited by P. M. Bardi, supported the Fascist version of rationalism. Meanwhile, some architecture of note did get built: the Fiat Works by Matté Trucco (1927) and Pagano's Casa Gualino, both at Turin; some houses by Lingeri on Lake Como; and Terragni's Novecomum at Como.

The position was soon clarified, however, by Edoardo Persico, a young critic who since 1929 had been the editor of Giuseppe Pagano's *Casabella*. He showed that rationalist architecture was essentially anti-nationalist, according to the tenets of the *Bauhaus, itself the most rigorous expression of it. Persico had to fight within the editorial board itself of *Casabella* against Pagano's Fascist illusions and his own noble errors, for which he ultimately paid with his life, dying at Mauthausen in 1943.

In 1933 Gio *Ponti took over the direction of the Vth Triennale. Ponti was of modernistic neoclassical provenance, but anti-monumental, and never taking his standpoint to extremes; this made him the

favourite architect of the Milanese bour-
geoisie. In a spirit of free experimentation,
and without any polemical intent, he
invited the 'rationalist' group of architects
to take a large part in the Triennale, and
published their work in his journal *Domus*,
thus paving the way to success for them.
Their contribution to the Triennale, a
series of villas and small houses erected in
the park, was of a splendid precision and
uniformity; but on the moral plane, though
they were not aware of it, the compromise
was grave. It was only with the war and
the end of Fascism that nearly everybody,
starting with Pagano, understood the cause
that Persico had defended: they understood,
that is to say, that a revolutionary architecture is incompatible with a reactionary
government, which is always willing to
exploit alliances and compromises. But by
that time, Piacentini, the leader of Fascist
architecture, and certain Novecentists like
him, such as Muzio in Milan, had already
sown their colonnades, lictoral towers and
'Roman' arches up and down the length of
Italy. It was the same with town planning:
Mussolini founded new cities, only one of
which had any architectural feeling:
Sabaudia (by Cancellotti, Montuori, Piccinato and Scalpelli); and it was only
Adriano Olivetti who called in some bright
young architects—*Figini and *Pollini—
to draw up a plan for the Val d'Aosta.
After the war, the reconstruction drive was
beginning to bear fruit, when Bruno Zevi,
back in Rome after many years' residence
in America (where he had not seen Italy's
difficulties and problems), thought he
recognized an error in the general alignment of Italian architects, victorious at last,
along the front of 'rationalist' aesthetics.
But although he performed a task of cultural value in spreading, with polemical
ardour, a knowledge of Frank Lloyd
*Wright and his campaign for 'natural', i.e.
*organic as opposed to 'rational' architec-
ture, he nevertheless helped to confuse
once more the ideas of Italian architects
who had only recently managed to sort
them out, and who in any case found
rationalism in architecture congenial.
Zevi had the greatest effect on the School
of Rome, which counted some of the best
architects in Italy amongst its members,
including Piccinato, Quaroni (who built
some experimental villages at Matera),
Montuori, the designer of the new station

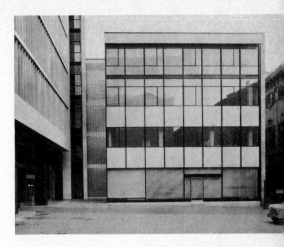

Gian Antonio Bernasconi, Annibale Fiocchi and
Marcello Nizzoli. Palazzo Olivetti. Milan, 1954

in Rome (1950, with Calini and others),
the whimsical Ridolfi, Moretti, Monaco and
Luccichenti. But above all, the architects
of Milan were disorientated. They had been
induced to re-think their architecture from
scratch, sometimes altering their whole
style, and it was this lack of ideological
clarity that later gave rise to the strange
form of the Torre Velasca (1957) and the
rising tide of 'neo-Liberty' (Art Nouveau
revival) which has almost drowned some
young architects and stirred up a scandal

Eugenio Montuori, Leo Calini, Massimo
Castellazzi, Vasco Fadigati, Achille Pintonello
and Annibale Vitellozzi. Main Railway Station.
Rome, 1950. Booking Hall

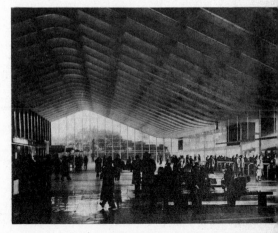

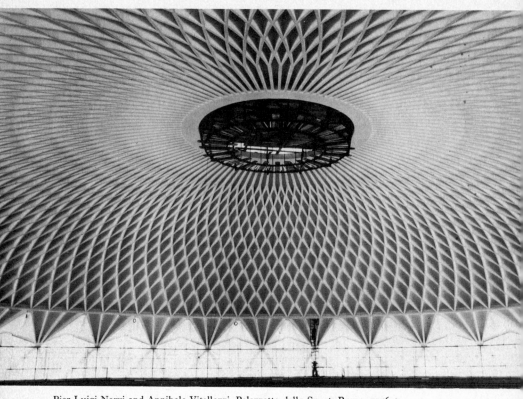

Pier Luigi Nervi and Annibale Vitellozzi. Palazzetto dello Sport. Rome, 1956–7

abroad out of proportion to the episode's size and significance.

In and around Milan however, innumerable buildings have arisen: workers' flats, factories, houses, office blocks, churches and a number of skyscrapers (the Pirelli Building by Gio Ponti; the much discussed Torre Velasca by *BBPR; the Torre Galfa by Bega; and the Torre al Parco by Magistretti). In addition to the architects of the first rationalist school, such as *Albini, Figini, Pollini, Sartoris, Lingeri, Belgioioso, Banfi (who died in a concentration camp), Peressutti, Rogers, *Gardella, Bottoni, Mollino, Astengo, Zavanella and *Nizzoli, may be named the younger generation of *Zanuso, Pagani, Castiglioni, Caccia Dominioni, Latis, *Fiocchi, Bernasconi, Morandi, Bassi, *Viganò and Mangiarotti (known for his 'glass church' at Baranzate) among others. But every city and every region is a centre where interesting architects are at work: Cocchia at Cosenza (Naples); Samonà at Minchilli (Bari); Michelucci, designer of the fine station in Florence (1936, in collaboration); the builders of the Market at Pescia in Tuscany (1951); *Scarpa in Venice, where the best school of architecture is situated; and Albini, himself a Milanese, in Genoa, where he has built the two splendid museums of the Palazzo Bianco (1951) and San Lorenzo (1954–6). Works of great interest may often be found in small towns, such as Terragni's Casa del Fascio at Como (1936), Gardella's buildings at Alessandria, those of Baldessari at Rovereto, Gellner's at Cortina, D'Olivio's at Trieste, Nervi's at Chianciano and Bologna, and those by Nizzoli, Fiocchi, Gardella, Figini and Pollini at Ivrea.

The nerve centre of the new Italian architecture is Milan, with its journals, its Triennali, its recently founded Museum of

Architecture, and the economic opportunities afforded by its industries. It was in Milan that culminated the activity of that generous and intelligent patron of modern Italian architecture, Adriano Olivetti; it is being continued by his son Roberto today. On the cultural plane, Rome competes for primacy; it is the home of the *Istituto Nazionale di Architettura*, headed by Bruno Zevi, who also edits *L'Architettura*, published in Rome. Architectural criticism, too, is very active in Italy, backed by an intelligent editorial policy (Argan and Zevi in Rome, Ragghianti in Florence, and Dorfles and Veronesi in Milan). Our general panorama may conclude on a positive note with the name of the greatest and best known amongst living Italian designers, the engineer Pier Luigi Nervi whose superb structures, which for the last thirty years have been rising throughout Italy and the world, have won for him universal renown.

Bibliography: Paolo Nestler, *Neues Bauen in Italien*, Munich 1954; Piero Bottoni, *Edifici Moderni in Milano*, Milan 1954; G. E. Kidder Smith, *Italy Builds*, London 1955; Carlo Pagani, *Italy's Architecture Today*, Milan 1955; Agnoldomenico Pica, *Architettura Italiana Recente*, Milan 1959.

GIULIA VERONESI

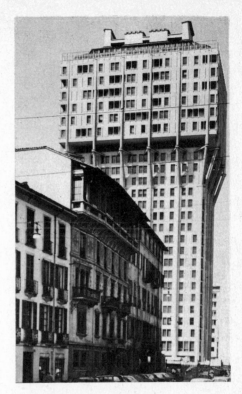

BBPR. Torre Velasca. Milan, 1957

Luigi Figini and Gino Pollini. Church of the Madonna dei Poveri. Milan, 1952–6

Jacobsen, Arne, b. Copenhagen 1902. Arne Jacobsen is an architect who has been to a notable degree open to new impulses without losing his attachment to the Danish tradition. The same sense for order, modular rhythms and natural proportions, which developed first in Danish half-timbered construction and later in the brick buildings of the classical revival, characterizes Jacobsen's architecture. Artistic discipline, together with an avoidance of sentimentality and theatric effects, led to a restraint which, combined with a sense for precision in detail and excellence in workmanship, pervades all Arne Jacobsen's later building.

Jacobsen grew up with *Functionalism. When he was a student *neoclassicism

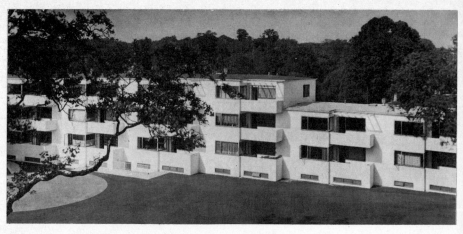

Arne Jacobsen. Bellavista Housing Estate near Copenhagen, 1933

still dominated Denmark and the architecture of about 1800 was greatly admired, in particular that of the architect Nicolaj Abildgård. But his encounter with the architecture of *Le Corbusier and *Mies van der Rohe in exhibitions at Paris (1925) and Berlin (1927–8) was important both for Jacobsen himself and for the whole development of Danish architecture.

Jacobsen was trained in the architectural school of the Academy of Arts, from which he graduated in 1928. He had already attracted notice with the first of a long series of single houses, reminiscent externally of Abildgård and his period, with yellow bricks and a tiled roof. The ease and flexibility of his talent enabled him at the same time to try his hand at Functionalism's cubist style. Together with Flemming Lassen he created a sensation at an exhibition in 1929 with a circular 'house of the future' with helicopter landing-place on the roof.

In his earliest Le Corbusier-inspired villas the smooth whitewashed walls concealed technical faults which followed from the over-hasty adoption of the new style. In 1930–5 he created a harmonious group of buildings in the Bellevue area near Copenhagen, beginning with the baths, whose cabins and kiosks were designed with elegance. These were followed by the three-storey Bellavista housing blocks, whose staggered perspectives gave all flats an equal share of sun and view. Finally

came the Bellevue Theatre, which was thought of primarily as a summer theatre and therefore given a sliding ceiling which could make the night sky serve as a roof. Unfortunately both the theatre and the adjoining restaurant have been altered beyond recognition.

It was through his friendship with the Swedish architect Gunnar *Asplund that Jacobsen reached maturity as an artist. From Asplund he learned what it is to *work* at a building, both technically and architecturally, and to respect detail. Asplund's influence shows clearly in Stelling House in Copenhagen (1937–8) and the town halls of Århus (1937) and Søllerød (1940–2), designed in collaboration with Erik Møller and Flemming Lassen respectively. Gradually Jacobsen was able to free himself from Asplund's imprint without forgetting the lessons he had learned from him.

Wartime isolation and the conditions prevailing until 1950 allowed Denmark no opportunity to make use of the new impulses arriving from abroad. Then with the Søholm housing scheme Jacobsen won back his position among the leaders of Danish architecture. In Munksgård's School (1952–6), a single-storey construction with numerous bays and courtyards, he combined a sense for total unity of design and quality with an atmosphere of intimacy. In a series of new offices and administrative buildings he tried to introduce the largely American-developed principle of construction with internal supporting columns and *curtain-wall façades. He appreciated the fact that the aesthetic qualities of so simple, almost anonymous, an architecture must be based on proportions and detail, and designed accordingly [Jespersen's Building in Copenhagen (1955); Rødovre town hall (1955); the SAS Building in Copenhagen (1959)].

Since the war Jacobsen has also constructed a series of handsome private houses, which show to a marked degree his ability to fit buildings into the landscape, such as the houses for C. A. Møller (1951) and Ruthwen Jürgensen (1956), lying in attractive surroundings near the Sound. Exclusive residences were constructed in Jægersborg and Gentofte and blocks of flats in Rødovre (1951). On the industrial side mention should be made of Odden Smokehouse (1943), built with traditional materials, the Massey Harris exhibition and works building (1952), which was awarded the grand prix in São Paulo, Brazil, and Tom's Factories (1961). Arne Jacobsen does not wish to be a specialist. Not only does he range over the entire field of architecture, but he is just as willing to plan silverware, gardens, furniture, and fabric patterns.

Jacobsen has been invited to take part in a number of international competitions [town halls of Marl (1957) and Cologne (1959), World Health Organization's building in Geneva (1960)]. He has received first prize in many Danish and Swedish competitions, including Denmark's National Bank (1961) and Landskrona town hall and sports hall (1957). Since 1959 he has been engaged on St Catherine's College, Oxford. He has been Professor of Architecture at Copenhagen Academy of Arts since 1956.

Bibliography: J. Pedersen, *Arkitekten Arne Jacobsen*, Copenhagen 1954.

TOBIAS FABER

Japan. It was in the year 1868 that a decisive new era dawned for Japan under the rule of Emperor Meiji, putting an end to the long feudal age of the Tokugawa Shogunates which had lasted for 260 years. The isolation policy of the Shogunates was abandoned and the country opened its doors to the world, absorbing Western civilization with eagerness.

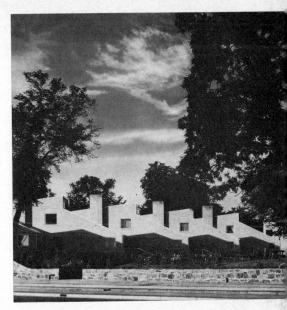

Arne Jacobsen. Housing. Søholm, 1950–5

Arne Jacobsen. Jespersen Offices. Copenhagen, 1955

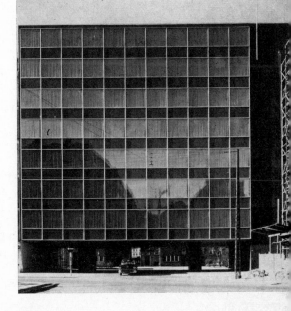

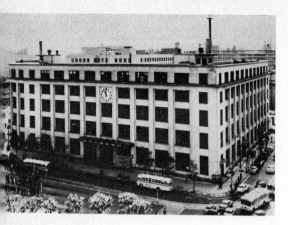

Tetsuo Yoshida. General Post Office. Tokyo, 1931

In Japan wood had always been the main building material. After the restoration the Japanese invited architects from Germany, England, Italy and the United States to help them build Western style architecture of stone and bricks. Japanese architects then copied these examples and soon began to give birth to a Japanese-European style, introducing elements of Renaissance, Gothic and Italian into the traditional native architecture.

Japan is naturally very receptive and liberal in adopting foreign cultures and has been much influenced by them. But she also

Hideo Kosaka. Post Office Savings Bank. Kyoto, 1954

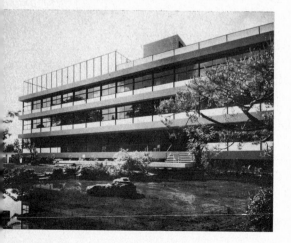

values and preserves her own age-old culture and blends it harmoniously with imported cultures, though the process of assimilation often takes a long time. The rapid introduction of Western architecture at the beginning of the Meiji period was a challenge to Japan's architectural circles. Scholars such as Professor Chuta Ito and Professor Tei Sekino turned their attention not only to the study of Western architecture but also to the traditions of their own country and other Asiatic lands.

Towards the end of the 19th century steel-framed structure and *reinforced concrete were introduced, bringing a rapid development in the Japanese building industry. Together with this innovation in building technique came the influence of modern movements in Europe such as *Art Nouveau and the Wiener Sezession. In 1920, under the prosperous conditions following the end of the war and with a call for humanism, the Japanese group Secession was formed by a number of younger architects, including Sutemi Horiguchi, Makoto Takizawa, Mamoru Yamada, Kikuji Ishimoto. In 1922 Japan's modern architecture was presented by this group at the Peace Exposition, Tokyo, for the first time. Of its members Mamoru Yamada designed the Central Telephone Office, Tokyo (1926); Kikuji Ishimoto, the Tokyo Asahi News Press Building (1927), and the Shirokiya Department Store, Tokyo (1929). Sutemi Horiguchi devoted his time to a re-examination of the traditions of Japanese architecture and received a doctor's degree for his thesis on Kundaikan-Sochoki, which is an historical document concerning interior decoration in 15th-century Japan.

Japanese modern style is best represented in works built for the Communications Services. Mamoru Yamada was first in this field. He was followed by Tetsuo Yoshida, *Functionalist in the best sense of the word, who designed the Tokyo General Post Office (1931); and later by Hideo Kosaka (Post Office Savings Bank, Kyoto, 1954).

The *International Style found its way into Japan through contacts made by her younger architects and critics with modern groups in Europe. Kenji Imai, a professor at the Waseda University, went to Europe in 1926 to study modern architecture and became personally acquainted with *Gropius, *Le Corbusier, *Mies van der Rohe, and others. On his return he published reports on their activities. Kunio *Maekawa went to Paris to work under Le Corbusier; Iwao Yamawaki and Takehiko Mizutani studied at the *Bauhaus in Dessau. About this time two foreign architects visited Japan who had a great influence on her modern movement. One of them was Frank Lloyd *Wright, whose famous Imperial Hotel (1915–22) had very much impressed Japan's architectural circles. The other was a German architect, Bruno *Taut, who travelled all over Japan, seeking out the wonderful treasures of her architectural tradition.

At this stage of their development Japanese architects were confronted with many difficult problems. They were not only concerned with the basic principles of modern building; they were also trying to find answers to the demands of modern living in a new age. In 1937 they founded the *Kosaku Bunka Renmai* (Japanese Werkbund) and issued a publication, *Kosaku Bunka*, in which they outlined their proposals and described the experiments they had made. Hideo Kishida, Shinji Koike, Sutemi Horiguchi, Yoshiro Taniguchi, Takeo Sato, Kunio Maekawa were the leading members of the group. But soon

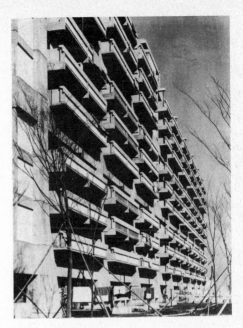

Kunio Maekawa. Harumi Flats. Tokyo, 1957

Kenzo Tange. Sogetsu Hall. Tokyo, 1960

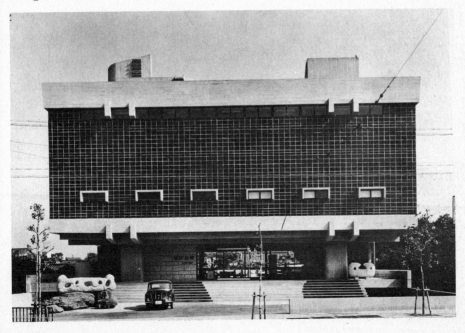

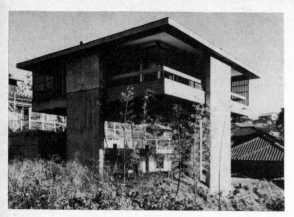

Kiyonori Kikutake. Sky House. Tokyo, 1958

the time became unfavourable to the growth of such a movement; with the rise of Fascism in Europe, militaristic nationalism took the lead in Japan, and finally the outbreak of war brought the activities of the Japanese Werkbund to an end. Their only chance lay in the rationalization which was necessitated during the war because of the shortage of material and labour.

After the signing of the San Francisco Peace Treaty in 1951 architecture began to develop again under the new democratic constitution. First came the construction of quarters for the occupation forces, then gradually the work of reconstruction in general. The leading architects were Mamoru Yamada, Kunio Maekawa, Kameki Tsuchiura, Kenzo *Tange, and Yoshiro Taniguchi, who had all formerly been connected with the Japanese Werkbund. Examples of their work are the Welfare Hospital by Mamoru Yamada (1953), the International House by Maekawa, Sakakura and Yoshimura (1955), the Peace Centre in Hiroshima by Kenzo Tange, and the Nagasaki Cultural Centre by Takeo Sato (1955). Isoya Yoshida, who remained deeply attached to the traditional styles of Japanese architecture, attempted a modern interpretation of these traditions in his building for the Japanese Academy of Art and several private houses. Kenzo Tange adopted a new curtain-wall technique for the Metropolitan Government Office in Tokyo. He also approached a traditional Jomon style in his use of reinforced concrete for the Sogetsu Hall and Kagawa Prefectural Office.

One of the most important problems for Japanese architects today is rationalization. They are encouraged by large-scale housing projects under the sponsorship of public corporations. Sky House, Kikutake's own house (1958), is an experiment pointing in the right direction for the future.

It is in the last ten years that Japan has given serious thought to the problems of her own cultural heritage. Younger architects such as Kiyonori Kikutake, Masato Otaka, Yoshinobu Ashihara are making great efforts to re-examine and revive Japanese architectural tradition and the Japanese way of living in terms of modern technology. The Kirishima Kogen Hotel, designed by Masachika Murata, is an attempt to achieve a harmony between the building and its natural environment, and the interior is perfectly in keeping with the traditional way of living (chopsticks and kimonos).

Bibliography: Shinji Koike, Contemporary Architecture of Japan, Tokyo 1953; Shinji Koike and Ryuichi Hamaguchi, Japan's New Architecture, Tokyo 1956; Udo Kultermann, New Japanese Architecture, London 1960.

SHINJI KOIKE

Jenney, William Le Baron, b. Fairhaven, Mass. 1832, d. Los Angeles 1907. Studied in Paris. He introduced the use of the steel frame in multi-storey buildings with his Home Insurance Building (Chicago, 1883–5), but the lavish mouldings of his masonry show no aesthetic consequences of his innovation. First Leiter Building (1879), second Leiter Building (1889–90), both in Chicago.

Johansen, John MacL., b. New York 1916. Studied at Harvard University under Walter *Gropius and Marcel *Breuer and worked in the offices of Breuer and *Skidmore, Owings and Merrill. Johansen is keenly interested in structural experiments: designs for a holiday house with a *reinforced concrete shell and a 'streamlined house' with walls of sprayed reinforced concrete. His design for the US Embassy in Dublin, a rotunda with circular courtyard and a façade of prefabricated, reinforced concrete frames, is based on the Irish round-tower tradition.

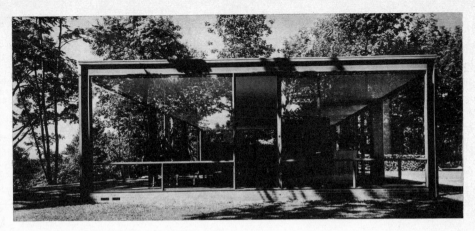

Philip Johnson. Johnson House. New Canaan, Conn., 1949

Johnson, Philip, b. Cleveland, Ohio 1906. Philip Johnson, the American architect, was the son of a prominent lawyer. In 1927, while studying classics at Harvard, he read an article on the modern movement in architecture by Henry-Russell Hitchcock which directed him towards his career: initially, in the thirties, as the first director of the pioneering architectural department of the Museum of Modern Art in New York; then, before the end of the forties, as a practitioner. During the period of his curatorship he distinguished himself as a propagandist and historian of the modern movement. In connection with the exhibition of modern architecture at the Museum in 1933, besides an influential catalogue, he wrote *The International Style* (1932) in collaboration with Hitchcock. It attempted an overall description of the aesthetic qualities of European modernism—and, incidentally, baptized the style with its generally accepted name (the suggestion of Alfred Barr, then Director of the Museum). Johnson's catalogue *Machine Art* (1934) was also influential, and the Museum's displays of industrial design under his aegis (while not exactly unprecedented in American museums) did much to stimulate museum interest in the exhibition of mass-produced objects. His catalogue for an exhibition of the work of *Mies van der Rohe (first edition, 1947; enlarged, 1953) was the first work on this architect.

Johnson's work as a propagandist for modern architecture whetted his appetite to become a practitioner. In the early forties, he left the Museum for Harvard, where he was strongly attracted by the teaching of Marcel *Breuer. But Mies, whom he had met in Europe in 1930, was his true mentor and he soon came to be known as Mies's most faithful disciple. His own 'Glass House' in New Canaan, Connecticut (1949) was derived from Mies's similar scheme for the Edith Farnsworth House in Fox River, Illinois (1950, but designed in 1946), and, more specifically, from the metal skeletal treatment of the buildings for the Illinois Institute of Technology. Despite these influences, the Glass House is a work of marked originality which instantly gained international recognition as among the masterpieces of the immediate post-war period. Unlike the austerely self-contained refinement of Mies's Farnsworth House, Johnson's Glass House possesses a romantic feeling for park-like landscape and a wealth of historical allusion (*Schinkel, *Suprematism, the diagram of the Acropolis from Choisy, for example). These qualities give an 18th-century quality of urbanity and wit to the play of the simple shapes on the terraced greensward: glass box, brick box and saucer pool diagonally opposed to one another around the axial vertical of Jacques Lipschitz's totemic *Figure.*

In a series of commissions for suburban houses Johnson elaborated the themes of the Glass House in various ways, and complicated them by the introduction of

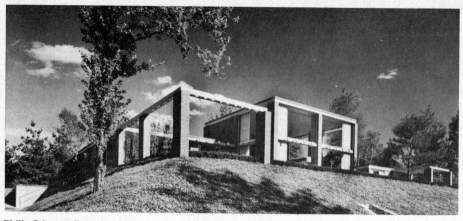

Philip Johnson. Boissonas House. New Canaan, Conn., 1956

courts. Notable among these early houses are the Hodgson and Wiley Houses in New Canaan (1951 and 1953 respectively), the Davis House in Wyzata, Minnesota (1954), and the Rockefeller Guest House in New York (now the property of the Museum of Modern Art, 1950). Meanwhile, Johnson's appreciation of both the architectonic and landscape values of the court led to what may well be the finest urban space designed during the decade and a half following the Second World War, the garden of the Museum of Modern Art (1953).

With his Temple Kneses Tifereth Israel at Port Chester, New York (1954–5), Johnson began to throw off his spiritual apprenticeship to Mies for more personal statements, although he was to collaborate with Mies on the Seagram Building (1957–), where his contributions are especially evident in the interior. In the Temple, the exposed Miesian metal skeleton is infilled with precast concrete slabs slotted with stained glass. The Ledoux-like ovoid entrance structure outside and the *Soane-like hung plaster vaulting within testify to his continued interest in bringing sophisticated historical allusions to bear on modern expression. Johnson's tentative use of precast concrete as a mural infilling in the Temple presages his increasing use of masonry in his recent buildings. In precast concrete or hand-carved masonry, he has reintroduced the classicist ideals of the portico and colonnade. His Sheldon Art

Gallery for the University of Nebraska in Lincoln (under construction) and the New York State Theater for the Lincoln Center (under construction) are major examples of this neoclassicism. Curvatures introduced at the juncture of column and 'entablature' of the Nebraska building are, by his own admission, also influenced by Gothic architecture. In his *béton brut* chapel for the Benedictine Priory in Washington, D.C. (designed in 1961), the relative weight of this combined classical/neo-Gothic inspiration shifts. If buttresses and vault are obviously medieval in feeling, the columnar character of supports alternating with the buttressing, together with the contained simplicity of the overall mass, are less evidently classicist. On the other hand, the specific design of the members is unimaginable without reinforced concrete construction.

Among the most convinced (and convincing) of modern 'traditionalists' (as Johnson has sometimes termed himself), his eclectic evocation of past architecture in his own work is far-ranging. For example, the domical forms of a nuclear reactor building for Israel (1960) and a shrine at New Harmony, Indiana (1960)—the first a gently gored shape in poured concrete, the second a bent wood and plywood structure thatched in wooden shakes—recall similar undulating domes in such a late Imperial Roman work as Hadrian's Villa or in Borromini's Baroque churches. But there are subsidiary recollections of Egyptian temple complexes in the one, of Indian *stupas* and Norwegian stave churches in the other. Meanwhile, both recall the austere containment of Ledoux's massing. Johnson's early interest in the steel skeleton appears in his campus complex for the University of St Thomas in Houston, Texas (two sections completed in 1959). He based the complex on Thomas Jefferson's scheme at the University of Virginia for an arrangement of separate buildings around a rectangular green, all linked by a covered colonnade. This interweaving of elemental building masses and covered colonnades with landscape also appears in his pavilion buildings, where the basic pavilion (supports and a roof) is repeated in plan as an irregular checkerboard. The Boissonas House in New Canaan (1956) and a garden pavilion for the Glass House (designed in 1961) variously call up classical, Islamic, and possibly Japanese prototypes, without specific reference to any of these.

The catholicity of his historical allusion notwithstanding, certain qualities generally characterize Johnson's urbane architecture: severely elemental massing, meticulous detailing and finish, a formal elegance of planning which disciplines even the casual environment, and, finally, a sensitivity to landscape values ranging from the well-manicured park to the planted terrace. As a teacher and critic he has magnified the influence of his buildings.

Bibliography: John Jacobus, *Philip Johnson*, New York 1962; 'Glass House', *Architectural Forum, 91*, New York November 1949; Henry-Russell Hitchcock, 'Philip Johnson', *Architectural Review, 117*, London April 1955; Philip Johnson, 'The Seven Crutches of Modern Architecture', *Perspecta 3*, Yale Architectural Journal; William H. Jordy, 'The Mies-less Johnson', *Architectural Forum, 111*, New York, September 1959; Ian McCallum, *Architecture USA*, London, New York 1959; Philip Johnson, *Perspecta 7*, pp. 3–8; Sibyl Moholy-Nagy, pp. 68–71; H.-R. Hitchcock, *Zodiac 8*, Milan 1961.

WILLIAM H. JORDY

Kahn, Albert, b. Rhaunen, Westphalia 1869, d. Detroit, Mich. 1942. Emigrated to America in 1881; 1928–32 in Russia (industrial building programme). Kahn's industrial buildings anticipated at an

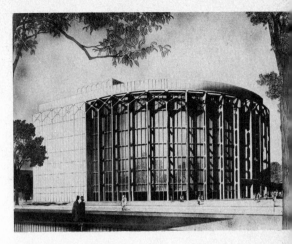

Philip Johnson. Theater of the Dance, Lincoln Center. New York, under construction. Project (first version)

early date the precise and slender cubic shapes of the fifties (*Mies van der Rohe, Eero *Saarinen). Ohio Steel Foundry Company at Limy, Ohio (1939); automobile works in Detroit.

Kahn, Louis I., b. Island of Osel, Estonia (Russia) 1901. Kahn came to the USA while young and received a traditional **Beaux-Arts* architectural education at the University of Pennsylvania, graduating in 1924. After various jobs and travel in Europe, he worked with an academic architect, Paul Cret, and during the depression did a project for the Philadelphia City Planning Commission. In 1941 he began an association with George *Howe, a pioneer in modern design in the USA who had created the earliest *International Style skyscraper outside Europe in the Philadelphia Savings Fund Society Building (with William *Lescaze) in 1932. Kahn's first work to attract any attention was the Carver Court War Housing Project, Coatsville, Pennsylvania (1942–3), in partnership with Howe and Oscar Stonorov. His independent practice dates from 1947. In 1950–1 he was resident architect of the American Academy in Rome, and subsequently became design critic at Yale. In 1955 he was named Professor of Architecture at the University of Pennsylvania.

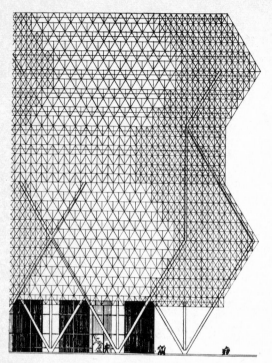

Louis I. Kahn. Building constructed from three-dimensional units. 1954. Project

Partly for lack of opportunity, partly because of an apparent reticence, Kahn did not emerge as a major creative figure until the mid 1950s. However, since that date he has been one of the most consistently discussed and admired of contemporary architects. Like all the undisputed masters of the 20th century, Kahn's mature style is the result of a dense fusion of many, sometimes contradictory, ideas and tendencies, all of which are brought together in a unique personal idiom. Unlike Philip *Johnson, Gordon *Bunshaft, and Eero *Saarinen, all of whom were drawing upon the industrial classicism of *Mies van der Rohe as a literal source for their designs of the early 1950s, Kahn, in his Yale Art Gallery, New Haven (1952–4), was already more self-reliant. The Miesian aspect of his first major building was not so much a matter of details and vocabulary as it was a question of creating large universal spaces for the gallery interiors (spaces which could be temporarily subdivided

according to need) and a simple cubic mass for the exterior. As for the details, the concrete frame and the tetrahedrons of the ceiling structure were a vigorous formal statement coming at a time when elegance and polished perfection were the fashion. Even the exterior, though aggressively simple in its contrast of brick and glass, avoided the classicizing smoothness of the then-popular Miesian envelope.

When the mid-20th-century wave of *neo-classicism and academicism at last overtook Kahn's design in the 1956 Trenton Bath Houses, his taste had already departed from the refined norms of Americanized modernism. At Trenton, the regular cross-axial plan with five square spaces, all but the central one being covered by pyramidal hipped roofs, revealed Kahn's early formed attachment to the plan-types favoured by the *beaux-arts* tradition, a tradition which, around 1895, had helped to focus the early development of *Wright, and which slightly later performed the same service in the orientation of *Le Corbusier's very different style.

This academicism, which was a literal aspect of Kahn's modest yet monumental Trenton building, aided in the creation of the more personally expressive Richards Medical Research Building, University of Pennsylvania (1958–60). Widely heralded by critics and architects as an unusually new departure in an age largely given over to imitations of the recent past, chic variations of historical styles, or irresponsible personal adventures, Kahn's Towers are equally, perhaps even more important as a major reinterpretation of several of the canonical aspects of the modern movement. Indeed, familiarity with this cluster of concrete and brick forms only underscores Kahn's reflexive utilization of his immediate roots, a utilization which is in no sense eclectic or narrowly cerebral. Some critics have noted that Kahn's perceptible separation of 'served' and 'servant' spaces parallels specific theorems in Wright's early work, notably the Larkin Building, Buffalo (1904); others are struck by similar instances of abrupt formal juxtaposition (caused by functional differentiation) that occur in works by Le Corbusier; while perhaps the most penetrating observation of all is that Kahn has, in this picturesque, red-brick conglomeration, found a road back to mid-19th-century

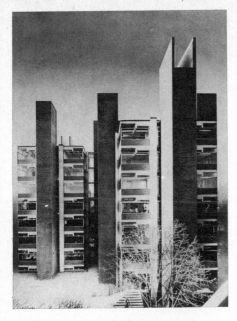

Louis I. Kahn. Richards Medical Research Building, University of Pennsylvania. Philadelphia, 1958–60

Victorian design principles, without, at the same time, sacrificing the gains of the modern movement. On the basis of this single building, Kahn has obtained a unique place in the annals of contemporary architecture, one which will certainly grow in the light of new constructions which have already begun to issue from his office.

JOHN M. JACOBUS, JR

Klerk, Michael de, b. Amsterdam 1884, d. Amsterdam 1923. Leading exponent of the generation of architects deriving from *Berlage, and centred round the journal *Wendingen* (*Netherlands). Residential buildings, especially in the suburbs of Amsterdam (*Expressionism).

Klint, Peter Vilhelm Jensen, b. near Skelskør 1853, d. 1930. Worked first as an engineer, then as a painter, and after 1896 as an architect. His best-known church is the Grundtvig Church in Copenhagen (1920–40), with its organ-shaped façade.

Kraemer, Friedrich Wilhelm, b. Halberstadt 1907. Studied at the Technical Colleges of Brunswick and Vienna. Private practice since 1935. Residential buildings, offices, schools, department stores, industrial buildings. Since 1946 he has been professor at Brunswick Technical College (Germany).

Labrouste, Henri, b. Paris 1801, d. Fontainebleau 1875. Trained at the *École des Beaux-Arts (Rome Scholar) which he later opposed with increasing vehemence. His epoch-making libraries employed steel frames encased in masonry. (Bibliothèque Ste Geneviève, Paris, 1843–50; Bibliothèque Nationale, Paris, 1858–68.)

Le Corbusier, b. La Chaux-de-Fonds, Switzerland 1887. Like few others of his generation, Le Corbusier (Charles-Edouard Jeanneret, called LC) had the opportunity while still studying of familiarizing himself with all the endeavours that led to the emergence of the new style. At his art school in La Chaux-de-Fonds reverberations reached him of Art Nouveau (in particular from the École de Nancy) and its search for organic, ornamental forms.

Le Corbusier

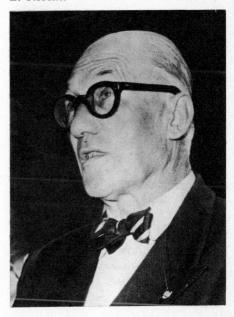

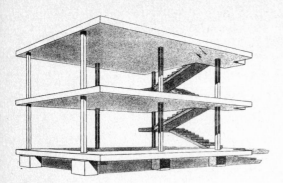

Le Corbusier. Dom-Ino system of construction. 1914

Then, in quick succession, he met nearly all the architects who had anything to give him: *Hoffmann in Vienna in 1907, *Garnier at Lyons and *Perret in Paris in 1908, and *Behrens in Berlin in 1910. He worked for a few months for both Perret and Behrens. In addition to his architectural and town planning studies, he was occupied from 1911 to 1912 with questions of mass-production and standardization in the circles of the *Deutscher Werkbund, which he had already been able to investigate under Perret, as far as they concerned the building trade. On extensive trips throughout Europe Le Corbusier, pencil in hand, analysed all possible architectural shapes and their settings from the Parthenon to a farmhouse, and from a Turkish summer house on the Bosphorus to Chartres Cathedral. After eventually settling down in Paris in 1917, he had his decisive encounter with Cubism. If we add that he

was occupied already before 1920 with the industrialization of building not only theoretically but practically, and that he exhibited a complete mastery of his profession in at least one executed design (Villa at La Chaux-de-Fonds, 1916), we shall come to the conclusion that the so-called amateur disposed of a knowledge and experience which no university training could have given him.

His preoccupation with painting, which he has never given up, and the founding, with Ozenfant, of Purism (*Après le Cubisme*, 1918) are far more than a mere episode. In attempting to determine the position of creative thought in the light of Cubism, Le Corbusier developed a theory of aesthetics which he published in the journal *L'Esprit Nouveau* in the form of 'Warnings to Architects'. In these articles, which appeared in 1923 in book form under the title *Vers une architecture*, followed in 1925 by *L'Art décoratif d'aujourd'hui*, *Urbanisme*, Le Corbusier has given the pithiest account of his architectural ideas. He himself demonstrated what he meant, first by models and drawings (Citrohan houses, 1920–2; 'A contemporary city of three million inhabitants', 1922), then by a series of houses (for Ozenfant, Jeanneret, La Roche, Cook, the Bordeaux-Pessac housing estate, 1922–6; Pavillon de l'Esprit Nouveau, 1925; Maison Stein at Garches, two houses at the Weissenhof Exhibition, Stuttgart, Villa Savoye at Poissy, 1927–31). These buildings, projects and writings are of threefold importance:

1. Every stylistic reminiscence is now rigorously removed from the vocabulary of

Le Corbusier. City of 3 million inhabitants. 1922. Project

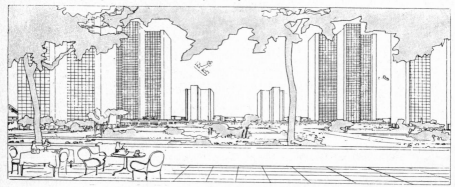

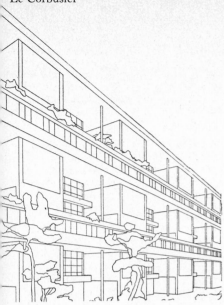

Le Corbusier. Immeuble-Villa. 1922. Project

form. In the uncompromising reduction of all buildings to the basic geometrical shapes of rectangle, plane surface, cube and cylinder may be recognized a transposition of purist pictorial composition. The architectural means employed are *pilotis* (free-standing columns at ground floor level), continuous strips of fenestration, glass walls, and flat roofs. The polychrome effects which Le Corbusier introduced at Pessac as a town-planning feature can also be traced back to insights gained when painting.

2. These distinctly provocative designs are meant to make clear the radically functional renovation of the house as an instrument of living; as is well known, Le Corbusier speaks of 'machines for living in'. After early studies of a more theoretical nature (Dom-Ino Houses, 1914; Monol Houses), Le Corbusier's investigations resulted in a prototype as early as 1922 (Second Citrohan House), which proved important for later developments. The living area available is newly distributed according to the way that domestic functions are grouped. The living-room runs through two storeys, and all parts of the dwelling are arranged *en suite*. The

house is enlarged by the open space which results from the flat roof garden and the *pilotis* (built at Stuttgart, 1927). Already in the same year, 1922, his project for Immeubles-Villas (multi-storey villas) illustrates the possibility of retaining meaningful living units in the only type of collective dwelling acceptable from the town planning point of view. The argument was supplemented by a full-scale model of such a living cell shown in the Pavillon de l'Esprit Nouveau in 1925. Instead of the ordinary type of furniture, use was made partly of built-in units, partly of standard industrial products chosen for their purist shape.

3. The multi-storey villas belong to that class of novel town planning device by which the structure of present-day metropolitan areas might be adapted to the requirements of modern life. The plan for a 'contemporary city of three million inhabitants' certainly springs from Garnier's *Cité Industrielle* and is also in many ways reminiscent of *Sant'Elia's drawings for the *Città Nuova*, but in essential points differs from both of them. Garnier had thought of a town limited to 35,000 inhabitants, all engaged in industry; Sant' Elia had only sketched highly suggestive but isolated views of the town of tomorrow. Le Corbusier, however, from the outset steered towards the problem of the 'change-over town', as he called it later, a metropolis with diverse functions, which must be

Le Corbusier. Maison Stein. Garches, 1929

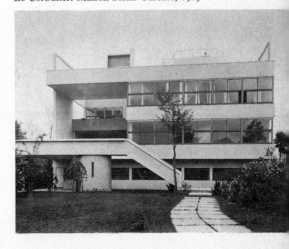

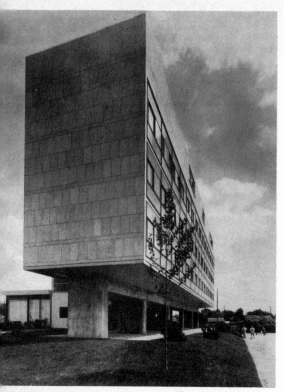

Le Corbusier. Maison Suisse. Cité Universitaire. Paris, 1930–2

disentangled. The Plan Voisin for Paris (1925) applies these theoretical studies to the particular case of Paris.

Le Corbusier is mainly concerned in the first instance to establish an orderly relationship between traffic lanes on the one hand and living and working zones on the other. Traffic must be classified, i.e. graded as to whether it is pedestrian or vehicular, through or delivery traffic. The tremendous loss of time occasioned by the incoherence of the present system may be reduced in this way. But 'traffic should not be allowed to develop'—the best way is to reduce distances to a minimum. If a metropolis is to be prevented from spreading out indefinitely, however, it must be built high: for residential areas multi-storey villas set in open parkland, instead of space-consuming, street-extending private houses; super-skyscrapers 1,300 feet apart,

surrounded by gardens, for business districts. This is the only way to unravel the present-day mix-up of traffic, work and living functions and to reduce the metropolis to human dimensions.

Owing to the economic crisis of the thirties, commissions by rich patrons of the arts, who were the main clients of modern architecture in France, were drastically reduced in number. Up to the outbreak of the Second World War, Le Corbusier devoted himself mainly to town planning projects (for Algiers, Nemours (Algeria), Barcelona, Buenos Aires, Montevideo, São Paulo, Zlín, Hellocourt, 'Paris 1937', 'Paris Ilot insalubre no. 6') and to refining the methods which he had only roughly defined: classified traffic lanes (the '7V' system), living units (design for the International Exhibition of 1937) and 'Cartesian' skyscrapers (design for Algiers, 1938). From the start (1927) Le Corbusier took an active part in the work of *CIAM. The *Athens Charter is entirely his idea and was also drawn up by him. His research, limited at first to restoring the urban body to health, was extended to country planning from 1934 onwards. In particular he interested himself in the renewal of production centres, agricultural ('radiating farm' and collective village, 1934) and industrial ('green factory', 1939–40). The synthesis of these ideas he ultimately summarized in 1945 in *Les Trois Etablissements Humains*, a book whose influence is still growing.

In the thirties, Le Corbusier also worked on his projects for monumental, large-scale buildings; in these he demonstrates his mastery in the organization and three-dimensional design of complex building programmes: competition design for the League of Nations Building in Geneva, 1927; plans for a museum with unlimited possibilities for extension (ultimately built in 1952–6 at Ahmedabad and Tokyo); the pensions office at Zurich; the Museum of Modern Art in Paris; a stadium and pageant arena for 100,000 spectators, etc. The only projects actually built were the Centrosoyus in Moscow, 1930; the Salvation Army Hostel and the Maison Suisse at the Cité Universitaire, Paris, 1931–2; and the Ministry of Education at Rio de Janeiro (in collaboration with *Costa, *Niemeyer and others, 1936–45). The ascetic geometry of his vocabulary of form which typified his

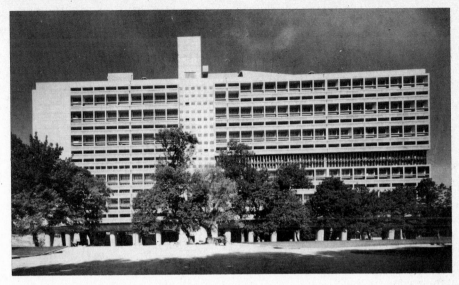

Le Corbusier. Unité d'Habitation. Marseilles, 1947-52

early work is enriched by new elements in these buildings and projects. White stucco gives way to an untreated finish (concrete or even stone in the Villa at Les Mathes, 1935). The abstract planary nature of the outer walls is superseded by a sculptural treatment, whose characteristic element is the 'brise-soleil' screen shading the glass wall (Ministry at Rio). This change is also noticeable on the 1938 model of a skyscraper.

Le Corbusier suggested 'Housing and Homes' as a theme for the 1937 International Exhibition, and as the main exhibit a completely furnished living unit, which could be let at the end of the exhibition. The idea to which he had constantly recurred since his multi-storey villas of 1922 was now ready for execution. This was how, after the war, the Unités d'Habitation at Marseilles (1947–52), Nantes-Rezé (1952–7), Berlin (1957) and Briey-la-Forêt (1960) came into existence. Here Le Corbusier's philosophy of domestic architecture seems to have found its final expression: vertical garden cities, which afford every family a maximum of privacy and independence (but also of communal services) combined with the utmost exploitation of space. These monumental structures, subtly proportioned on Le

Corbusier's *Modulor system, function impeccably as 'machines for living in' and belong, without any doubt, to the grandest architectural creations of the century. That they have found no imitator so far can only be explained, apart from the prejudice that still continues, by the unadmitted feeling that only Le Corbusier can play with such vast masses (350 flats in eight double-storeys) without being crushed by them.

Le Corbusier. Supreme Court. Chandigarh, 1950–6

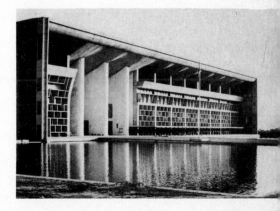

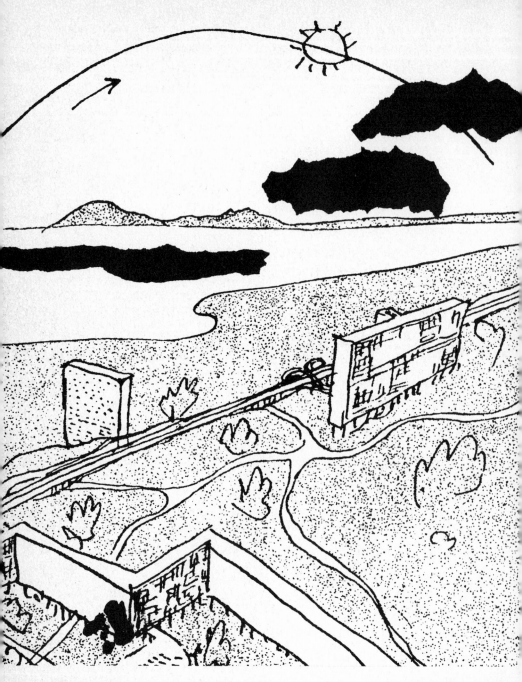

Le Corbusier. Project for Algiers Heights, 1942

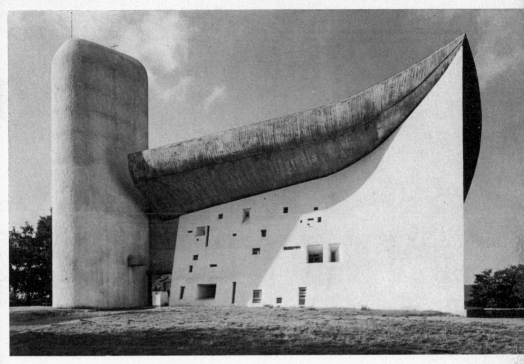

The other main projects of the fifties are as monumental as the 'Unités' and as likely to discourage any possible imitators. The capitol of Chandigarh (from 1950) is an approximately lyrical enhancement for the new metropolis of the State of Punjab of the idea for a community centre which Le Corbusier had worked out for the small town of St Dié in 1945–6. The symbolic significance of the composition, stressed by the dramatic treatment of the individual buildings, has been combined with astonishing ease into a harmonious whole with the practical functions that the law courts and the ministries have to fulfil, while making use of whatever local building resources were available. In the development and circulation plans for the city itself, Le Corbusier was able for the first time to realize his theories on zoning and traffic separation, practically without restriction. The grid-type layout, which some critics beforehand had called inhuman, has in practice proved excellent.

The pilgrimage church of Notre-Dame du Haut at Ronchamp (1950–4) strikes one at first as a wilful piece of sculpture, as

Le Corbusier. Notre-Dame du Haut. Ronchamp, 1950–4

Le Corbusier. Monastery of La Tourette. Eveux, near Lyons, 1957

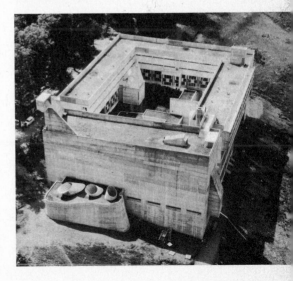

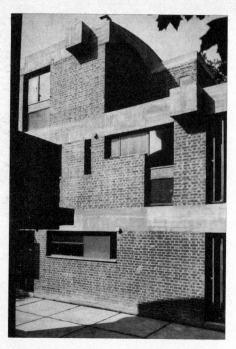

Le Corbusier. Maisons Jaoul. Neuilly, 1954–6

unsuitable for the fulfilment of any function as for instance F. L. *Wright's spiral shape for the Guggenheim Museum, built at roughly the same time. On closer examination, however, it proves to be an organism which (as previously with the living unit, the museum, the multi-storey offices, or even the farm) had been newly thought out in all its details and consequently completely altered in outward appearance. That the curved surfaces of Ronchamp were not just an impulse to which Le Corbusier had succumbed when he was confronted for the first time with a religious theme, has been proved by the Dominican novitiate monastery of La Tourette, at Eveux near Lyons (1957). The rectangle to which Le Corbusier had dedicated the 'Poème de l'angle droit' in 1955, is now only reserved for what Le Corbusier calls 'phénomènes d'espace indicible', 'phenomena of ineffable space', which he regards as the highest perfection in architecture.

Such ideas, in which his work has always abounded, give even his secular buildings of the fifties an unforgettable, special note,

whether they are 'Unités', museums, the Brazilian House at the Paris Cité Universitaire or smaller intimate buildings such as the Textile Industry Club, Shodhan House at Ahmedabad, and the Maisons Jaoul at Neuilly, or projects in which Le Corbusier's rich experience of architectural space has proved itself on difficult subjects such as the model for a multi-storey hotel at the Gare d'Orsay, Paris, or the design for a college building at Harvard (1961).

However diverse the shapes may be that Le Corbusier has employed—whether in the possibly most perfect example from his first creative period, the Villa Savoye at Poissy, or later at Ronchamp or Chandigarh, his architectural work nevertheless displays an amazing unity. It can only be called 'classical', if this is taken to mean not a repertoire of forms and massing, but a sense of the right form. The traditional modules and orders represented a harmonious link between the human body and the dimensions of ancient buildings and articles of use. In our contemporary civilization, however, whose towns, machines and equipment create completely new dimensions of space and time, they are no longer adequate. Their endless repetition is stifling, their extension emphatic and false. By a completely new, all-embracing system of measurement, by abandoning the scale imposed through dividing an elevation into storeys, but even more by an unprecedently sure instinct for proportion Le Corbusier has made his buildings examples of classical massing which contrasts sharply with the inhuman disorder of so many pseudo-modern buildings. Le Corbusier is the purest exponent of the French tradition in building, in whose noblest creations logic and lyric become one in the service of mankind.

Bibliography: Le Corbusier, *Oeuvre complète*, 1910–57, at present 6 volumes, Zurich 1929 ff.; Le Corbusier, *Mon Oeuvre*, Paris 1960; Maximilien Gauthier, *Le Corbusier*, New York 1945; Stamo Papadaki, *Le Corbusier*, New York 1948; J. Alazard, *Le Corbusier*, Florence and Paris 1950; Anton Henze, *Le Corbusier*, Berlin 1957; Françoise Choay, *Le Corbusier*, New York 1958; Boesiger/Girsberger (editors), *Le Corbusier, 1910–60*, Zurich and Stuttgart 1960.

MAURICE BESSET

Lescaze, William, b. Geneva 1896. Pupil of Karl *Moser. Architect of the Philadelphia Savings Fund Society Building (1932) in collaboration with George *Howe.

Lewerentz, Sigurd, b. Bjärtrå near Sundsvall, Sweden 1885. After graduating from Göteborg Technical College (1908), he lived in Germany. Residential buildings and housing estates. Crematorium at Malmö (1943), church at Skarpnäck near Stockholm (1960).

Lissitzky, Eliezer (El) Markovich, b. Polshinotz near Smolensk 1890, d. Moscow 1941 (or 1947). Studied at Darmstadt Technical College, 1909–14. Teacher at Moscow Academy, 1921. Emigrated to Germany and Switzerland, back in Russia 1928. Collaborated with the avant-garde of Central European architects (van *Doesburg, *Mies van der Rohe) and was a co-founder of *Constructivism. At the same time as *Tatlin's Memorial to the Third International, Lissitzky's office designed a speaker's platform (1920) in the form of a sloping steel structure of great expressiveness. In 1924, together with Mart Stam, he designed the 'Cloud Props' project, an extensively cantilevered office block on immense piers.

Lods, Marcel, b. Paris 1891. Collaborated with Eugène *Beaudouin. Designed buildings for the French Ministries of Education and War. Housing estate at Marly-le-Roi near Paris (with Honegger and Beuté), buildings in Guinea.

Loos, Adolf, b. Brno 1870, d. Vienna 1933. A keen admirer both of vernacular and Roman architecture, Adolf Loos was a great pioneer of the modern movement in Europe, and, at the beginning of the 20th century, one of the first architects to react against the decorative trends of *Art Nouveau.

Loos was the son of a stone-cutter. He attended classes at Reichenberg Polytechnic before studying architecture at Dresden technical college. On the conclusion of his studies he was anxious to broaden his outlook and in 1893 made a journey to the United States; he remained in America for three years, working by turn as a mason, a floor-layer and even as a dish-washer. During this time he was able to observe the innovations made by the young School of *Chicago: the expressive steel-frame structures Le Baron *Jenney introduced for office buildings, the austere blocks of *Burnham and *Root, and the uncompromising severity which *Sullivan was displaying in his famous Guaranty Building (Buffalo, 1894–5). Sullivan it was who, after providing American architecture with an original and personal style of floral surface decoration, wrote in 1892 in an article entitled 'Ornament in Architecture': 'It would be greatly for our esthetic good if we should refrain entirely from the use of ornament for a period of years, in order that our thought might concentrate acutely upon the production of buildings well formed and comely in the nude.'

This attitude was to provide Loos with a conception of major significance for his work. On his return to Europe in 1896, he settled in Vienna, a cosmopolitan centre with a culture typified by elegance of thought and sophisticated manners. In this milieu, Loos showed himself forthwith an

Adolf Loos. Kärntner Bar. Vienna, 1907

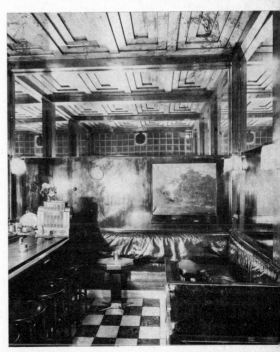

ardent and aggressive doctrinarian. In a first series of articles published chiefly in the *Neue Freie Presse* between 1897 and 1898, he took up arms against the stylistic and aestheticizing tendencies preached by the painter Klimt and the architects *Olbrich and *Hoffmann to the Wiener Sezession, which they had founded in 1897. Basing himself partly on Sullivan's purist argument, and partly on the functionalist doctrine which Otto *Wagner had expounded to the Vienna Academy in 1894, Loos set out to show that the type of ornament inculcated by Art Nouveau is unworthy of our culture; that a work divested of ornament is symbolic of pure and lucid thought and a high degree of civilization; that good form must find its beauty in the degree of usefulness it expresses, and in the indissoluble unity of its parts; and that consequently all ornamentation must be systematically rejected.

Loos was to resume and develop this thesis in a major essay published in 1908 entitled 'Ornament und Verbrechen' ('Ornament and Crime'). To spread his theories, he had founded a Free School of Architecture in 1906. His rationalist philosophy underlies his rare and very puritanical architectural works: the Villa Karma (Montreux, 1904); Steiner house (Vienna, 1910), one of the first private houses to be built in reinforced concrete, and a turning point in the history of modern architecture (reshaping of plan, new method of condensing and articulating internal space, purity of the straight line, flat roof, horizontal fenestration, dominance of solids, cubic style); the imposing Goldman commercial block on the Michaelerplatz (Vienna, 1910), where the arrangement of levels foretells the complete expression of the 'plan of volumes' achieved by the Rufer house (Vienna, 1922).

From 1920 to 1922 Loos was in charge of municipal housing in Vienna, where he drew up some bold development schemes, such as the Heuberg model estate. In 1923 he settled in Paris, where he established contact with the leading figures of the *Esprit Nouveau*. He frequented Dadaïst circles and built a house for Tristan Tzara (1926). Returning to Vienna in 1928, he built the Moller house at Pötzleinsdorf; the Khuner house at Payerbach (1930); and also in 1930, his finest work, the Müller house in Prague.

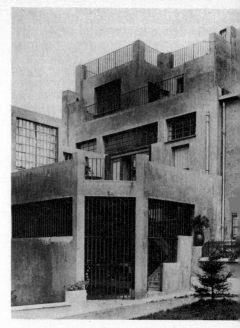

Adolf Loos. Maison Tristan Tzara. Paris, 1926

Bibliography: Adolf Loos, *Ins Leere gesprochen, 1897–1900*, Paris 1921; 2nd edition, Innsbruck 1932; Adolf Loos, *Trotzdem, 1900–1930*, Innsbruck 1931; Heinrich Kulka, *Adolf Loos*, Vienna 1931; Franz Glück, *Adolf Loos*, Paris 1931; Ludwig Münz, *Adolf Loos*, Milan 1956.

ROBERT L. DELEVOY

Luckhardt, Hans and Wassili. Wassili Luckhardt b. Berlin 1889. Hans Luckhardt b. Berlin 1890, d. Bad Wiessee 1954. Their first designs were in the Berlin *Expressionist style, characterized by the precision of their rectangles (Schorlemer Allee experimental estate, Berlin, 1927; private houses at Rupenhorn, Berlin, 1928) or dynamically curved blocks divided up by continuous strips of fenestration (projects for the new layout of the Alexanderplatz, Berlin, 1929). Berlin Pavilion at the Constructa Exhibition, Hanover (1951); Regional Government Offices, Munich (1957).

Bibliography: Udo Kultermann, *Wassili und Hans Luckhardt, Bauten und Entwürfe*, Tübingen 1958.

Lundy, Victor A., b. Los Angeles 1921. Studied at Harvard under *Gropius. Timber churches with large curved roofs (First Unitarian Church at Westport, Connecticut, 1961), Motel with reinforced concrete awnings at different heights (Warm Mineral Springs Inn at Venice, Fla., 1958). Exhibition pavilion of the US Atomic Energy Commission, a 'pneumatic' structure (1962).

Lurçat, André, b. Paris 1892. His houses typify the style of the late twenties and early thirties in France (Villa Hefferlin at Ville D'Avray, 1931–2). School at Villejuif (1931–3).
Bibliography: André Lurçat, *Oeuvres Récentes I*, Paris 1961.

Lyons, Eric Alfred, b. 1912. Architect whose schemes have set a new standard for private-enterprise housing in *Great Britain, where he controls the planning and landscaping of entire estates. His layouts feature simple buildings that display an eye for textures, and the highly repetitive use of structural elements and equipment in dispositions which largely avoid streets by creating courtyards and varying patterns of 'external enclosures'; this he considers to be the secret of urbanity. Flats at Ham Common, near Richmond; at Blackheath; and West Hill, Highgate (for the Soviet Trade Delegation). Houses, flats and maisonettes at Cambridge; housing for old people at Bognor Regis, with certain shared accommodation.

Lyons, Israel and Ellis. Edward Douglas Lyons, Lawrence Israel, Thomas Bickerstaff Harper Ellis. Partnership that has developed a powerful and expressive style in reinforced concrete: Peckham Comprehensive School (reinforced concrete frame); Wolfson Institute, London University; theatre workshops for the Old Vic Company, with constant expression of function by exposed reinforced concrete frame, inside and out; Trescobeas Secondary Modern School, Falmouth; Finchley Town Hall.

Mackintosh, Charles Rennie, b. Glasgow 1868, d. London 1928. Mackintosh, a resolute adversary of historic revivalism, was one of the most brilliant precursors of 20th-century rationalist architecture. As leader of the *Art Nouveau movement in Great Britain this Scottish architect made, a contribution of fundamental importance in reappraising the rôle of function in building, expressed via a style based on ancient Celtic ornament and the cultural traditions of Japan.

When he was barely sixteen, Mackintosh entered John Hutchinson's office as an articled pupil; from 1885 he attended evening classes at the Glasgow School of Art. In 1889 he was engaged as a draughtsman in the building firm of J. Honeyman and Keppie, where he met the architect J. Herbert McNair, his future brother-in-law. He stayed with the firm until 1913, having become a partner in 1904. In 1890 he was awarded a scholarship which enabled him to make a study-tour in France and Italy. His first executed work, the corner tower of the Glasgow Herald Building (1894), reveals Mackintosh as about to emancipate himself from academic trammels. He participated (December 1895) in the opening exhibition of the Maison de l'Art Nouveau in Paris with a number of posters which already clearly displayed the linear symbolic style of the Glasgow School. In 1897, at the age of twenty-nine, he won the competition for an extension to the Glasgow School of Art. These buildings were erected between 1898 and 1909 and made a profound impression on the Continent at the time. In 1898 he drew up a bold scheme for a concert hall on a circular plan, covered by a parabolic dome, which was not however premiated at the Glasgow Exhibition of 1901.

At the same time Mackintosh was interested in the decorative arts and in furniture. The pieces he designed are notable for their character, which is at once exquisite and austere, based on the straight line and the right angle, and set off in light tones (ivory). The upswing of their slim parallels elongates their forms beyond any functional requirement, as Mackintosh's aesthetic fancy turns to mannerism. This is the style he adopted when commissioned in 1897 to design the furniture and decorations for Cranston's chain of tea-rooms. The Buchanan Street Tea-room (1897–8) illustrates the curvilinear style of this first period (1894–1900) most completely: the walls are dominated by two-dimensional figures, tall and graceful, enclosed within a network of vertical

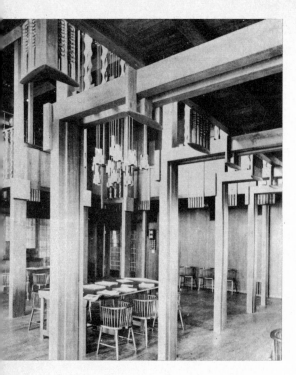

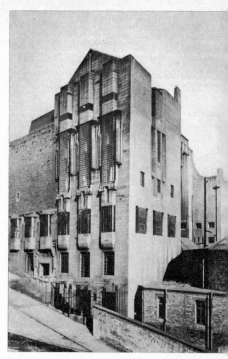

Charles Rennie Mackintosh. Library of the
Glasgow School of Art, 1907–9. Reading room

Charles Rennie Mackintosh. Library of the
Glasgow School of Art, 1907–9

lines and entwined by circular waves that
evoke the manner of Klimt. This style first
became known on the Continent through
the illustrations published in 1897 by *The
Studio*, followed the year after by the
showing of a suite of furniture at Munich,
and in particular by the contribution
Mackintosh sent to the annual exhibition
of the Wiener Sezession in 1900. The
furniture and panels he showed at Vienna
emphasize the close links between the
Scottish trends and the Viennese School.

In the same year Mackintosh had married
a former student of the Glasgow School of
Art, Margaret Macdonald, an interior
decorator and metalworker, whose sister
Frances had married the architect Herbert
McNair in 1899. These ties helped to knit
together more closely a little group united
since 1890 by similar professional and
aesthetic interests, which had already won
an international reputation under the name

of The Four. It was as the leader of this
group that Mackintosh entered a competition in 1901, organized under the auspices of the *Zeitschrift für Innendekoration*
of Darmstadt by its editor, A. Koch. The
subject was a house for a connoisseur,
including its interior decoration. Mackintosh was awarded second prize. His scheme
envisaged a revolutionary use of space, with
an arrangement of large, simple volumes
distinctly cubic in appearance, stripped, in
elevation, of any kind of ornament or
moulding, and marked by an asymmetrical
predominance of solids over voids: it
was a harbinger of the purist style of
*Loos.

If the country houses Mackintosh built in
the environs of Glasgow (Windy Hill at
Kilmacolm, 1899–1901; Hill House at
Helensburgh, 1902–3) still show external
stylistic affinities with the Scottish baronial
tradition (angle towers with conical caps,

huge double-pitch roofs, massive chimneys), their internal layouts evince great boldness in the handling of space. The hall of Hill House (1903) is a masterpiece where light, colour, openwork partitions, cage-type lamps and light furniture combine in a spatio-dynamic composition that anticipates Russian *Constructivism and Dutch *Stijl.

The superb library which Mackintosh built as an addition to the Glasgow School of Art (1907–9) shows similar stylistic trends. The straight line reigns supreme, and the subtle arrangement of horizontal beams and rectangular pillars which support the galleries punctuate space in a manner hitherto unknown, raising architecture to the level of poetic abstraction. Similar principles are at work, with equal effect, in Mackintosh's last masterpiece, the Cranston Tea-room in Ingram Street (1907–11). Apart from this, in his short architectural career, the Scottish Pavilion

at the Turin Exhibition of 1902 may be noted, which Mackintosh built and furnished.

He moved to London in 1913, where his activities were limited to designing furniture and printed fabrics. In 1920 he retired to Port-Vendres to devote himself exclusively to water-colour painting.

Bibliography: Hermann Muthesius, *Haus eines Kunstfreundes*, Darmstadt 1902; Nikolaus Pevsner, *Ch. R. Mackintosh*, Milan 1950; Thomas Howarth, *Charles Rennie Mackintosh and the Modern Movement*, London 1952.

ROBERT L. DELEVOY

Maekawa, Kunio, b. Niigata-shi, Japan 1905. Studied at Tokyo University; worked for *Le Corbusier; on his own since 1935. Maekawa's investigations into the structural possibilities of reinforced concrete (stimulated by Pier Luigi *Nervi) led to buildings in a sculptural idiom: Town Hall at Fukushima (1958), Community Centre at Setagaya (1959). His Harumi flats in Tokyo (1957) carry over Japanese domestic traditions into the dimensions of a modern skyscraper. Maekawa has had a considerable influence on the younger Japanese architects; Kenzo *Tange joined him on finishing his studies.

Maillart, Robert, b. Berne 1872, d. Geneva 1940. After studying from 1890 to 1894 at Zurich Technical College (ETH), where he graduated as structural engineer, Maillart worked in various engineering offices until he became an independent partner in the building firm of Maillart and Co., Zurich, in 1902. In 1911 he was appointed a lecturer at Zurich Technical College. In 1912 he left Switzerland to build in Russia, whence he returned penniless after the Revolution. In 1919 he started an engineering office in Geneva followed in 1924 by others in Berne and Zurich.

Maillart has not only built bridges but has also designed the structural details for a large number of multi-storey buildings. The intrinsic character of his constructions shows up particularly clearly, however, in his bridges: these are the outcome of his ability to think through a problem in its entirety and to look for the specific solution to each specific instance, based on his own specially developed methods of construction. In 1901, Maillart built the first of his

Charles Rennie Mackintosh. Glasgow School of Art, 1898–1909

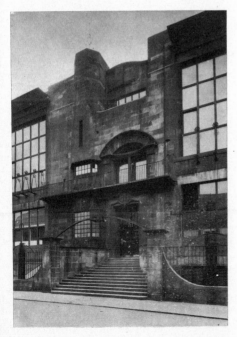

forty or so reinforced concrete bridges at Zuoz in the Engadine. It already displays some of the essential features of that concept of his which does away with the old principle of separation between the functions of bearing and loading. All parts of a bridge are integrated in their structural function; the roadway is no longer a load carried by the bridge vaults but is incorporated as a structure element. Economy of means, structural strength and harmonious balance make Maillart's bridges works of art to the extent that anything may be considered as art which is perfect of its kind.

Maillart's most important bridges are those built according to the principle he developed of the triply articulated box girder; they include the Rhine bridge at Tavanasa (1905, destroyed 1927) and the Salginatobel bridge near Schiers (1929–30, 295 feet long), both in Graubünden; the Rossgraben bridge near Schwarzenburg in the Canton of Berne (1932, 269 feet long); the Arve bridge near Versey, Geneva (1936); and the overpass between Altendorf and Lachen, Canton Schwyz (1940), the last project personally supervised by Maillart.

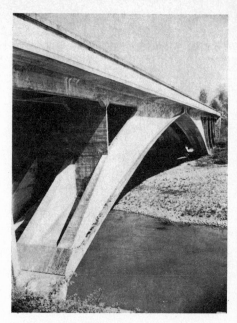

Robert Maillart. Bridge over the river Thur at Felsegg, 1933

Robert Maillart and Hans Leuzinger. Cement Pavilion at the Swiss Provinces Exhibition. Zurich, 1939

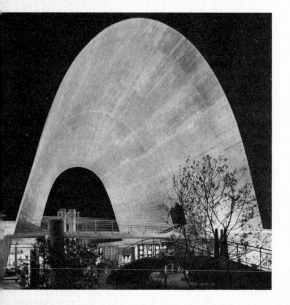

Another of his structural systems was the so-called stiffened bar arch which he used among others on the following: the Val Tschiel bridge (1925), and the curved Landquart railway bridge at Klosters (1930), both also in Graubünden; the Schwandbach bridge between Hinterfultigen and Schönentannen in the Canton of Berne (1933), also on a curve; and finally the Aire bridge at Lancy, Geneva, with an arch-span of 167 feet, designed in 1938 and built 1952–4. A number of his boldest bridge designs were never carried out.

Among the multi-storey buildings for whose architectural form Maillart's contribution was essentially responsible, the following may be mentioned: the entrance hall of a warehouse at Chiasso (1924–5) and the barrel-vaulted Cement Pavilion at the Swiss Provinces Exhibition, Zurich, 1939, a show building of the Swiss cement industry. His most important invention in the field of high structures was made in 1908 with mushroom slab construction, which he used for the first time on a large scale in 1910. In this method, columns, beams and floors are no longer treated as separate units as in timber or steel structures, but the

column passes organically into the beamless floor slab. Here again, a structural system that is economical in the use of materials permits flexibility in application and helps to ensure a light and elegant appearance.
Bibliography: Max Bill, *Robert Maillart,* Zurich 1949; 3rd edition 1962.
MARGIT STABER

Malevich, Kasimir, b. Kiev 1878, d. Leningrad 1935. In his early days, he was strongly influenced by the paintings of the Post-Impressionists, the Fauves, and later the Cubists. Transition to geometric (*Suprematist) painting between 1913 and 1915. His 'suprematist architectures' are architectural sculptures made of wood, in which he investigates the interrelation of simple cubes. Visited the *Bauhaus (1927).

Mallet-Stevens, Robert, b. Paris 1886, d. 1945. Exponent of French avant-garde architecture in the late twenties and early thirties. His buildings, in particular private houses, are often characterized by over-emphasis of cubic form.

Markelius, Sven, b. Stockholm 1889. Graduated in 1913 from Stockholm Technical College and from the Academy of Fine Arts in 1915. Influenced by *Le Corbusier. Flats and offices, concert hall at Hälsingborg (1932). First won international recognition with his Swedish Pavilion at the World Fair in New York (1939). Responsible for the establishment of the satellite town of Vällingby near Stockholm (commenced 1953) in his capacity as head of the town-planning department.

Matthew, Robert Hogg, b. Edinburgh 1906. Studied at Edinburgh College of Art School of Architecture. From 1946 to 1953, he was architect to the London County Council, during which period his department emerged as one of the most progressive forces in the architecture of *Great Britain, and his Royal Festival Hall (1950) was acclaimed as the first modern building to achieve a feeling of monumentality. Appointed Professor of Architecture at Edinburgh University, 1953; in private practice with Stirrat Johnson-Marshall since 1957. University buildings for Dundee, Aberdeen and Edinburgh; Turnhouse Airport, Edinburgh, 1956; New Zealand

House, Haymarket, London; seventeen-storey flats in the Gorbals, Glasgow; power station at Killin; Commonwealth Institute in Holland Park, London, with an ingeniously planned exhibition layout under a hyperbolic paraboloid roof. Far-reaching town- and country-planning proposals for the Government of Northern Ireland, 1963.

May, Ernst, b. Frankfurt 1886. Studied at Munich Technical College under Thiersch and *Fischer. Was City Architect at Frankfurt am Main between 1925 and 1930 (suburban development with extensive rationalization of building processes). In Russia (1930–4), later practised in East Africa. After the war served as town planner for several German towns.
Bibliography: J. Bueckschmitt, *Ernst May, Bauten und Planungen,* Stuttgart, in preparation.

Maybeck, Bernard Ralph, b. New York 1862, d. Berkeley, Calif. 1957. Studied at the École des Beaux-Arts in Paris. Was much impressed by the restoration work of *Viollet-le-Duc. Eclectic, especially Far Eastern motifs, which always played an important part on the west coast of America, were combined by him with structural experiments such as the employment of prefabricated units (Christian Science Church, Berkeley, 1910). Private houses, clubs. Fine Arts Building, San Francisco (1915) in neoclassic style with romantic trappings.

Mendelsohn, Erich, b. Allenstein, East Prussia 1887, d. San Francisco 1953. Among the architects of the 20th century who have used the new methods of construction made possible by steel and concrete with originality and imagination and have been successful in imparting to their buildings the quality of organic unity Erich Mendelsohn must hold a notable place. He received his architectural training at Berlin and Munich. In 1912 he started practice and for the first two years was engaged chiefly in stage designing, painting, and on projects for various buildings. During this period he became interested in the *Expressionist movement, and its influence can be seen in some of his early work. During the First World War he served in the German army, first on the Russian front and later on the Western front.

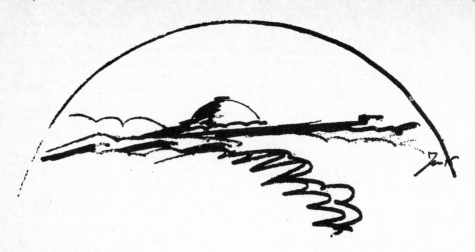

Erich Mendelsohn. Synagogue. Cleveland, Ohio, 1946–52. Project

Shortly after the war he held an exhibition in Berlin of architectural sketches which attracted considerable attention. They were designs of a wide variety of buildings: factories, grain elevators, observatories, religious buildings, in which steel and concrete were used expressively and in which the purpose of the building was suggested by the symbolism of its forms, thereby showing the influence of Expressionism.

One of his first buildings was the Einstein Observatory at Potsdam (1920) which caused a sensation. This was followed by a very large number of buildings that he designed during the twenties, including several departmental stores such as the Petersdorff Store at Breslau (1927), and

the Schocken Stores at Stuttgart (1927) and Chemnitz (1928); a group of buildings adjoining Kurfürstendamm which included a cinema with a dramatic interior with horizontal emphasis (1928); and the Columbus House (1931), a large block of offices and shops in the Potsdamerplatz, which together with the Schocken Store at Chemnitz represent Mendelsohn's best work in Germany. The façades of both have long bands of fenestration alternating with opaque bands, and the whole effect is one of lightness combined with grandeur, the effect of lightness being achieved by a cantilevering of the walls beyond the structural supports.

Owing to the racial persecution which accompanied the rise to power of the

Erich Mendelsohn. Schocken Department Store. Stuttgart, 1927. Project

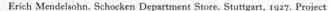

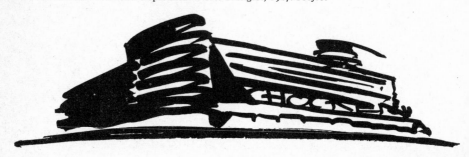

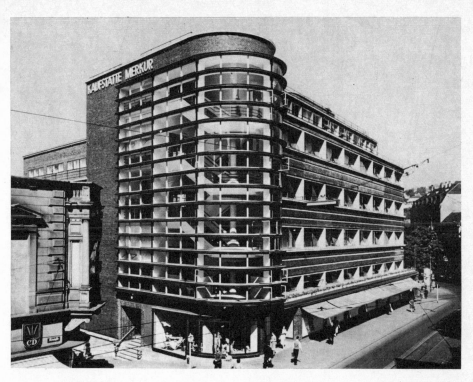

National Socialist Party, Mendelsohn left
his native land in March 1933 and went
first to Brussels, and then to London,
where he began practice in partnership
with Serge Chermayeff in the summer of
that year. For the next six years Mendelsohn divided his practice between England
and Palestine. His principal work in
England was the now famous De la Warr
Pavilion, Bexhill (1934). His work in
Palestine was more considerable and included two large hospitals, that at Haifa
(1937) and the University Medical Centre
on Mount Scopus, Jerusalem (1937–9); the
Palestine Bank, Jerusalem (1938); several
large houses, a college and library.

In 1941 Mendelsohn went to America, and
after the war he started practice in 1945
in San Francisco. His principal work in
America was the Maimonides Hospital in
San Francisco (1946) and a series of large
synagogues and community centres, some
of which remained only projects. Those
completed are at St Louis, Missouri
(1946–50); Cleveland, Ohio (1946–52),
which includes a large dome 100 feet in

Erich Mendelsohn. Schocken, later Merkur,
Department Store. Stuttgart, 1927

Erich Mendelsohn. Columbus House. Berlin, 1931

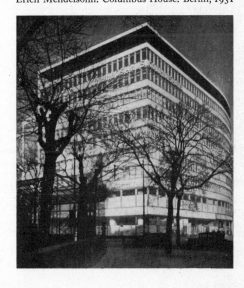

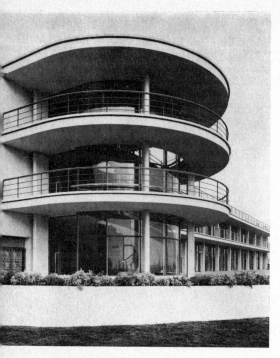

diameter; Grand Rapids, Michigan (1948–52); and St Paul, Minnesota (1950–4).

Mendelsohn's work was characterized by a sympathetic and original use of materials, steel, concrete and glass, and by an expression of purpose through the forms of his building, seen in such works as the Observatory at Potsdam, the departmental stores in Germany, the Bexhill Pavilion, and the hospitals in Palestine. His designs were always actuated by the principles of organic unity, so that each part by its character denotes its relation to the whole, and each building is closely wedded to its site. The synagogue at Cleveland, where the forms of the building harmonize so well with the contours of the undulating site, is a notable example.

Bibliography: Mario Federico Roggero, *Il contributo di Mendelsohn alla evoluzione dell'architettura moderna*, Milan 1952; Bruno Zevi, 'Eric Mendelsohn', in *Metron*, Nos. 49–50, Rome 1954; Arnold Whittick, *Eric Mendelsohn*, London 1956, New York 1956, Bologna 1960.

ARNOLD WHITTICK

Erich Mendelsohn. De la Warr Pavilion. Bexhill, 1934

Erich Mendelsohn. House on Pacific Heights. San Francisco, 1950–1

Messel, Alfred, b. Darmstadt 1853, d. Berlin 1909. Flats and commercial buildings, in particular department stores (Wertheim department store in Berlin, 1896), with extensive use of glass on façades and basically functional design.

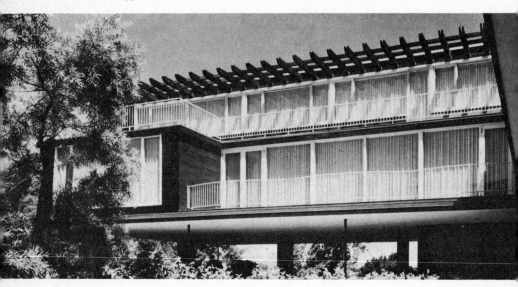

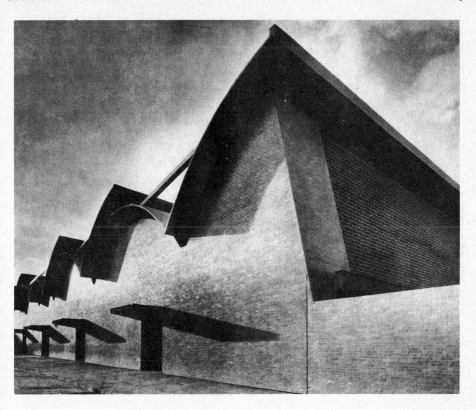

Mexico. Mexico was the first of the Latin-American countries to come to terms with the claims of the *International Style. The revolt against the senseless imitation of inherited building forms in the mid-twenties, i.e. a decade before the building of the Ministry of Education at Rio de Janeiro, found expression first in the teaching of the architect José *Villagrán Garcia and in his early works and those of his pupils Legorreta, *O'Gorman, de la Mora and Yáñez. The hospitals, houses and schools designed by this group took the Functionalism of *Le Corbusier's *Vers une architecture* literally, and thus presented the starkest contrast to the popular love of decoration. During the two subsequent decades, modern architecture made uninterrupted progress in Mexico. The economic advantages of the purism that went hand in hand with the new structural methods, account for only a part of its rapid success. In the main it was due to the fact that the

Enrique del Moral. 'La Merced' Market Hall. Mexico City, 1957

Pedro Ramírez Vázquez and Rafael Mijares. Ministry of Labour and Social Welfare. Mexico City, 1953

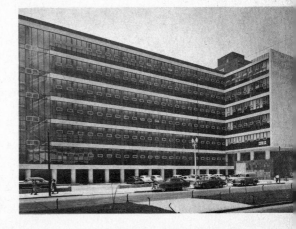

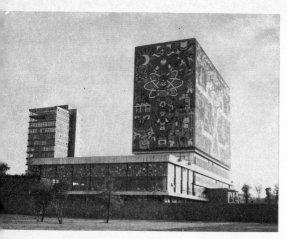

Juan O'Gorman, Gustavo Saavedra and Juan Martínez de Velasco. University Library. Mexico City, 1952

government held the modern style to be an adequate expression of its progressive administration and social building programme, and used it for numerous buildings, thus helping it to secure general approval. At the beginning of the fifties this development reached its peak in the building of the University City (to a layout by Mario Pani and Enrique del Moral) for 20,000 students, a number which has doubled in ten years. With the collaboration of approximately one hundred young architects and engineers, the extensive complex was finished in three years.

Mexico's building tradition, which in contrast to the *USA has strong roots in the centuries before and after its conquest by Europeans, has left its mark on the modern architecture of the country. In the University City this influence is immediately obvious in the extraordinary dimensions of its open spaces and in the ever-recurring passion for decoration. In the name of integrating art and architecture, the restraint of the last twenty years was abandoned and all available surfaces were covered with murals, mosaics and reliefs in an idiosyncratic social-realist style. In some cases, as for instance the main library (Juan° O'Gorman) and the stadium (Diego Rivera), this kind of façade decoration may be considered successful. But its unfettered use, as for example on the Ministry of Transport

building, has reduced this tendency to the absurd.

In the capital today, offices and hotels with *curtain walls reign supreme in the North American manner (architects: Alvarez, Marcos, Kaspé, Sordo Madaleno, Villagrán García and others). State-backed housing schemes are currently being promoted in increasing measure, and large, integrated complexes—whole districts even of apartment houses—are being built (architects: Felix Sánchez, Alejandro Prieto, Mario Pani). Private houses have a more distinctive personality, especially those in the new suburb of Pedregal, built on a foundation of lava in the southern part of Mexico City (architects: Barragán, Cetto, Greenham, Artigas, Attolini Lack, Rosen, Castañedo and others).

Mexico's contribution of the greatest significance to modern architecture lies in the most recent development of shell vaulting by *Candela. Often, in collaboration with other architects, he has built factories, warehouses, filling-stations, market halls, pavilions, restaurants and churches in free organic shapes, from which a new sculptural quality emerges. It was with similar intentions, based however not so much on structure as on a mannerist attempt to broaden the frontiers of architecture, that the sculptor Goeritz fashioned his 'emotional' casing for the Eco nightclub (1953) and the group of non-functional towers at the entrance to a satellite town under construction (1958). The painter-architect

Juan O'Gorman. O'Gorman House. San Angel, 1956

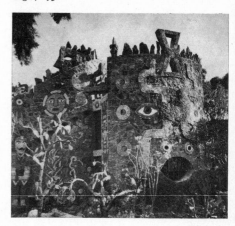

Juan O'Gorman peopled his fantastic dream cave inside and out with creations made of coloured stones and seashells.

The school building programme of the present government, which will take till 1970 to complete, deserves the international regard which was given it at the XII Triennale at Milan. Its essential core is a school unit made up of prefabricated parts by the architect Ramírez Vázquez and his collaborators, which solves the urgent problem of Mexican village schools both economically and functionally.

Bibliography: I. E. Myers, *Mexico's Modern Architecture*, New York 1952; Henry-Russell Hitchcock, *Latin-American Architecture since 1945*, New York 1955; Max Cetto, *Moderne Architektur in Mexico*, Stuttgart 1960.

MAX CETTO

Meyer, Adolf, b. Mechernich, Eifel 1881, d. on the island of Baltrum, in the North Sea 1929. Trained as a cabinet-maker. Attended the Art School at Düsseldorf and worked as an architect with *Behrens and Bruno Paul. He taught at the *Bauhaus from 1919 to 1925 and worked as city architect in Frankfurt from 1926 to 1929. Meyer was a collaborator of *Gropius (Fagus Works at Alfeld, 1911, and Jena Municipal Theatre, 1925), then flats, schools, the planetarium of the Zeiss Works in Jena (1925–6), and municipal buildings in Frankfurt.

Meyer, Hannes, b. Basle 1889, d. Crocifisso di Savosa, Switzerland 1954. Appointed lecturer and studio master at the *Bauhaus, Dessau, and succeeded *Gropius as director (1928–30). Competed (with Hans Wittwer) for the League of Nations Building, Geneva (1927); German Trades Union School at Bernau (1928–30), a school laid out in separate blocks. Worked in the Soviet Union from 1930 to 1936, then in Switzerland; from 1939 to 1949 in Mexico. Meyer rejected architecture that depended on aesthetic principles of form: 'Architecture is not the individual, emotional activity of an artist. Building is a collective activity.'

Michelucci, Giovanni, b. Pistoia 1891. Took his architect's diploma at Florence in 1914. Joint architect of the S. Maria Novella Station at Florence (1933–6). Savings Bank, Florence (1953).

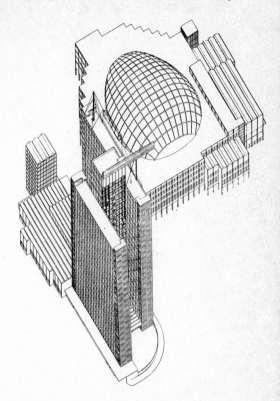

Hannes Meyer and Hans Wittwer. League of Nations Building, Geneva, 1927. Project

Mies van der Rohe, Ludwig, b. Aachen (Aix-la-Chapelle) 1886. Ludwig Mies van der Rohe, German-American architect, is generally acknowledged as one of the four most influential architects working during the first half of the 20th century—the others being Frank Lloyd *Wright, *Le Corbusier, and Walter *Gropius. He was born Ludwig Mies, later compounding his surname with that of his mother. Without formal training as an architect, his initiation into building and the superb craftsmanship for which his architecture is famous, came initially from his father, who was a master mason and the proprietor of a stone-cutting shop. Mies learned to draw as a designer for stucco decoration. In 1905 he went to Berlin where he worked briefly for a minor architect who specialized in wooden structures. Better to master this

material, he apprenticed himself for two
years to Bruno Paul, a leading furniture
designer. In 1907 Mies set up briefly on
his own as an architect, but the following
year he joined Peter *Behrens, at the time
the most creative architect in Germany.
While Mies worked in the office, Walter
Gropius was among the chief designers,
and Le Corbusier passed a few months
there.

The three years which Mies spent with
Behrens (until 1911) provided his most
valuable training. In a sense Behrens's
career anticipates Mies's. On the one hand,
as the designer for the Allgemeine Elek-
tricitäts Gesellschaft (AEG), Behrens not
only designed the factory buildings of
the German electrical combine but its
products as well. More than any other
architect of his generation, he therefore
anticipated the ideal of the architect as a
comprehensive designer for the modern
industrial society. Behrens's product design in metal reinforced the training which
Mies had received in cabinet making from
Paul, while both contributed to Mies's
achievement in furniture design. Moreover, Behrens's Turbine Factory in Berlin
(1909), with its bold exposure of the metal
structural frame infilled with glass, is
astonishingly prophetic of Mies's much
later development of an architecture
austerely dependent on the naked metal
skeleton. But Behrens's factory production
represented one aspect only of his *œuvre*.
He also brought the neoclassicism of Karl

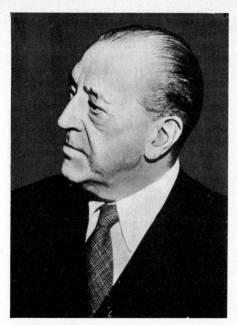

Ludwig Mies van der Rohe

Mies van der Rohe. Kröller House. The Hague,
1912. Project

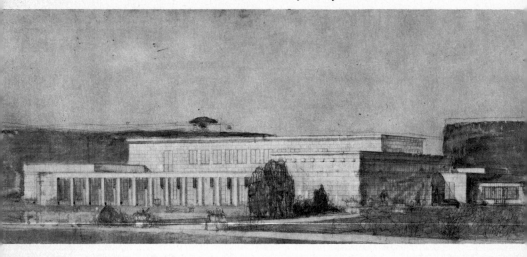

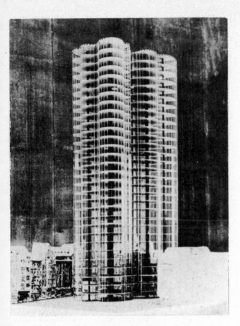

Mies van der Rohe. Glass skyscraper. 1920-1.
Project

Friedrich *Schinkel to his architecture—
especially to his monumental and domestic
commissions, although Schinkelesque neoclassicism occasionally appears in the
severe masonry piers and simplified pedi-
ments of some of his factories as well. To
create a modern architecture with a neoclassical severity of means, purity of form,
perfection of proportions, elegance of detail
and dignity of expression is the underlying
preoccupation of Mies's career. For this
ideal he owed much to the imperfect
synthesis of industrialism and neoclassicism in Behrens's work.

Initially, Mies was more overtly influenced
by the neoclassical rather than by the
industrial aspects of Behrens's work, in
large part perhaps because he had served
as the supervisor of construction for one
of Behrens's most monumentally neoclassical edifices, the German Embassy in
St Petersburg (1911–12). Leaving Behrens
in 1911, Mies designed several houses in
a neo-Schinkelesque style akin to Behrens's
work. The most notable design of the
group (and superior to the neoclassicism
of his mentor) was a projected house and

gallery for Mme H. E. L. J. Kröller (1912),
the owner of the famed Kröller-Müller
Collection. This went as far as a full-scale
mock-up of the house in canvas and wood,
built on the site at The Hague. For the
Kröller commission, Mies went to Holland.
There he came to know the work and
philosophy of Hendrik Petrus *Berlage,
who was the Dutch counterpart to Behrens.
Where Behrens was primarily concerned
with form, however, Berlage derived his
architectural philosophy from the 19th-
century moralistic theory of the 'honest'
expression of structure and materials,
which was Gothic rather than neoclassical
in inspiration. Taken together, Behrens's
emphasis on neoclassical form, Berlage's
on revealed structure and materials, and
their joint desire for a new architecture
somehow expressive of modern conditions,
might be said to stake out the territory
which Mies would explore.

His romantic neoclassicism continued up
to the war. After this interruption to his

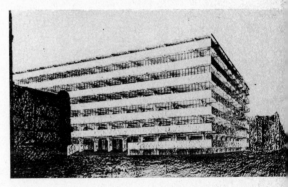

Mies van der Rohe. Reinforced concrete office
building. 1922. Project

career, there was, in 1919, one last post-
war project in the Schinkelesque vein.
Whereupon Mies's career in modern architecture was abruptly launched in a series of
projects from 1919 to 1924 which are
astonishingly varied and original. They
reflect the sense of liberation in post-war
Berlin which suddenly felt the impact of
native *Expressionism, of De *Stijl from
Holland, of *Constructivism and *Suprematism from Russia. Mies was active in
this ferment, not only as a designer, but as
a propagandist too. He was among the

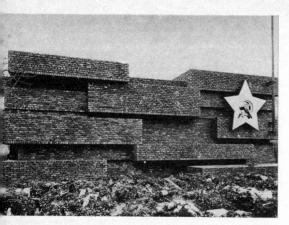

Mies van der Rohe. Memorial to Karl Liebknecht and Rosa Luxemburg. Berlin, 1926

founders of the magazine *G* (for *Gestaltung*, or creative force) which was devoted to modern art. He joined the *Novembergruppe*. Founded in 1918, and named after the month of the Republican Revolution, this organization too publicized the modern movement. Mies directed the architectural section from 1921 until 1925. It was principally in the annual exhibitions of the *Novembergruppe* that his early modern projects appeared.

In two glass skyscrapers, the first (1919) of triangular forms, the second (1920–1) of curved free forms, Mies sought to dramatize the reflective qualities of glass in

Mies van der Rohe. Wolf House. Guben, 1926

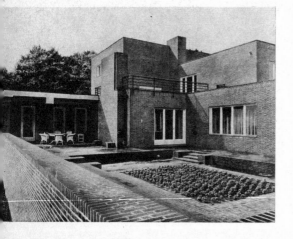

faceted shapes. In fact, the free form curvature of the second of these skyscrapers was specifically determined by the shape which produced the greatest play of light over the building. A project for a reinforced concrete office building (1922) was even more prophetic. Cantilevered slabs closed by a parapet permitted continuous inset window bands with the lightest of metal mullions. Although not widely known until much later, this project, among the first ribbon window designs, uses the ribbon motif so logically and purely that, as a consummate expression of what became a familiar element in modern architecture, it has remained unsurpassed. The initial series of projects is concluded by two houses. One, that of 1923 for a brick country house, uses De Stijl principles. Brick panels in slab, L and T shapes, infilled where necessary with floor-to-roof window panels, modulate a spatial continuity through their arrangement in a tense asymmetrical equilibrium in space. For the first time in architecture, the wall by its placement and shape actually generates the plan. Although the design is schematic only, it nevertheless represents the first truly architectural achievement employing De Stijl principles of composition, since earlier ventures had arbitrarily intermixed De Stijl with Cubist elements. The second project for a country house, this time for a concrete structure, is a spreading structure in a pinwheel composition around a multi-terraced site. Both the horizontality of the house and the determination of the irregular mass in accordance with the major elements of the plan run counter to the compact *prisme pur* enclosure of space which dominated the *International Style at the time. Mies's concrete country house in this respect looks rather ahead to later developments of the International Style after 1930. On the whole these five projects are among the most creative architectural conceptions of the early twenties, and remain among the least dated.

The latter half of the twenties finally sees a few (very few) executed buildings in Mies's modern style. Notable among them are the Monument to Karl Liebknecht and Rosa Luxemburg in Berlin (1926, and demolished by the Nazis). A textured brick slab, faceted with horizontal, box-like projecting and receding elements and emblazoned at one end by the hammer and sickle with a flagstaff, it is among the few significant memorials erected in the 20th century. Two brick houses—the Wolf House in Guben (1926) and the Hermann Lange House in Krefeld (1928)—reveal how far Mies had come from his pre-war neo-Schinkelism, and how much his early neoclassicism continued to influence his work. Both possess a solidity and rootedness at variance with current practice in the International Style. Their elegance of detail and proportioning are such as Schinkel himself would have admired. The Wolf House is especially fine in the extension of the beautiful precision of the brick walls (a material which Mies had come to appreciate during his interlude in Holland) and in an abstract arrangement of brick terracing reminiscent of the Liebknecht-Luxemburg Monument. Meanwhile, during the late twenties, too, Mies continued to be interested in the glass office building, and he projected no less than four different schemes, none of which came to fruition. His early work in planning the exhibitions of the *Novembergruppe* prepared him to design several such exhibitions in which products are displayed with a restrained elegance that enhances their visual qualities.

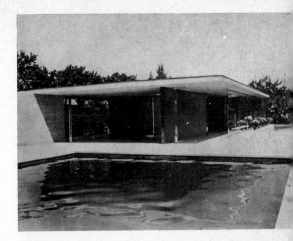

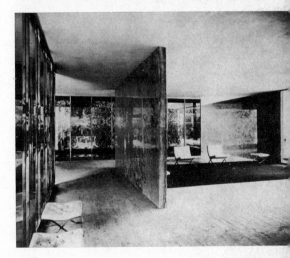

His work at this time, however, is climaxed by two major works. One, the Weissenhof-siedlung in Stuttgart (1927), was a large-scale outdoor exhibition of housing of various types with designs by most of the leading modern European architects. Sponsored by the *Deutscher Werkbund and directed by Mies, this outdoor exhibition contained no less than twenty-one permanent buildings, ranging from one-family villas to Mies's dominating apartment structure, together with an adjunct of temporary exhibits. The most comprehensive group endeavour of the International Style, it clearly revealed the unifying characteristics of European modernism, An even more impressive work qualitatively, and indeed among the masterpieces of modern architecture, was Mies's German Pavilion for the International Exhibition in Barcelona (1929). It continues the De Stijl experiment of Mies's project for a country house of 1922, but with a simplification of elements and a breadth of treatment far surpassing the complications of the earlier design. Over a portion of a

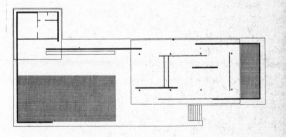

Mies van der Rohe. German Pavilion at the International Exhibition. Barcelona, 1929

raised podium, Mies lightly supported a reinforced concrete slab on cross-shaped, chrome-plated steel columns. He placed vertical slabs of travertine and panels of glass of various kinds well under the spreading slab of the roof. Partially enclosing the roofed area, and partially sliding from under it, these panels in their right-angled asymmetrical arrangement loosely, but firmly, ordered the space while preserving its continuity. Two pools completed the complex: the larger on the open terrace; the smaller at right angles to it at the opposite end of the podium. The smaller is enclosed in a semi-court created by the slide of the travertine panels from under the slab of the roof. The sculpture of a female figure by Georg Kolbe placed in the water serves as a tenuous point of destination within this scrupulously chaste pavilion, otherwise occupied (so far as the standard photographs tell us) only by some of Mies's furniture. It was in this pavilion that he displayed his famous 'Barcelona Chair'. Among the classics in modern furniture design, this was the culminating piece in a series of distinguished designs which Mies realized during the late twenties. Although relatively little noted during the summer of its existence, the photographic record of the modest structure—truly 'almost nothing' in Mies's own aphorism on his architecture—has made it

among the most influential buildings of the 20th century.

Immediately after the Barcelona Pavilion, Mies designed the most important house of his European career, the concrete-surfaced Tugendhat House at Brno, Czechoslovakia (1930). Built on a gentle slope, the house presented a closed one-storey front to the street, with two storeys to the rear. The continuous space of the lower living floor with its chrome-plated columns and freestanding panels (one a semicircle of Macassar ebony) recalled the treatment of the Barcelona Pavilion. Here an even richer display of Mies's furniture completed an elegance, every detail of which (down to the curtain tracks) was meticulously custom-designed.

The Tugendhat House was Mies's last important executed building in Europe. Among the projects of the early and mid thirties the designs for houses within walled courts are the most interesting. Although the surrounding brick walls occasionally opened on to a distant view, for the most part these houses were wholly bounded by their rectangular frame, while in one instance several houses of various sizes, walled from one another, shared the same enframement. Inside the enclosure there was the usual Miesian spatial continuity interrupted here and there by carefully placed glass walls and solid panels, partially roofed (again slabs on metal supports), and partially open overhead. Indoors and out, ceiling and sky, solid and transparency are brought into intimate play with one another in these characteristically dynamic but serene spaces which are here adapted to a type of residence ideal for urban living.

On Gropius's recommendation Mies succeeded him as the Director of the *Bauhaus in 1930. Immediately thereafter, however, Nazi pressure forced Mies to move the school from Dessau to Berlin. There it had a tenuous existence, until Mies finally decided to close it in 1933. The hostile political environment made it increasingly impossible to work in Germany and, in the summer of 1937, when just past fifty, he emigrated to the United States. There, in 1944, he became an American citizen.

Whereas Mies had built relatively little in Europe and his work was known to a discriminating few, his practice and influence grew rapidly in the United States. It

Mies van der Rohe. Tugendhat House. Brno, 1930

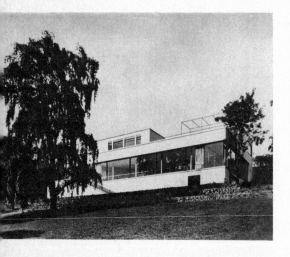

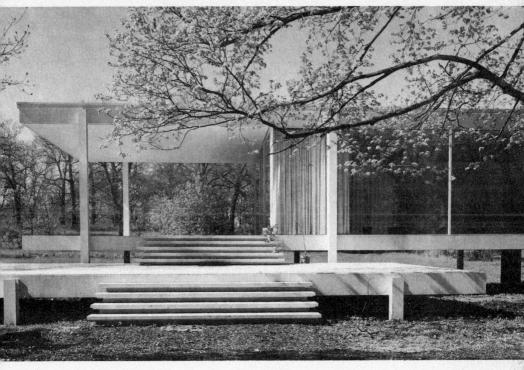

Mies van der Rohe. Farnsworth House, Fox River, Ill., 1946–50

was here, precisely a decade after his arrival, that Mies had his first large retrospective exhibition at the Museum of Modern Art in New York. For this exhibition his principal disciple, Philip *Johnson, published the first book on Mies's work—at a time when, as he notes in the preface, only two articles wholly devoted to Mies's work had appeared. This publicity and the importance of his American commissions established Mies's popular fame. In 1938 he had been called to teach at the Illinois Institute of Technology (then known as the Armour Institute) in Chicago, as Gropius had been somewhat earlier called to Harvard. His first major American commission, a campus plan (1940) and buildings (the first in 1942–3) for IIT, immediately established the central theme of his American work: the exposed metal frame as it reticulated neutral rectangular volumes. He viewed the cleared site, which consisted of a number of city blocks in a scrubby area of the Chicago South Side,

as an idealized space, much like the podium of the Barcelona Pavilion. On this he arranged rectangular and slab-shaped blocks in accord with a modular grid for the entire project, such that semi-courts and corridors of space were created in a manner analogous to (but more formal than) his conditioning of interior space by slabs from the Barcelona Pavilion onward.

The revealed metal frame in his American buildings is rarely the structure itself, since fire regulations demand that most steel must be covered. Hence the visible 'structure' is more often symbolic of the reality beneath, much as pilasters symbolized columns in Renaissance buildings—except that Mies's pseudo-structure more convincingly resembles and more intimately relates to the real thing within. From the standard alphabet of the steelmaker's catalogue (the I-shaped beams, the H's, L's, the plates, and channels), he welds mouldings as the metallurgical equivalent of the carved mouldings of the past. The careful proportioning of his frame, the gradation of components from heavy to light, the firm elegance of his profiling and the subtleties of transitions where corners occur or one material butts another: this intensity of effort and artistry expended on the image of the structure has been unexcelled and all but unmatched by his numerous followers, most of whom have taken his image as a mere convenience for prefabrication.

Even as the first buildings were going up on the IIT campus, Mies designed (1946, completed 1950) a glass and metal house for Dr Edith Farnsworth in Fox River, Illinois. Three floating slabs—a terrace slab, and behind it floor and roof slabs— are all lifted from the ground on metal I-beam supports. The welding of the supports to the sides of the slabs, as though magnetism kept the frame intact, enhances the floating quality of the spreading slabs. Smaller slabs, also seemingly floated, serve as stairs, from the ground to the terrace and from the terrace to the entrance porch of the rectangular glass-box living area. It is so apparently simple that the subtleties of this extraordinarily elegant frame are readily missed on casual inspection, as are the subtleties of a composition in which the evident asymmetry is countered by hidden symmetries.

In his American work especially Mies has

Mies van der Rohe. Crown Hall, Illinois Institute of Technology. Chicago, 1952–6. Staircase

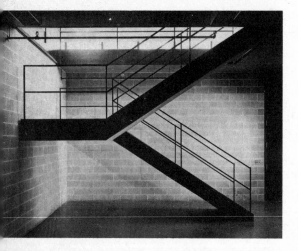

repeatedly taken a basic building type—in this instance the open pavilion lightly supported around the perimeter—and worked variations on the theme. Thus he enlarged the pavilion theme of the Farnsworth House by suspending the roof slab from exposed girders in a series of projects which was eventually realized in Crown Hall for the School of Architecture and Design at IIT (1952). Again the floating stair slabs rise to the floating terrace, and more stairs rise to the floor slab, which is lifted a few feet above the ground much as that of the Farnsworth House. Despite appearances, however, the Crown Hall floor slab is conventionally supported from the basement beneath. Where the earlier glass box was completely open beneath its floor slab, this is glazed, so that Design can be crowded into the basement, while Architecture reigns in the all but uninterrupted space of the glass box above. Again, the openness of this space is enhanced by the suspended nature of the two slabs hanging or abutting (rather than resting) on their supports. In so far as Mies has been concerned with space at all in his American work, it has tended towards the universal box of Crown Hall and not towards the further development of the subtly modulated spaces of his European work after the Barcelona Pavilion.

Enlarged again, the pavilion becomes the project for a convention hall on the Chicago lake-front (1953). The roof slab of this unbuilt pavilion is a three-dimensional structure of interwoven trusses built on a cubic module of 30 feet in each direction and 30 feet deep. Mies designed this heroic structural slab to span 720 feet (or roughly two city blocks) so as to provide a column-free interior space with a height of 112 feet for a capacity audience of 50,000. Diagonal bracing extended from the outside edges of the three-dimensional ceiling trusses makes a two-dimensional truss of the exterior walls. This bracing brings the entire structure down on low reinforced concrete columns spaced 120 feet apart, with the area between available for entrances wherever needed. Finally, a pattern of triangles in light and dark metal panels not only dramatizes the triangulation of the structure, but also provides a compelling visual

Page 197. Mies van der Rohe. Crown Hall, Illinois Institute of Technology. Chicago, 1952–6

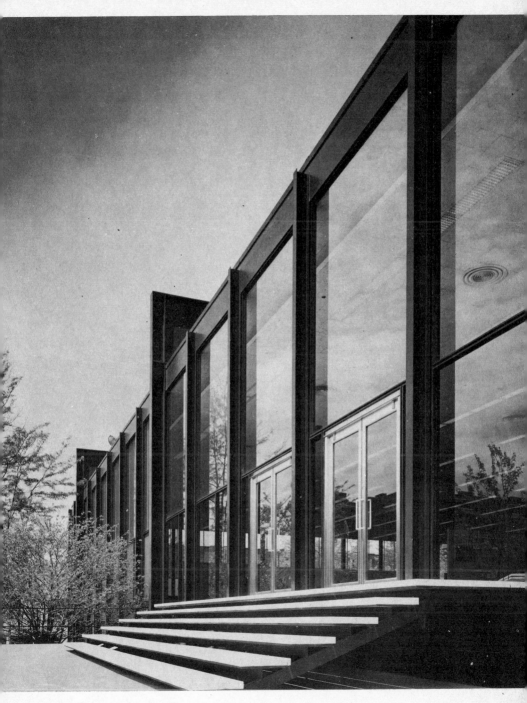

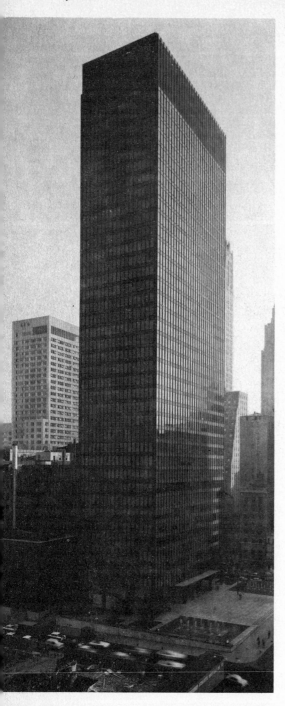

entity for what Arthur Drexler in 1960
termed 'the most monumental image 20th-
century architecture has yet produced'.

As the basic pavilion could be proliferated
into a series of buildings, so could the
skeletal skyscraper. Mies's two classic skyscrapers, 860 Lake Shore Apartments
(1957) and the Seagram Building in New
York (1958) are in a sense exactly the same
building creating different experiences,
much as the Greek Temple of Poseidon at
Paestum and the Parthenon are at once the
same building and different buildings.
Relative to one another, the Paestum-like
severity of Lake Shore contrasts with the
Parthenaic refinement of the Seagram. In
the Lake Shore Apartments, vertical blocks
are set at right angles to one another across
a narrow interval of space in such a manner
that their static shapes are always in tension with one another. As we circle the
complex, we find that it possesses neither
a true 'front' nor a true 'back'. We always
see the narrow side of one block against
the broad side of the other in a constantly
changing relationship. The I-beam projec-
tions from the walls appear to close over
the windows seen obliquely and open over
those seen head-on, while in moving so as
to open those which closed we automatically close those which were open. The
Seagram Building, on the other hand,
reconciles the Lake Shore paradox of static
elements in perpetual disequilibrium. The
bronze building rises like a dense, dark
cliff behind the absolute void of its entrance
plaza. The axis of the *plaza* culminates in
the formal grandeur of the entrance with
its two-storey stilts each backed by the
pylons of the elevator shafts. Where, in the
window grid of the Lake Shore Apartments, horizontals constantly challenge the
verticals, this tension too is reconciled in
the Seagram by the clear affirmation of
verticality. In the Lake Shore, then, a
perpetual tension; in the Seagram, the
reconciliation of tension in a formal climax.
To cite Mies's famous axiom, 'Less is more.'
As he has extracted architecture from
the 'almost nothing' of the brick or the
I-beam considered as ultimate 'things in
themselves', so he has used elemental
building types to squeeze different buildings from the same one. His approach is

Mies van der Rohe. Seagram Building. New
York, 1958

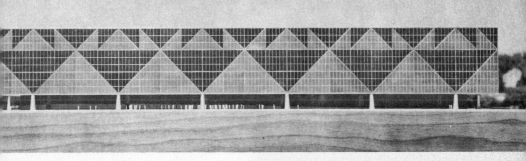

Mies van der Rohe. Convention Hall. Chicago, 1953. Model

Mies van der Rohe. Lake Shore Apartments. Chicago, 1957

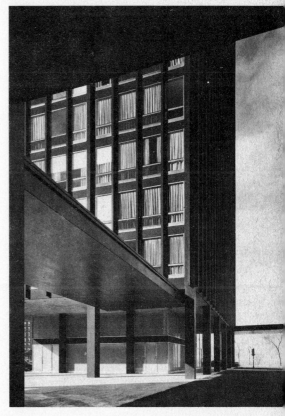

narrow, and his austerity can lead to dryness where the problem has already been so substantially resolved that only refinement is left. But the narrowness of approach permits his passionate integrity and purifying artistry to come to focus. In his greatest works, the 'almost nothing' contains the paradoxical plentitude of an elemental demonstration.

Bibliography: Philip Johnson, *Mies van der Rohe*, 2nd edition, New York 1953; Ludwig Hilbersheimer, *Mies van der Rohe*, Chicago 1956; Arthur Drexler, *Mies van der Rohe*, New York 1960; Peter Blake, *Masters of Modern Architecture*, New York 1960; Ian McCallum, *Architecture USA*, London, New York 1959; 'Farnsworth House', *Architectural Forum, 95*, October 1951; Arthur Drexler, 'Seagram Building', *Architectural Record, 124*, July 1958; Lewis Mumford, 'Skyline: the Lesson of the Master', *New Yorker, 33*, 13 September 1958; William H. Jordy, 'Seagram Assessed', *Architectural Review, 124*, London December 1958; William H. Jordy, *Zodiac 8*, Milan 1960.

WILLIAM H. JORDY

Mills, Edward David, b. 1915. Studied at Polytechnic School of Architecture, London. In private practice since 1937; churches, schools, industrial buildings, research centres, flats and houses. Designed the British Industries Pavilion and the Britannia Inn at the Brussels International Exhibition, 1958.

Modular Coordination. It is, perhaps, unfortunate that the words 'module' and 'modular' were adopted by the pioneers of modular coordination and given a restricted sense after having been current in a wider meaning for several thousand years. 'Module' is the English, or French, form of the Latin *modulus,* which meant a small unit of measure, being the diminutive of *modus.* In classical architecture the modulus is half the diameter of the column at its base and is the unit for proportioning the classic order of column and entablature. Its actual size is not determined in advance, but prescribed for each particular design.

In modular coordination the module is not a unit of proportion, but a predetermined standard size used for coordinating the dimensions of components for building (doors, windows, panels, beams) with the dimensions of the spaces in a projected building into which they are intended to fit. The modular size (or basic size) of the component is expressed in the same whole number of modules as the size of its space in the building. The actual size of the component, the size found by measuring it, will be less than the modular size, by an allowance for the width of joint and for tolerances (manufacturing and positional). The confusion between 'module' as a unit of standardization and its ancient use as one of architectural proportion persists, for example, in a misunderstanding of the use of Le Corbusier's 'Le Modulor'. This is, in fact, a method of applying the Golden Section proportion and has nothing to do with modular coordination. Modulor has nothing in common with Modular.

The module in modular coordination is sometimes referred to as the 'Basic Module', to distinguish it from its multiples which are used as 'Planning Modules', 'Derived Modules', 'Design Modules' and so on. The best usage, however, is to confine the term 'module' to the Basic Module and to find other expressions, such as

'Planning Grid' for its multiples. This is because the size of the Basic Module has been fixed internationally as 10 centimetres for metric countries and 4 inches for countries using inches and feet, after a long process of debate and experiment. The logic behind the choice of this size as the Basic Module does not, by analogy, support the use of any other size, larger or smaller, repetitively as a module. In short, there is only one module (10 centimetres or 4 inches).

The international 10 centimetres/4 inches module is the resultant of two forces pulling against each other: the pull from manufacturers was to make it as large as possible in the interests of simplification and mass-production; that from architects was for it to be as small as possible for the greatest freedom of aesthetic and functional design. That this resultant should have been the same in all parts of the world, where the problem has been tackled, is a significant reassurance of its validity. National standards have been published for modular coordination in the following countries, on the 10 centimetres module unless otherwise stated:

1942 France	1954 USSR
1945 USA (4 in.)	1955 Chile
1948 Belgium	1955 Poland
1949 Italy	1956 Portugal
1951 Germany (10	1956 Roumania
cm. and 12.5 cm.)	1957 Austria
1951 Norway	1958 Denmark
1951 Hungary	1958 India
1952 Sweden	1959 Canada (4 in.)
1953 Argentine	

The promulgation of a national standard for modular coordination does not by itself achieve the savings in cost and in construction-time that are expected to derive from the use of the modular method. Much development work is required, by manufacturers in the choice of modular sizes for particular sets of components, and by architects in the application of the method to building design so as to incorporate standard modular components to the best advantage. In this process of development a vicious circle has constantly to be broken: manufacturers are reluctant to change their production to modular sizes until there is a clear demand for them from architects, whilst architects maintain that it is of no use to design modular buildings until ample ranges of modular components are available on the market. This vicious circle even appears in the 'planned economy' of Socialist countries, as is reported by a contributor from Poland to *The Modular Quarterly* (1963/1, p. 16).

In most of the countries named above, and in others, e.g. New Zealand and the Central American Republics, where modular coordination is under study but where a standard has not yet been issued, the development of modular method is entrusted to the Standards institutions or other agencies of government. In some, however, the initiative has been taken by private organizations.

In the USA there is the Modular Building Standards Association, Washington, D.C.; in Australia there is the Australian Modular Society, based at Sydney with branches in other states; and, in the United Kingdom, the Modular Society, London. Besides these three national societies (though the UK Modular Society has many overseas members) there is the International Modular Group, with its headquarters at the housing ministry in Copenhagen.

Finally, a few words on the situation in the United Kingdom at the time of writing (February 1963). It has not yet been possible to get the unanimous support from all sections of the building industry that is required for the issue of a British standard for modular coordination. Nevertheless, the Ministry of Public Building and Works has published a first statement on 'Dimensional Coordination for Industrialized Building', which in effect adopts the 4-inch module and the modular method for the whole of the government building programme, although for tactical reasons it adopts a somewhat off-beat terminology. This statement is expected to break the vicious circle and to create the demand from architects that will fill the *Modular Catalogue* of the Modular Society with ample ranges of modular components.

Bibliography: Modular Coordination—Second Report, EPA Project 174, OEEC., HMSO, London 1961; E. Corker and A. Diprose, 'The Modular Primer' in *Architects' Journal* 1.8.62 (reprinted by Modular Society); *Scandinavian Modular Coordination in Building*, Ministry of Housing, Copenhagen 1960; *The Modular Quarterly* (journal), London.

MARK HARTLAND THOMAS

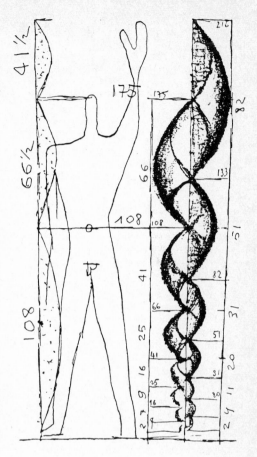

Le Corbusier. Modulor

Modulor. A scale of proportions laid down by *Le Corbusier and his colleagues, 'which makes the bad difficult and the good easy' (Albert Einstein). The Modulor is based on two lines, arrived at via the Golden Section and related to the proportions of the human body. The initial dimension is 7 ft 5 in. (226 cm.) (an upright man with his hand raised) and half that, viz. 3 ft 9 in. (113 cm.). A man's height is taken as 6 ft (183 cm.).

Bibliography: Le Corbusier, *The Modulor: A harmonious measure to the human scale, universally applicable to architecture and mechanics*, London 1954. Continued in: Le Corbusier, *Modulor 2, 1955 (Let the user speak next)*, London 1958.

Morris, William, b. Walthamstow 1834, d. Kelmscott, Oxfordshire 1896. In 1861, together with artists from the Pre-Raphaelite Brotherhood, he founded the Morris Company whose products (furniture, textiles, metalwork, stained glass and wallpapers) sought to convey honesty and decency in the crafts. This attitude and the example set by the Red House at Bexley Heath, Kent, which Philip *Webb built for him, exerted a strong influence on the architecture of the times. Morris, who had trained under the architect G. E. Street, never built anything himself.

Moser, Karl, b. Baden, Switzerland 1860, d. Zurich 1936. Studied at Zurich College of Technology and later at the École des Beaux-Arts, Paris; 1887–1915 architect at Karlsruhe, 1915–28 taught at Zurich. Moser, whose reinforced concrete Church of St Anthony, Basle (1926–7) was the counterpart to *Perret's Church at Le Raincy (1922–3), taught many modern Swiss architects.

Muthesius, Hermann, b. Gross-Neuhausen 1861, d. Berlin 1927. Studied at Berlin Technical College; worked in Wallot's office. Period in Japan; attaché at the German Embassy in London (1896–1903), with a brief to study English architecture and design. His book *Das englische Haus* (Berlin 1904–5) by spreading a knowledge of the works of *Voysey and his contemporaries stimulated a renaissance in domestic architecture on the Continent. Founder-member of the *Deutscher Werkbund.

Nash, John, b. London 1752, d. East Cowes 1835. After a varied career, he worked as an architect in London from 1796. Built partly in classic, partly in Gothic style. His friendship with the Prince of Wales, later King George IV, led to many important commissions: town planning, public buildings, landscaping, country estates, churches, buildings and designs for the Royal House, including the eccentric Brighton Pavilion (1815–23). *Bibliography:* Terence Davis, *The Architecture of John Nash*, London 1960.

Nelson, George, b. Hartford, Connecticut 1908. Designer (in particular furniture and advertising) and architect who faces the problems of modern industry in his architectural designs. Factories, private houses. The model of his experimental house (1957) incorporates a flexible arrangement of square room units.
Bibliography: George Nelson, *Problems of Design*, New York 1957.

Neoclassicism. In the German-speaking countries of Europe the new architecture of the 20th century was born under the sign of the Doric Column, which appears in *Behrens's Mannesmann Building, Düsseldorf, in *Mies van der Rohe's Perls House, Berlin, and in Adolf *Loos's 'Looshaus' in Vienna. At the same time, Loos, like Hermann *Muthesius and others, was acclaiming K. F. *Schinkel as 'the last great architect'. In the same years Julien Guadet, professor at the *École des Beaux-Arts in Paris, taught a system of architecture that had hardly changed from that taught eighty years earlier by J. N. L. Durand and contrived to impose its concepts even on students as radical as Auguste *Perret and Tony *Garnier. Thus, all the fathers of the modern movement in architecture were soundly grounded in neoclassicism, and—even while they protested their disgust at the academies—they took over into their own work the academic neoclassical apparatus of trabeated structure, the preference for simple geometrical forms and smooth surfaces, and the concept of 'elementary composition', i.e. design, as the assembly of a number of disparate volumes, each dedicated to a single identifiable function.
In this way a durable neoclassical tradition was built into modern architecture from the beginning and was the basis for most concepts of 'order' and 'discipline' current in the first thirty years of the century. Since technology was also seen as one of the enemies of disorder, the mechanistic enthusiasms of the Futurists were early assimilated to the neoclassical tradition—in the writings and designs of Antonio *Sant'Elia in 1914, the rhetoric of a Marinetti is allied to an architectural vision more classically pure than even that of Loos. In *Le Corbusier's *Vers une Architecture*, nine years later, parallels between machinery and classical architecture are openly drawn, and the author equates Phidias with the designer of modern sports cars.

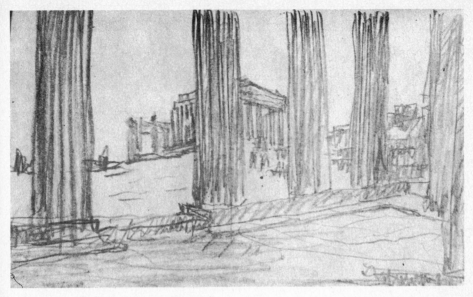

Le Corbusier. The Parthenon. 1911. Sketch

By about 1930, however, a new generation of critics and historians who had attached themselves to modern architecture as its mouthpieces (e.g. Sigfried Giedion) began to offer an account of modern architecture that relied exclusively on a supposed *'Functionalist' origin, and by 1936 another historian, Nikolaus Pevsner, could offer an account of the rise of modern architecture in which the academic and neoclassical contributions were not discussed at all. Rapidly, and especially after the disastrous competition for the League of Nations headquarters in Geneva, classicism came to be regarded as the enemy of modern architecture. But this was classicism in the superficial and debased sense of 'ornamented with Greek and Roman detail', for the planning of Le Corbusier's unsuccessful entry in the competition was fully as academic and neoclassical as that of the preferred designs. Similarly one finds, in Italian modern architecture, *Terragni praised for his 'rationalism' and Piacentini damned for his classicism—though a comparison of the façade of Terragni's Casa del Fascio at Como reveals it to be fully as classicist as Piacentini's arcading at EUR42 (Terza Roma) which is fully as rational as Terragni's space-games.

This facile and purely stylistic opposition between modern and classical, this growing ignorance among modern architects of the origins of their own design techniques, was to lead to profound intellectual confusions in the years after the Second World War. On the one hand, Bruno Zevi was to point out, with justice, how neoclassicism was the outstanding weakness of much second-rate modern architecture, but at the same time many Anglo-Saxon critics failed to see that the supposed modernism

Mies van der Rohe. Perls House. Berlin. 1911

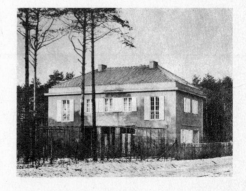

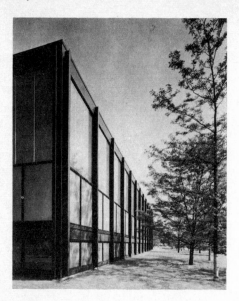

Mies van der Rohe. Crown Hall, Illinois
Institute of Technology. Chicago, 1952–6

of the Italian buildings then in vogue was
little more than a frank exhibition of a
neoclassicism that they no longer recognized as their own, an error that left them
entirely unprepared for the abandonment
of the moral and functional imperatives of
modern architecture by the *neo-Liberty
faction in Northern Italy.

A similar confusion can be seen in the
various valuations placed upon the architecture of Mies van der Rohe in the years
after 1950. The English radical functiona-

list Llewelyn Davies read Mies's repetitive
façades at the Illinois Institute of Technology as 'endless' and believed that their
complex corners implied the continuation
of the planes of the façades beyond the
ends of the buildings. But a younger
generation of English writers (e.g. Colin
Rowe) rendered consciously classicist by
the influential writings of Rudolf Wittkower (such as his book, *Architectural
Principles in the Age of Humanism*) preferred
to read the façades as closed, symmetrical
compositions, and the complex corners as
emphatic visual terminations, comparable
to the doubling of pilasters at the corners
of buildings, such as had been regular
classical practice since the time of
Bramante.

Among the intellectuals of Anglo-Saxon
architecture the rediscovery of the roots of
the classical tradition through the works
of scholars like Wittkower had a profound
influence and was seized upon as a welcome
source of order in a modern architecture
that, deprived of its classical origins, had
lost its way in the formless currents of
Functionalism. Under such names as
neo-Palladianism or the New Formalism,
it visibly affected the design of monuments
as diverse as Marchwood II power station
(England), designed in the office of
*Farmer and Dark, the Goodyear House
in Connecticut, designed by John *Johansen, and even the first major building of the
*Brutalist movement: Hunstanton School,
by Alison and Peter *Smithson. But here
the Anglo-Saxon stream of development
divides; in *Great Britain the native preference for a functionalist solution, aided, no

Philip Johnson. Sheldon Art Gallery. Lincoln, Neb., under construction

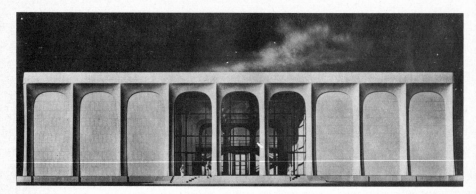

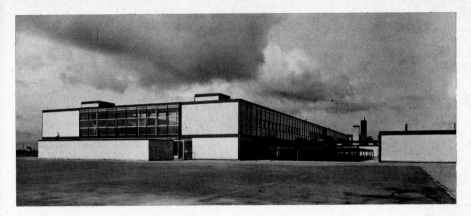

Alison and Peter Smithson. Hunstanton School. Norfolk, 1954

doubt, by the example of the anti-classicism of Ronchamp and the absence of a strong *beaux-arts* tradition, produced a situation in which neoclassicism was absorbed back into a kind of rational functionalism, and became little more than a modular discipline for the design of structures (e.g. *CLASP schools).

But in the *USA neo-Palladianism rapidly struck root in a *beaux-arts* tradition that had been only thinly buried by the dominance of *Gropius, *Sert, *Breuer and Mies. Philip *Johnson progressed rapidly from the Miesian classicism of his own house at New Canaan to the revival of the vault-forms of Sir John *Soane in the adjoining guest-pavilion, and from there to the vaulting and axial planning of the Port Chester Synagogue, the clearest and most justifiable example of the neoclassical revival in the USA. A more subtle and guarded neoclassicism is seen in the work of Louis *Kahn: the concealed axiality of the Yale Art Centre (1955); the use of elementary composition in the planning of the Philadelphia laboratories; the Laugieresque primitivism of the Trenton bathhouse (1955); and the pure *Prix-de-Rome* planning of the Torrey Pines Biological Institute.

This reawakening to the neoclassical roots of modern architecture coincided with a general relaxation of functionalist discipline, with rising standards of affluence and the retirement of Gropius from Harvard. The result, on the east coast at least, has been a slow recrudescence of *beaux-arts* academicism, with contrived symmetrical plans and even Doric columns such as could be seen in a number of designs that received awards from the magazine *Progressive Architecture* in 1962. In countries other than the USA, however, neoclassicism seems not to have proceeded any further than various forms of Miesian symmetry and rectangularity. But it does seem to be firmly entrenched as an essential part of the mental substructure of modern architectural design-practice, a geometrical discipline common to both classicizing formalists and prefabricating functionalists.

REYNER BANHAM

Louis I. Kahn. Baths. Trenton, N.J., 1956. Plan

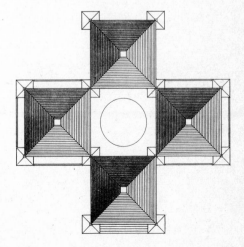

Neo-Liberty. Reversion of post-war Italian architects to *Art Nouveau (Italian: Stile Liberty) forms, in particular to its last geometrical phase, as practised in Vienna and Scotland. Attempts to justify this movement have sparked off heated controversies between English and Italian architectural writers.

Neoplasticism. Piet Mondrian's term for his own painting, developed from Cubist prototypes. The artists and architects of De *Stijl were the protagonists of neoplasticism's clear, geometric order and transferred its concepts to architecture.

Nervi, Pier Luigi, b. Sondrio, Lombardy 1891. Nervi graduated in engineering at Bologna in 1913. He lives in Rome and since 1946 has lectured on structural engineering in the Faculty of Architecture at Rome University. He was awarded an honorary degree by the University of Buenos Aires in 1950.
This great builder ranks with *Freyssinet and *Maillart in his prodigious ability to derive beauty from the results of calculations, and form from the nature of his materials and techniques, which he has made the instruments of his vision. He takes his place in the history of architecture above all for the absolute aesthetic value of some of his buildings, where technology and aesthetics combine to determine dimensions and proportions, based on the same structural rationale that presided at the birth of the pyramid and the column. He himself, on the other hand, has many times laid down the principle in his writings, which he firmly believes in, that the process of creating form is identical, whether it is the work of technicians or of artists: the principle, that is, whereby the beauty of a structure, for example, is not just the outcome of calculations, but of an intuition as to what calculations to use, or with which it is to be identified. This perfect identification has clearly not been achieved in all his works, but where it has the architecture of the 20th century is ideally symbolized.
The material Nervi has adopted is reinforced concrete, which he moulds and works with an understanding of its possibilities which allows his imagination free rein. His first structures (for a theatre in Naples) date from 1927, the year in which

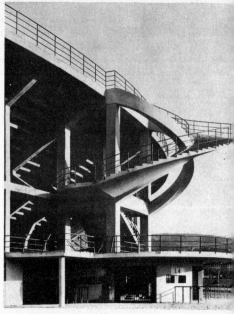

Pier Luigi Nervi. Communal Stadium. Florence, 1930–2

the *Movimento Italiano per l'Architettura Razionale* was founded, and the Weissenhof estate built at Stuttgart. The idea was gaining ground (the source of much subsequent misunderstanding) that 'form follows function', and it was this idea that brought the engineer Nervi into architecture forthwith. His first important work, the Communal Stadium at Florence (1930–2), consisting of nothing but exposed structural elements, was published straightaway in the most controversial journals as an example of modern architecture, which could be compared, in its dramatic exploitation of structure, with certain designs of *Le Corbusier and strikingly highlighted the expressive possibilities of the raw material, concrete.
Projects followed for viaducts, bridges, silos, tanks and even small revolving houses on a circular plan, which were never built. In 1935, however, Nervi designed a military hangar (of which versions were built, from 1936 to 1941, at Orvieto, Orbetello, and Torre del Lago) which started him on the study of roofs built up from a network of loadbearing joists. These were to prove the object of constant and

even deeper research on his part, in an infinite variety prompted by his taste for creation and experiment. In the hangars which he built (now destroyed) Nervi achieved a great step forward in the process of lightening his structures, at which he has been aiming all his life, for aesthetic as much as for technical reasons.

In the same period, around the year 1940, he brought to a successful conclusion the studies and experiments he had been carrying out to obtain 'strength through form' in buildings, i.e. strength in surfaces alone; this is at once the most technically interesting and the most aesthetically satisfying of his achievements. He went on to design a series of immense roofs for warehouses, factories, aircraft hangars, stations and pavilions of various kinds. In 1947 he built the swimming baths at Leghorn, and in 1948–9 the fantastic roof of the great hall of the Exhibition Building in Turin, which remains one of his masterpieces, although due to a misunderstanding on the part of those responsible for the actual erection an important internal detail was altered, thus depriving it of the perfection which Nervi's design had attained. The enormous building consists in effect of a single roof structure, made up of undulating prefabricated units; Kidder Smith has called it the finest exhibition building in Europe since *Paxton's Crystal Palace, and ranks it with Le Corbusier's Unité d'Habitation at Marseilles as the two most important buildings in post-war Europe.

A number of smaller buildings followed, based on the same principle of roofing in reinforced concrete which leaves the space below completely free; some are on a circular plan, such as the halls at Rome Lido and Chianciano Terme (1950–2). Sometimes Nervi works in conjunction with architects, but not always. In 1953 he planned a huge Sports Palace for Vienna on a circular plan, which carried his experience at Turin a stage further; it was not built, however, nor was a smaller, but equally impressive design for a hangar at Buenos Aires.

At the same time as the above works, Nervi was carrying out research on improved systems of reinforced concrete prefabrication, using small ferroconcrete moulds for on-site manufacture, in conjunction with a movable type of staging patented by

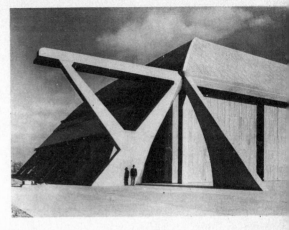

Pier Luigi Nervi. Aircraft hangar. 1935

Pier Luigi Nervi. Exhibition hall. Turin, 1948–9

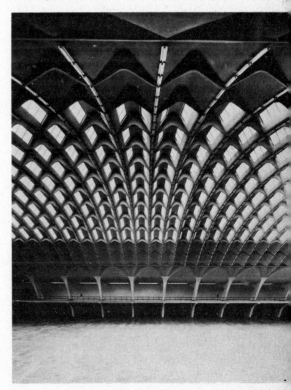

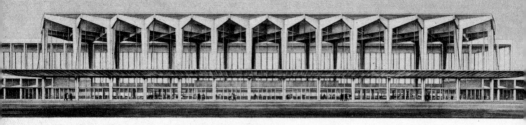

Pier Luigi Nervi. Main Railway Station. Naples, 1954. Project

himself, Bartoli and Angeli. This device per-mitted a great variety of designs based on a ribbed structure, making de *Baudot's boldest and most utopian designs now seem capable of realization. Another important invention of Nervi's in the technical field is his system for the hydraulic pre-stressing of reinforced concrete. But none of these researches is an end in itself. The ever greater liberty which these technical im-provements bestow, by making work simpler and quicker, has led Pier Luigi Nervi to deeper researches of another kind, e.g. on rhythm as an element of beauty, as may be seen in his design for the concourse building of the new Main Railway Station in Naples (1954), in the Palazzetto dello Sport in Rome (1957), and above all in the conference hall of the Unesco Building in Paris (1953–7, jointly with Breuer and Zehrfuss).

With its overtones of barbaric monu-mentality reminiscent of some ancient temple, combined with extreme technical and aesthetic modernity, the Unesco Building is one of Nervi's most interesting

structures, one of the most interesting examples, in fact, of recent European architecture generally. The system of 'strength through form' has contributed to produce this splendid result. Strength was in fact achieved by corrugating the surfaces, and Nervi has studied the principle on the corrugated surfaces of shellfish, insects and flower calixes; the magical perfection of infinite smallness in nature seems to be transferred with the same qualities of strength and beauty to his own works.

In the construction of the Pirelli Skyscraper in Milan (1958, with Gio *Ponti and the architects of his office), the principle on which its strength is based is derived from nature too, viz. from the example of a tree. This is the prototype of the building's sectional development, with its four main stanchions growing ever more slender to-wards the top, as might have been seen more clearly if a lighter cladding had been used. Nervi's creative mastery of structure may also be seen in the most recent pro-jects for which he has acted as the engineer: in the sail-like roof of the exhibition hall for the Centre National des Industries in Paris (1955), in the circular exhibition building in Caracas (1956), and in the enormous columns, shaped like palm trees, of the Palazzo del Lavoro at Turin (1961).

Bibliography: Pier Luigi Nervi, *Arte o scienza del construire?*, Rome 1954; Pier Luigi Nervi, *El lenguaje arquitectonico*, Buenos Aires 1950; Pier Luigi Nervi, *Costruire correttamente*, Milan 1954; G. C. Argan, *Pier Luigi Nervi*, Milan 1955;

Pier Luigi Nervi and Annibale Vitellozzi. Palazzetto dello Sport. Rome, 1956–7

Jürgen Joedicke, *The Works of Pier Luigi Nervi*, London 1957; Ada Louise Huxtable, *Pier Luigi Nervi*, New York 1960; Ravensburg 1961; Pier Luigi Nervi, *Neue Struckturen*, Stuttgart 1963.

GIULIA VERONESI

Netherlands. Modern architecture in the Netherlands undoubtedly begins with H. P. *Berlage, whose classic work is the Amsterdam Stock Exchange, completed in 1903. His immediate predecessor and contemporary was P. J. H. *Cuijpers, who as a follower of the romantic school was an enthusiastic adherent of *Viollet-le-Duc. His numerous works, including the Rijksmuseum (1885) and main railway station (1889) in Amsterdam, mark the close of eclecticism, and the neo-Gothic phase in particular, in the Netherlands. Despite his predilection for this style and the French neo-Renaissance, Cuijpers too, like Berlage, helped to promote the trend back to an architecture based on craft traditions. Nearly all the Dutch practitioners of arts and crafts around the year 1900 were graduates from Cuijpers's studio. From that time onwards, we can speak of a 'school of Berlage' also often referred to at the time as the Amsterdam School.

For the younger generation, Berlage was the leading personality of his time in the fields of art, architecture and handicrafts. His many lectures and articles exerted great influence. Breaking completely free from the eclecticism of the 19th century, he took as his starting point a consideration of the demands of reason and logic in the use of materials and in structure. As reinforced concrete was virtually unknown as an architectural medium at this time, he chose to work in brick. In his later works, however, he made an equally 'logical and honest' use of concrete.

Around 1910, a diametrically opposite movement began in Dutch architecture; its leading figure became Michael de *Klerk (1884–1923) together with P. L. Kramer and M. van der Mey. The best known example of this new *Amsterdam School is the Marine Terminus Building in Amsterdam (1914). This trend was basically anti-Berlage: individual artistic design was seen as the highest goal, and personal idiosyncrasies of detail were

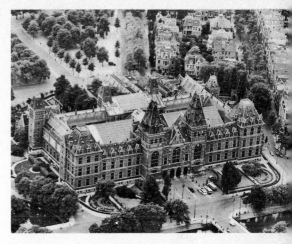

P. J. H. Cuijpers. Rijksmuseum. Amsterdam, 1885

Hendrik Petrus Berlage. Stock Exchange. Amsterdam, 1897–1903

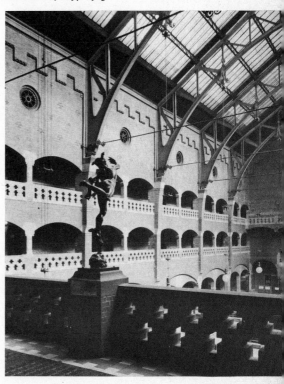

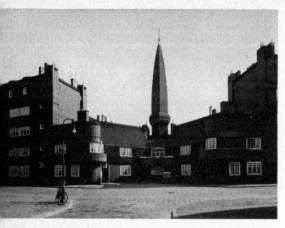

Michael de Klerk. Eigen Haard flats.
Amsterdam, 1921

realized, where necessary, at the cost of
logical construction and the right use of
materials.

This period, which lasted from about
1912 to 1926, is characterized by a form
of *Expressionism, comparable to that
which was developing in *Germany;
international interest was drawn to Dutch
architecture, and to the new housing in
Amsterdam in particular. A typical
Expressionist façade-architecture developed at this time, which left the real
problems of modern mass-housing untouched. The new estates in South

Willen Marinus Dudok. Town Hall.
Hilversum, 1928–30

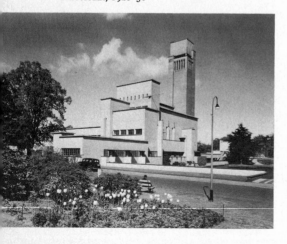

Amsterdam built in the years around 1922
all exhibit the influence of this romantic
school, which has become identified
today with the name of de Klerk, undoubtedly an architect of great gifts. The
influence spread into the provinces,
where it was long active, leaving its mark
on numberless second- and third-rate
buildings. Even Berlage was not wholly
immune from it as his flats on the Mer-
catorplein in West Amsterdam show.

A new tendency emerged with the founding of De *Stijl, which set itself against
both the unaffected outlook of Berlage and
the romantic architecture of de Klerk and
his circle. A violent struggle ensued,
which led to the ultimate defeat of the
romantic cause. In addition to J. J. P.
*Oud, De Stijl attracted to its side such
figures as Robert van't Hoff, Jan Wils and
Gerrit Thomas *Rietveld. It was chiefly
concerned with basic problems of space
and colour. In principle, colour has no
'additional' decorative function, but acts
rather as a space-moulding element. In
practice, however, it turned out that
spatial and decorative functions often
overlapped.

After his break with van *Doesburg,
Oud went his own way, while still adher-
ing to De Stijl ideology, and became a
leading figure in West European *Functionalism. His circle included J. B. van
Loghem, J. A. and L. C. van der *Vlugt,
B. Bijvoet, J. *Duiker, Cor van *Eesteren,
B. Merkelbach, Ch. J. F. Karsten, Rietveld, Mart Stam, J. G. Wiebinga, Jan
Wils and B. Groenewegen. This powerful
upsurge of functionalism again focused
the attention of the architectural world on
Holland, while simultaneously marking
the end of the romantic Amsterdam
School. The platform for functionalism
was provided by the controversial journal
De 8 en Opbouw, in whose pages the
advanced spirits of Amsterdam and
Rotterdam made common cause. It stood
in opposition to the ethically and aesthetically orientated journal *Wendingen.
The fact that, since 1912, every new
building in Holland required the official
approval of a 'vetting' committee, explains why it took till 1930–2 for a pioneer
building such as Duiker's open-air school
in the Cliostraat, Amsterdam to get
built, and then only in the face of numerous protests from the experts.

A completely independent part was played by Willem Marinus *Dudok. Though showing himself an admirer of Berlage in his early works, he gradually developed an extremely personal style, of which Hilversum Town Hall (1928–30) is a typical example. The 'Dudok Style' found many imitators in Holland up to about 1935, especially in the provinces.

Another turning point in Dutch architecture was reached in 1925, with the appointment of Professor G. M. Granpré Molière to Delft Technical College. His philosophy and system of aesthetics, based on the Roman Catholic religion, made a strong appeal to many students. The first building to appear which bore his stamp was the Town Hall at Enschede (1933) by his pupil G. Friedhoff; it also shows Scandinavian influence. With the professor from Delft, Dutch architecture became subject to ever more philosophical considerations. Granpré Molière was opposed to a so-called technical and materialistic outlook. He was against the undermining of religion, and against functionalism and humanism, which he considered the common denominator of everything Oud and his circle stood

for. In the pre-war atmosphere of political unrest and increasing malaise towards the tendencies of modern culture and technology, the Delft theories fell upon fertile ground.

The School of Delft, which was historically orientated, especially in regard to church building and town planning, seemed to dominate Dutch architecture until about 1955. Architects and town planners from this group were entrusted with the reconstruction of bombed cities during and after the Second World War. Functionalism and De Stijl seemed to be played out. Granpré Molière exerted particular influence on the development of Dutch church architecture, and not only amongst his fellow-Catholics, but on Protestant architects, too. The character of the Delft School was chiefly determined by the real or supposed tradition of Dutch building, and the maintenance and romantic perpetuation of craftwork in the manner of Berlage. This led to the evocation of great interest in comparable architectural trends in the Scandinavian countries and Germany (Tessenow, *Muthesius). Four years of German occupation also naturally left their mark.

Johannes Andreas Brinkmann and L. C. van der Vlugt. Van Nelle tobacco factory. Rotterdam, 1928–9

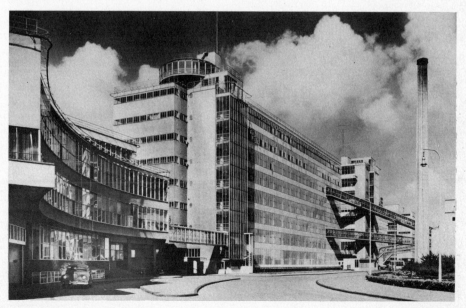

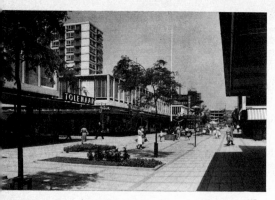

J. H. van den Broek and Jacob B. Bakema.
Lijnbaan pedestrian precinct. Rotterdam, 1953

The situation changed around 1950. It was in particular the badly damaged city of Rotterdam that led the way. The traditional type of reconstruction scheme that had been originally planned was abandoned and a new one adopted. Rotterdam became a centre of architectural and town-planning activity, thanks chiefly to the work of van den *Broek and *Bakema. The former was appointed professor at Delft Technical College in 1948. He and Bakema challenged the concepts of the Delft School, and in this they were supported by Oud

Aldo van Eijck. Municipal Orphanage.
Amsterdam, 1955

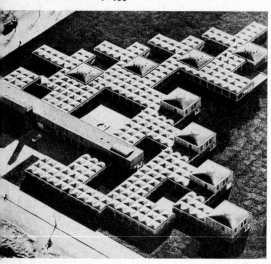

and a small group of fellow spirits. Functionalism began to develop again, but it was of a clearly different type from that which had flourished from 1925 to 1935. In Amsterdam itself however, few buildings of note have been erected, save for the large town extension schemes in West Amsterdam. A scheme for a new town hall by the architects Berghoef and Vegter encountered stiff opposition both from the profession and the public. The two architects were convinced disciples of Granpré Molière.

The general impression made by Dutch architecture a few years after the Second World War was chiefly one of diversity and vigour. The works of architects in Sweden, Italy and North and South America (*Breuer, *Gropius, *Mies van der Rohe) were making their influence felt, as was the ever-increasing number of publications. The *CIAM idea was revived, and its meaning for our time was critically reassessed. The desperate housing shortage focused particular interest on this sphere of building. The well-nigh impregnable bastion of the romantic Delft School was being progressively undermined in practice. After c. 1955 even its most zealous adherents became converted—some hesitantly, others out and out—to a new and in many respects modern form of functionalism. A comparison of the highly ornate Provincial Authority Headquarters at Arnhem (1955) with the Town Hall at Groningen (1961), both by J. J. M. Vegter, illustrates this change. Delft School concepts held out longest in the sphere of Catholic church building, especially in the predominantly Catholic provinces of North Brabant and Limburg, in the south, where the so-called 'Hertogenbosch School' clung on to the North Italian type of Early Christian basilica. But here too, in Catholic lay and architectural circles, loud protests have been voiced against this trend, and attempts are being made to exploit new methods, as in Protestant church architecture, where reinforced concrete is no longer rejected out of hand as an ignoble material.

By the side of good contemporary design, a vast amount of building has gone up in what is no more or less than bread-and-butter modern. This is especially the case with housing. The few notable figures include van den Broek, Bakema and later, Aldo van *Eijck; Rietveld's work is greatly admired by most of the younger generation. Dissatisfaction with CIAM's doctrinaire outlook led to the setting up of Team X, whose views have been appearing in the Dutch press since 1959, especially in the journal *Forum*, and have given rise to sharp controversy. 'Architecture is the three-dimensional expression of human behaviour' (Bakema).

An attempt to carry some new ideas into effect may be seen in the Municipal Orphanage, Amsterdam (1955), by Aldo van Eijck. The transitions from exterior to interior, and the spatial relationships of this building make it one of the most important of its time. Van Eijck and his circle have been able to realize their theories to a certain extent in planning for the village of Nagele, in the southeast Polder. Van den Broek and Bakema's proposals for the Kennemerland region of Noord-Holland also herald some new developments in the field of town planning. The same architects' design for a civic centre at Marl, currently under construction, will no doubt give ample expression to the new theories of the *Forum* group.

Bibliography: J. P. Mieras and F. R. Yerbury, *Dutch Architecture in the 20th Century*, London 1926; J. J. Vriend, *Nieuwere Architectuur* Amsterdam 1957; J. J. Vriend, *Reflexen*, Amsterdam 1958; J. J. Vriend, *Algemeen Overzicht Architectuur van deze eeuw*, Amsterdam 1959; G. M. Granpré Molière, *Woorden en Werken*, 1949; H. L. C. Jaffé, *De Stijl 1917–31. The Dutch Contribution to Modern Art*, Armsterdam 1956; R. Blijstra, *Netherlands Architecture since 1900*, Amsterdam 1960.

J. J. VRIEND

Neutra, Richard Joseph, b. Vienna 1892. Neutra was trained at the Technische Hochschule, Vienna, receiving his diploma in 1917. He met Adolf *Loos in 1910 and was influenced by the elder architect's work (e.g. the Steiner House, 1910), by his strictures against the use of ornament in architecture and by his admiration for American design (which Loos knew at first hand from a stay in the USA in 1893–6). Neutra was also impressed with the novel character of Otto *Wagner's Vienna subway entrances, dating from before 1900.

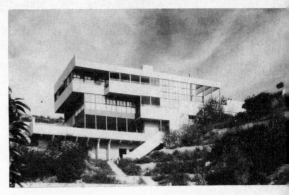

Richard Neutra. Lovell House. Los Angeles, 1927–9

Richard Neutra. Sidney Kahn House. San Francisco, 1940

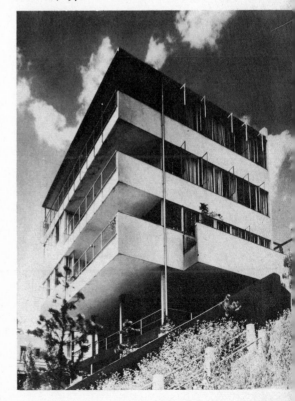

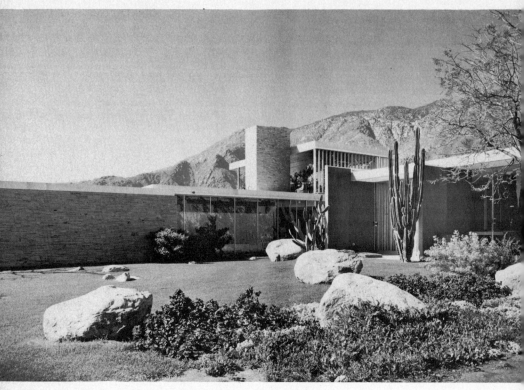

Richard Neutra. Kaufmann Desert House. Palm Springs, Cal., 1946–7

In 1911 his interest in American architecture was broadened through the discovery of the work of Frank Lloyd *Wright
which had just been extensively published
in Europe. Many of the motifs that dominate Neutra's architecture today, a half-
century later, can be traced to this familiar
and influential source.

Immediately after the First World War
Neutra worked in Switzerland, gaining
experience in the fields of landscape and
city planning. Employed in the Municipal
Building Office, Lukenwalde, Germany, in
1921, he subsequently became associated
with Erich *Mendelsohn in 1922. The
following year Mendelsohn and Neutra
were awarded a First Prize for a Business
Centre in Haifa. Neutra moved to the
USA in 1923, and for the next few years
he worked alternately in Chicago, with the
large commercial firm of *Holabird and
Roche, and at Taliesin, Spring Green,

Wisconsin, with Frank Lloyd Wright. In
1926 he settled in Los Angeles, beginning
his practice in the office of another Vienna-
born architect, Rudolph *Schindler.

Schindler had been an assistant of Wright
in the construction of several houses in
Los Angeles in the early 1920s, and in
1926 was building the concrete-framed
Lovell House, Newport Beach, in a
striking, liberated style reflecting his
origins, both in the proto-*International
Style of Central Europe and in the more
romantic architecture of Wright. In 1927
Schindler and Neutra collaborated in a
project for the League of Nations competition.

Under these several influences Neutra's
personal style rapidly came into focus in
the late 1920s. The key work in his early
maturity was the rambling, quasi-pictur-
esque Lovell House (1927–9) built for
Schindler's former client on a steep,

challenging Los Angeles hillside site. A contemporary (albeit geographically isolated) of *Le Corbusier's noted Villa Stein, Garches, France, and *Mies van der Rohe's Barcelona Pavilion, Neutra's steel-framed Lovell House, with its slabs and balconies supported from above by steel cables, differs in certain structural details from these European masterworks, but is stylistically identical in terms of its thin, weightless forms which only partly enclose a series of fluidly juxtaposed interior spaces. Neutra developed and expanded this International Style into a more pronounced personal idiom throughout the 1930s in such houses as the one built for Josef von Sternberg, San Fernando Valley (1936), and these simple forms were often realized in novel or unusual materials. Always interested in large-scale planning, with implications of social welfare, Neutra found a wartime opportunity in the Channel Heights Housing Project, San Pedro, California (1942–4), where out of necessity redwood was substituted for the more familiar materials of the machine age. At the same time he worked on numerous projects for schools and health centres in Puerto Rico.

The apogee of Neutra's career occurs in the immediate post-war era with the construction of the Kaufmann Desert House, Palm Springs (1946–7), and the Tremaine House, Santa Barbara (1947–8). Here the elegant restatements of the by now traditional International Style themes reach a degree of elegance and precision that is not present in the earlier work, and these features are further enhanced by sensitive siting and landscaping. In 1949, with an expanding practice, he formed a partnership with Robert E. Alexander. Since that time domestic work has had to vie with more sizeable projects in Neutra's œuvre. While his houses of the 1950s have almost invariably maintained the suavity of those of the 1940s, the designs have tended towards the rhetorical in their repetition of earlier motifs. In general, in the most recent phase of his career, Neutra's customarily sensitive works have appeared to have less and less relevance with the constantly changing direction and interest that is to be found in the main stream of building design in the late 1950s and early 1960s.
Bibliography: Richard Neutra, *Survival through Design*, New York 1954; W. Boesiger, *Richard Neutra, 1950–60, Buildings and Projects*, Zurich 1959; Esther McCoy, *Richard Neutra*, Ravensburg 1962.

JOHN M. JACOBUS, JR

Niemeyer, Oscar, b. Rio de Janeiro 1907. The leading exponent of modern architecture in Brazil, by virtue of the extent, the scope and the character of his work, Oscar Niemeyer Soares Filho, as his name is written in full, has had a rich and varied career. He graduated in 1934 from the National School of Fine Arts, Rio, and a few years later stepped into a position of effective leadership when he succeeded Lúcio *Costa as the head of the design team for the new building of the Ministry of Education and Health. Since then he has always been in the front line of architectural development in Brazil, setting trends and opening up new avenues of plastic expression, as well as influencing students and fellow architects to a very noticeable degree.

Niemeyer himself was decisively influenced by *Le Corbusier, with whom he worked on the design for the Ministry of Education and Health during the master's short stay in Brazil, in 1936. He began by applying Le Corbusier's basic ideas, as in the Day Nursery, Rio de Janeiro (1937). Very soon, however, he branched out in a personal direction, adding to such ideas an element of adaptation to local conditions, an imaginative and creative exuberance, and a typical lightness of touch, which to this day distinguishes all his work, even when it is apparently massive or heavier than usual.

Disregarding the tenets of orthodox *Functionalism whenever they seemed to him to run counter to the ideal of architecture as a great art of expression and of social purport, Niemeyer has consistently striven for beauty and harmony, grace and elegance in an enriched formal vocabulary as the legitimate goals of architectural creation in opposition to merely technical and functional refinements. Unafraid of the curved line, for which he found good precedent in Brazilian Baroque architecture, Niemeyer has used it with an instinctive lyrical touch and an uninhibited spontaneity throughout his career—free-flowing and seemingly arbitrary in the earlier phases, subtly distilled and sophisticated in his later work, where conciseness of expression is equally

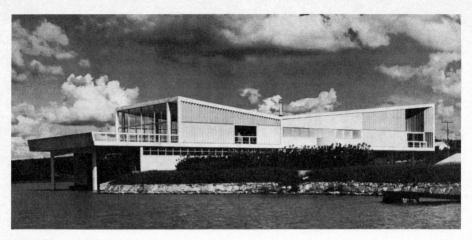

Oscar Niemeyer. Yacht Club. Pampulha, 1943

stressed in the straight and in the curved lines of the composition. This use of the curved line, however, is but one aspect of Niemeyer's most characteristic contribution to modern architecture, his genuine inventiveness, always blossoming in beautifully expressive new forms, or in the revitalized use of consecrated ones. In this connection, his collaboration with numerous structural designers must be mentioned, starting with Emilio Baumgart in the early days and reaching supreme fulfilment with Joaquim Cardoso, from Pampulha to Brasilia.

Oscar Niemeyer, Zenon Lotufo, Helio Uchôa and Eduardo Kneese de Mello. Palace of Industry, Ibirapuéra Park, São Paulo, 1951-4

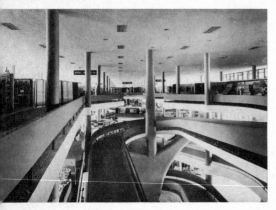

The extent and variety of Niemeyer's significant work, both the executed jobs and the relatively fewer unrealized projects, defeat any attempt to shorten their list. If four larger ones may be thought to highlight Niemeyer's career—Pampulha (1942), São José dos Campos (1947), Ibirapuéra (1950-4), and Brasilia (1956-61)—a great many others have to be taken into account in the intermediate periods. Prior to Pampulha, besides the Brazilian Pavilion at the New York World's Fair in 1939, with Lúcio Costa, three others must be noted: the Hotel Ouro Preto (1940); the architect's own house in Rio (1942); and his competition design for the National Stadium (1941); the first for its fusion of old and new in the traditional setting of the colonial town, the second for its open interior plan, on three levels, and its pioneering use of an inside ramp, the third as a first example of large-scale planning.

The Pampulha group of buildings, famous for its display of new forms, different yet kindred, its gay interplay of light and shade and its deliberate integration of architecture with painting and sculpture—the Casino with the ovoid prism well joined to the crisply rectangular block, the circular Dance Hall with its freely flowing marquee, the Yacht Club with its inverted double slope roof, and the St Francis Chapel with its several parabolic domes—also marks the beginning of the close collaboration between Niemeyer and Juscelino

Kubitschek, then Mayor of the City, later Governor of the State of Minas Gerais, and finally, as President of the Republic, the creator of Brasilia.

The period from 1942 to 1947, to which belong the Boavista Bank, Rio (1946), distinguished by its unassuming openness and its light undulating glass-brick wall in the main banking hall, the Municipal Theatre in Belo Horizonte and the Cataguazes Academy for Boys (1946), as well as the Peixoto residence (1943), is important because of a number of projects which, though never carried out, led Niemeyer into an intensive study of residential architecture. He discovered new possibilities in the interplay of volumes, planes and levels, and better relationships with the site and the view. These conceptions were realized in the Staff Housing units for the São José dos Campos Aeronautical Technical Centre (1947), built as part of an overall scheme which had won first prize in a competition. Later in 1947 Niemeyer joined the international team entrusted with the design of the United Nations' Headquarters in New York, strongly influencing the final scheme, derived from Le Corbusier's and Niemeyer's proposed solutions.

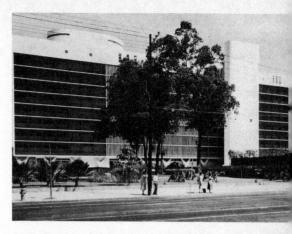

Oscar Niemeyer. Sul America Nursing Home. Rio de Janeiro, 1953

Then follow a series of projects exploring the use of reinforced concrete in the development of complex curved surfaces, such as the twin-theatre Annexe for the Ministry of Education and Health esplanade (1948), the proposed shell-like dome for a monument to Rui Barbosa (1949), or

Oscar Niemeyer. President's Palace. Brasilia, completed 1959

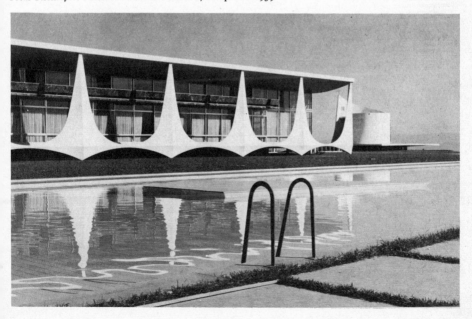

the Duchen Factory (1950, with Helio Uchôa), a 300-metre-long block dramatized by a row of double-span curved rigid frames, spaced 10 metres apart, carrying a roof slab designed to improve the distribution of light; and several equally important jobs emphasizing the possibilities of long straight lines, in wide overhangs or in variously designed sloping supports, as in both the Club and the School at Diamantina (1951), or in the Governor Kubitschek Building in Belo Horizonte (1951), a huge apartment unit complex of two tall simple towers contrasting with the flowing lines of the supporting single storey, which covers almost two city blocks.

All this led to the Parque Ibirapuéra exhibition buildings for the Fourth Centennial of the City of São Paulo, a rare instance of integrated planning of a group of permanent fair buildings over a wide area. Niemeyer unified the scheme by the spreading irregular marquee which links the various blocks to each other; two low ones, 140 metres long, Palace of Nations and Palace of States, with their tilted concrete brackets; the three-storey Palace of Industry, 250 metres long, with its various interior levels capriciously silhouetted by the outline of the mezzanine slab; and the dome-like Palace of the Arts, with its spectacular and almost surrealist interior. All these were designed in 1951 (with Zenon Lotufo, Helio Uchôa and Eduardo Kneese de Mello as associate architects, Gauss Estellita and Carlos Lemos as collaborators).

The sweep and imaginativeness of the Ibirapuéra job, dramatizing and stressing the simplicity of the scheme and of the general concept, in contrast to the hodge-podge usually found in exhibition grounds, seems an appropriate stepping-stone for Niemeyer's crowning achievement, the design of the main public buildings of Brasilia (1950–60). In the intervening

Oscar Niemeyer. Museum with Congress Building in the background. Brasilia, completed 1960

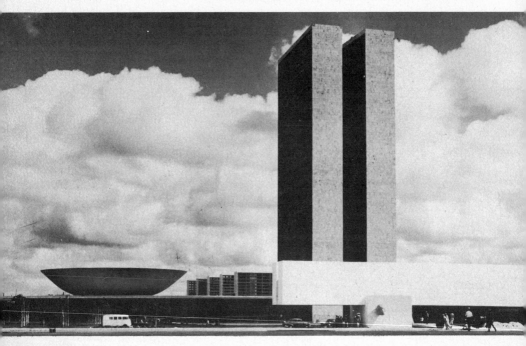

period he is working on the Sul America Hospital (1953); his own house at Gavea (1953), a leaf-like slab inserted in a gorgeous sub-tropical site; the High School at Belo Horizonte (1954), with its striking eye-like auditorium; a project for a museum at Caracas in the form of an inverted pyramid (1954); and an apartment building in the Hansa district of Berlin (1955).

In Brasilia, however, where he was given the task of designing all the main public buildings, Niemeyer was able not only to express the symbolic content of each job and of the whole, implicit in Lúcio Costa's sophisticated general plan, but also to achieve it within a restrained vocabulary, in which poetic flights of imagination, severely disciplined, only highlight, where the artist considers necessary, the particular significance of one or another element in the general context: for example, the beautiful colonnade of the Palace of Dawn, an original theme whose variations may be found in the Supreme Court Building or in the Highland Palace; the startling flower-like design for the Cathedral; the concave and convex dome of the Congress Building in contrast to the soaring twin towers and the horizontal expanse of the base block; farther away, the truncated pyramid of the Opera House; all of them unforgettable accents underlining, against the backdrop of Brasilia's wide horizon, the essential quietness, the coherent simplicity and dignity of all the other architectural elements.

Bibliography: Oscar Niemeyer, *Minha Experiencia em Brasilia*, Rio de Janeiro 1961; Stamo Papadaki, *The Work of Oscar Niemeyer*, New York 1950; Stamo Papadaki, *Oscar Niemeyer—Works in Progress*, New York 1956; Stamo Papadaki, *Oscar Niemeyer*, Ravensburg 1962. Also most of the issues of *Modulo*, which document Niemeyer's later work, especially with regard to Brasilia.

HENRIQUE E. MINDLIN

Nizzoli, Marcello, b. Boretto, Reggio Emilia 1895. Architect, painter and designer. Housing at Ivrea (together with Annibale *Fiocchi and Mario Oliveri), Palazzo Olivetti in Milan (together with Gian Antonio Bernasconi and Annibale Fiocchi, 1954).

Nowicki, Matthew, b. 1910, d. 1949 in a plane crash on the way from India to the United States. He was the architect of the arena at Raleigh, N.C. (1952–3), together with William H. *Deitrick and Severud. Together with Albert Mayer, he produced the first town plan for the new capital of the Punjab, Chandigarh, but this was not executed.

Noyes, Eliot, b. Boston 1910. Architect and designer. Studied at Harvard Graduate School of Architecture, latterly under *Gropius and *Breuer. Sometime director of the Department of International Design at the Museum of Modern Art. His balloon house at Hobe Sound, Florida, was made by spraying concrete on an immense inflated balloon, to produce a hemispherical shell.

O'Gorman, Juan, b. Coyoacán, Mexico 1905. Pupil of José *Villagrán García. His private houses at San Angel (1929–30) are amongst *Mexico's first buildings in the *International Style. Mosaics on the University Library, Mexico, 1952. O'Gorman's own house, a fantastic dream castle in a mannered style, takes advantage of a natural grotto in the rocks.

Olbrich, Joseph Maria, b. Troppau 1867, d. Düsseldorf 1908. Architecture, arts and crafts, book design. Pupil of Otto *Wagner,

Joseph Maria Olbrich. Hochzeitsturm. Darmstadt, 1907

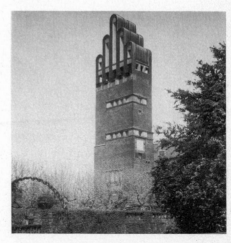

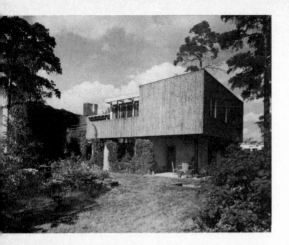

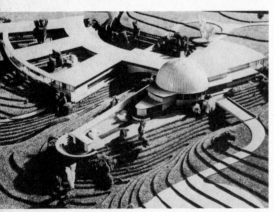

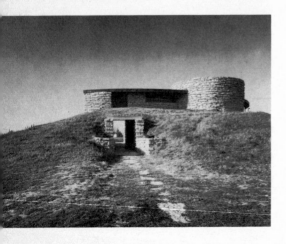

co-founder of the Vienna Sezession, whose exhibition building he designed in 1898–9. Olbrich was the architect of nearly all the buildings for the exhibitions on the Mathildenhöhe in Darmstadt. His Hochzeitsturm ('Wedding Tower') at Darmstadt (1907) is one of the most distinguished pieces of civic adornment in modern architecture.

Organic Architecture. That architecture should in its appearance have a character similar to a natural organism and give the same impression of unity has actuated the work of some of the most important architects of the age, of whom Henry van de *Velde and Erich *Mendelsohn are notable examples in Europe and Louis *Sullivan and Frank Lloyd *Wright in America.

Different theories of organic architecture have been advanced and there is some confused thinking on the subject. It is therefore important to try to dispel this confusion. Some writers have confused the idea of organic architecture with functional building according to social needs, so that if a house is designed in stages according to changing needs, rooms being added as the family grows, that is regarded as organic. It might be regarded as organic building for social needs, but it is too simple and elemental an idea to cover the meaning of organic architecture as conceived by the famous architects mentioned and by others who have been influenced by the idea.

The theory derives from ancient Greek and Roman architecture, and was further developed during the Renaissance. The Greeks based the proportions that should determine the design of temples on the proportions of the human figure. This is recorded and developed by Vitruvius, and many artists of the Renaissance inevitably adopted the theory. Vasari remarked that architecture must appear organic like the body, and Michelangelo held that a knowledge of the human figure led to a comprehension of architecture. Later writers have

Alvar Aalto. Aalto House. Helsinki, 1935–6

Erich Mendelsohn. Synagogue. Cleveland, O., 1946–1952. Model

Frank Lloyd Wright. Jacobs House. Middleton, Wis., 1948

seen in the theory of *Einfühlung*, whereby bodily feelings are projected into the forms of a building, the basis of a modern theory of organic architecture. Although there is a kinship between the two they are not identical. One is the recognition that our bodily existence and bodily feelings must be the measure of the world around us, the other is the application of the principles of that organic life to design.

The nature of organic structure indicates these principles. We find in all natural organisms a certain harmony of parts in relation to the whole which appears to be conditioned by the work the organism is designed to perform, and we find in nature that the plan of an organism influences the character of the subordinate organisms. Transferred to a building this means the integration of the parts with the whole, so that the design of the whole controls the design of the subordinate parts. In addition it would appear to mean that the forms of a building integrated into an harmonious whole shall express a purpose similar to the conditioning of the forms of an organism by the work it is created to perform. This purpose may be to express the structure, such as emphasis on the lines of stress, of thrust and support, and in this there is again the link with *Einfühlung*. The application could not legitimately be extended further to include the social purpose of the building, for this enters the realms of symbolism and departs from the physical context of organic architecture.

We find the theory controlling the work of many modern architects. It was a consistent aim with van de Velde and Mendelsohn, and the latter was pleased when Einstein remarked of his Observatory building at Potsdam that it was Organic. Most architects who are guided by the theory of organic unity do not limit it to the building but insist that the building should be a unity with its surroundings, especially with the site, with the earth on which it stands. Frank Lloyd Wright was especially insistent on this, and he said that a building should not be *on* a hill, but *of* a hill, that it should appear to grow out of the earth. With domestic architecture he said that house and garden should be one, and that it should be difficult to discern where the house ends and the garden begins, a characteristic found in much Japanese architecture. Mendelsohn in many of his buildings let the contours of the ground control the design of his buildings. In brief, organic architecture is not only the complete harmony of the parts of a building with the whole but an integration of the building with its site and surroundings. In a theory of organic architecture, building and town planning should conform to the unity, to the integration of parts, found in the natural world.

Bibliography: Walter Curt Behrendt, *Modern Building*, London 1937; Frank Lloyd Wright, *An Organic Architecture— The Architecture of Democracy*, London 1939; Bruno Zevi, *Towards an Organic Architecture*, London 1950.

ARNOLD WHITTICK

Otto, Frei, b. Siegmar near Chemnitz 1925. Designs for suspended roofs and inflated plastic structures. Marquees at the Federal Flower Shows in Kassel (1955) and Cologne (1957).
Bibliography: Frei Otto, *Über zugbeanspruchte Konstruktionen*, Berlin 1962.

Oud, Jacobus Johannes Pieter, b. Purmerend 1890, d. 1963. Oud received his education at the Quellinus School, the State School of Draughtsmanship in Amsterdam, and Delft Technical College, which awarded him an honorary doctorate after the Second World War. He worked for the architects Jan Stuijt and Theodor *Fischer in Munich for a time, and

Jacobus Johannes Pieter Oud. Workers' housing estate. Hook of Holland, 1924

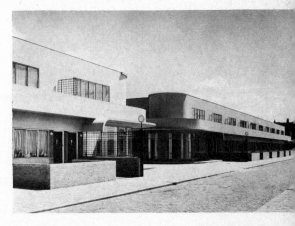

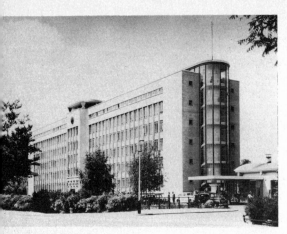

Jacobus Johannes Pieter Oud. Shell Building.
The Hague, 1938

became City Architect of Rotterdam in
1918, where he was responsible for
the Spangen and Tussendijken housing
estates (1920). Oud played a leading part
in the development of *Functionalism
in Western Europe, from the stage of
Neue Sachlichkeit to the emergence of the
*International Style.
Round about the year 1916, Oud came
into contact with Theo van *Doesburg,
and was an active participant in the new
De *Stijl movement. Like most of his
generation, Oud was a great admirer of

Jacobus Johannes Pieter Oud. Bio-Children's
Convalescent Home near Arnhem, 1952–60

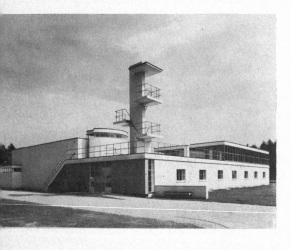

*Berlage, as his early works clearly show.
Berlage's honest handling of materials and
structure was to influence Oud's functionalist architecture strongly, despite its
complete difference of form. Oud was
faced with the difficult task of translating
De Stijl's often all too theoretical ideas
into practical building terms. Examples
of his De-Stijl-type architecture include
the Café de Unie in Rotterdam (1924–5,
destroyed 1940), a project for terraced
housing on the promenade at Schevenin-
gen (1917), and a design for a factory at
Purmerend (1919). After a few years,
Oud broke with van Doesburg, who laid
too much stress on the rôle of abstract
painting in modern architecture. The
housing schemes at Oud-Mathenesse
(1922), Hook of Holland (1924–7) and
Kiefhoek, Rotterdam (1925–7) demonstrate the transition to Neue Sachlichkeit.
From about 1935 onwards, Oud renounced the strictly functionalist style
(Shell Building, The Hague, 1938, and
several post-war office blocks in Rotterdam). This defection drew on him some
sharp criticism, which still affects the
estimation of his oeuvre. His competition
design for the South Holland Local
Government offices at the Hague (1952,
not premiated), and more recent buildings
such as the Bio-Children's Convalescent
Home near Arnhem (1952–60), demonstrate, however, that the Shell Building
belongs to a transitional period influenced
by the general tension in Europe on the
eve of the Second World War. The same
malaise in orthodox Functionalism, albeit
differently manifested, is clearly implied
in the developments of the last ten years
(*CIAM, Otterlo, 1959).
In his book Mijn Weg in De Stijl (1961)
Oud wrote: 'The desire for abstraction
requires melody. Pure abstraction is like
religion without humanity. Humanity
means living in the flowing continuum of
daily existence. The flow and rhythm of
daily existence demand melody from
architecture.'
Bibliography: J. J. P. Oud, Holländische
Architektur (Bauhausbücher 10), Munich
1926; J. J. Pieter Oud, Mijn Weg
in De Stijl, Rotterdam 1961; Henry-
Russell Hitchcock, J. J. P. Oud, Paris
1931; Giulia Veronesi, J. J. Pieter Oud,
Milan 1953.

                                        J. J. VRIEND

Paxton, Joseph, b. Milton-Bryant, Bedfordshire 1803, d. Sydenham 1865. A farmer's son, Paxton was trained as a gardener and became head gardener to the Sixth Duke of Devonshire at Chatsworth, Derbyshire, in 1826. Subsequently he became the Duke's land-agent, business adviser and friend. Paxton had no training as an engineer or architect, but had a gift for shrewd observation and deduction; he proceeded empirically in all his ventures, which stemmed from his own knowledge of natural phenomena.

Paxton had started experimenting with horticultural building at Chatsworth in 1828, and in 1831 hit upon the idea of the 'ridge and furrow' roof. This was refined in detail to become a sloping glass roof without rafters, with very light sash-bars and with the Paxton gutter, which collected both internal and external moisture as well as being a structural member. This roofing was entirely of wood and glass, the wooden parts being produced by machinery which Paxton himself had designed. Hollow cast-iron columns were introduced to support longer spans, serving also for drainage of the roofs. This principle was followed in the curvilinear Great Conservatory at Chatsworth (1836–40), the curved members being of laminated wood, the house being 277 feet long, 123 feet wide and 67 feet high. From curved roofs Paxton moved to a flat roofing system, still with ridges and furrows, for the Lily House of 1849. This was essentially the same system —except for a necessarily larger iron framework—as that used by Paxton in his design for the Great Exhibition Building of 1851, erected in concert with the contractors, Fox and Henderson, and the glass-maker R. L. Chance. This, the largest building ever erected up to that date, was a completely prefabricated structure of standardized, mass-produced parts, based on a module of 24 feet, covering a ground area of over 770,000 square feet. The materials were used afterwards in the erection of the Crystal Palace at Sydenham (1852–4, destroyed by fire 1936), a more elaborate design with three arched transepts and a vaulted nave. Amongst other designs by Paxton for glass buildings were the projects for Crystal Palaces in New York and Paris, the latter being as long as the 1851 building but with three great circular domes in front.

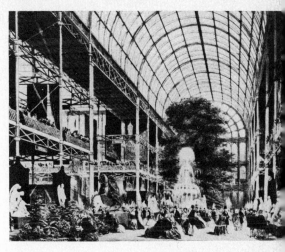

Joseph Paxton, Crystal Palace. London, 1851

At the same time as he was developing his glass structures, Paxton was building conventional masonry houses in accepted styles, including the mansions of Mentmore, Buckinghamshire; Ferrières, near Paris; and Lismore Castle in Ireland. As a landscape architect he designed the grounds of the Crystal Palace, modified the gardens at Chatsworth and laid out a number of public parks, notably that at Birkenhead. He experimented successfully with hydraulic engineering, constructing the highest fountain jet in the world at Chatsworth,

Joseph Paxton. Crystal Palace. Sydenham, 1852–4

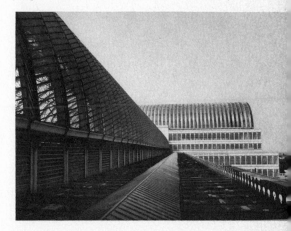

and in heating and ventilating. His interests as a railway promoter, contractor and Member of Parliament led him to advocate important town-planning schemes, of which the most important were the Thames Embankment (1864–70) and his project for the Great Victorian Way (1855). The latter was to be an eleven-mile-long 'girdle' around central London, to solve its traffic problems, combining a glass-roofed road lined by houses, shops and public buildings with railways on upper tiers.

Bibliography: Violet Markham, *Paxton and the Bachelor Duke*, London 1935; G. F. Chadwick, *The Works of Sir Joseph Paxton*, Architectural Press, London 1961.

G. F. CHADWICK

Pei, Ioh Ming, b. Canton, China 1917. Studied at the Massachusetts Institute of Technology and at Harvard. Office blocks, department stores, town planning projects. The Mile High Center at Denver, Col. (1956) has an attractive façade design featuring two intersecting systems: columns and beams with dark cast-aluminium cladding; the air conditioning ducts are sited

Auguste Perret. Apartment Block, Rue Franklin. Paris, 1903

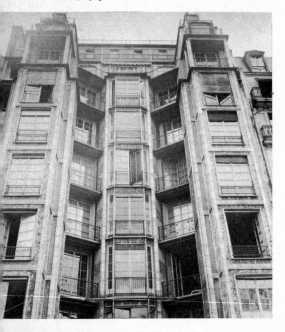

behind strips of bright enamelling. Has worked on the development plans of Washington, Chicago and Philadelphia.

Perret, Auguste, b. Brussels 1874, d. Paris 1954. Perret had his first architectural training at the Paris *École des Beaux-Arts, which he left, however, before sitting his finals. He entered his family's building firm, which had early specialized in reinforced concrete construction; the first building he himself designed dates already from the year 1890.

Perret is frequently reproached with having, on the one hand, applied reinforced concrete methods that were still in their infancy at the time of his first sensational buildings (apartment house in the Rue Franklin, Paris, 1903; Garage Ponthieu, Paris, 1906; Théâtre des Champs-Elysées, Paris, 1910–13) to a system of columns and beams taken over from carpentry, hence depriving architecture for decades to come of freedom in employing the new material. On the other hand it is said that in his old ago he grafted neoclassic features onto this monolithic material which were in no ways a logical outcome of its use (Mobilier National, Paris, 1931; Musée des Travaux Publics, 1937; atomic research station, Saclay, 1947; reconstruction of Le Havre). The reproach of neo-Academic formalism is justified as regards Perret's late work. His talent for structurally lucid design peters out into empty trifling. It can hardly be claimed, however, that Perret's early intervention in the history of reinforced concrete construction has had negative consequences. Not only did Perret make it possible to use *reinforced concrete in architecture, which none of his contemporaries succeeded in doing to the same extent, he was also the only one among the pioneers of modern architecture who did not simply preach 'honest building' but practised it as well. His system of columns and beams, the essence of the whole method of framed structures, accords exactly with the demand for economy of formwork. The fruit of his mature years displays a perfection of craftsmanship which is only to be encountered elsewhere in *Mies van der Rohe, who, incidentally, has not a little in common with Perret. But Perret was not just a consummate structural designer who paved the way to architecture for reinforced concrete. His consistent use of the material resulted in a number of buildings still considered exemplary today, among them that masterpiece of 20th-century architecture, the Church of Notre-Dame at Le Raincy (1922–23). There the neoclassicist Perret has paradoxically been successful—uniquely in his time—in reviving the Gothic church lunette. His numerous villas and studio-houses of the next decade are characterized by precision and delicacy of proportion and detailing. The sharp distinction made between framework and infill is raised to the point of dogma and leads to a new conception of form reminiscent of the purest creations of a Gabriel or *Schinkel. Thus both traditions of French rationalism are perpetuated in Perret's reinforced concrete style, that of the neo-Gothic, as significantly formulated by *Viollet-le-Duc, and that represented by the classicism of Perret's teacher Guadet.

The freest expression of Perret's structural genius is to be found in his industrial commissions where he is relieved of the frustrating task of achieving monumentality (warehouses at Casablanca, 1915; clothes factory and scene painting studio, Paris, 1919; workshops for steel or aluminium rolling mills at Montataire, 1920 and Issoire, 1939; watch factory at Besançon, 1939; aircraft hangar at Marseilles, 1950). Unhampered by decorative details, these purely functional buildings however lack those amazing effects achieved by *Maillart, *Nervi, or *Freyssinet through the use of novel structural shapes. And yet they have an elegance and dignity, attained by their unparalleled lucidity of construction and harmony of rhythm and proportion. Perret's industrial buildings, from the Garage Ponthieu to the marine laboratories on the Boulevard Victor, Paris (1928), like those by Saarinen and Mies, rank amongst the most important architectural efforts to stress the 'nobility of the industrial age'.

Finally, Perret's research into the standardization and industrialization of building components should be mentioned, which apart from anything else was not without influence on his sometime pupil *Le Corbusier.

Bibliography: Auguste Perret, Contribution à une Théorie de l'Architecture, Paris 1952; P. Jamot, A. et G. Perret et l'Architecture du Béton Armé, Paris and Brussels 1927; Ernesto N. Rogers, Auguste Perret, Milan

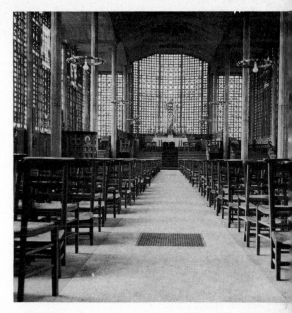

Auguste Perret. Notre-Dame. Le Raincy, 1922–3

1955; Bernard Champigneulle, Auguste Perret, Paris 1959; Peter Collins, Concrete —The Vision of a New Architecture, London 1959.

MAURICE BESSET

Auguste Perret. Place de l'Hôtel de Ville. Le Havre, commenced 1947

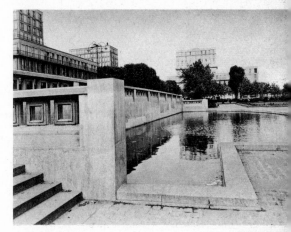

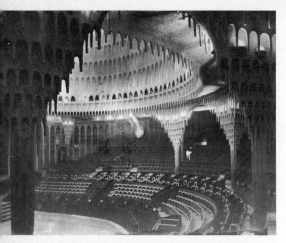

Hans Poelzig. Grosses Schauspielhaus. Berlin, 1919

Gio Ponti. Pirelli Building. Milan, 1958

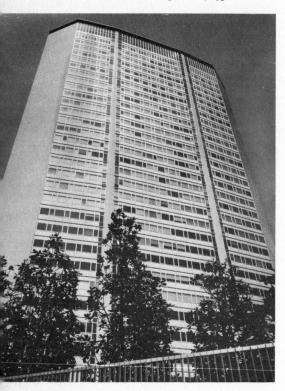

Poelzig, Hans, b. Berlin 1869, d. Berlin 1936. Poelzig exerted great influence in Germany both as an architect and as a teacher (Professor at the Charlottenburg Technical College). His office building, Breslau 1911, anticipates the favourite motive of the twenties, fenestration in horizontal strips. Industrial buildings such as the Luban chemical factory near Posen (1911–12) and the water tower at Posen (1911) are the forerunners of Poelzig's Expressionist phase. His designs just after the First World War (Project for the Salzburg Festival Theatre, 1920–1) are of visionary imagination. The rebuilding of the Schumann Circus into Max Reinhardt's Grosses Schauspielhaus was based on these designs (Berlin 1919): a 'space-cave' masked by stalactite-shapes, which made acting on an arena stage feasible. Towards the end of the twenties, Poelzig went over to buildings of a monumental straightforwardness. (Administrative block for IG-Farben, Frankfort on the Main, 1928–31).
Bibliography: Theodor Heuss, *Hans Poelzig, Lebensbild eines deutschen Baumeisters,* Tübingen 1955; *Architectural Review,* June 1963.

Polk, Willis Jefferson, b. near Frankfort, Kentucky 1867, d. San Mateo, Calif. 1924. Pupil of *Maybeck. The Hallidie Building (San Francisco, 1918) by Polk and Co. is one of the first buildings with a fully glazed, non-loadbearing outer wall (*curtain wall).

Pollini, Gino, b. Rovereto, Trentino 1903. Graduated Milan 1927. Founder-member of *gruppo 7. Works in collaboration with Luigi *Figini.

Ponti, Gio, b. Milan 1891. Ponti is the best known Italian architect today. He graduated in Milan in 1921, and already had some professional experience when the foundation of the *Movimento Italiano per l'Architettura Razionale* in 1927 presented Italian architects with radically new problems and new responsibilities, at a period when the *Novecento Italiano's* neoclassic revivalism was triumphant.
In this current, which saw the end of *Futurism, Gio Ponti practised an elegant 'modernism', derived partly from the Viennese style of the time, mixed with neoclassic motifs and rationalist lucidity. In

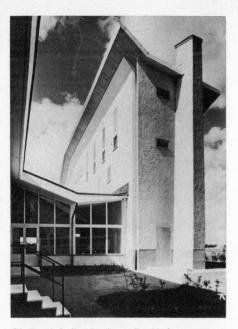

Gio Ponti. Italian Institute. Stockholm, 1959

contrast to the other architects of his generation, who relied on the classical effects of arches and columns and took no account of the new developments in building technology, Ponti adhered in general to the tenets of the rationalist and functionalist school; but he stayed clear of the controversies, perilously conducted by Persico and Pagano, nor did he join the revolt of the younger architects (banded together as *gruppo 7) against revivalism, the historic styles and the abuse of decoration.

Ponti founded the journal *Domus* in 1928. Now the most widely read publication in the field of interior decoration, it proved a very effective instrument at the time in improving the taste of the Italian middle classes. In 1933, before he had discarded his neoclassicist leanings, Ponti was appointed to the executive committee of the V Milan Triennale, then known as 'Ponti's Triennale'. Its great merit was that it opened the doors of this famous international exhibition to the young 'rationalists' of the Milanese avant-garde, who had now become the most representative archi-

tects of the modern movement. During these years Ponti did a good deal of work in the field of industrial design, to new criteria; built flats, churches and factories; and wrote articles and books (e.g. *La casa all'Italiana*, 1933) in which he put forward the viewpoint that architecture must always preserve some national characteristics.

Ponti's long series of buildings began in 1923. In 1934 he designed the Institute of Mathematics for the University of Rome; but it was only in 1936, with his scheme for the Catholic Press Exhibition in Vatican City, one of his happiest creations, that he gave up the strict symmetry and conventions of neoclassicism. Again in 1936 he designed the first office block for the Montecatini Company in Milan (the second dates from 1951), in which he combined *Novecento* elements (e.g. maximum plastic evidence of volumes) with others of the rationalist system of aesthetics. This imposing building remains one of his most important and lasting works. After a series of projects carried out in every part of the world save in Italy, from São Paulo to Caracas, and from Paris to Stockholm, he achieved his masterpiece in 1958 with the Pirelli Skyscraper in Milan (with *Nervi as structural engineer), whose outline is now universally familiar. This building, with its hexagonal plan and its sides tapered like a ship's bows, has affected the town planning layout of the whole surrounding zone, itself partly designed by the same architect.

Among the buildings he has currently under construction may be mentioned a new hospital for Milan, with an interesting surface treatment; two churches; offices for the Bagdad Planning Board; and eight ministry buildings for Islamabad, the new capital of Pakistan. Since 1936 Gio Ponti has lectured in the faculty of architecture at Milan Polytechnic, and has held courses in the Universities of São Paulo, Paris, Delft, Istanbul, Barcelona, Caracas, Zurich, Stockholm, Madrid and Gothenburg. He was the first president of the International Museum of Modern Architecture, founded in Milan in 1961.

Bibliography: Gio Ponti, *Amate l'Architettura*, Milan 1957; Edoardo Persico, 'Giovanni Ponti', in *L'Italia Letteraria 29*, April 1934; James S. Plaut, *Espressione di Gio Ponti*, Milan 1954.

GIULIA VERONESI

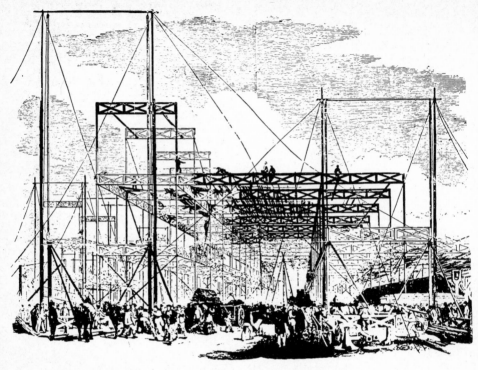

Joseph Paxton. Crystal Palace. London, 1851. Assembling prefabricated units

Powell and Moya. Philip Powell and John Hidalgo Moya. Studied at the Architectural Association School of Architecture, London, and founded their partnership in 1946, two years after graduating, to carry out the Pimlico Housing Scheme, London, which they had won in competition against sixty-four entrants with a design that proved a significant landmark in the attempt to establish a post-war vernacular. Vertical feature ('Skylon') at the South Bank Exhibition, London, 1951; Mayfield Comprehensive School, Putney, 1956, 'subtle, elegant, humane' (Ian Nairn); Princess Margaret Hospital, Swindon; undergraduates' rooms at Brasenose College, Oxford; hexagonal theatre with an arena stage, Chichester, 1962.

Prefabrication. Prefabrication is the attempt of modern building technology to increase building productivity. Many variations of this idea and its realization are feasible and are already being developed

today. Even traditional building consists of a large number of parts previously fabricated in factories, but they rarely exhibit common principles of design, structure or manufacture. Besides raising productivity by the use of rationalization on the building site, the logical aim of prefabrication must be the factory-made building, turned out by industrial production techniques. The method still in use today of craft prefabrication is imperfect and must be supplemented by the complete interposition of industrial manufacturing processes. Entire dispensation with site work, however, is only possible in the case of smaller private houses (prefabricated houses). That is why the greatest efforts are being concentrated on turning out this type of building in factories.

These attempts to produce a prefabricated or even an industrially manufactured house have so far not evinced any conclusive results. Many prototypes and some production models of certain series are available, however. Examples—some already of historical interest—include the Acorn House, the Dymaxion House (*Fuller), the General Panel House (*Gropius, *Wachsmann), the Lustron House and the TVA-Trailer, to mention but a few. Another large field of application that has opened up is that of filler units, internal and external wall panels, and roof and floor slabs; other typical products include *curtain walls, infill panels and movable partitions.

The various materials and the industrial processes connected with them have rendered novel structural methods possible and a number of countries have already turned out some excellent products. Fundamentally light structural systems, light forms of building with light or even heavy materials show the greatest progress as compared with traditional building. Integral structures, *space frames and *suspended roofs are particularly progressive developments of this method of building. Other branches of industry, such as aircraft and vehicle production, have strongly influenced the ideas of architects and structural engineers.

The hazards of prefabrication and the industrial manufacture of buildings lie on the sociological plane. Heavy structural systems are particularly unsuitable as they lack adaptability to the multifarious natural patterns of population and their ways of living. That is why adaptability in building

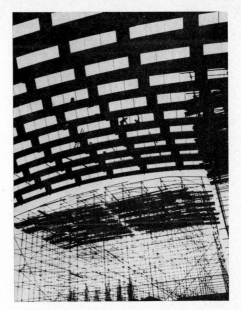

Pier Luigi Nervi. Exhibition hall, Turin, 1948–9. Erecting prefabricated reinforced concrete units from a mobile staging

Below left. Richard Buckminster Fuller. Dymaxion House, 1927. Elevation and isometric view

Walter Gropius. Type series house, with various methods of combining the individual components. 1923. Project

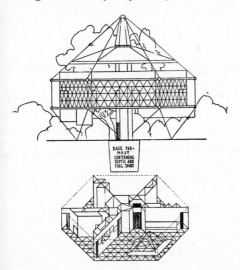

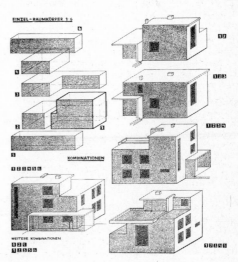

is given special consideration when prefabricated structures and components are designed: hence the emergence of 'building block' systems that can be combined to meet different circumstances, together with the reduction of the total number of building types, effected by standardization. Modular coordination, which has long been recognized as a prerequisite for rational manufacture and planning, has been introduced in many countries and is proving an indispensable rule in the design of these new building products.

The achievements of individual countries have been helped by the conscious co-operation of industry, government departments and large planning and construction teams. In the *United States, the mass-production of family houses has made great headway, while *curtain walling in

Kaija and Heikki Siren. Terraced housing on the Tapiola estate, 1954–5. Erecting a prefabricated façade unit

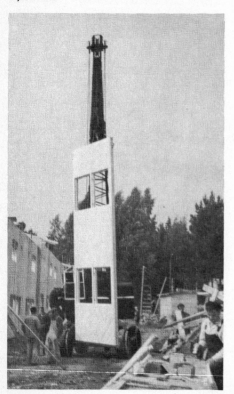

particular has been developed for multi-storey buildings. In *Great Britain, after the Second World War, a systematic development of various methods of light prefabricated construction for school buildings has taken place, which have not only quickly solved a technological problem but have also made an indirect contribution to education for free and contemporary living. In *France, Scandinavia and the USSR likewise since the Second World War numerous prefabricated heavy structural systems, based on concrete units, have been devised for multi-storey blocks of flats. Examples, however, which are functional and economic in their countries of origin are not necessarily suitable for export elsewhere without modification. Another interesting development towards complete prefabrication has taken place, again in the United States. In 1960, for example, twice as many caravans, i.e. mobile houses, have been manufactured as prefabricated stationary houses. Thus for the first time we have a building completely prefabricated in the factory, from raw material to final assembly.

With the introduction of prefabrication and the aim of industrial manufacture the demands on architects, planners and engineers have risen. The traditional methods of architectural design are no longer sufficient. These new requirements and the increased responsibility that goes with them make it essential today to transfer the methods of applied science and industrial engineering to architecture. Architecture is thus becoming more and more of an applied science.

Bibliography: Buckminster Fuller, *Brief Building Construction*; Robert W. Marks, *The Dymaxion World of R. Buckminster Fuller*, New York 1960; Konrad Wachsmann, *Wendepunkt im Bauen*, Wiesbaden 1959.

HERBERT OHL

Prouvé, Jean, b. Nancy 1901. What Jean Prouvé, constructor in light metal, has in common with the great ironwork engineers of the 19th century, apart from a sure feeling for his material and a wealth of technical and design ideas, is a dynamic conception of the interplay of the different components and functions of a structure, regardless of whether he is designing a prefabricated façade element, a living unit, a school or a desk. Jean Prouvé is a son of the painter Victor Prouvé, who played a leading part in the École de Nancy, one of the most important centres of Art Nouveau. A trained art-metalworker, Prouvé tackles the formal problems of construction in the 'organic' spirit of this school. For him, form can develop only from a synthesis of all structural and functional components, which in their turn must be considered as parts of a unique constellation. At the same time he is fully aware that the road to the architecture of the future inevitably leads via the thoroughgoing industrialization of building methods, and that industrialization without sweeping standardization of forms is unthinkable.

Prouvé escapes this dilemma by an empirical attitude which abolishes all formalism. As early as 1934 he developed *curtain walling, which he employed in 1936 for a club house at Buc airport and in 1937–9 at the Maison du Peuple at Clichy (architects *Beaudouin and *Lods). But while this type of structure often becomes a purely graphic pattern, Prouvé has created a number of variants that constitute a series of very acceptable formal innovations, conceived from a need to achieve the best possible adaptation to particular technical and functional requirements: Building Industry Association Headquarters, Paris, 1950 (with Lopez); Exhibition Hall, Lille (with Herbé); CNIT Exhibition Hall, Paris (with *Zehrfuss, Camelot and de Mailly) and the French Pavilion at Brussels (with Gillet), 1958; block of flats, Paris, 1954 (with Mirabaud); hall for the *100 Years of Aluminium* exhibition in Paris, 1954; Technical College, Lyons (INSA with Perrin-Fayolle); Central Research Institute of Grenoble University, 1959. Prouvé considers that all building components, from roof slabs to built-in cupboards, and from the columns to the essential services (kitchen, bath, w.c.) can be factory-made, ready for assembly in the same way as façade units, and put into service structurally as well as functionally at the same time. As a result of decades of research, which led to the extensive redesigning of all these elements, Prouvé began to mass-produce prefabricated buildings of all types (houses, schools, offices, canteens, workshops, laboratories, holiday camps), among which the shell type houses (estate at Meudon, 1949), the Abbé Pierre

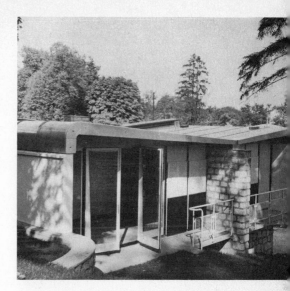

Jean and Henri Prouvé, André Sive. Experimental houses. Meudon, 1954

House, the isothermal living quarters for Sahara conditions and the schools deserve special mention.

Despite the extreme economy of their method of production and their standardization, these buildings possess an almost luxurious character and retain a high degree of individuality. This is in contrast to the usual dreary monotony found in prefabricated buildings and recalls instead the affluent architecture of *Mies van der Rohe.

Jean Prouvé and Maurice Novarina. Refreshment room. Evian, completed 1957

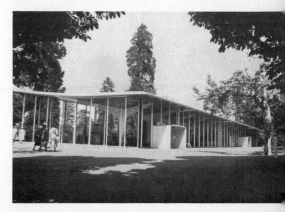

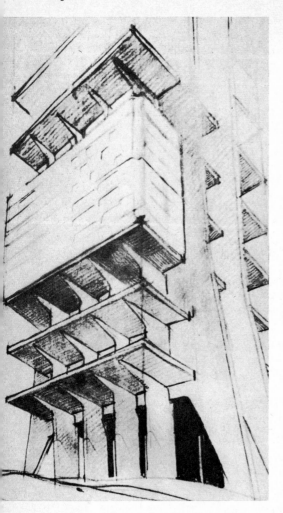

Jean Prouvé, Belmont and Silvy. Point block of flats for lecturers, Cité Universitaire. Nancy. Project

The reason is not so much the precise finish and the carefully planned equipment but the feeling of freedom bestowed by the elegance of proportions and forms and the generous distribution of space. In some buildings (villas at Nancy and on the Côte d'Azur, school at Villejuif, refreshment room at Evian) Prouvé's artistry in structure reaches a point of perfection, where the building seems to be weightless. Although the shell of such buildings is

exclusively of glass, they do not appear to be mere glass boxes. Tensile stresses which infuse the structural forms with a lively excitement, hinged stanchions with asymmetrically cantilevered arms, intersections which are not rectangular but acute or quite gradual, even with curved transitions, and finally a spatial flow which is never unnecessarily interrupted, all these combine to lend his buildings a clear, gay character which is unique in the architecture of today. These designs, which originated in the laboratory and the factory, have nothing artificial or schematic about them; on the contrary, they are alive and unfold with a surprising spontaneity, like organisms friendly to man.

Bibliography: Special issue of the journal *Architecture*, Nos. 11/12, Brussels 1954; Françoise Choay, 'Jean Prouvé' in *L'Oeil*, Vol. X, No. 46, Paris 1958; G. Gassiot-Talabot, 'Jean Prouvé' in *Cimaise*, Vols. VII-VIII, No. 54, Paris 1961.

MAURICE BESSET

Rainer, Roland, b. Klagenfurt 1910. Trained at the Vienna Technical College. Began teaching 1953; professor at the Vienna Academy of Fine Arts (1956). Since 1958 town planner at Vienna. Schools, housing (prefabricated housing estate for Vienna XIII, together with Auböck, 1954), municipal halls for Vienna (1954–8), and Bremen (under construction).

Reidy, Affonso Eduardo, b. Paris 1909, d. Rio de Janeiro 1964. Reidy graduated at the Escola Nacional de Belas Artes, Rio, in 1930. Before joining the design team of the Ministry of Education Building, he had produced a significant job in the 'Home of Good Will', a charitable institution for old people (1931–2), and when Lúcio *Costa appointed *Warchavchik Professor of Architectural Design at the School of Fine Arts (1931) had served as his assistant. Subsequently, his work developed in a subtly personal manner, characterized not only by the apparent casualness with which he embarked upon the most daring formal or structural scheme but also by a pioneering research into new architectural and technical solutions, noticeable, to a greater or lesser degree, in all his projects and finished work. Among others, in the designs for the City Transport Service

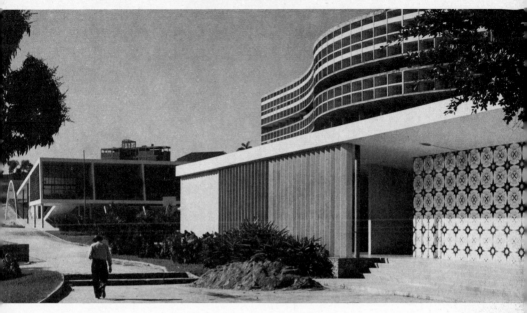

Affonso Eduardo Reidy. Pedregulho Estate. Rio de Janeiro, commenced 1947

Offices and Workshops, Rio (1939), with double saw-tooth roofs over the workshops area; for a pumping station in Rio (1949), a service installation transformed into an attractive spot in a park by the sculptural integration of all the elements of the programme; the design for a Museum of Visual Arts, São Paulo (1951), a clean-cut triangular prism sitting on an expressive base structure, on a highly irregular site; or for a Student Theatre, Rio (1955), with the structural supports of the auditorium roof almost floating in mid-air, cantilevered from the massive stage block. And again, in such finished work as the 'Pedregulho' Housing Development, Rio (begun in 1947), with its 260-metre-long apartment block, following the winding contour of the hillside, and its imaginatively designed school, gymnasium, clinic, laundry and

Affonso Eduardo Reidy. Museum of Modern Art. Rio de Janeiro, commenced 1954. Sketch

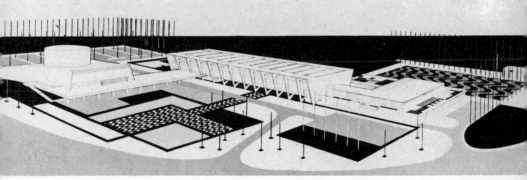

market; or the Marechal Hermes Community Theatre, Rio (1950), a precise and pleasant application of the inverted double slope roof; or the private houses built for Miss Carmen Portinho (1952-4) or Dr Couto e Silva (1955) as well as his latest country house near Petropolis. These same qualities find expression in several important projects still under construction: the 'Gavea' Housing Development, in Rio (1954-), an extension of the principles first applied in the 'Pedregulho' project; the Experimental School in Asuncion, Paraguay (1953-), and the Museum of Modern Art of Rio de Janeiro (1954-), two limpid groupings of various different volumes, underlined by serene rows of concrete ribs enclosing and supporting roof and floor slab, and characterized by freely flowing wide spaces as well as by the novel ways in which natural daylight is combined with artificial lighting; the headquarters for the Rio City Employees Insurance Fund (1957-), with its striking *brise-soleil* façade arrangement.

Reidy's superb plan for the development of Santo Antônio Hill, in the centre of Rio (1948), still under way, has unfortunately suffered the impact of bureaucratic antagonism in many important respects.

Bibliography: K. Franck, *The Works of Affonso Eduardo Reidy*, London 1960.

HENRIQUE E. MINDLIN

Reinforced Concrete. In 1895, François Hennebique completed the Charles VI Mill at Tourcoing. Its loadbearing structure in reinforced concrete was clearly expressed in the elevations; designed without any straining after decorative effects, it fulfilled the functional and technical requirements of its industrial programme admirably, achieving a formal equilibrium and a new vocabulary of style without recourse to traditional solutions. Two years later, Anatole de *Baudot, with the technical collaboration of Contamin, finished building the Church of St Jean-de-Montmartre, Paris—the first conscious exploitation of the new material for architectural and compositional ends as compared with purely technical ones.

It was in this way, at the end of the 19th century, that the design possibilities of a new material were demonstrated in the first buildings to use it, though it had been discovered, experimented with and its basic technical properties established over the course of the previous fifty years. Reinforced concrete is an artificial monolithic material, derived from the union of steel and concrete, when the latter hardens after the mix has been poured in a fluid state into specially prepared shuttering. The concrete itself is obtained from mixing cement, water and aggregate (sand and gravel) in proportions that vary with the technical results required. The steel reinforcement consists of a cage of steel bars, normally round, though other special sections are sometimes used to increase the degree to which the reinforcement is anchored in the concrete. The size and disposition of the bars is determined in accordance with the particular static and technical requirements involved. The shuttering which holds the mix in its liquid state until it has set, determines the shape of the concrete. Shuttering, or form-work as it is sometimes called, is made up of timber boards, metal panels or units of other material; structural, economic, architectural and decorative factors influence the choice. The two components of reinforced concrete perform the static functions appropriate to their respective properties: basically, the concrete takes up the compressive stresses, and the steel absorbs those of tension.

The idea of assigning different but complementary stress-resistant functions to different materials within the same static system, was first developed and applied many centuries ago; examples may be found in the use of chains for tying in vaults in Byzantine, Islamic, Italian Gothic, Renaissance and Baroque architecture, for which iron, and more anciently wood, was employed. Working to different formal standards, static systems were also evolved, especially after the Late Renaissance, in which the device for resisting tensile stress (chain or hoop) was masked. In Paris, from the 17th century onwards, stressed reinforcements were incorporated and interposed between single elements of the same masonry structure (colonnade at the Louvre by Claude Perrault, 1665-80; portico of the Church of Ste Geneviève (later the Panthéon) by Germain Soufflot, 1757-90). At the Panthéon in particular, the iron ribs, disposed in a more complex manner than hitherto, specifically absorb the forces of tension and shear, thus

achieving empirically the typical layout of
the bars in reinforced concrete and antici-
pating intuitively the results that were to
be reached a hundred years later by the
processes of scientific calculation.

The first instances of the employment of
iron in conjunction with concrete, however,
only go back to the first half of the 19th
century: these consist of wrought-iron
I-section floors with thin curved metal
plates running between the girders, filled
in on top with concrete; the engineer
William Fairbairn built an eight-storey
refinery at Manchester in 1845 using such
a system, patented in 1844. A number of
basic experiments were carried out between 1849 and 1878: in 1849–50 the
French gardener Joseph Monier made
some concrete tubs for orange-trees in
which he embedded a mesh of iron rods;
J. L. Lambot exhibited a boat in concrete
on a frame of iron flats at the 1855 Paris
Exposition; in 1861, the French builder
François Coignet improved the strength
of his concrete structures by inserting a
metal mesh in them; a British immigrant
to America, Thaddeus Hyatt, outlined the
theory of reinforced concrete in 1877 on
the basis of tests with beams, made for him
at a laboratory in London. Between 1867
and 1878 Monier took out a series of patents
for various applications, showing a clear
appreciation of the different stress-resistant
properties of iron and concrete respectively.
Theoretical and experimental research
carried out chiefly by Wayss, Bauschinger,
Contamin, Bordenave, Hennebique, E.
Coignet and De Tedesco succeeded between 1880 and 1900 in fully establishing
the main characteristics and the static
behaviour of the new material, and the
theoretical bases for calculating structures
in it. The use of reinforced concrete began
to spread at the beginning of the 20th
century in projects of ever-increasing
importance; official standards and codes of
practice were called for, and these were
published in various countries in the first
decades of the century.

The young French architect Tony *Garnier in his scheme for a *Cité Industrielle*
(1901–4) made sytematic use of reinforced
concrete and other modern materials,
adopting the unadorned grid system even
for housing and offices, which Hennebique
had employed for the first time in 1895 for
the Charles VI Mill. He thus anticipated

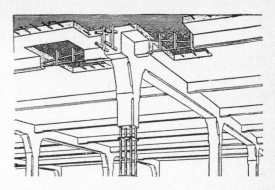

Hennebique's reinforced concrete system, 1892

by almost twenty years an architectural
idiom that was first to become widespread
only in the period of the *International
Style.

At the same epoch, Auguste *Perret, at the
beginning of his career as an architect and
builder, erected a house in the Rue Franklin,

Anatole de Baudot and Contamin. Church of
St Jean-de-Montmartre. Paris, 1894–7

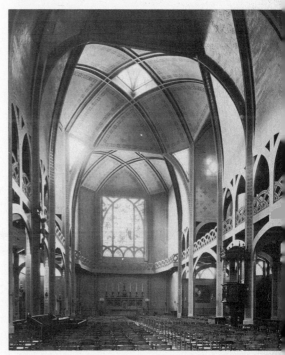

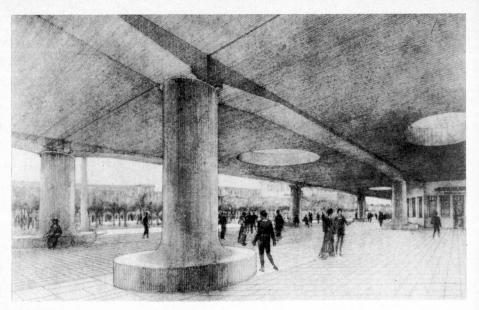

Tony Garnier. Town Hall. Cité Industrielle. 1901–4. Project

Paris, in which he exploited the technical possibilities of a reinforced concrete-framed structure (smaller size of stanchions and greater freedom of manoeuvre with them) to resolve a difficult planning problem, basing the architectural treatment of the façade on the contrast between the loadbearing frame and the infill panels. Meanwhile, in the villa he built himself at Bourg-la-Reine in 1904, Hennebique demonstrated the static possibilities of reinforced concrete in controversial fashion with such structural novelties as an octagonal tower carried on 13-foot cantilevers. The architectural idiom employed is still traditional and eclectic, but Hennebique, perhaps unconsciously, opened up new prospects of three-dimensional design.

The first, almost contemporary, works of the Swiss engineer Robert *Maillart, on the other hand, are the result of a far-reaching attempt to achieve absolute stylistic purity by deliberately aiming at unity of form and static behaviour in his structures. In his bridge over the Rhine at Tavanasa (1905) carriageway and structural framework are intimately fused to produce a structural and plastic unity. The first example of mushroom slab construction occurs in a warehouse he built in 1910 at Zurich, where beams are eliminated and the floor slab itself is designed in such a way as to take over their static functions.

The problem of large-span roofs, hitherto dealt with by using steel-frame structures, was now finally tackled and solved in reinforced concrete. In his Centenary Hall at Breslau (1912–13), Max *Berg roofed the central area of the assembly hall with a dome made up of huge concrete ribs 213 feet in diameter. Eugène *Freyssinet covered his two airship hangars at Orly (1916–24) with a barrel vault consisting of a thin membrane of reinforced concrete, pleated to give the necessary rigidity, and parabolic in overall section to reduce tensile stresses to a minimum.

The employment of reinforced concrete for large industrial complexes became a regular practice. In 1915, the engineer Matté Trucco began building the Fiat-Lingotto works at Turin, with an area of over a hundred acres. He adopted reinforced concrete for every type of structure, solving technical problems of great difficulty in the automobile testing track he sited on the roof of a five-storey factory, and the access ramp that leads up to it.

It was during these years, too, that *Le Corbusier, not yet thirty, was working out the premises of his architectural manner. Reinforced concrete seemed to him to be the most appropriate medium for realizing them in. With his project for the Dom-Ino houses (1914), based on a modular grid in reinforced concrete, he set forth the theoretical preconditions for designing a free plan. America, too, whose architecture had developed during the 19th century via the habitual adoption of the steel frame, began to accept the use of reinforced concrete (albeit not without controversy), especially for large-scale industrial buildings (warehouse for Montgomery, Ward & Co., Chicago, by Schmidt, Garden and Martin, 1908; silos at Fort William, c. 1900). *Gropius published these buildings in 1913 in the Annual of the *Deutscher Werkbund, acknowledging them as creations of modern architecture.

The commission to design the Einstein Observatory-Tower at Potsdam in 1920 gave Erich *Mendelsohn his first opportunity of bringing to actual realization the architectural vision which had been maturing in his sketches from 1914 to 1919

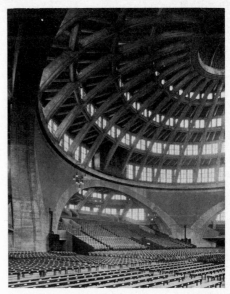

Max Berg. Centenary Hall. Breslau, 1912–13

Auguste Perret. Garage Ponthieu. Paris, 1906

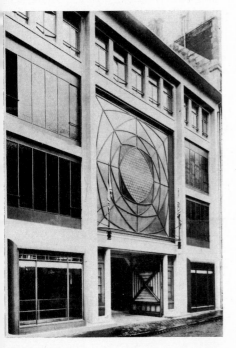

(*Expressionism). Reinforced concrete is the material theoretically best adapted for modelling a form that has to be rendered as a fluid, homogeneous and continuous mass, and for creative works of architecture freed from the traditional schematism of horizontal and vertical lines. It was impossible to make use of the new material, however, because no curved shuttering was available: the tower had to be built in brick and rendered over. The full exploitation of the plastic possibilities of concrete was achieved shortly afterwards, in the German Expressionist manner, with the War Memorial at Weimar by Gropius (1921) and the Goetheanum at Dornach by Rudolf Steiner (1925–8).

Inspired by the climate of research and experiment of the early post-war years, *Mies van der Rohe prepared a scheme for the Novembergruppe Exhibition in 1922 for a reinforced concrete office block in which the stanchions are set back from the façades and support the floors, which project out all round, by a cantilever arrangement. The external walls assume the character of a series of horizontal strips, one on top of the other. In the years that followed, this architectural idiom became the common property of the rationalist movement, and may be met with in the works of many architects before the Second World War, modified to accord with personal styles (Boots' Factory at Beeston, by Sir E. Owen *Williams, 1932; Open-Air School, Amsterdam, by J. *Duiker, 1930–2; tobacco factory at Linz, by P. *Behrens, 1930–5).

Perret, meanwhile, had carried his architectural use of reinforced concrete further. In the Church of Notre-Dame, Le Raincy (1922–3), a limited budget favoured the elimination of many of the frills usual in ecclesiastical work. The reinforced concrete frame supports a system of vaults and forms the bell-tower. The walls are perforated concrete panels set with coloured glass. The decorative result is indubitably rich, despite the poverty of materials and the rough appearance of the concrete left completely exposed. Karl *Moser's Church of St Antony, Basle (1926–7) is an organic structure in frankly exposed reinforced concrete which derives its inspiration from the contemporary works of Perret.

Walter Gropius adopted reinforced concrete construction in 1925–6 for all the buildings of the Bauhaus. The individual

Le Corbusier. Unité d'Habitation. Nantes-Rezé, 1952–7

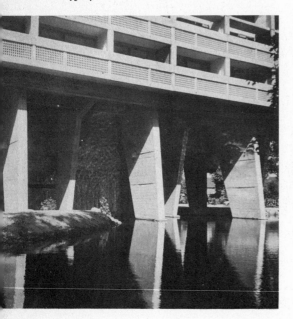

character of the various structural elements, however, was not stressed by underlining their physical consistency and technical properties, but static and formal design was rigorously conditioned by architectural and functional requirements. Henceforth reinforced concrete became a structural element of great versatility, capable of responding to all the demands made on it by the compositional freedom of modern architecture, without having to assume major status as a source of expression. In Le Corbusier's Pavillon Suisse (1930–2) the reinforced concrete substructure, consisting of six huge piers over which the steel frame of the upper storeys is cantilevered, provides an airy and welcoming portico that is imposing in appearance while effecting a happy transition between the external surroundings and the inside of the building. The surface of the concrete is left in the state it was when the shuttering was struck, the irregular impressions made by the timber creating a kind of decorative effect.

Thus began a long series of works in which Le Corbusier was to interpret with extraordinary freedom the technical, architectural and decorative possibilities of reinforced concrete, thereby setting a trend that found many followers amongst the practitioners of modern architecture in Europe and beyond (Ministry of Education, Rio de Janeiro, by *Costa, *Niemeyer, *Reidy and Vasconcellos, 1936–43; consultant architect: Le Corbusier). In the Unité d'Habitation at Marseilles (1947–52), reinforced concrete is systematically employed for the main framework of the building, cladding on the façades and 'interior roads', sun-breaks and emergency stairs. In the Church of Notre-Dame du Haut, at Ronchamp (1950–4), the inventive plan for Chandigarh (1950 onwards) and the Dominican Convent of La Tourette (1957) Le Corbusier has finally freed himself of rigid geometrical schemes, relying on reinforced concrete for a type of three-dimensional creation that is not limited to single elements but comprises the total scope of the architectural organism.

Frank Lloyd *Wright, too, has employed a strongly personal and at times unprecedented style in the projection of bold, if

Page 239. Pier Luigi Nervi. Exhibition Hall. Turin, 1948–9

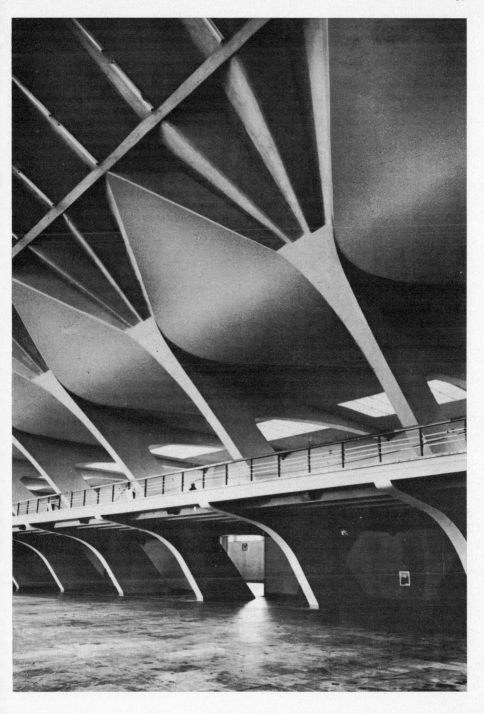

not always strictly pertinent, structural schemes in the field of residential and commercial building. Notable examples of his use of reinforced concrete include the Imperial Hotel, Tokyo (1916–22), an earthquake-proof design with projecting floor slabs; 'Falling Water' House at Bear Run, Pa. (1937–9) with its cantilevered balconies; the Johnson Wax Building, at Racine, Wis. (1936–9), featuring umbrella-type columns; the laboratory tower at the same site (1949), where the upper floors are cantilevered out from a central core; the Guggenheim Museum, New York (1956–9), based on a spiral ramp; and the Price Tower at Bartlesville, Okla. (1955).

The reconstruction of Le Havre (1947–54) gave Perret the opportunity at last for a great experiment in the employment of reinforced concrete on an urban scale, making extensive use of heavy *prefabrication. Methods like these had been successfully tried out in the inter-war period (Le Corbusier, at the Pavillon Suisse; *Beaudouin and *Lods at La Muette, 1933); they have since been developed further in *France and many other European countries, including the Soviet Union.

Besides these experiments in coordination aimed at industrializing the building trade in the service of vast housing projects, further refinements of technique were worked out and gained currency in the field of multi-storey structures. Pier Luigi *Nervi employed undulating prefabricated reinforced concrete units on a vast scale in his Exhibition Hall at Turin (1948–9), considerably reducing the self-weight of the structure while greatly increasing its elasticity and tensile strength. In the Unesco Building, Paris (1953–7, with *Breuer and *Zehrfuss), he stresses the correspondence between the way the structure is modelled and the development of bending moments by varying the depth and profile of the undulations in the roof of the Conference Hall.

Nervi's vaults; Maillart's bridges, and his barrel-vaulted pavilion for the cement industry at the Swiss Provinces Exhibition in Zurich (1939); the structures of Eduardo *Torroja and the recent emergence of *shell structures (*Candela), all show the current tendency in engineering to transcend the orthogonal system of beams and girders in order to attain a structural unity in the whole building. For their arena at

Raleigh, N.C. (1952–3), *Deitrick, *Novicki and Severud adopted reinforced concrete for the anchorage structure of the tension cables of the *suspended roof. Opportunities for using reinforced concrete have been multiplied still further by the introduction of pre- and post-stressing, in which the steel reinforcement is placed in stress either before or after the concrete is poured.

Reinforced concrete is now being used for tower blocks of flats or offices, achieving parity of esteem in a sector which for many decades had been the exclusive prerogative of steel. In Mies van der Rohe's design for the Promontory Apartments, Chicago (1949) and *BBPR's scheme for the Torre Velasca, Milan (1957), two structural solutions were drawn up and compared, one using reinforced concrete, and the other steel. The choice fell in both cases to reinforced concrete, Mies keeping to the strict grid system he had envisaged for either solution, and BBPR, on the other hand, opting for a more continuous and unitary scheme which the choice allowed. The Pirelli Building by Gio *Ponti and others (1958) and the Torre Galfa by M. Bega (1959), both at Milan, make use of great reinforced concrete piers, sited orthogonally, as the bases of their support structures. In their departure from the usual grid pattern they open up new possibilities for attaining variety and freedom in design.

Bibliography: C. Cestelli-Guidi, *Cemento armato precompresso*, Milan 1960; R. Gabetti, *Origini del calcestruzzo armato*, Turin 1955; R. Morandi, *Strutture di cemento armato e di calcestruzzo precompresso*, Rome 1954; P. Collins, *Concrete: The Vision of a New Architecture*, London 1959.

GIUSEPPE VARALDO
GIAN PIO ZUCCOTTI

Revell, Viljo, b. Vaasa, Finland 1910, d. 1964. Studied at a time when Functionalism had its first flowering in *Finland. His studies, during which he also worked as an assistant to Alvar *Aalto, were completed in 1937. Already before then he had built the so-called 'Glass Palace' with two colleagues, Kokko and Riihimäki, a department store which introduced a bold piece of modern architecture into the then very conservative scene at Helsinki. For his diploma design, Revell characteristically chose a real subject: a building for a small manufacturer; and he dealt with the problem in a logical way, as a rationalist would. An eye for the practical solution, a propensity for systematic thought and a talent for organization fitted him for the directorship of the Reconstruction Office, founded by the Association of Finnish Architects during the war, and later for the chairmanship of the Finnish Standards Committee.

Revell's first important design was for an office block with a hotel, Teollisuuskeskus at Helsinki (1952, in collaboration with Keijo Petäjä). His studio had meanwhile become a kind of headquarters for the new Rationalism in Finland, and the way up for many of today's leading young architects led through Revell's office. Revell often confined himself to critical advice when training his assistants, who were allowed much freedom. An impressive number of competition prizes and completed buildings are the visible achievement of this constantly rejuvenated team (Meilahti Primary School, Helsinki, 1953, together with Osmo Sipari; experimental housing at Tapiola; luxurious private villas, terraced houses).

The clear layout, the externally simple but effective shape and the precise planning of the Kudeneule Textile Works at Hanko (1955) are immediately obvious. Revell does not stress the repetition of secondary elements but presents a unified formal theme. He prefers to work with large structures and wide spans. This conception is also apparent in some of his unbuilt competition designs (Sininen Nauha housing estate, planned for Helsinki, 1954; Tasa, planned for Tampere, 1953) in which Revell's ideal becomes obvious: wide open spaces, whose only boundary is the horizon.

Together with H. Castrén, B. Lundsten and S. Valjus, Revell won the competition for Toronto City Hall in 1958. The design arose out of an attempt to emphasize the significance of this public building by giving it a shape that would mark its difference from the commercial skyscrapers. At the same time, the building is an expression of Revell's striving after free form, which has also been apparent in other rationalists towards the end of the fifties. Revell's generalizing, international and industrially orientated outlook is in

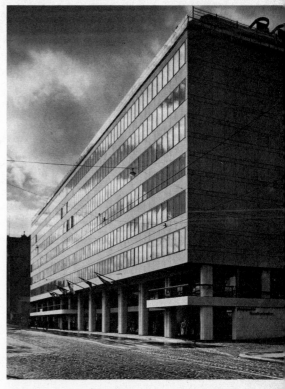

Viljo Revell and Keijo Petäjä. Teollisuuskeskus Hotel and offices. Helsinki, 1952

Viljo Revell. Kindergarten. Tapiola, 1954

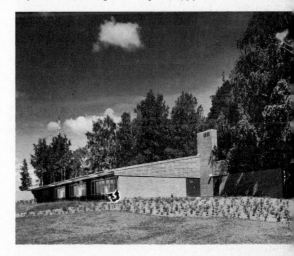

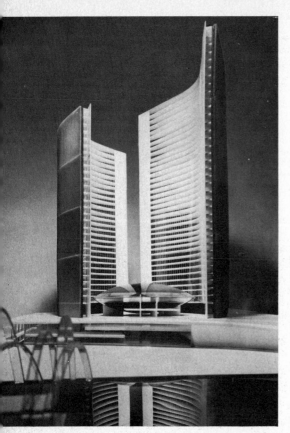

Viljo Revell. Toronto City Hall. 1958. Model

contrast with the rest of Finnish architecture, which mostly shows a preference for individual building on a small scale and in a style that tends to betray a craft approach. But it is exactly because contrasts are conducive to development that Revell's influence is so fruitful.

KYÖSTI ÅLANDER

Richardson, Henry Hobson, b. St James Parish, La., 1838, d. Boston 1886. Richardson studied at the École des Beaux-Arts, Paris and worked in the studio of Henri *Labrouste. Returned to the States in 1865. Housing, offices, churches and public buildings. Richardson, who commanded nation-wide respect, developed a characteristically heavy style with reminiscences of the Romanesque. His Marshall Field Warehouse in Chicago (1885-7),

with massive masonry, has a slab-like unity despite its enormous arched windows. His taut monumentality long influenced the School of *Chicago.
Bibliography: Henry-Russell Hitchcock, *The Architecture of H. H. Richardson and his Times,* 2nd edition, Hamden, Conn. 1961.

Riemerschmid, Richard, b. Munich 1868, d. Munich 1957. Architect and designer. Riemerschmid, like many artists of the *Art Nouveau, progressed from painting to the applied arts. In 1897 he was a founder-member of the United Workshops for Art in Craft; 1901, interior decoration of the Munich Theatre; 1910, factories at Hellerau.

Rietveld, Gerrit Thomas, b. Utrecht 1888, d. 1964. Worked as an apprentice from 1899 to 1906 in his father's joinery shop, and then ran his own cabinet-making business in Utrecht (1911–19). His first architectural studies were carried out under the architect P. J. C. Klaarhamer in Utrecht (1911–15); Rietveld was also an admirer of *Berlage. In 1918, chiefly through the agency of Robert van't Hoff, he came into contact with the founders of the *Stijl movement, of which he remained a member till 1931. His early furniture designs (from 1918) were primarily three-dimensional compositions. In 1921 he began collaborating with the interior decorator Tr. Schröder-Schräder (Rietveld-Schröder House, Utrecht, 1924). Work with van *Doesburg and van *Eesteren followed in 1923. Rietveld was one of the founders of *CIAM at La Sarraz in 1928. From then on he worked as an architect in the Netherlands (terraced housing, Utrecht, 1931-4; Vreeburg Cinema, Utrecht, 1936), Germany, Austria, Italy (Venice Biennale, 1953), Curaçao, France and Belgium.
After his difficult start, which brought him, however, international fame, the number of Rietveld's commissions began to dwindle (shops for the Wessels company, Utrecht 1923, now altered). From 1931 onwards, when *De Stijl* ceased publication and the group broke up, modern architecture passed through a difficult period in the *Netherlands, having to sustain a running battle with the historicizing 'national' style. This trend

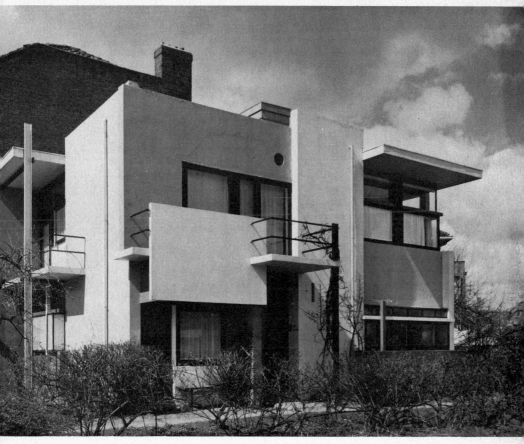

Gerrit Thomas Rietveld. Schroeder House. Utrecht, 1924

received a particular fillip in the years 1945–55, and its practitioners considered Rietveld's work to be completely superseded. His reputation began to revive with the new interest shown in America, and later Europe, in the work of Mondrian and De Stijl. Since then Rietveld has received an increasing number of important commissions, and achieved complete recognition by the younger generation of architects (country houses; Soonsbeek Pavilion, near Arnhem, 1954, since demolished; De Ploeg Textile Works, Bergeijck, 1956; housing development, Hoograven, 1954–6, with other architects).

One of the main characteristics of Rietveld's work is his three-dimensional handling of space, which has developed from De Stijl practice without ever becoming fixed in rigid attitudes. This also explains his consistent interest in interior decoration and furniture design. Rietveld has always been receptive to anything new, whether in materials or methods, while making no concessions to the merely fashionable. His use of the primary colours red, blue and yellow still testifies to his close allegiance to De Stijl. But the natural colours of his materials have gained the upper hand, and together with a restrained palette of

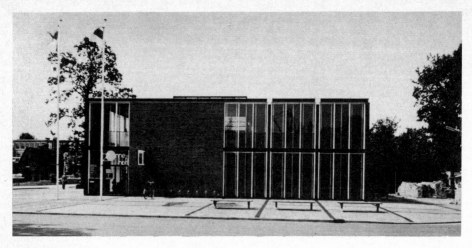

Gerrit Thomas Rietveld. Zonnehof Museum. Amersfoort, 1959

white, grey and black, help to set off the
ever-cubistic forms of his architecture.
Bibliography: Th. M. Brown, *The Work
of G. Th. Rietveld*, Utrecht 1958; *Architectural Review*, December 1964.

                                          J. J. VRIEND

Ring, Der. Berlin architects' association
founded in 1925. Among its members
were such eminent German architects as
*Bartning, *Behrens, Döcker, *Gropius,
*Häring, Haesler, *Hilberseimer, the

brothers *Luckhardt, *May, *Mendelsohn,
*Mies van der Rohe, *Poelzig, *Scharoun,
and the brothers *Taut.

Rogers, Ernesto N., b. Trieste 1909.
Graduated Milan 1932. Belongs to the
architectural team *BBPR. Publisher of
the architectural journal *Domus*, then
(since 1954) of the architectural journal
Casabella Continuità.
Bibliography: Ernesto N. Rogers, *Espe-
rienza dell'Architettura*, Turin 1958.

Gerrit Thomas Rietveld. House. Ilpendam, 1959

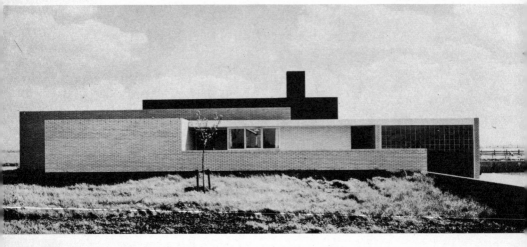

Root, John Wellborn, b. Lumpkin c. 1850, d. Chicago 1891. Partner of Daniel Hudson *Burnham.

Rotterdam, School of. *Stijl, De.

Rudolph, Paul, b. Elkton, Ky. 1918. Studied at Harvard University under Gropius. Since 1958 Chairman of the Department of Architecture at Yale University, New Haven, Conn. Rudolph developed an astonishingly wide range of design features ('new freedom') in his search for an individuality appropriate to the function of each building: Cultural Centre with resemblance to the neighbouring older neo-Gothic buildings of Wellesley College, Mass. (1955–9); schools at Sarasota, Fla.; a scheme featuring closely interlocking blocks for a motel at Waverly, N.Y., and students' quarters at Yale University, New Haven (both started in 1960); an elegant cantilevered concrete structure for a multi-storey garage at New Haven (started 1959); a building radiating in many directions as a chapel at Tuskegee, Ala. (started in 1960).

Saarinen, Eero, b. Kirkkonummi, Finland 1910, d. Birmingham, USA 1961. Eero Saarinen was the son of the architect Eliel *Saarinen. He came to the USA with his family in 1923, and received his degree from Yale University in 1934. He travelled in Europe in 1934–6, and subsequently entered into partnership with his father at Cranbrook. Although Eero's influence is certainly to be seen in his father's work from the late 1930s onward, it was the winning of the Jefferson Memorial Competition, St Louis, 1949 (which he had entered by himself), that established the younger man as a separate personality.

His first major work, the General Motors Technical Center, Warren, Michigan, completed in 1955, was for a client who had originally engaged his father for the task. Eero Saarinen and his associates responded to the demands of this remarkable challenge with considerable distinction. The numerous buildings of simple, cubic shape are spaced irregularly around a central lagoon in a manner reminiscent of the master plan of *Mies van der Rohe for the Illinois Institute of Technology, Chicago (1940). However, the shapes of the Saarinen buildings are more individualized in scale and surface modulation, and are more varied in colour than is the case with Mies's inveterately regularized 'industrial classicism'. Together with the contemporary works of Philip *Johnson and of *Skidmore, Owings and Merrill, Saarinen's General Motors designs determined the trends that would dominate American architecture until the late 1950s.

In the light of his subsequent development, and of the evolution of architecture that has taken place since then, this General Motors 'style' already seems at least superficially antiquated. Two 'central plan' edifices for the Massachusetts Institute of Technology, Cambridge, Mass., finished in 1955, the shell-domed Kresge Auditorium and the Chapel, indicate a multiple heritage as well as a diverse future for Saarinen's architecture. The simple domical form enclosed a complexly shaped

Eero Saarinen. General Motors Technical Center. Warren, Mich., completed 1955

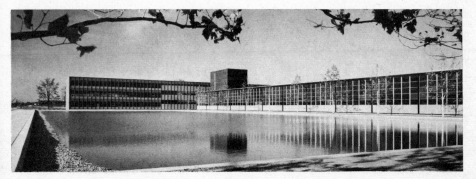

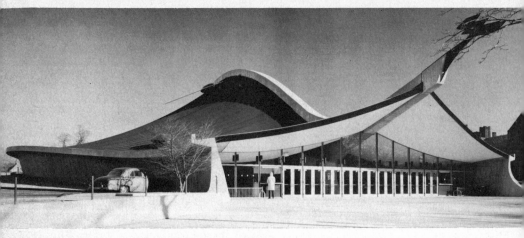

Eero Saarinen. Yale Hockey Rink. Yale University, New Haven, Conn., completed 1958

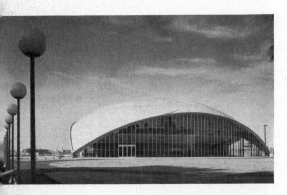

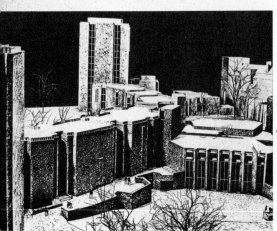

auditorium with a single, sweeping curve in a way that provoked much criticism, especially from those who felt that the arbitrary-seeming form of the exterior was not suited to the varied requirements of the interior space. There is indeed a paradox in the outer forms and the interior workings of the Kresge Auditorium, and it tends to underscore one of the most challenging problems in recent architecture. The difficulty comes about from the recurring effort to reconcile a style appropriate to the exact programme of the building and the technological nature of modern construction with the desire to use forms of a pure, simplified character, indeed forms with pronounced classicizing overtones. In their late styles, both Mies van der Rohe and *Le Corbusier have found eminently successful personal means of reconciling the paradoxical demands of the machine age with their latent predilections for inventing shapes whose ancestry lies in classic or pre-classic Mediterranean architecture.

Eero Saarinen. Kresge Auditorium, Massachusetts Institute of Technology. Cambridge, Mass., completed 1955

Eero Saarinen. Yale Colleges, Yale University. New Haven, Conn., under construction. Project

Page 247. Eero Saarinen. Yale Hockey Rink, Yale University. New Haven, Conn., completed 1958

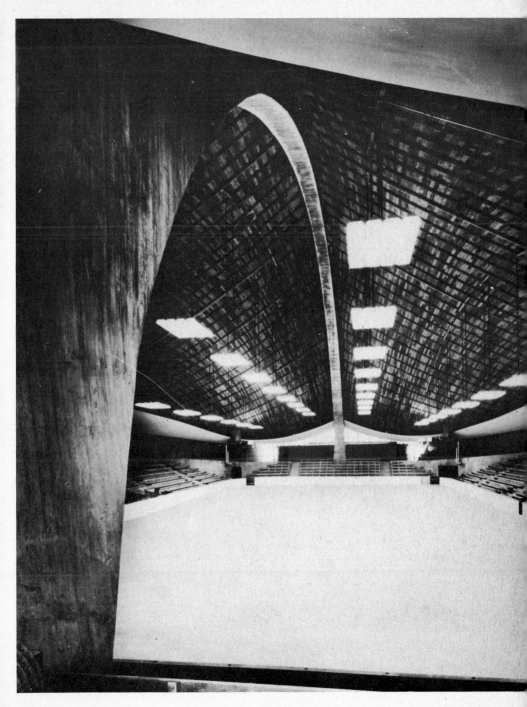

Saarinen's difficulty—and, for that matter, the difficulty encountered by many of his contemporaries—is that his reconciliation seems tentative and insecure. It is made to seem even more unconvincing in the Kresge Auditorium with the presence near by of the more romantic, subjective form of the Chapel, a work which seems to be a devout evocation of his father's stylistic conceptions. The lack of *rapport* between these two MIT structures, which, in itself, is thought-provoking, sounds a warning as to the shifting nature of Eero's later development until his untimely death in 1961. Subsequent designs for large interior spaces, such as the Ingalls Hockey Rink, Yale University, the TWA Terminal, Idlewild, New York, and the Dulles Airport, Washington, D.C., show a more comprehensible relationship between interior space and exterior form. However, while the spaces themselves seem to indicate a common spirit of dynamic coordination, the forms are heterogeneous. The spaces may be expressive or appropriate in a dramatic way, yet one wonders whether there is a justifiable relation between these inventions and the material demands of the programme and of structural technology. Only the future will be in a position to bear out the validity of these designs, as well as such 'neo-academic' designs for government structures as the American Embassies in London and in Oslo, buildings which represent other efforts at creating distinctive and unique-seeming forms at the expense of allowing a more personal, idiomatic style to evolve. The London Embassy was intended to harmonize with the vernacular architecture of London, but failed to accomplish this aim. The residential colleges at Yale are yet another effort to harmonize with tradition, or, more exactly in this case, with the neo-traditionalism of 'collegiate Gothic', while at the same time maintaining the imprint of modernism. We cannot be sure that Eero Saarinen developed a new method for the design of contemporary buildings; indeed, it can almost be said that he did not produce an individual, consistent style. None the less, he produced a sequence of influential if not organically related buildings that have been much discussed, and which surely illuminate the direction taken by modernist architecture in the 1950s.

JOHN M. JACOBUS, JR

Saarinen, Eliel, b. Rantasalmi, Finland 1873, d. Michigan 1950. Saarinen studied painting at the University and architecture at the Polyteknisk Institut, Helsinki (1893–7). In 1896 he formed a partnership with Herman Gesellius and Armas Lindgren, and in 1899–1900 they received international recognition with the Finnish Pavilion at the Paris Exposition. Significantly, their somewhat neo-medieval design indicates a possible influence from American architects such as H. H. *Richardson and Louis *Sullivan, and at the same time reveals the spirit of the *Art Nouveau in certain decorative touches.

In 1902 Gesellius, Lindgren and Saarinen began work on a joint residence and studio, Hvitträsk, in the wooded countryside outside Helsinki. Certainly one of the most important examples of domestic architecture at the turn of the century, and, in spite of its somewhat indigenous appearance, worthy of comparison with contemporary houses in various parts of the world by *Wright, *Voysey, *Mackintosh and *Hoffmann, Hvitträsk also demonstrates that its architects were familiar with the new spirit in interior design that was then centred in Vienna and Glasgow. Equally, this studio-house reveals an awareness of the progressive domestic designs of such late-19th-century masters as Philip *Webb, Richard Norman *Shaw and Richardson. A similar awareness is to be found in the Saarinen design for the Helsinki Railway Station of 1904, constructed from 1910 to 1914. A typical eclectic monument of the period, its boldly articulated and simply detailed masonry masses sum up a variety of academic, romantic and rational influences that were common at the time. More important, however, is the individual character which Saarinen has wrought from these multiple inheritances of the early modern tradition, and the personal infusion which makes this design unique in the railway architecture of the period. Its creative spirit is equalled only in the more severe romanticism of *Bonatz's nearly contemporary Stuttgart Station.

The scope of Saarinen's architectural practice continued to expand during this decade with his involvement in a number of city planning schemes, one of which was a project for Canberra, Australia. His participation in the competition for the Chicago Tribune Tower, 1922 (for which

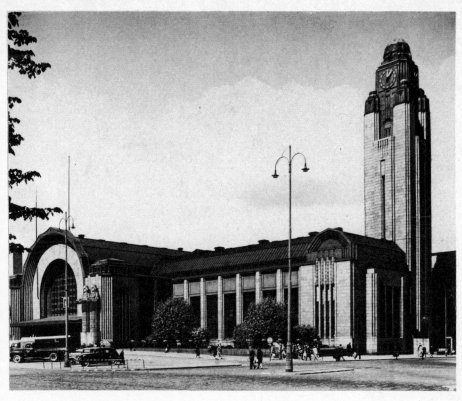

Eliel Saarinen. Main Station, Helsinki. Designed 1904, built 1910–14

he received a second prize), led to further work in the USA, to which he moved permanently in 1923. In 1925 he began work on what was destined to become a group of schools at Cranbrook, Michigan. In 1928 he built his own house in Cranbrook, a simple pale brick structure which seems closer in appearance to the bland 'collegiate Gothic' of 20th-century American architecture than to the more pronounced modelling and incisive detail of Saarinen's earlier and more overtly romantic style. Other features at Cranbrook are distantly suggestive of Wright's characteristic use of horizontals, with sheltered loggias, etc. By way of contrast the Cranbrook Academy design of 1940 possesses a dry, neoclassic solemnity, and although its plans and elevations are not perfunctory they are similar in appearance to the simplified, modernized academic tradi-

tionalism that was a feature of monumental architecture throughout the world in the 1930s. Comparison of the Cranbrook buildings of the 1920s and 1930s with the earlier Helsinki Station reveals little or no intensification or development of a personal style, but instead only an overall simplification or generalization of forms that are ultimately derivative.

In 1937 Eliel Saarinen formed a partnership with his son, Eero *Saarinen, and many of his last works must be considered as fundamentally collaborative designs. The Kleinhans Music Hall, Buffalo, New York (1938), clearly indicates an awareness of the new European architecture of the 1920s and early 1930s, which had blossomed after Saarinen's departure from Finland. Here and in a series of churches culminating in Christ Lutheran, Minneapolis, Minn. (1949–50), there is an effective

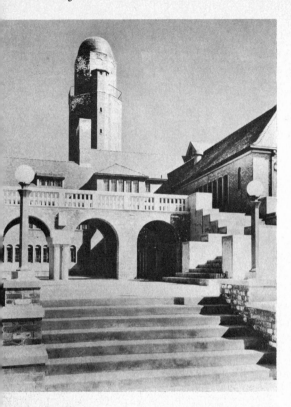

blend of the half-century-old romantic, craftsman-like approach in both decoration and constructive elements, along with a new spirit of design that is more decisive in its geometric simplicity, bolder in the abstract handling of spatial and lighting elements, and even outwardly functional in the sense of the word as then understood. The first Saarinen projects for the General Motors Technical Center were done in 1945, but the definitive designs were not completed until after his death in 1950. The final result was a group of buildings in a severe, industrial, *Mies van der Rohe style that in certain ways is foreign to the more genteel, occasionally unobtrusive personal manner of Eliel Saarinen.

Bibliography: Eliel Saarinen, *Search for Form*, New York 1949; Albert Christ-Janer, *Eliel Saarinen*, Chicago 1949.

JOHN M. JACOBUS, JR

Sant'Elia, Antonio, b. Como 1880, d. Monfalcone 1916. Sant'Elia studied architecture at Milan and later at Bologna, where he graduated at the age of twenty-four. He then began to work for other architects, and to design for himself in the manner of Otto *Wagner's Vienna School. He was greatly attracted by many features of North American civilization, not those realistic and rational aspects of it which had impressed Adolf *Loos, but the romantic aspects of its technical development and the progressive expansion of an industrial metropolis. The new city, the city of the future, thus appeared to him a reality that could be achieved in Italy too, but an Italy shaken from her long sleep and aroused to life once more. He set himself to work out a grandiose project for a *Città Nuova*, both in general and in detail, which was shown in 1914 at the first exhibition in Milan by the *Nuove Tendenze* group, of which he was a member. Designs for 'Structures of a modern metropolis' were displayed at the same exhibition by Sant'Elia's fellow student, the architect Mario *Chiattone, who shared his ideals.

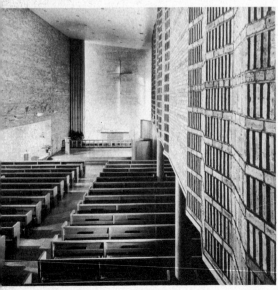

Eliel Saarinen. Cranbrook School for Boys. Bloomfield Hills, Mich., 1925

Eliel and Eero Saarinen. Christ Lutheran Church, Minneapolis, Minn., 1949–50 did not have much time to think out his position as an architect vis-à-vis Marinetti, for he was called up in 1915 on Italy's entry into the war and was killed a year later leading an assault.

Sant'Elia's architecture had very little affinity with the beginnings of the modern movement that was currently stirring in *Germany and *Austria; it remains an isolated phenomenon in Europe, although it introduced a number of motifs to Italian culture and a stylistic formula that had much in common with Russian *Constructivism. Its main influence was on the architecture of the great international exhibitions and their pavilions. But it is due to him that Italian culture, shaken by his words, looked for the first time at the problem of the new architecture as a problem, albeit a limited one, of a new life and new customs, in an age that witnessed the triumph of the petit-bourgeois mentality.

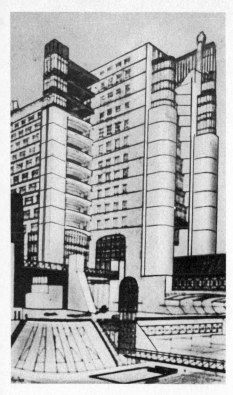

Antonio Sant'Elia. Città Nuova. 1914. Project

Antonio Sant'Elia. Skyscraper. 1914. Project

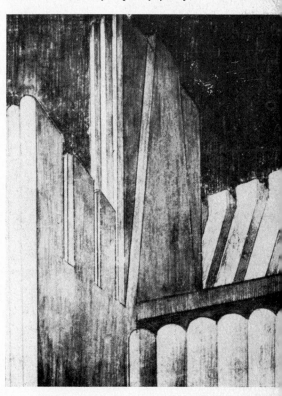

In the catalogue to this exhibition Sant' Elia published a diffuse manifesto on the need for breaking with the past in order to create in Italy too, where 'everything had to be revolutionized', a new architecture, as new as 'the state of mind' of the younger generation; this alone could give valid form to the city of men freed from the bonds of traditions and conventions. Thus, for Sant'Elia, it was eminently a case of historical necessity.

His text was published again a few months afterwards by Marinetti, who had modified it on a number of points. Henceforth one speaks of *Futurist architecture, and Sant' Elia himself is referred to as a Futurist. In reality Sant'Elia was a Socialist, who had joined Marinetti's movement without enthusiasm, for it was of an outspokenly nationalist character and ended up a few years later by going along with Fascism completely. Sant'Elia, however,

Hundreds of Sant'Elia's designs have come down to us; one of them was actually built posthumously at Como, although altered in too many details. A recurrent theme in them is the architecture of a metropolis, derived from a mechanical and industrialized civilization: towering buildings with external elevators, multi-level road bridges, enormous stations, and imaginary factories: monuments of the city of the future, seen through the vision of Sant'Elia, and raised by their unreal dimensions and perspectives to the level of symbols. A permanent exhibition of Sant'Elia's works has been opened at the Villa Olmo near Como.

Bibliography: Giulio C. Argan, 'Il pensiero critico di Antonio Sant'Elia', in *L'arte*, Rome September 1930; Alberto Sartoris, *Antonio Sant'Elia*, Milan 1930; Gherardo Dottori, *Sant'Elia e la nuova architettura*, Rome 1933; Francesco Tentori, 'Le origini liberty di Antonio Sant'Elia' in *L'architettura*, Rome July/August 1955 and January/February 1956; Umbro Apollonio, *Antonio Sant'Elia*, Milan 1958; *Architect's Journal*, 15 January 1964.

GIULIA VERONESI

Scarpa, Carlo, b. Venice 1906. Pavilions for the Biennales at Venice, new fittings and extensions of museums in Florence, Palermo, Possagno, Venice, Verona. Organic architecture in the manner of Frank Lloyd *Wright.

Scharoun, Hans, b. Bremen 1893. Scharoun grew up in Bremerhaven until he took his school certificate; he studied from 1912 to 1914 at Berlin Technical College, and during his military service worked as an architect on reconstruction in East Prussia, whence he established contact with Bruno *Taut and the circle of young architects round him in Berlin. In 1925 Scharoun accepted an appointment through Oskar Moll at Breslau Academy of Art and Crafts. Here he met Rading and they collaborated on schemes in Breslau and Berlin. For the WUWA (Home and Work Exhibition, Breslau, 1928) he built an apartment block with set-back floors, roof gardens and communal services on the ground floor; and a private house in 1927 on the Weissenhof estate of the *Deutscher Werkbund at Stuttgart, co-ordinated by *Mies van der Rohe.

As a member of the Berlin architectural association *Der *Ring*, Scharoun designed the layout of the large Siemensstadt estate. There in 1930 he built a number of blocks of flats, standing set back from the street, with living-rooms extending the entire depth of the block from wall to wall. In the twenties in Berlin, Scharoun participated in numerous town planning schemes and competitions under the leadership of Martin *Wagner. He built blocks of flats at the Kaiserdamm, Hohenzollerndamm and Flinsberger Platz in an attempt to keep the business of renting flats an economic proposition for private enterprise by carefully thought-out planning.

For the exhibition '*Sun, air and houses for all*' at the Berlin Funkturm in 1932, Scharoun built a 'growing house'. His design is based on the grid system to give the builders a precise synopsis of costs during the whole process of erection, together with the necessary extensions. In the same year, he built a house for an industrialist by the name of Schminke at Löbau in Saxony, a steel-frame structure that seems to be freely suspended amidst the scenery.

Under the Nazis, Scharoun was cut off entirely from all chance of executing major schemes. He was merely allowed to build private houses in and around Berlin. In these years of enforced inactivity, he worked on numerous drawings and designs whose ideas he drew on in later work. After the end of the war in 1945, he was appointed by Berlin Corporation head of the Department for Building and Housing. He prevented the complete demolition of many factories and offices in the shattered city and set up the planning group called the 'Berliner Kollektiv', which presented a revolutionary plan for the rebuilding of Berlin in 1946. This plan was an application and development of theoretical work by Miljutin and Soraja y Matyas, and a realization and continuation of Martin Mächler's theories: 'not a land-use plan but a dynamics plan' His work on the centre of Berlin was continued in 1958 in the *Metropolis Berlin* competition, 'the first design that deserves to be taken seriously in the rebuilding of the city centre'. While working on detailed plan analyses for the Havel area (Spandau, Potsdam) in his capacity as head of the Building Institute at the German Academy of Sciences from 1947 to 1950, he was also (until 1960) lecturer in town planning at Berlin Technical

University, of which he was one of the re-
founders in 1946.

In this post-war period, he carried out many
important competition designs: the rebuilding of the island of Heligoland, the
Liederhalle in Stuttgart, the American
Memorial Library and an old-people's
home in Berlin. Prize-winning and world
famous designs such as the theatre at
Kassel and the National Theatre at Mannheim were never built; they were based on
a far-reaching analysis of theatrical problems. An analysis of the principles affecting
the spatial problems of school buildings
led to a design for a primary school at
Darmstadt on the occasion of his Darmstadt lecture on 'Man and Space' in 1951.
Scharoun's design marks an important
advance in his work as well as in the
development of modern architecture. In
1955 he was commissioned to build the
Geschwister Scholl High School at Lünen,
Westphalia, completed in 1962. The classrooms in this girls' school have been
arranged as a 'flat', in order to humanize
the division between school and home in
modern education. 'Scharoun is the
guarantor of a continuity between post-
1918 and post-1945 Germany.' (*L'Architettura*).

This continuity is expressed particularly
in his residential buildings. In 1947
Scharoun designed a suburb south of the
Stalinallee, as it later became, his first
attempt to combine some ideas of Ludwig
*Hilberseimer's with the experience he had
gained on the Siemensstadt scheme in the
1930s, and to create a design team. In
1954 he submitted plans and models for
the rebuilding of the Hansa district, which
he was commissioned to do by the revived
Ring. He also built 'homesteads' in Charlottenburg-Nord (1955–61), a further
development from linear building in its
social aspect, as evaluated by the most
recent research. At Stuttgart, Scharoun
built Romeo and Juliet point blocks in
collaboration with Wilhelm Frank, whose
penthouses and studios must be understood as the completion of a design which
had hitherto featured only low buildings.
These blocks show a connection with the
idea that underlies the Breslau Exhibition
flats of 1928. They may similarly be associated with the concept of townscape, as
are the 'Salute' block at Stuttgart and the
concert hall for the Berlin Philharmonic

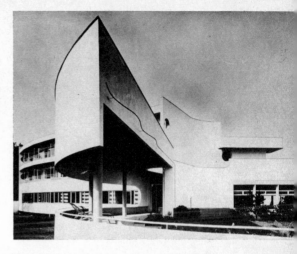

Hans Scharoun. Apartment house at the Home
and Work Exhibition. Breslau, 1928

Hans Scharoun. Schminke House. Löbau, 1932

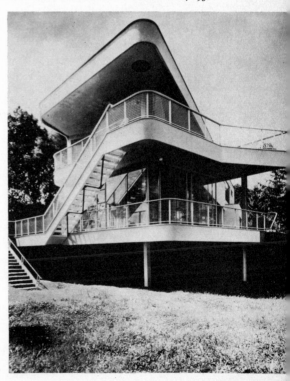

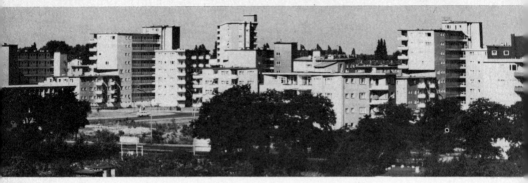

Hans Scharoun. Charlottenburg-Nord housing estate. Berlin, 1955–61

Orchestra, both of which are currently under construction.

Scharoun was awarded the commission for building the new Berlin Philharmonic Concert Hall as a result of a prize-winning competition design which condenses the unity of music and space into three-dimensional form.

Bibliography: Margit Staber, 'Hans Scharoun. Ein Beitrag zum organischen Bauen', in *Zodiac 10*, Milan 1962.

KLAUS-JAKOB THIELE

Hans Scharoun. Concert Hall for the Berlin Philharmonic Orchestra. Berlin, opened 1963, nicknamed 'Circus Karajani'. Section

Schindler, Rudolph M., b. Vienna 1887, d. Los Angeles 1953. Studied at the Vienna Academy of Art, strongly influenced by Otto *Wagner; 1913 emigrated to Chicago; 1916–21 worked in Frank Lloyd *Wright's office. In Schindler's buildings the relationship of horizontal and vertical, solid and void appear as an American parallel to De *Stijl (Lovell Beach House, Newport Beach, 1926).

Schinkel, Karl Friedrich, b. Neuruppin 1781, d. Berlin 1841. Architect and painter. Pupil of David and Friedrich Gilly. Extensive journeys in Italy and France; worked

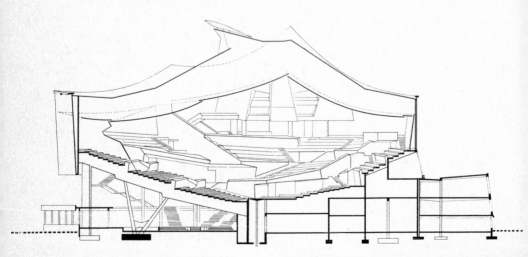

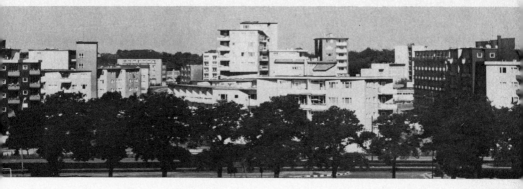

in Berlin. Schinkel combined classical forms with a romantic spirit in his dignified designs: New Guard House, Unter den Linden (1815–16), Theatre (1818–31), Old Museum (1823–8), all at Berlin. Early Gothic Revival work in his Memorial to Queen Louise (1810) and his Werdersche Church in Berlin (1824–30). Schinkel influenced *Mies van der Rohe and through him 20th-century architecture with his designs for a shop (1829) whose façades consist of glass areas divided by masonry piers, and with his country-house projects. *Bibliography:* Paul Ortwin Rave, *Karl Friedrich Schinkel, Das Lebenswerk*, 1942–56.

Schwarz, Rudolf, b. Strasbourg 1897, d. Cologne 1961. Pupil of *Poelzig. His ecclesiastical buildings form an important contribution to modern Catholic church design. Schwarz sought to create with them 'high inhabitable pictures like life-size parables'. Fronleichnam Church, Aachen (in collaboration with Hans Schwippert, 1928), St Anne, Düren (1951–6), St Michael, Frankfurt (1953–4).
Bibliography: Rudolf Schwarz, *Kirchenbau*, Heidelberg 1960.

Seidler, Harry, b. Vienna 1923. Studied at Harvard University, Cambridge, Massachusetts, and Manitoba, Canada. Collaborated with *Breuer and *Niemeyer. Since 1942 independent practice in Sidney, Australia. Houses and offices; Olympic Stadium at Melbourne (1956), a suspended roof structure for 125,000 spectators.

Bibliography: Harry Seidler, *Houses, Interiors and Projects*, Sidney 1954.

Harry Seidler. Lend Lease House, Sydney

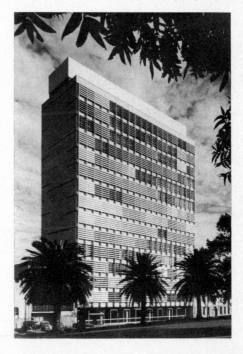

Semper, Gottfried, b. Hamburg 1803, d. Rome 1879. From 1834 in Dresden which he left for political reasons in 1849. Stayed in Paris and London. In Zurich (1855), Vienna (1871). His work is removed from the romantic classicism of *Schinkel, who was a friend of his. His adaptations of Romanesque, Gothic and Renaissance features are typical examples of 19th-century historicism. Semper's originality lies in his massing, where the building's function stands out sharply. (The projecting curvature of the auditorium in the Dresden Opera House, 1837–41, rebuilt in 1878 following the fire of 1871). Dresden Art Gallery (started 1847); Burgtheater in Vienna (rebuilt differently, 1874–88). His theoretical writings stress the influence of structure on style and recommend the use of colour in architecture.

Bibliography: Gottfried Semper, *Der Stil in den technischen und tektonischen Künsten,* Frankfurt 1860–3; *Architectural Review,* July 1964.

Sert, José Luis, b. Barcelona 1902. Studied at the Escuela Superior de Arquitectura in Barcelona; 1929–30 worked for *Le Corbusier and Pierre Jeanneret in Paris.

Richard Norman Shaw. Old Swan House. London, 1876

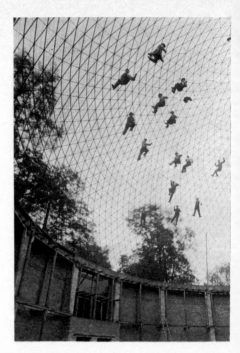

Walter Bauersfeld, Grid for the shell dome of the Planetarium in the Zoological Gardens. Berlin, 1926

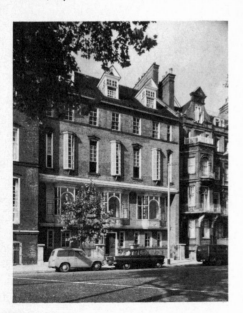

Emigrated to the United States in 1939; 1947–56 President of *CIAM at whose instance he published among other writings *Can our Cities Survive?* (3rd edition, Cambridge, Mass. 1947). Since 1958 Dean of the Harvard Graduate School of Design. US Embassy, Bagdad (commenced 1955); Harvard University Health Center, Cambridge, Mass. (1957–61); Maeght Museum, St Paul-de-Vence (work still in progress). Extensive town-planning projects.

Shaw, Richard Norman, b. Edinburgh 1831, d. Hampstead 1912. Studied at the Royal Academy, London. Shaw, who synthesized numerous influences and styles in his own work, exercised a strong influence on his contemporaries with his churches, offices and in particular with his tasteful private houses. Among the latter, the Old Swan House, London, is especially distinguished by its delicate and slightly mannered proportions.

Shell structures. Support features formed from a singly or doubly curved surface and consisting of tension- and compression-resistant material (i.e. material resistant to bending) are called shell structures; the thickness of the shell is slight in relation to its surface area. The most important properties of a shell are that it is not straight but curved, and it is thin. Hence the designer also calls the shell a plane support structure. A girder on the other hand is called a beam-type support structure. In a plane support structure, two dimensions (length and width) are considerably greater than the third (thickness); in a beam-type support structure, however, two dimensions (depth and width of section) are decidedly smaller than the third (length).

Beam-type support structures and plane support structures are different with regard to their stresses. A girder which is loaded at right angles to its axis is acted on by bending moments and sheer stress, whereas an ideal shell has neither bending moments nor sheer stress, only normal stresses uniformly distributed over its thickness. A girder resists loading by its strength, a shell by its shape. A simple test will explain the structural properties of a shell. A piece of paper, spread out flat and held along its two edges, will bend. It cannot even carry its own weight, let alone additional loads. But if the same piece of paper is curved and held along its edges, it develops a surprising rigidity. In nature we find many forms comparable to our new shell structures. We may mention diatoms, single-cell creatures consisting of siliceous algae; eggs, sea-shells and snails. These shapes are built on the principle that a firm casing may be formed from the minimum of material. Their rigidity does not depend on the firmness of the material or its thickness, but on the casing's curved shape.

The engineers Walter Bauersfeld and Franz Dischinger deserve the credit for having established the theoretical and practical advantages of shell construction. It is true that early attempts to calculate similar structures can be found in the literature of the end of the 19th century and the beginning of the 20th, but no practical use was made of this theory. Bauersfeld and Dischinger in the early twenties were the first to tackle the problem both in theory and in practice and thus laid the foundations

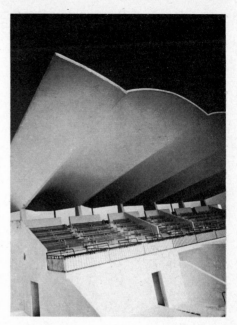

Eduardo Torroja. Grandstand. Zarzuela race course, near Madrid, 1935

for one of the most interesting developments in the field of structural engineering. Since that time development has been rapid and constant. In the twenties the first barrel and dome shells were constructed by the Zeiss-Dywidag process, invented by Bauersfeld and Dischinger, (Dome shells: experimental structure near Jena, 1922; factory for Schott and Gen., 1923–4; Jena Planetarium, 1925. Barrel shells: roof of the exhibition halls at the GESOLEI, Düsseldorf, 1926; market hall, Frankfort on the Main, 1926–7. Intersecting barrel shells in the shape of cross-arched vaults: market hall, Leipzig, 1927–9; market hall, Basle, 1929). *Freyssinet built the market hall at Rheims in the shape of a barrel vault (1928–9) and the repair workshop at Bagneux as a conoidal one (1928–9). As early as 1934 G. Baroni built the first shell in Milan in the shape of a hyperbolic paraboloid (iron foundry at Milan) and in 1938 the first shell in the shape of an upturned umbrella (warehouse at Ferrara). Bernard Lafaille has been working with shell structures since 1929. Between 1931 and 1933 different types of hall structures

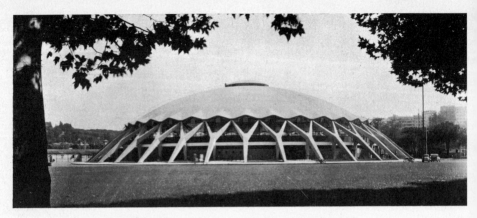

Pier Luigi Nervi and Annibale Vitellozzi. Palazzetto dello Sport. Rome, 1956–7

were put up on a grid system, where the shell thickness for spans between 98 and 164 feet was a mere 2 to 2¾ inches. A little later, Konrad Hruban worked on similar structural shapes. After 1940 his shells developed in the form of hyperbolic paraboloids began to be used and are employed in many ways for industrial buildings. Eduardo *Torroja designed the roof of the market hall at Algeciras (1934), the racecourse at Zarzuela (1935) and the ball-games hall, Madrid (1935). Dischinger constructed a number of large-span aircraft hangars in the thirties (Bug/Rügen hangar 1936–7). *Maillart's Cement Hall for the Swiss Provinces Exhibition, Zurich, 1938–9, may be called a model instance of the structural and sculptural possibilities of shell construction.

It is at first amazing that up to the present time the knowledge of these structures and their application has remained confined to a small circle of architects. Neither *Le Corbusier, nor *Gropius, not *Breuer concerned themselves during the twenties or thirties with shell structures. It is only now, in a changing architectural world, that architects regard shell construction as a suitable means for realizing their ideas. Frequently, however, they restrict themselves to accepting shapes designed by structural engineers. The task that lies before architects of employing this form of construction as an architectural medium is only being achieved step by step.

The application of shell construction is now reaching every type of architecture. Among the most important examples are the airport reception buildings at St Louis, Mo. by Hellmuth, Leinweber and Yamasaki, engineers Roberts and Schaefer Co. (1953–5); exhibition hall of the Centre National des Industries et Techniques at Paris by Camelot, de Mailly and *Zehrfuss, engineer Esquillan (1957–8); Palazzetto dello Sport, Rome, by A. Vitellozzi, engineer *Nervi (1956–7); Palazzo dello Sport, Rome, by Piacentini, engineer Nervi (1958–60); TWA airport reception building at Idlewild, New York, by Eero *Saarinen and Associates (1961–2); Windward City Shopping Centre at Kaneohe, Hawaii by Wimberley and Cook, engineer Bradshaw (1957); buildings by Félix *Candela; market hall at Royan by Simon, Morisseau, engineer René Sarger (1955).

Bibliography: Jürgen Joedicke, *Schalenbau* (= Dokumente der Modernen Architektur 2), Stuttgart 1962.

JÜRGEN JOEDICKE

Sheppard, Richard Herbert, b. 1910. Studied at the Architectural Association School of Architecture, London; in private practice since 1938, latterly with Geoffrey Robson and other partners. Wide range of buildings, especially educational ones; awarded RIBA Bronze Medal for Harrowfield Boys' School, Harold Hill, Essex (1954). Winner of the limited competition for Churchill College, Cambridge (1959) with a design featuring twenty courts grouped informally round a library and

Page 259. George Francis Hellmuth, Joseph William Leinweber and Minoru Yamasaki. Airport reception building. St Louis, Mo., 1953–5

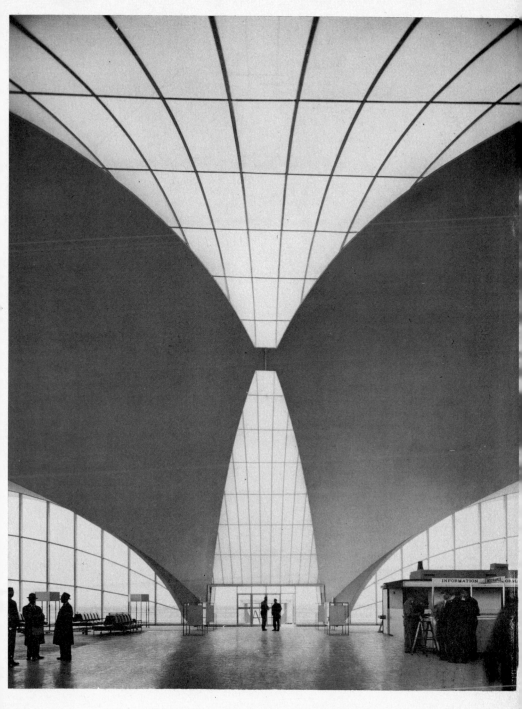

clerestory-lit reading room in the centre.
Students' hall of residence, Imperial College, London; pithead bath, Dudley Colliery, Northumberland. Created OBE, 1964.

Siren, Heikki and Kaija. Heikki Siren, b.
Helsinki 1918, Kaija Siren, b. Kotka 1920.
Studied at Helsinki Technical College.
Since 1946 this married couple have had
an office of their own. Schools, housing (in
part prefabricated), office blocks. Small
auditorium of the Finnish National Theatre,
Helsinki (1954); Chapel, Otaniemi Technical College (1957).

Skidmore, Owings and Merrill (SOM)
(Louis Skidmore, b. 1897, Nathaniel A.
Owings, b. 1903, and John O. Merrill,
b. 1896).

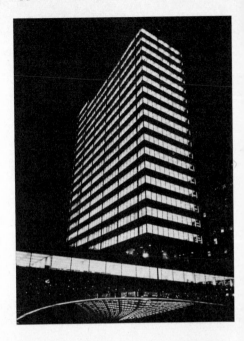

Skidmore, Owings and Merrill. Lever House.
New York, 1952

Skidmore, Owings and Merrill. Connecticut
General Life Insurance Building, Hartford,
Conn., 1957

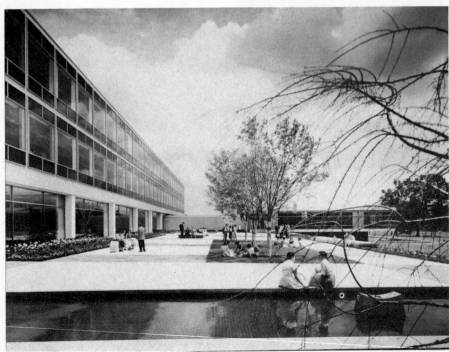

This American architectural firm was founded by Messrs Skidmore and Owings in 1935 and the partnership was expanded to include Mr Merrill in 1936. Although the two founders had been associated with the 'modernistic' designs of the Chicago 'Century of Progress' Exposition (1933), the impact of the firm upon the course of recent architecture was not significant until after the Second World War. Its leadership dates from the completion of the Lever Building, Park Avenue, New York City (1952), the design of Gordon *Bunshaft, a partner in the firm who has been largely responsible for the establishment and direction of the SOM style. The Lever design was one of the very first successful commercializations of the *Mies van der Rohe geometry of metal and glass; so successful that by the end of the 1950s imitations of this specific office block could be found in London, Copenhagen, Caracas and elsewhere.

Since that date SOM, with offices in Chicago, San Francisco and Portland, Oregon, as well as in New York, has proceeded to refine the original model in a series of increasingly simple yet elegant glass towers, notably those for Inland Steel, Chicago (1954), Pepsi Cola (1959), Union Carbide (1960), and Chase Manhattan Bank (1957–61), the last three in New York City. Their style has been imitated at one time or another, albeit usually in a coarsened form, by almost every large American architectural firm, irrespective of location or previous taste. This largely SOM-created image of expensive efficiency became, by the end of the 1950s, the most universally admired quality in large-scale architectural schemes. Their abstractly classicizing contemporary idiom, with all of its carefully proportioned urban restraint, was even applied in large-scale offices constructed in artfully landscaped rural sites, notably in the entirely glazed three-storey blocks of the Connecticut General Life Insurance Company, near Hartford, Conn. (1957). Similar elements were utilized on a vaster scale and in a more dramatic, mountainous setting in the Air Academy, Colorado Springs, Colo., finished 1959. This huge complex heralded the momentary establishment of the SOM modernist idiom as the semi-official architectural style of the day. However, at the exact moment of the

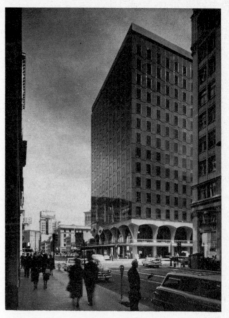

Skidmore, Owings and Merrill. John Hancock Building. San Francisco, 1960

greatest success of this mirror-like purist style, which was the ultimate and most academic manifestation of the taste established by the masters of the *International Style of the 1920s, new tendencies were to be discerned in other SOM projects and realizations. The John Hancock Building, San Francisco (1960), rather self-consciously rejected the glass *curtain wall in favour of a bay system of separate windows and load-bearing external walls. A vigorous, structurally expressive touch was provided by the flaring concrete piers which formed the Expressionistic 'order' of the ground floor and mezzanine. In other projects, such as the Banque Lambert, Brussels (1958), or in the Rare Book Library, Yale University, New Haven, Conn., still other design innovations appear, all of which represent divergences from the established orthodox modernism of the glass box. In the Yale design the rectangular cubic form of the building is carried upon a huge Vierendeel truss which is supported by four concrete pylons at the corners. Hence while the bulky mass is dramatically elevated from the ground, it

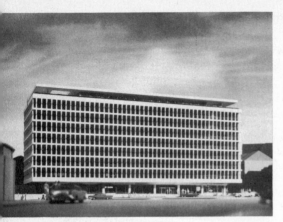

Skidmore, Owings and Merrill. Banque Lambert. Brussels, 1958. Model

does not float gracefully or hover above the site in the characteristically contemporary fashion of the Lever Building, nor are its forms sheathed in the seemingly weightless glass surfaces first employed by the International Style. Instead the external surfaces are divided into emphatic grid patterns by precast concrete elements of a marble aggregate.

SOM is not the largest of American architectural firms; neither is it truly typical of the building design industry in the USA, if only because of its superior taste and understanding of the stylistic requirements of contemporary commercial and monumental architecture. However, its finest work does represent in a particularly elevated fashion the aspirations of a major segment of today's architectural profession. *Bibliography:* Ernst Danz, *SOM: Architecture of Skidmore, Owings and Merrill 1950–1962*, London 1963.

JOHN M. JACOBUS, JR

Smithson, Alison and Peter. Alison Smithson, b. Sheffield 1928. Peter Smithson, b. Stockton-on-Tees 1923. The Hunstanton School, Norfolk (1954), ranks as the first example of *Brutalism. Their design for the Berlin City competition (third prize) provides for a closed pedestrian precinct on a second level. Economist Building, London (started 1962). Commissioned to design British Embassy for Brasilia 1964.

Soane, Sir John, b. Goring-on-Thames 1753, d. London 1837. Appointed architect

to the Bank of England in 1788, for which he carried out alterations and new additions from 1788 to 1833. Numerous government commissions; from 1806 professor at the Royal Academy. Churches, private houses, villas. His composition with abstract shapes reminiscent of the French revolutionary architects, the broad disposition of his volumes and masses, as well as the exposed cast-iron construction of his cupolas have earned Soane the reputation among modern architects of being contemporary in feeling. *Bibliography:* J. N. Summerson, *Sir John Soane*, London 1952; Dorothy Stroud, *The Architecture of Sir John Soane*, London 1961.

Soleri, Paolo, b. Italy 1920. Since 1947 in the United States. Influenced by Frank Lloyd *Wright for whom he worked. Admirer of Antoni *Gaudí. Advanced designs such as the tubular bridge (1947) and the project for a 'town on a table mountain' with two million inhabitants (since 1959). Among his few executed designs is the House in the Desert (Cave Creek, Ariz., 1951, together with Mark Mills) which is roofed by two movable hemispheres, and a ceramics factory at Vietri sul Mare near Salerno (1954), a five-storey hall with spiral ramps.

Sommaruga, Giuseppe, b. Milan 1867, d. Milan 1917. Studied architecture at the Brera, Milan. He was the main exponent of Italian *Art Nouveau, together with D' *Aronco and *Basile. Sommaruga employed floral Art Nouveau details, particularly in his decorative friezes, which contrast with the bare masonry. Palazzo Castiglioni, Milan (1900–3), Mausoleum Faccanoni, Sarnico (1907).

Space Frames. The development of space frames is a challenging task for engineers and architects. The traditional concept of a linear progression of stresses in structures has been extended by a system involving the spatial dissolution of the stresses, with all the load-bearing members working together. Thus structures could be devised that are remarkable for stability and load-bearing capacity despite their low weight. A wealth of possibilities for the dissolution of tensile and compressive stresses in space grids has already been examined.
The different systems are principally distinguished by the geometric form of the

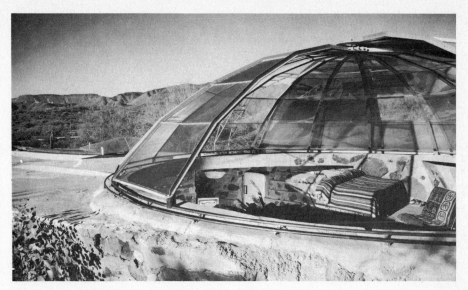

Paolo Soleri and Mark Mills. House in the Desert. Cave Creek, Ariz., 1951

Konrad Wachsmann. Structural system for halls. 1950–3. Model

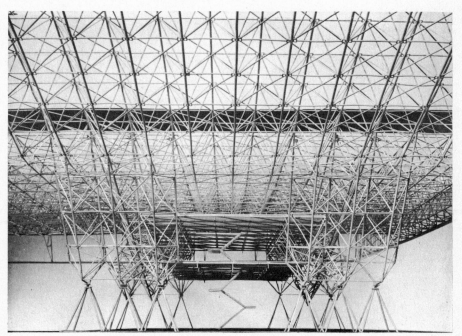

grid module they use, which often already constitutes a stable element. Further distinctions result from the uniform use of tension and compression members or surfaces, or by a clear differentiation between tension and compression members. The most extreme, efficient and fascinating structures are undoubtedly the continuous tension-compression systems made up of cables and struts by Buckminster *Fuller.

The natural requirement that buildings should afford protection from the elements leads to the development of closed surfaces. These surfaces are integrated into the space frame as tension or compression components and become an effective part of the structure. This method of construction affords further important advantages in that even plastics can be employed as structural building materials. In this instance, the low modulus of elasticity of these materials is of no effect due to the extraordinarily advantageous spatial distribution of stresses and the geometrical stability of the structure as a whole.

Space frames are particularly suitable for prefabrication, due to their multitude of modular components. That is why all space frame structures so far known are made of standardized prefabricated building components which can be quickly erected by simple methods such as the Unistrut, Mero and Space-Deck systems. Outstanding schemes made possible by this development include: the aircraft hangar built as early as 1946 by *Wachsmann and the different types of geodesic domes by *Fuller. Makowski and Le Ricolais have made further important advances towards a full theorectical and practical understanding of the distribution of stresses in these systems.

These structures will become ever more important in the future, as their current applications already indicate. The freedom of uninterrupted space and spans which they afford, even of the largest dimensions, and their almost unlimited adaptability to changing and diverse requirements, permit functional solutions of a completely new type.

The architectural expression of these structures is leading to a new aesthetic dimension. In a way that compares with the composition of matter itself, they provide direct spatial models of their theoretical content in their dematerialized multiformity.

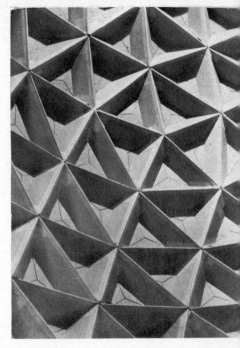

Richard Buckminster Fuller. Geodesic Dome. 1954. Individual units of cardboard

Bibliography: Buckminster Fuller, *Brief Building Construction*; Z. S. Makowski, *Space Structures*; Konrad Wachsmann, *Wendepunkt im Bauen*, Wiesbaden 1959; Robert W. Marks, *The Dymaxion World of Buckminster Fuller*, New York 1960.

HERBERT OHL

Spence, Sir Basil, b. India 1907. Studied at the Schools of Architecture of London and Edinburgh Universities. Assisted Lutyens on the Viceroy's House, New Delhi. In private practice since 1930. Won the competition for Coventry Cathedral (1951); Sea and Ships Pavilion, at the South Bank Exhibition, *Festival of Britain; university buildings at Durham, Exeter, Liverpool, Newcastle, Nottingham and Southampton. His design for Sussex University is a Piranesian fantasy of flat arches and barrel vaults. Housing estates at Dunbar, Selkirk and a premiated

Page 265. Basil Spence. Coventry Cathedral. 1954–62

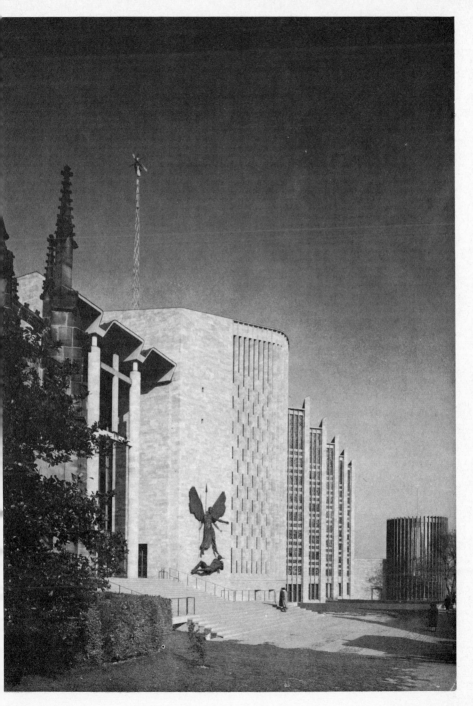

scheme at Sunbury-on-Thames (1951); tall blocks of flats in the Gorbals, Glasgow and Basildon Town Centre. Churches, theatres, factories and office buildings, including Thorn House, St Martin's Lane, London (1959). His most celebrated design, that for Coventry Cathedral (1954–62), represents an attempt to express a traditional layout in a contemporary idiom. As such it may be considered to have achieved a fair measure of success, though it does not display any radical re-thinking from the point of view of the liturgical movement, or the modern movement in architecture. *Bibliography:* B. Spence, *Coventry Phoenix*, London 1962.

HAROLD MEEK

Steel. In the second half of the 18th century the first steps were taken in England which opened up the way for the industrial manufacture of iron products at Abraham Darby's Coalbrookdale foundry: coke was used in 1747 for smelting iron ore instead of charcoal, and by 1750 they were able to produce malleable pig-iron in bars. Up to then iron had only been worked by the elementary methods of artisan production, and was used for two main purposes in building: for structural members, mostly in tensile stress (tie-rods, chains, tie-bars for arches and vaults), and for wrought-iron.

The first of the new manufactured products used in building construction were cast-

Matthew Boulton and James Watt. Cotton Mill. Salford, 1801

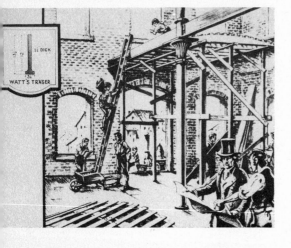

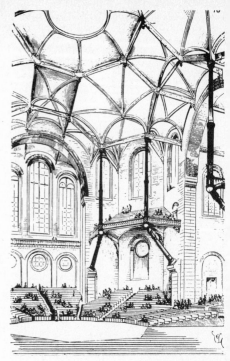

Eugène Emmanuèle Viollet-le-Duc. Assembly Hall. 1863–72. Project

iron girders, beams and columns. The first known use of cast-iron columns in England is in St Anne's Church, Liverpool, by a certain Dodd (1770–2). Matthew Boulton and James Watt built a seven-storey cotton mill in Salford (1801) with an internal framework of cast-iron columns and inverted T-section beams with external walls of solid masonry. In the following decades this type of construction was frequently adopted for factories and warehouses (mills in Derbyshire and Lancashire; warehouses at St Katherine's Docks, London, by Thomas Telford, 1824–8 and at Liverpool Docks by J. Hartley, 1824–45). In an eight-storey refinery built in 1845, William Fairbairn adopted an analogous system, but for cast-iron beams substituted wrought-iron I-sections, and instead of the shallow brick arches running between girders employed in the previous factories he used thin curved metal plates, filled in with concrete. Meanwhile John Cragg had built three churches at Liverpool, St

George's, St Michael's and St Philip's (1813–16) to designs by Thomas Rickman, using cast-iron frames throughout.

Taking advantage of the ease with which different types of section could be obtained in cast-iron, Humphrey Repton designed a pheasant-house for the Royal Pavilion at Brighton in 1808, fanciful in its general lines and decorative details. The Pavilion itself was built by John Nash in 1818 in the 'Indian Style', and made use of cast-iron on a grand scale for the first time in a prestige building (columns, girders, dome structure, decorative elements).

In France, the roof of the Théâtre Français, Paris, was built on an iron frame to the designs of Victor Louis (1786), and Bélanger and Brunet rebuilt the dome of the Halles au Blé, destroyed by fire, in iron and copper (1811). This rapid and widespread recourse to iron is due to its properties of adaptability to complex profiles by means of casting, its fire-resistance, ease of use and ability to span large areas with slender members at distant centres. Works involving particular technical difficulties were faced from the outset and solved. The earliest cast-iron bridge was built over the Severn at Coalbrookdale between 1775 and 1779. It spans 100 feet and consists of five ribs subdivided into two series of half-arches, each cast in a single piece by the Darby Foundry. An experiment of great boldness was completed in 1796 with the Sunderland Bridge, spanning 236 feet, erected by Rowland Bourdon over the Wear to a design of Tom Paine's. This structure was built up from ribs consisting of openwork cast-iron voussoirs and wrought-iron straps, laid upon timber centering. The same technique, derived from masonry construction, was proposed by Telford in 1801 for a bridge across the Thames with a span of 600 feet, which was never realized, however, due to difficulties in acquiring the land on either bank for the abutments. In France, too, iron was used in 1801–3 for a bridge that still exists and is in use: the Pont des Arts, Paris, a multiple arch structure by de Cessart and Dillon.

The technique of constructing suspension bridges had been developed from the end of the 18th century, firstly with chains and later with wire ropes (Conway Castle Bridge, by Telford, 1822–6; Rhône Bridge, by Séguin, 1824). In 1836, I. K. Brunel

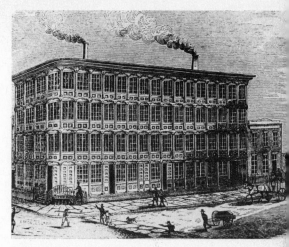

James Bogardus. Cast-iron foundry. New York, 1848–9

commenced building the Clifton Suspension Bridge over the river Avon, at Bristol, which with its span of 700 feet is one of the masterpieces of 19th-century engineering. Brunel, a naval architect, pursued the experiments begun around the year 1825 on the application of iron to shipbuilding. In 1843, he launched the first screw steamer to cross the Atlantic; it had an iron hull, and initiated the technique of self-supporting riveted shell structures. Similar techniques were adopted for other major engineering projects, as instanced by Robert Stephenson's Britannia Bridge over the Menai Straits (1846–50) which features pairs of huge rectangular wrought-iron tubes which run between massive masonry towers.

Simultaneously with these developments improvements were being made in the technology of iron manufacture. The production of puddle iron entered the industrial stage in 1840; steel production with Bessemer converters began in 1856, followed by the open-hearth process in 1864 and the basic converter process in 1878. The *glass industry had made great strides, too, from the second half of the 18th century onwards, and the combination of glass and iron opened up new possibilities in architecture: galleries, conservatories, exhibition buildings such as Joseph *Paxton's Crystal Palace in London and

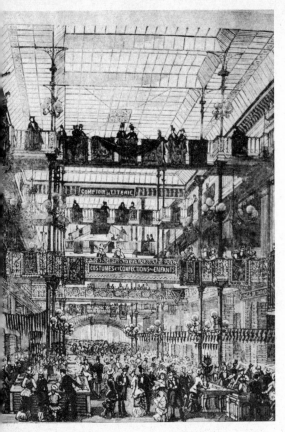

Gustave Eiffel and L. A. Boileau. Bon Marché
Department Store. Paris, 1876

buildings at the various Paris Exhibitions,
culminating in Dutert and Contamin's
Machinery Hall (1889), whose nave is
roofed via a series of three-hinge portals
with a span of *c.* 380 feet.
An important rôle in the gradual perfecting of structural methods and components
was played by Gustave *Eiffel; the designer
of many bridges, viaducts and the Eiffel
Tower, he pursued an architectural ideal
that sought to make the essential lines of a
structure correspond with its static functions. The architect Henri *Labrouste, who
founded a private school of architecture in
Paris with the aim of teaching strict
adherence to the demands of function and
structure, designed the Bibliothèque

Ste Geneviève (1843) and the Bibliothèque
Impériale (1855) using a system of cast-
iron columns and arches to give greater
space, though retaining eclectic or traditionally academic forms for the walls that
formed the outer shell and for the decoration. In his Bibliothèque Nationale (1858–
68), while employing the same structural
and decorative schemes as in the Bibliothèque Impériale for the reading room, he
adopted a system of stanchions, girders and
floor grilles for the book stacks that allowed
the daylight, coming in from above, to
filter down to the lower floors; the structural elements are exposed to view without
any decorative trimmings, and conspire to
produce novel spatial effects of a high
order. Another important contribution to
the handling of internal spaces was made
by the Bon Marché department store in
Paris (1876), by Boileau and Eiffel, who
achieved their effects by an airy system of
foot-bridges, supported by slender columns
and lit by the large glazed roof.
The years around the middle of the 19th
century saw the beginnings of framed construction as we know it now. A decisive
step in this direction was the replacement
of solid external walls by columns and
beams or arches in cast-iron. The first
evidence of the new technique may be seen
in the work of James *Bogardus, who is
considered the inventor of this method of
construction, on the basis of his designs
(New York World's Fair, 1853) and
executed projects (five-storey factory, New
York, 1848; Harper and Brothers Building,
New York, 1854). The system underwent
notable developments, including those in
quality, in the United States (riverfront
buildings at St Louis) and England
(commercial buildings in Liverpool). All
the formal elements of these cast-iron
façade structures, however, were taken
from the traditional repertory of 19th-
century historicism.
One of the first buildings to use a framed
construction throughout was the Chocolat
Menier factory built at Noisiel-sur-Marne,
near Paris by Jules Saulnier in 1871–2. The
iron frame, with diagonal struts clearly
showing on the façade rests on four hollow
iron girders supported by four masonry

Page 269. Ferdinand Dutert and Contamin.
Machinery Hall at the International Exhibition.
Paris, 1889

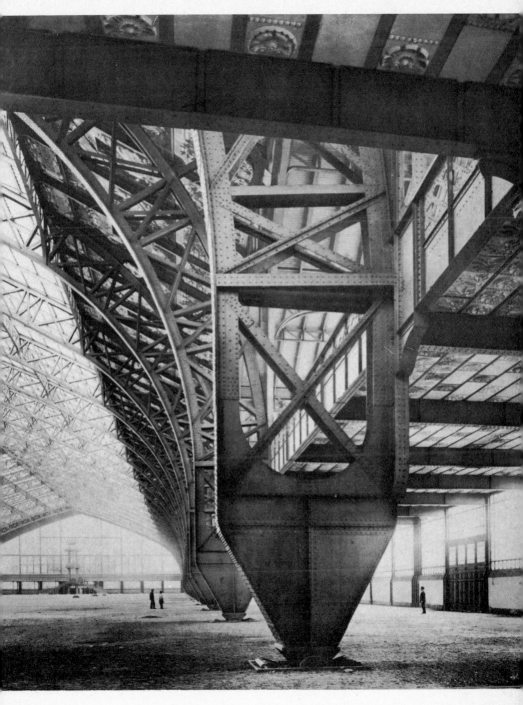

piers built up on the bed of the Marne. The reconstruction of Chicago, growing rapidly after the fire of 1871, provided the impulse for exploiting the possibilities of frame construction (hitherto only used for industrial buildings) in multi-storey commercial blocks, with their need for fireproofing and broad areas of glass. William Le Baron *Jenney, having used the by now usual internal structure with iron columns in his first Leiter Building (1879), employed a complete metal framework for the Home Insurance Building (1883–5), though the surrounding masonry wall shared part of its loadbearing functions. With the second Leiter, Manhattan and Fair Buildings, he refined his structural system, reducing the façades to a form of light cladding carried on a uniform metal frame, thus achieving the prototype of the modern office block. In the spirit of Le Baron Jenney, the architects of the *Chicago School perfected the system, and in the Loop district defined the original

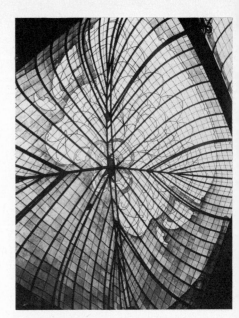

Victor Horta. Hôtel Aubecq, Brussels, 1900. Dome over the stair well

Hans Poelzig. Water tower. Posen, 1911

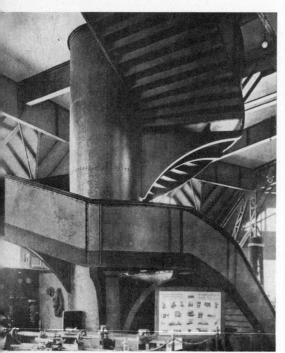

architectural physiognomy of the first centre of the modern movement. Having passed through a phase of attempting to interpret the new structures by adapting traditional stylistic details, they began to derive their forms logically from the framed structure, and abandoned superimposed decoration (Marquette Building by *Holabird and Roche, 1894; Reliance Building by *Burnham and *Root, 1890–5; Carson, Pirie and Scott Building by *Sullivan, 1899). After the 1893 Columbian Exposition in Chicago, American architecture underwent a period of stylistic eclipse with the return of eclecticism and academicism. Meanwhile however, steel frame techniques for skyscrapers were making progress—sometimes sensationally so—throughout America (Woolworth Building [58 storeys] 1912; Empire State Building [85 storeys] 1931, both in New York).

The main exponents of progressive architecture in Europe at the turn of the century approached the use of steel without any preconceptions, and employed it freely in their schemes in conformity with their own styles and the possibilities they saw for applying it. Victor *Horta in the Hôtel

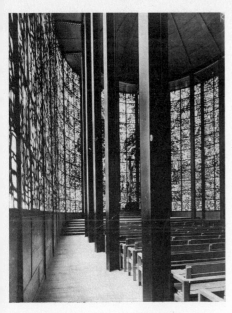

Otto Bartning. Steel Church. Cologne, 1928

Tassel (1893) and the Maison du Peuple (1896-9) in Brussels achieved a perfect unity between structure and decoration. H. P. *Berlage obtained unusual effects in his Amsterdam Stock Exchange (1897-1903) by exposing the structural elements. Otto *Wagner in the hall of the Post Office Savings Bank in Vienna (1904-6) aimed at unity of composition by reducing the individual structural elements to their simplest formal expression. Peter *Behrens in his AEG Works, Berlin (1908-9) revealed that steel, too, had a secret form of expression that lay within the material itself. Hans *Poelzig infused a unitary character into the variegated structures that went to make up his water tower at Posen (1911), derived from his *Expressionist type of sensibility.

The modern movement, in the period after the First World War, took the steel-frame structure for granted, as an indispensable instrument for achieving freedom and rationality in design. In the Weissenhof Estate at Stuttgart (1927) and in other more or less contemporary works, the masters of the modern movement (*Neutra, *Le Corbusier, *Mies van der Rohe, *Mendelsohn) presented a substantially unified panorama to the public, in which a joint purpose and a broad measure of agreement were more in evidence than any personal differences. A common denominator was the principle of the pure expression of function by structural elements. Around 1930, modern architecture began to gain ground in America, and the *International Style was applied uncompromisingly to the skyscrapers, too, where the severity of the modern method brought a notable measure of lucidity to the traditional treatment (Philadelphia Savings Fund Society Building by *Howe and *Lescaze, 1932).

The outburst of building activity after the Second World War helped to perfect and spread the methods of steel frame construction to the most diverse of building types. The need to make savings in time, cost and upkeep led the industry to prefabricate various versions of *curtain walling, which afford numerous possibilities for architectural expression. Outstanding contributions in these fields of research have been made by Mies van der Rohe, whose theoretical studies go back to the year 1919.

Parallel to the work of perfecting the steel frame construction, other forms of structural technique have been studied and applied: *suspended roofs, hung from stressed steel cables; *shell structures in welded plate (water tower at General

Skidmore, Owings and Merrill. Manufacturers Trust Company. New York, 1953-4

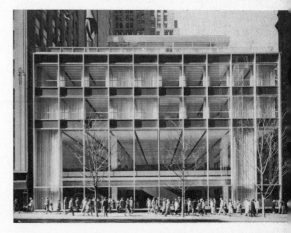

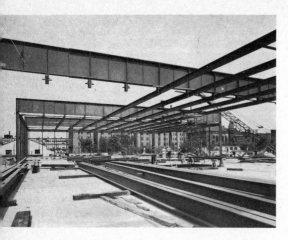

Ludwig Mies van der Rohe. Crown Hall, Illinois Institute of Technology. Chicago, 1952–6. Steel-work in course of erection

Motors Technical Center, Detroit, by Eero *Saarinen, 1955); wide span cantilever roofs of ribbed flats on reinforced concrete piers (hangar at San Francisco airport, by Goldsmith, 1959; Palazzo del Lavoro, Turin, by *Nervi, 1961); reticulated *space frames of prefabricated modular units (geodesic domes by Buckminster *Fuller and studies by K. *Wachsmann). These new techniques, which provide the opportunity and means for bold architectural experiments, may be considered the bases for developing new forms of expression and design.

Bibliography: John Gloag and Derek Bridgwater, *A History of Cast Iron in Architecture*, London 1948; O. Johannsen, *Geschichte des Eisens*, Düsseldorf 1953; *Construire en acier, Bauen in Stahl,* Zurich 1956; V. Zignoli, *Costruzioni metalliche,* Turin 1956–7; *Ponti stradali in acciaio,* Milan 1958; Konrad Wachsmann, *Wendepunkt im Bauen,* Wiesbaden 1959; H. R. Hitchcock, *Early Victorian Architecture in Britain,* London 1954; T. K. Derry and T. I. Williams, *A Short History of Technology,* Oxford 1960.

GIUSEPPE VARALDO
GIAN PIO ZUCCOTTI

Stijl, De. A group of artists and architects, formed in Leiden in 1917, which published a journal of the same name; its members included Vilmos Huszar,

Antonie Kok, Piet Mondrian, Jacobus Johannes *Oud and Theo van *Doesburg. They were subsequently joined by the architects Robert van't Hoff, and Gerrit Thomas *Rietveld, the painter Bart van der Leck and the sculptor and painter Georges Vantongerloo.

The type of design associated with De Stijl was very much determined by the neoplasticism of the painters Piet Mondrian and Theo van Doesburg; it implied, in every respect, a break with tradition. Like neoplasticist painting, De Stijl architecture was influenced by Cubism, too. Right angles and smooth walls were almost exclusively the order of the day; the demand for unmistakably spotless surfaces excluded the use of bricks, which

Theo van Doesburg and Cor van Eesteren. Studies for a private house. 1923

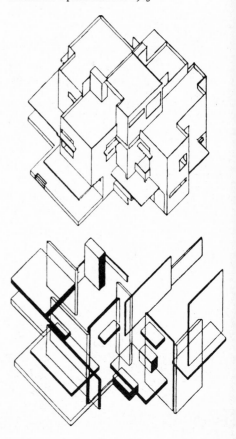

gave too graduated and imprecise a colour-effect. The cube or parallelopiped served as the point of departure, but the cubic shape, as an elementary expression of space, was not felt as something static, but as part of an infinite environment, into which the internal walls continued. Hence every circumscribed definition of a building by front, side or rear elevations was rejected. The designed space, i.e. the room, opened out on all sides into the universal space, conceived of as a crystal.

New attitudes emerged with regard to the use of colour, both as regards external surfaces and interior decoration. Colour no longer served as an element of decoration, but helped to define space. Following Mondrian's example, the primary colours, red, blue and yellow, were used exclusively; white, black and grey were admitted as contrasting tones. All other colours were regarded as impure, in stark contrast to the picturesque brown tones that had prevailed in late-19th-century interiors. Typical examples include Rietveld's Schröder House in Utrecht (1924) and the Café de Unie in Rotterdam by Oud (1924–5, destroyed in the 1940 blitz).

Its cubistic design, simplicity and austerity of line are the reasons why the architecture of De Stijl is often confused with the concept of 'Neue Sachlichkeit', a term that was applied to German painting around 1925. De Stijl architecture certainly exerted great influence, and set the type for developments in the later twenties (*Functionalism, *International Style) with its new attitude to space.

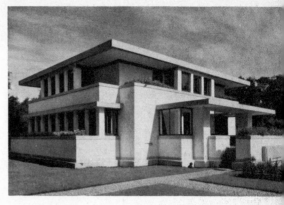

Robert van't Hoff. Huis ter Heide. Utrecht, 1916

But despite the contrary asseverations of its supporters, De Stijl was to a great extent an aesthetic theory. In this respect it differed from later developments, since Functionalism and the International Style rejected all fixed notions of aesthetics, believing in the unity of form and function.

The translation of De Stijl's theories into architectural practice was not accomplished without a measure of conflict. After an initial period of collaboration, the partnership between Oud and van Doesburg broke up, since Oud's solid expertise in architecture was confronted by the brilliant dilettantism of a painter and theoretician, who, as an architect, was self-taught. Oud developed his

J. J. P. Oud. Factory at Purmerend. 1919. Project

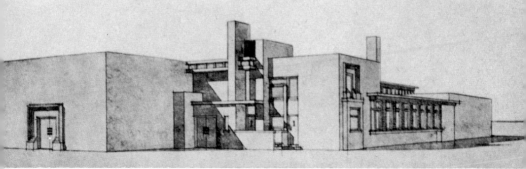

architecture from the tentative essays of De Stijl, and went on to exert a leading influence on Functionalism in W. Europe. Reminiscences of De Stijl features are still discernible in Rietveld's buildings, especially in the décor; his work, and with it the significance of De Stijl, were rediscovered by the younger generation of architects after 1945.

Bibliography: De Stijl, Internationaal Maandblad voor de Nieuwe Kunst, Wetenschap en Kultuur, Leiden 1917–31; *De Stijl*, Catalogue 81 of the Stedelijk Museum, Amsterdam 1951; Bruno Zevi, *Poetica dell'architettura neoplastica*, Milan 1953; H. L. C. Jaffé, *De Stijl 1917–1931, The Dutch Contribution to Modern Art*, Amsterdam 1956.

J. J. VRIEND

Stillman and Eastwick-Field. John Cecil Stillman and John Charles Eastwick-Field. Miscellaneous practice including houses, hospitals and farm buildings. Point block of flats at Hide Place, Westminster, for the local authority, with extensive use of precast concrete techniques. Authors of a valuable study on joinery practice.

Stirling and Gowan. James Stirling, b. Glasgow 1925, and James Gowan, b. Glasgow 1923. Partnership producing work of distinctive plastic effect. Housing at Ham Common (1958) with imaginative use of untreated concrete detailing to give rich sculptural quality; rehousing scheme at Preston with powerful visual patterns of fenestration evoking *Constructivist imagery. See *Architectural Review*, April 1964.

Hugh Stubbins. Congress Hall. Berlin, 1957

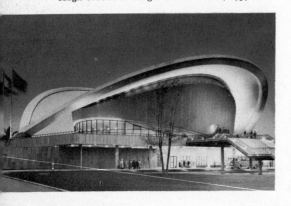

Stone, Edward Durell, b. Fayetteville, Ark. 1902. Stone, who was called 'a young man with a brilliant future' by Frank Lloyd *Wright, first built clearly defined square blocks with smooth white surfaces, punctuated by strips of fenestration (Mandel House at Mount Kisco, New York, 1930; Museum of Modern Art, New York, 1939, together with Philip L. Goodwin). Commissions abroad, especially in tropical and sub-tropical countries, may have led to his now characteristic screen walls, non-loadbearing partitions in front of or behind the real structural members. These pierced walls of tiles, profilated bricks or metal grilles, which provide shade and ventilation, and which Stone employs in all buildings, appear as huge, carpet-like patterned areas and often go together with classically symmetrical plans and façades: Medical Centre at Palo Alto, Calif. (1957–60); US Embassy at New Delhi (1958). Stone used them also for the circular US pavilion at the Brussels Exhibition of 1958, where the roof structure rested on a compression ring more than 328 ft in diameter.

Stubbins, Hugh, b. Powderly, Ala. 1912. Became Walter *Gropius's assistant at Harvard Graduate School of Design in 1939. Private houses, schools, office blocks, churches. The stage of the Loeb Theatre at Harvard (1957–60) can be changed from a proscenium type to an arena. The Congress Hall in Berlin, which was erected for the Interbau Exhibition, comprises auditorium, conference rooms, exhibition hall and theatre. Its saddle-shaped roof, whose weight is partly carried by walls and internal columns, partly by two anchors, is a bold feat of engineering.

Subtopia. Term coined by Ian Nairn to connote 'the world of universal low density mess . . . an even spread of abandoned aerodromes and fake rusticity, wire fences, traffic roundabouts, gratuitous noticeboards, car-parks and Things in Fields' extending out from suburbia to the country 'and back into the devitalized hearts of towns, so that the most sublime backgrounds, urban or rural, English or foreign, are now to be seen only over a foreground of casual and unconsidered equipment, litter and lettered admonition. . . . Within the town the agents of Subtopia

are demolition and decay, buildings replaced by bijou gardens, car-parks and
underscale structures, reduction of density
where it should be increased (and the)
reduction of vitality by false genteelism,
of which Municipal Rustic is the prime
agent.'
Bibliography: Ian Nairn, *Outrage*, London
1955; Ian Nairn, *Counter-attack against
Subtopia*, London 1957.

Sullivan, Louis H., b. Boston 1856, d.
Chicago 1924. Sullivan's fame is based

upon the refinements that he introduced in
the design of large metal-framed commercial buildings, and upon the development
of an organic theory of architecture. In
1873 he attended architectural classes at
the Massachusetts Institute of Technology
and subsequently worked for the Philadelphia architect, Frank *Furness. Afterwards he spent a few months at the *École
des Beaux-Arts, Paris (1874), and in 1875
went to Chicago to seek employment. After
several routine positions, he joined the staff
of Dankmar *Adler and rapidly displayed

Louis H. Sullivan. Auditorium Building. Chicago, 1886–9

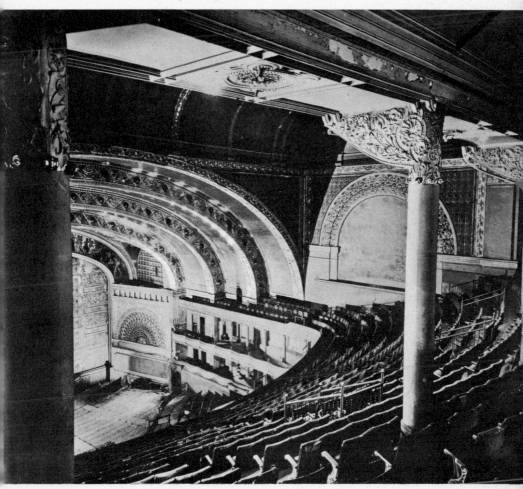

his talents as a designer. Two years later, in 1881, the partnership of Adler and Sullivan was formed, Adler devoting his energies to technical and business problems while Sullivan carried the burden of responsibilities with respect to design. The early work of this partnership is outwardly utilitarian, though its style remains somewhat tentative. It is only with the design of the Auditorium Building, Chicago (1886–9) that Sullivan's talent comes into focus. The monumental, round-arched vocabulary which dominates the exterior sheath of the Auditorium Building (which was an hotel and office building as well as a theatre) derives from the example of *Richardson, notably his Marshall Field Warehouse,

Louis H. Sullivan. Wainwright Building. St Louis, 1890–1

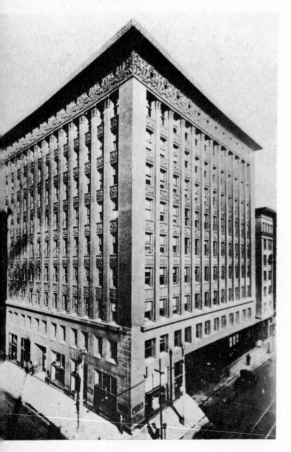

Chicago (1885–7). On the other hand, the interior, and notably the proscenium of the auditorium, is one of the most original instances of planning and decoration in American architecture.

Office buildings—skyscrapers—were the stock-in-trade of the Chicago architectural profession, and Sullivan accommodated himself to such programmatic limitations during a decade (the 1890s) of extremely successful commercial design before a combination of personal and business problems deprived him of major commissions. After 1900, and the nominal close of the earlier portion of his career, most of his works were modest-sized edifices for clients in small mid-western farming communities.

Sullivan's Chicago skyscrapers of the 1890s reflect his sensitivity with respect to the adjustment of external detail to the rhythms and proportions of the building's structural core, the steel frame. Contrary to the implications of his oft-quoted epithet, 'Form follows function', Sullivan used the building's material and structural requirements as a point of departure for his creation, rather than conceiving of functional expression as a fixed, limited goal. The Wainwright Building, St Louis (1890–91) and the Guarantee Building, Buffalo (1894–5), represent the maturing of this attitude, which is well expressed by the title of an article by Sullivan of 1896, 'The Tall Office Building Artistically Considered'.

After the termination of Sullivan's partnership with Adler, he was sometimes engaged to design the façades of commercial buildings that were built by other architects, as in the Bayard Building, New York (1897–8), and the Gage Building, Chicago (1898–9). The adjustments of proportion and the expressive clarity of detailing in the cornices and vertical members of these two façades are not equalled by their general shape, over which Sullivan had no control; it is regrettable that he did not have an opportunity in this period to build the kind of free-standing skyscraper that is so common today. Not even the corner site of his Carson, Pirie & Scott Store, Chicago (1899), his last major commercial building, suggests what he would have done on an

Page 277. Louis H. Sullivan. Auditorium Building. Chicago, 1886–9. Stair well

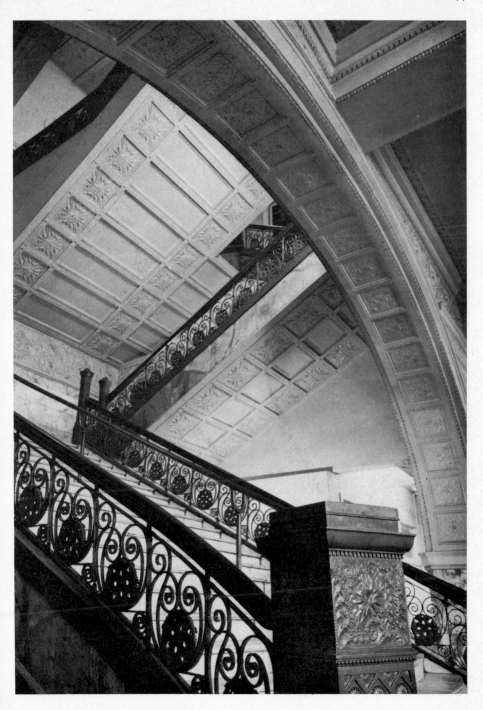

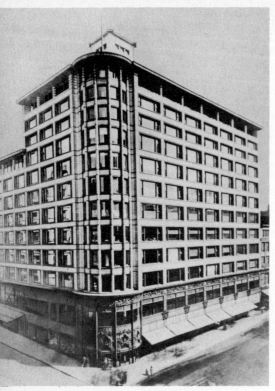

Louis H. Sullivan. Carson, Pirie and Scott. Chicago, 1899

open site, since the client insisted upon the round corner element and the mass of the building was subsequently extended by D. H. *Burnham, albeit using Sullivan's elevation. Thus his genius is apparent here only in the adjustment of detail to the bay system imposed by the steel frame.

Under the circumstances it is understandable that Sullivan's gift for inventive ornament, ultimately of a quasi-Art Nouveau, organic quality, developed to such a remarkable extent. This interest almost dominates his formal, monumental work, notably the Wainwright Tomb, St Louis (1892), and the Transportation Building at the Chicago World's Columbian Exposition of 1893. This latent urge towards the fusion of elaborate ornament with rhetorical, monumental forms is developed in his late, post-1900 work, notably in the National Farmers Bank, Owatonna, Minn.

(1907–8), and in the Farmers and Merchants Union Bank, Columbus, Wis. (1919). Critical appraisal of these buildings has tended towards condescension as they are supposed to represent a falling off of creative force and functional cogency. However, an objective consideration of these small but major designs amply demonstrates Sullivan's continued development and creative maturity, albeit in a direction that is not immediately related to the more revolutionary strains of contemporary architecture.

In contrast to these almost traditional buildings, Sullivan's writings, notably *Kindergarten Chats* (1901) and *The Autobiography of an Idea* (1922–3), contain flashes of wisdom and insight into the evolution of contemporary architecture. However, these thoughts, occasionally beautifully expressed, are buried in texts which are turgid and unnecessarily repetitious. Contrary to accepted opinion, the very best of Sullivan's late work is to be found consistently in his buildings, and only occasionally in his writings.

Bibliography: Hugh Morrison, *Louis Sullivan, Prophet of Modern Architecture*, New York 1952; Willard Connely, *Louis Sullivan as he lived*, New York 1960.

JOHN M. JACOBUS, JR

Suprematism. A term invented by Kasimir *Malevich for purely abstract art, of the kind he first exhibited in 1915. Suprematism meant for Malevich the 'Supremacy of pure sensation in the fine arts'. The simple elements of form in his paintings are also applied to abstract architectonic compositions.

Suspended Roofs. Suspended roofs originated from the discovery that a structure consisting of tensile members involves little self-weight yet is capable of supporting relatively great loads. Tents and suspension bridges are early examples. As distinguished from these is an essentially new principle which consists in providing complete rigidity of form by the use of saddle-shaped surfaces (especially hyperbolic paraboloidal planes or lattices). Any deformation of shape such as buckling, oscillation or vibration caused by wind force or by self-weight can thus be avoided.

The hall at Raleigh by *Deitrick and *Nowicki (1952–3) is one of the first known

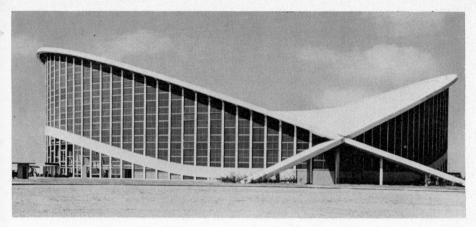

Matthew Nowicki, William H. Deitrick and Fred Severud. Arena. Raleigh, N.C., 1952–3

examples of this type of construction and the new kind of architecture to which it has given rise. It served as a pointer to the future of the new building method; apart from its logical use of stressed cable lattices, it also employs extremely light-weight prefabricated slab units for cladding purposes. Simultaneously with the new saddle-shaped suspended roofs, cable lattices or *shell vaults, methods of supporting compressive stresses via optimum stress arcs or modified thrust collars were developed. New shapes for roofs and halls and in particular a methodical system of foundations were developed by Le Ricolais, in theory and experimentally, as an extension of these principles. Inspired by the possibilities of traditional tent shapes and the new knowledge about suspended roofs, Frei *Otto has produced a wealth of forms in which he has used the roofing material itself as a structural component.

Suspended roof systems have introduced new possibilities to modern architecture, which question the whole principle of the use of rectangular shapes, while considerably enriching the contemporary idiom at the same time.

Bibliography: Frei Otto, *Über Zugbeanspruchte Konstruktionen*, Berlin 1962.

HERBERT OHL

Sweden. Industrialism came rather late to Sweden. In the late 19th century the economy of the country was still mainly based on agriculture, mining and forestry. Architecture followed the general European development on rather a moderate scale. The tendency of the 1880s was a combination of stylistic eclecticism and realistic treatment of the materials. In the following decade a German-influenced neo-Baroque played an important part. This was the background for the rise of modern Swedish architecture.

Its key figure was Ferdinand Boberg (1860–1946). Under the influence of the American H. H. *Richardson he began about 1890 to design a series of buildings such as the fire station at Gävle and the old Stockholm electricity works, which are characterized by a functionalist grouping of massive, block-like volumes. In his subsequent work the cubic heaviness is developed, but set off against concentrated elegant ornaments, in which the inspiration of *Sullivan is evident.

Towards the turn of the century the influence of *Art Nouveau was beginning to be felt in Sweden. It was, however, of rather a well-balanced and moderate character. An important part was played by the painter Carl Larsson, whose blond interiors from his own home greatly influenced interior architecture. In the bank buildings of Gustaf Wickman (1858–1916) neo-Baroque and Art Nouveau are skilfully mingled in sculpturally expressive forms. The desire to discard historical forms is especially evident in an interesting group

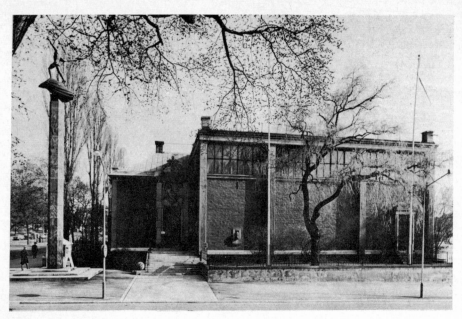

Carl Bergsten. Liljevalch Gallery. Stockholm, completed 1916

of office buildings in Stockholm designed by different architects. The façades all show a pronounced vertical treatment, often with very big glass areas between narrow pillars. Internally skeleton construction is used. Outstanding are a couple of buildings created by Ernst Stenhammar (1859–1927) and Erik Josephson (1864–1929).

Most important of the architects who tried to get away from the old forms were Carl Bergsten (1879–1935) and Georg A. Nilsson (1871–1949). The radical ideas of Bergsten reflect the influence of the Vienna Sezessionists, but in his tendency to regard the building as made up of geometrical planes he is also strongly reminiscent of *Berlage and Frank Lloyd *Wright. This is shown in his remarkable competition project for the Stockholm City Hall of 1905. The Norrköping Exhibition of the following year and the Hjorthagen Church in Stockholm gave him opportunities to realize his ideas. Nilsson's production as a whole is much more moderate, but some of his works show an evident affinity with the Anglo-Saxon modernists. His finest work is the iron-skeleton office building in Stockholm, Regeringsgatan 9, the final culmination of this modern school.

Other tendencies had by then become dominant. A group of architects had taken up Boberg's cubic forms and combined them with a new interest in materials of a rich, living texture, such as red brick or traditional Swedish timber. This 'national realism' derived partly from *Morris and his successors in England and the Nyrop circle in Denmark, but old Swedish architecture came to be of increasing importance as a source of inspiration. Nevertheless the character of the movement was not reactionary. The stress on traditional techniques and constructions was rather natural in a country where industrialism had not yet advanced very far. But what was modern was the social awareness of the leading architects. For perhaps the first time low-cost housing was seen as a task worthy of first-rate architectural treatment. The building which is generally regarded as the first work of this school is the one completed for the Medical Society in Stockholm in 1905 by Carl Westman (1866–1936). He used the traditional forms

Page 281. Erik Gunnar Asplund. Stockholm Exhibition. 1930

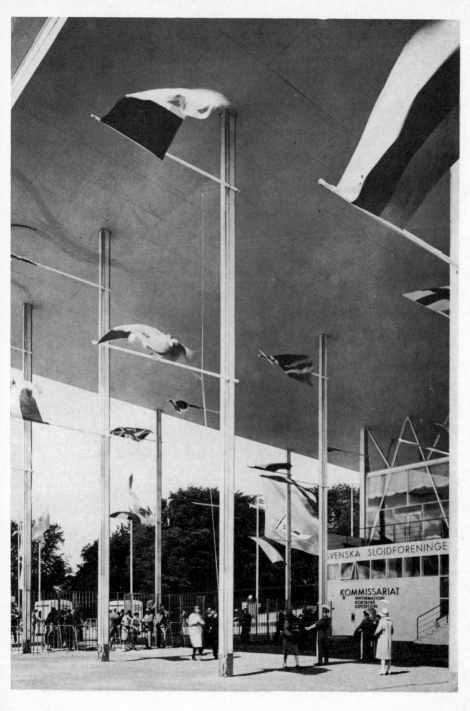

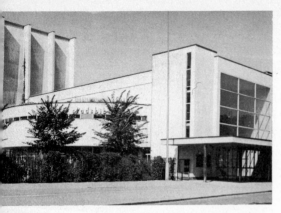

Sven Markelius. Concert Hall. Hälsingborg, 1932

in a realistic and rational way, as is shown expecially in his Stockholm Law Courts Building ten years later. The functional ideals of the period were even more stressed in the work of Erik Hahr (1869–1944), for many years city architect of Västerås, where he carefully preserved the old character of the town but also added industrial buildings and workmen's houses; these are remarkably advanced for their day, but nevertheless clearly show the links with tradition. Hahr's work also illustrates a very important feature of the architecture of this time, namely the strong feeling of relationship between buildings and town planning.

The artistic possibilities of this architecture of volumes and materials were exploited to the full by Ragnar Östberg (1866–1945), the supreme artist of the period. His greatest work, the Stockholm City Hall, was a source of inspiration to others during the long history of its design and erection, but by the time it was completed in 1923 other ideas had taken the lead. Romantic in a way, similar to Östberg's buildings, but more freely modern in its details, was the Engelbrekt Church in Stockholm by Lars Israel Wahlman (1870–1952). Quite different is Wickman's great wooden church at Kiruna, a remarkably powerful synthesis of form and structure. These are the two most important works in the religious architecture of the period.

About 1910 the school of national realism had become dominant in Swedish architecture. But at the same time the first signs

of a reaction began to appear among the younger architects. They started to look for geometrical precision, for the nuances of lines and shadows and for materials of a more abstract character. Instead of heavy blocks they wanted to create a lighter impression. It was natural that their interest began to turn towards classicism. The first of the leading architects to develop these tendencies was Ivar Tengbom (b. 1878), who had been one of the foremost theorists among the national realists. Gradually he introduced a more restrained way of handling the materials and a simplification of forms—a typical example of the progressive, in no way revolutionary development towards a completely new architecture that has characterized so many Swedish architects.

But the greatest of the modernists, Carl Bergsten, saw clearly that classicism was only a stage in the search for pure new forms. In his Liljevalch Art Gallery in Stockholm, completed in 1916, he had covered quite a good bit of the way. The block character is gone, exterior and interior have been put in close relation to one another. One of the central ideas behind 20th-century architecture, the continuity of space, is appearing.

In the development of modern architecture as we see it today no generation has played a greater part than those born about the middle 1880s, the generation of *Gropius, *Le Corbusier, and *Mies van der Rohe. Three very important Swedish names belong to this group: Osvald *Almqvist Gunnar *Asplund and Sigurd *Lewerentz. They started within the bounds of national realism. When Lewerentz designed a group of holiday houses in the Stockholm archipelago in 1914, he used the forms of Swedish tradition, but in such a timelessly functional way that these little houses are extremely difficult to date. Through Kay *Fisker they came to exercise a considerable influence on Danish architecture. A couple of years later Almqvist created the 'Bergslagsbyn', a village for the workmen and employees of the Domnarvet iron works, where the red wooden houses and the carefully studied town plan make up a model housing scheme which must be counted as one of the best Swedish examples from this century. Asplund at the same time was developing a feeling for space which was fundamentally related to

modern international tendencies, only that
he worked with more traditional forms. But
it became increasingly clear that his classicism was only a superficial, artistic game
and that his real development lay deeper.
With the 1920s industrial architecture came
to be of real importance. On the merits of
his water-power stations Almqvist must be
counted one of the great pioneers in the
field, judged from an international point of
view. The mighty Forshuvudforsen of 1921
still remains in the functional tradition, but
with Hammarforsen and Krångforsen, both
designed and built in 1925–8, he had cut
all ties with the past. These buildings,
extremely pure and simple, have nevertheless a very strong dynamic expression,
conveying something of the idea of water-
power. Chenderoh in Malaya, completed
in 1930, is perhaps even finer in its bright,
calm clarity.
Almqvist had developed into 'the first
Swedish functionalist' practically independently of all influences from abroad. At
about the same time, however, Le Corbusier's theories got an intelligent and

far-seeing interpreter in the person of Uno
Åhrén (b. 1897). Of first-rate importance
also was the founding in 1925 of the
Co-operative Society's architects' office,
with Eskil Sundahl (b. 1890) as chief
architect. The factories, shops and other
works sponsored by this office came to be
known for a purist quality with strong
social, and one might even say moral,
aspects, which became of decisive importance for the whole Swedish architecture
of the 1930s.
In 1930 Asplund was finally ready to
discard the cloak of formalism under which
he had been carrying out his studies of
space problems and room relations during
the whole of the 1920s. In the Stockholm
Exhibition he exploited to the full the
artistic possibilities of the 'new architecture' with a refinement and an elegance
probably unsurpassed to this day. Within
a very short time functionalism then became generally accepted in Sweden. The
ground had been well prepared. The
progressive political atmosphere favoured
the social consciousness which had for so

Sven Backström and Leif Reinius. Gröndal Estate. Stockholm, 1944–5

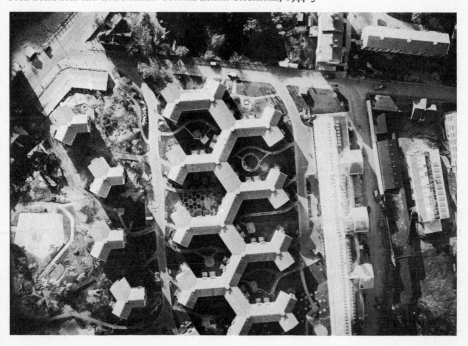

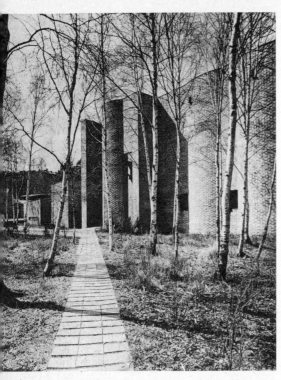

Sigurd Lewerentz. Björkhagen Church. Skarpnäck near Stockholm, 1960

Sven Backström and Leif Reinius. Town centre with cinema and assembly rooms in background. Satellite town of Vällingby, near Stockholm, commenced 1953

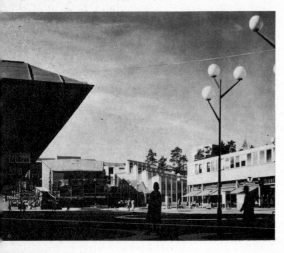

long been part of the architectural programme; on the formal side, the more abstract line in the classicism of the 1920s had been gradually leading up to pure *Functionalism. Of course there were differences of opinion and heated debates, but hardly worth mentioning if we compare the situation in most other countries where the new ideas had to fight hard against official resistance. In this way Sweden became the 'model country' of modern architecture in the 1930s. But to a considerable extent the real strength lay on the side of the social programme. Much of what was built seems in retrospect rather dry and schematic. This concerns especially the town plans with their parallel blocks, where a correct orientation was valued higher than the creation of outdoor rooms between buildings.

Nevertheless there were many buildings of high artistic value. The leading name was Asplund, who was now softening the abstract character of the pioneer works by his exquisite feeling for different materials. The Gothenburg Concert Hall by Nils Einar Eriksson (b. 1899) shows similar qualities. Le Corbusier's influence is evident in the works of Sven *Markelius, especially in his private houses. But the strongest personal note is to be seen in the very limited production of Lewerentz, who shows a deep feeling for all the technical and aesthetic aspects of building, accepting no ready-made solution but working until the problems are mastered. Thus, while Lewerentz's buildings are always technically right, as independent works of art they also stand on a level above most contemporary architecture and show a continuous personal development. In 1937 he built a remarkable private house at Falsterbo; the landscaping of the Stockholm Forest Cemetery round Asplund's crematorium is chiefly his work, and in 1943 he completed his own crematorium in Malmö in the cemetery which he had begun to plan already in 1920.

In the 1940s a reaction started against international Functionalism. This was partly caused by the war, which cut off contacts with other countries and also restricted the use of certain building materials. Swedish architecture turned provincial. The clarity of the 1930s gave way to a superficial play with forms and materials. This romanticism could, however, sometimes lead to fine results, as in the Karlskoga Town Hall and Hotel by Sune Lindström (b. 1906), where it was combined with strongly disciplined volumes. A new tradition in brick building was formed. A really positive contribution of the decade was the abandoning of the stereotyped housing schemes in favour of differentiated plans, where the architects sought to create more 'home-like' surroundings and the plans of the houses themselves were very thoroughly studied. The partners Sven Backström (b. 1903) and Leif Reinius (b. 1907) are the most important architects of such projects.

With the 1950s a new wave of international influences swept over Sweden. This time, however, it was less surely handled than in the 1930s. There was no artist of Asplund's calibre to take the lead. Perhaps the general level might be called quite good, but there were no highlights. The really important things still happened on the programme side, above all in civic planning, where such projects as the Vällingby scheme, with its much-studied social and commercial centre, saw the light. The rebuilding of the central parts of Stockholm is another gigantic project which has attracted much interest. But here again uncertainty in the treatment of volumes, materials and details has often been manifest.

A new reaction began to appear at the end of the 1950s. Interest in the truly three-dimensional aspects of architecture has awakened again, but it has not taken the form of any wild experimentation. The liking for the simple cube is coming back, combined with a tendency to strong individualization. Not seldom colourful materials such as bricks are used. There are certain parallels to the tendencies of about 1910. These ideas have come to light most vigorously in church architecture. The works of Peter Celsing (b. 1920) offer a good field for study. But most remarkable is Lewerentz's church at Skarpnäck near Stockholm, a group of low brick volumes that seem to be in some way naturally grown on their site. There is nothing radically new in such a way of building, but it has here been given the timeless quality of a great work of art. And continued progress has always been more popular than revolution in Sweden.

Bibliography: G. E. Kidder Smith, *Sweden Builds*, 2nd edition, New York 1957; *New*

Swedish Architecture, Stockholm 1939; *Swedish Housing of the 'Forties*, Stockholm 1950; *New Architecture in Sweden*, Stockholm 1961 (all published by SAR, the National Association of Swedish Architects).

BJÖRN LINN

Switzerland. Long before the term modern architecture could be used with regard to Switzerland, Robert *Maillart (from 1901 onwards) constructed his reinforced concrete bridges which were as technically audacious as they were aesthetically perfect. Karl *Moser, whose Church of St Anthony at Basle (1926–7) was the first ecclesiastical building in Switzerland built entirely of reinforced concrete, taught the next generation of architects while he was professor (1915–28) at Zurich Technical College (ETH). At the same time, Hans Bernoulli by his writings awakened their

Karl Moser. Church of St Anthony. Basle, 1926–7

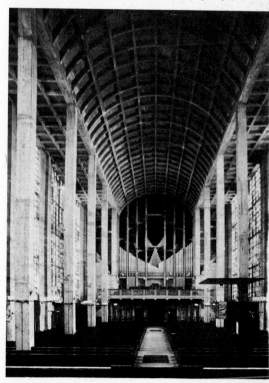

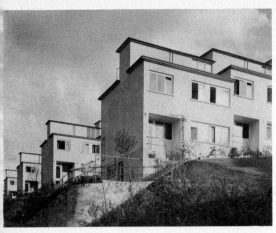

Paul Artaria, Hans Schmidt, Max E. Haefeli, Carl Hubacher, Rudolf Steiger, Werner M. Moser and Emil Roth. Neubühl Estate. Zurich, 1930–2

sense of responsibility for civic design and town planning; he, too, was a professor at the ETH (Chair of Civic Design, 1919–39). The younger generation gave their point of view in the journal *ABC* (1924, Hans Schmidt and Mart Stam). Moser's successors to the professorship were O. R. Salvisberg and Hans Hofmann.

Above all, *Le Corbusier's ideas exerted great influence. The Weissenhof houses at Stuttgart (1927) and the developments in

Hermann Baur. School on the Bruderholz. Basle, 1938–9

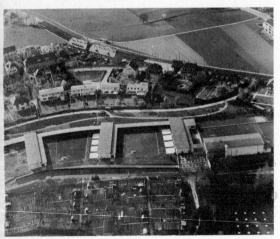

Holland were studied. The *Bauhaus, directed in 1928–9 by the Swiss architect Hannes *Meyer, after Gropius's resignation, made its effects felt in Switzerland, too. Meyer's Trade Union School at Bernau (1928) was one of the first examples of a purely functional building; his design for the League of Nations Building at Geneva (1927), awarded the third prize, was the antithesis to Le Corbusier's scheme, which came first. *CIAM was founded at La Sarraz in 1928 and the *élite* of the world's architects joined it. In the ideological struggle against 'vernacular style', the new buildings erected between 1930 and 1940 achieved the homogeneity of functional thought: precise, objective and unpretentious, adapted to the rich local tradition of burgher and peasant culture and to the variety yet compression of the landscape within the framework of a federally constituted democracy. A high standard of housing was achieved, backed by perfection of structure and workmanship. Switzerland built excellent housing estates, hospitals and schools; her theoretical contributions, publications and exhibitions were influential. Paul Artaria, Ernst F. Burckhardt, Karl Egender, Max Ernst Haefeli, Werner M. Moser, Emil and Alfred Roth, Hans Schmidt, Otto Senn and Rudolf Steiger began to work at this time; Max *Bill and Hans Fischli came from the Bauhaus.

The National Provinces Exhibition at Zurich in 1939 (chief architect Hans Hofmann) aimed at showing a cross section of all that had been built since 1914. One of its positive results was the foundation of the Swiss Town and Country Planning Association (1943). The next National Provinces Exhibition to be held in Lausanne in 1964 will itself be an example of modern planning, and will make a fundamental attempt to tackle the planning problems of our time (chief architect: A. Camenzind; divisional architects: Max Bill, Zurich; Fréderic Brugger, Lausanne; Tita Carloni, Lugano; Jean Duret, Geneva; Marc-J. Saugey, Geneva; Florian Fischer, Basle; Jakob Zweifel, Zurich).

The Neubühl estate by the Werkbund at Zurich (1930–2) became a prototype of its kind: it featured differentiation of living requirements, standardization of units, and provision of open spaces by arranging the blocks at angles to each other (Artaria and

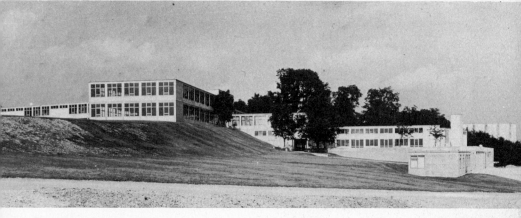

Max Bill. College of Design (Hochschule für Gestaltung). Ulm, 1953–5

Schmidt; M. E. Haefeli; C. Hubacher; R. Steiger, W. M. Moser and E. Roth). The housing scheme for Prilly near Lausanne went even further (1947; M. E. Haefeli, W. M. Moser, R. Steiger, M. Hottinger—not built) in envisaging a mixed development, including point blocks. The Gellert district at Basle (general layout by H. Baur, 1956) adopted the same principle but different means of execution. The estate at Halen near Berne (1957; Atelier 5, Berne, and Niklaus Morgenthaler) is a group of detached houses set close together in the manner of a village and rationalized by the use of prefabricated concrete units.

Hospital and school buildings were freed from schematism. At the cantonal hospital, Zurich (started 1942; M. E. Haefeli, R. Steiger, W. M. Moser, H. Weideli, J. Schütz, H. Fietz) spatial unity has been achieved in accommodating the most modern therapeutic knowledge, with its facilities in a constant state of renewal and extension. The current level of this development may be seen in Zurich Dental Institute, by the same architects. The school on the Bruderholz at Basle by Hermann Baur (1938–9) gave the lead to this type of district school, freely laid out amidst greenery. There is a large number of excellent examples of this kind today everywhere in Switzerland. The school building programme of Zurich in particular is remarkable for its far-sighted planning for anticipated requirements under the direction of progressive architects. Larger

schools are best represented by the technical colleges: Zurich, Karl Egender, (1926–32); Berne, Hans Brechbühler, (1937–9); and Basle, H. and H. P. Baur, F. Bräuning and A. Dürig (1956–61). As an example of the organization of a complex group of buildings in a natural setting, on the basis of uniform elements, the College of Design (Hochschule für Gestaltung) at Ulm by Max Bill may be cited (1953–55). A similar problem arose at Zurich, where the Freudenberg cantonal school by Jacques Schader (1958–61) had to combine two types of schools on a limited site.

Rudolf and Peter Steiger. 'Cern' Laboratory. Geneva, 1954–60

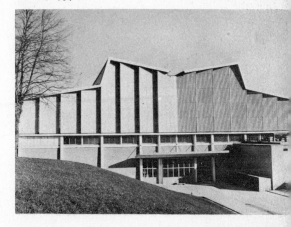

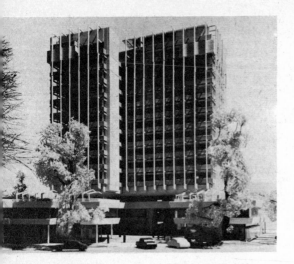

Max E. Haefeli, Werner M. Moser, Rudolf Steiger, O. Caretta and André Studer. Multi-storey office block 'zur Palme'. Zurich, under construction. Model

Since 1945, new buildings in Switzerland have assumed a multitude of shapes. Typical examples include the churches that followed Le Corbusier's experiment at Ronchamp. The multi-storey office building 'zur Palme' in Zurich by M. E. Haefeli, W. M. Moser, R. Steiger, O. Caretta and A. Studer (under construction) attempts a form of three-dimensional modelling inspired by Frank Lloyd *Wright. The terraced layouts at Zug by F. Stucky and R. Meuli (1957–60) and at Zurich-Witikon by C. Paillard and Peter Leemann (1959–60), with flats stacked above each other in self-contained living zones, are all distinguished by the utmost economy in the exploitation of the site. Large blocks of flats with a high standard of comfort have appeared, particularly in Geneva (Denis Honegger, Arthur Lozeron, Marc-J. Saugey). The construction of the 'Cern' Research Centre near Geneva by R. and P. Steiger (1954–60) successfully coped with spatial requirements of a hitherto unknown category for nuclear research. In French Switzerland modern architecture has made a late start, although the famous Swiss architect Le Corbusier, who has been living in Paris since 1917, came from this region. The Italian part of

Switzerland has started even later to let modern architecture in; but there Italian influence is unmistakable.

Bibliography: Max Bill, *Moderne Schweizer Architektur 1925–1949*, Basle 1949; G. E. Kidder Smith, *Switzerland builds*, London and New York 1950; Hans Volkart, *Schweizer Architektur*, Ravensburg 1951.

MARGIT STABER

TAC (The Architects Collaborative), founded in 1946, an architectural association in which Walter *Gropius joined with architects of the younger generation (Norman Fletcher, John Harkness, Robert McMillan, Louis McMillen, and Benjamin Thompson). Gropius here realized his conception of 'teamwork by individualists' in such large TAC schemes as the Harvard Graduate Center (1949–50), the US Embassy in Athens (1961), and the project for Bagdad University.

Tange, Kenzo, b. Imabari City in Shikoku 1913. Tange spent his high school days at Hiroshima. Imabari and Hiroshima are both located facing the Inland Sea, which is said to be the Mediterranean Sea in Japan. Being fascinated since his early days by *Le Corbusier, whose works are based on Mediterranean traditions in Europe, Tange entered the Tokyo Imperial University and took architectural courses in the Department of Engineering from 1935 to 1938. Immediately after his graduation, he entered Kunio *Maekawa's architectural office, and later with Maekawa he joined the Japanese Werkbund. While he was working there, he was almost entirely responsible for the planning of the Kishi Memorial Gymnasium. Later, in 1941, he re-entered the Tokyo University and took a post-graduate course. In 1942 he was awarded first prize in a competition for the design of a Far East memorial building sponsored by the Japanese Architectural Institute. A year later he won a prize for the plan of a Japan-Thai cultural centre to be built in Bangkok. However, none of these projects were realized. His first building to be erected was a Pavilion of Local Products for the Kobe Industry and Trade Fair (1950), which was removed after the fair was over.

Page 289 Kenzo Tange. Town Hall of the Kagawa Prefecture, 1958

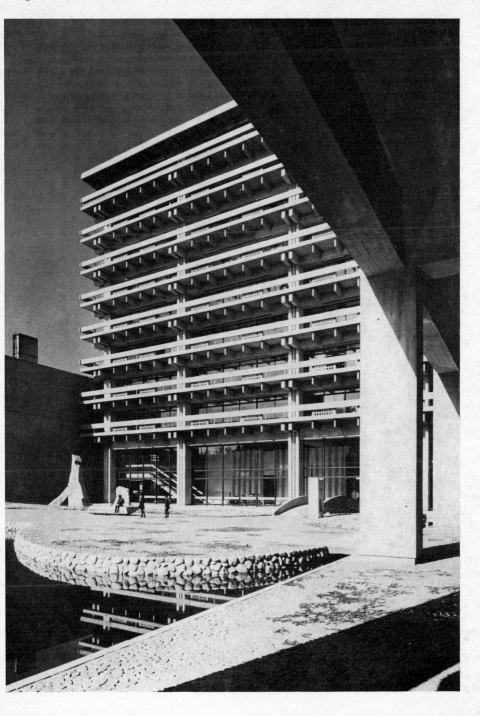

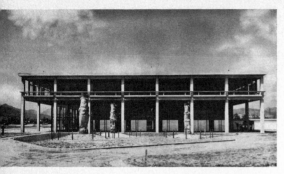

Kenzo Tange. Peace Centre. Hiroshima, 1955–6

From that time Tange's creative talent rapidly increased. He designed the Ehime Convention Hall and his own house in 1954 as well as the Shimizu Town Hall. The Kurayoshi Town Hall was built in 1956, and the Tokyo Metropolitan Government Office was completed in 1957. Other important buildings were the Peace Centre in Hiroshima, a library for children which reveals his originality in space vision, and the small but carefully planned Tsuda College Library in Tokyo.

Tange's aim has always been to integrate Japan's architectural traditions with the needs of modern society, and he sought an answer to this problem through the planning of a series of buildings for local communities; he reached a successful solution in the Kagawa Prefectural Office completed in 1958. The realization of the project owed a great deal to the influential governor, Kaneko, who appreciates Tange's

Kenzo Tange. Town Hall. Shimizu, 1954

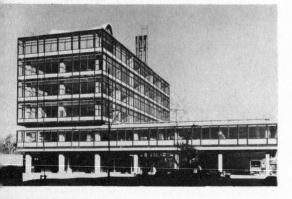

work. The building marks a peak in his career. Versatility and creative power have characterized Tange's work from the time he participated in the prize competition up to the present with his design for the Sogetsu Hall in 1960. If he succeeds in establishing his architectural philosophy on a firmer foundation, he should be one of the leading architects of the future.

He has written an essay on the 'Relation between Regional Planning and Architectural Design in Big Cities', and received his doctor's degree. At present, he is a professor at the Tokyo University and gives lectures on City Planning in the Engineering Department.

Bibliography: Robin Boyd, *Kenzo Tange*, New York 1962.

SHINJI KOIKE

Tatlin, Vladimir E., b. Moscow 1885. Graduated 1910 from Moscow Academy. First Constructivist type of work 1913–15. His design for a memorial to the Third International (1920) was a leaning spiral made of steel and wire and anticipates the buildings and designs of *Constructivism; Tatlin imagined the memorial as a 1,300-ft-high structure with large rooms.

Taut, Bruno, b. Königsberg 1880, d. Ankara 1938. Pupil of Theodor *Fischer. Erected a 'Monument of Steel' at the Leipzig Building Exhibition of 1913, and a glass pavilion at the 1914 Cologne Exhibition, which demonstrated in a most imaginative way the potentialities of *glass as a building material. During the First World War produced designs for Utopian *Alpine Architecture* (published Hagen 1919). Worked as City Architect at Magdeburg. Housing estates in Berlin in the *International Style. Taut went to Moscow in 1932, to Japan in 1933, and to Istanbul in 1936.

Bibliography: Bruno Taut, *Die neue Baukunst,* Berlin 1929; Bruno Taut, *Frühlicht,* ed. U. Conrads, Frankfurt and Vienna 1962; U. Kultermann, *Die Gläserne Kette,* Leverkusen 1963.

Taut, Max, b. Königsberg 1884. Private practice since 1911. Schools, housing and office buildings (in particular for trade unions; headquarters for the German Printers' Union, Berlin, 1928); 1945–53 Professor, Berlin College of Fine Arts.

Tecton. Architectural team founded in 1931 by Berthold Lubetkin, with Anthony Chitty, Lindsey Drake, Michael Dugdale, Val Harding, Godfrey Samuel and Francis Skinner. Later Denys Lasdun was a member for a short time. Highpoint Flats, Highgate (1933), Finsbury Health Centre, London (1938). The work of this group received popular recognition with their buildings for the London Zoo, in which *reinforced concrete was used in an imaginative way.

Telford, Thomas, b. Westerkirk, Dumfriesshire 1757, d. London 1834. Scottish architect and engineer. Stone buildings with large areas punctuated by projecting planes, not by ornaments, with Romanesque touches (St Catharine's Dock, 1824–8). Bold designs for bridges making use of cast iron (design for a Thames bridge, London, 1801; Conway Castle Bridge, 1822–6).

Terragni, Giuseppe, b. Meda near Milan 1904, d. Como 1942. Terragni is one of the most complex and at the same time most consistent figures of the early modern movement in Italy. His work covers a period of only thirteen years, from his graduation in Milan in 1926 to the time of his call-up in 1939. He fought on the Greek and Russian fronts, was repatriated to Italy, and died of the after-effects of exhaustion in January 1942. In this short span he was responsible for some of the most significant buildings produced during the period, beset with so many difficulties and reverses, that brought Italian architecture from its neoclassical and eclectic backwaters to join the mainstream of the modern European style.

Terragni originally adhered to the *Novecento Italiano* group, which set out on a rationalist basis to restore plastic values and a sense of volume to modern architecture, in opposition to the new *International Style, which depended for effect on the manipulation of surfaces. In 1926 he helped to found the *Movimento Italiano per l'Architettura Razionale*, which unleashed the whole weight of the academic opposition against the young members of *gruppo 7* (Terragni, *Figini, *Pollini, Frette, Larco, Rava and Libera); he kept up the lively controversy which ensued to the very end of his life, writing his last article from the Russian front. The debate was a difficult and bitter one, since the protagonists on both sides were Fascists, consequently the movement's ideology ended in an impasse of opinions, tastes and interests.

Terragni's best arguments were his buildings, however. His first design to be carried out was a block of flats at Como (1927), called Novecomum, a typically 'novecentist' design which caused a considerable stir. A series of shops and interior decoration schemes followed, with various contributions to the Monza Biennali and the 1933 Milan Triennale. In 1932 he designed a hall for the Exhibition of the Fascist Revolution in Rome. In the same year he drew up plans for the Casa del Fascio at Como (completed in 1936), which remains the purest and most interesting monument of the *Novecento Italiano*, standing as it does on the verge of *Functionalism. The building is a cube devoid of any movement or ornament, in which solids and voids, by virtue of the violent contrasts they afford of light and shade, create a dramatically punctuated architectural dialogue. This austere and interesting building is the only

Giuseppe Terragni. Novecomum. Como, 1927

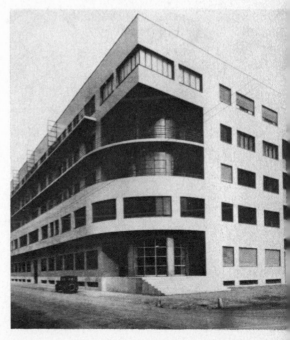

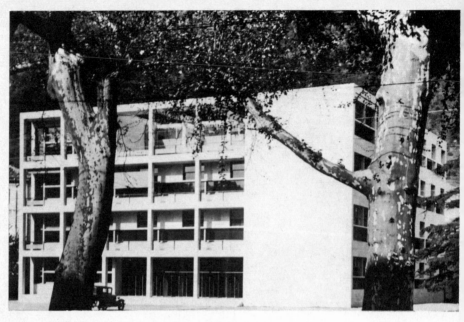

Giuseppe Terragni. Casa del Fascio. Como, 1936

one to have conferred a European validity on that typically Italian phenomenon, the *Novecento*. It was denounced however by Giuseppe Pagano in the pages of *Casabella* as an example of '17th-century affectation applied to Functionalism', since he feared that the younger generation of Italian architects might be diverted by it from their true objectives.

In his next work, however, a kindergarten at Como (1937), Terragni abandoned the *Novecento* line to create, within the framework of European Functionalism, the most elegant and lucid of his projects. Three houses dating from the same year (Villa Bianca at Seveso, Villa Bianchi at Rebbio and the Casa Pedraglio at Como) restate the problem in strictly geometrical terms, while pointing somehow to a specifically 'spatial' type of solution. With his last important work, the Casa Frigerio at Como (1939), the volumetric cube is broken up, although a freely articulated plan is not achieved. Among his other works may be mentioned four houses in Milan (1935–6, in collaboration with Pietro Lingeri) and the Casa del Fascio at Lissone (1939, with Carminati).

Terragni left behind him a large number of architectural and town-planning schemes; also a collection of controversial writings which reveal that intellectual honesty and sensitivity which led him, on the eve of his death, to renounce his great political error in despair.

Bibliography: Giuseppe Pagano, 'Tre anni di architettura in Italia', in *Casabella*, February 1937; Mario Labò, *Giuseppe Terragni*, Milan 1947; Attilio Podestà, 'Omaggio a Terragni' in *Emporium*, Vol. CVII, No. 640, April 1948; Giulia Veronesi, *Difficoltà politiche dell'architettura in Italia, 1920–1940*, Milan 1953.

GIULIA VERONESI

Torroja, Eduardo, b. Madrid 1899, d. 1961. Studied civil engineering in Madrid. He was director of the Instituto Técnico de la Construcción y del Cemento, and an honorary doctor of numerous universities.

Torroja belongs to the great creators of architectural form in the 20th century. As his many works built in Europe, Africa and America strikingly demonstrate, he possessed great imaginative powers, capable of stating surprising problems and devising unexpected solutions for them, together with an immense technical capacity for solving these problems and actually carrying out the solutions. His views may be found in essence in his book *Philosophy of Structures*, where we see how different he is from the usual mathematical type of engineer when he asserts from the outset the rights of the imagination and declares that calculations only serve to show whether what has been imagined will stand.

According to Torroja, there are three classes of structure: those which serve to contain a volume, those which carry loads and those which resist thrusts. The architectural problem centres round his system of four equations with four unknowns. The equations are those of ultimate purpose, static function, aesthetic qualities and economic conditions. The unknowns are the materials, the structural types, the critical shapes and sizes and the actual building process. In determining structural types, Torroja started by considering the conditions of stress. The networks set up by the systems of stress, namely the

lines of tension and compression, allowed him to emphasize the way each form works. As regards materials, recognizing the truth of *Wright's assertion that each one of them speaks its own language, he concentrated on exploiting the great properties of reinforced and pre-stressed concrete, which was his favourite means of expression.

In considering the question of aesthetic expression, Torroja believed that truth alone was not enough and that a psychological factor in the material supervened which might lead to the possibility of structural jests, surprising absurdities and a gratuitous playfulness. Notwithstanding this, he considered simplicity a virtue. In regard to the architectural forms of his times, he used to speak with a certain sadness about materialism, and about those who disclaim nature on anti-romantic grounds while assigning excessive value to rhythm. He accepted an essentially baroque principle in maintaining the idea that the eye is deceptive, and in preferring psychological phenomena to material reality. Although regular geometrical forms exist

Eduardo Torroja. Grandstand at Zarzuela race track, near Madrid, 1935

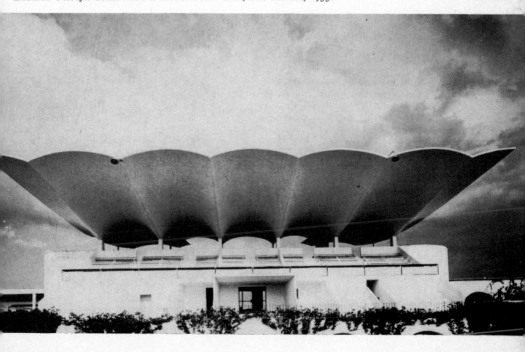

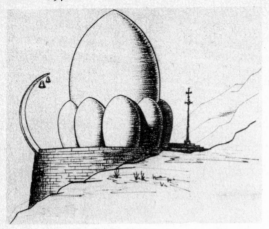

Eduardo Torroja. Church of the Ascension.
Xerralló, 1952. Sketch

1942; in the following year, the great roof over the entrance to the Campo de Les Corts in Barcelona, with its sinuous outline, is the first of Torroja's major works to feature organic asymmetry; its final flowering is to be seen at the Táchira Club at Caraças (1957).

Torroja's churches at Xerralló, Sant Esperit and Pont de Suert (1952) are the first examples of modern religious art to be found south of the Pyrenees since the Civil War.

Bibliography: Eduardo Torroja, *Philosophy of Structures*, California 1958; Eduardo Torroja, *The Structures of Eduardo Torroja*, New York 1958; Fernando Cassinello, 'Eduardo Torroja' in *Cuadernos de Arquitectura*, Barcelona 1961; Eduardo Torroja, *Logik der Form*, Munich 1961.

ALEXANDRE CIRICI-PELLICER

in some of his works, such as the twelve-sided concrete coal bunker he built for the Instituto Técnico de la Construcción y del Cemento (Madrid, 1951), most of his designs employ folded, undulating or warped shapes.

In 1928, *Freyssinet took out the first patent for pre-stressed concrete. A year later, Torroja was using it for the Tempul bridge, where the longitudinal girders were pre-stressed. His ribless roof for Algeciras Market Hall (1933) was Torroja's response to the ribwork of Basle Market Hall (1929). For the Zarzuela race track near Madrid in 1935 he designed a system of fluted grandstand roofs with a very extensive cantilever, counterbalanced by vertical tie rods behind the stanchions. In the same year he built the shell roof of the Frontón Recoletos, whose form derives from the penetration of two barrel vaults of different dimensions running parallel to each other. The hyperboloid form of a reservoir for Madrid (1936) was the forerunner of the great hyperboloid dome of the water tower at Fedala, Morocco (1956).

Torroja's Aldoz aqueduct (1939), with X-shaped pipeline supports, broke new ground in this type of structure. His Martín Gil bridge over the Esla (1940) with its 623-foot span, broke the world record for a single arch. It is currently (1963) the third largest in the world in absolute span, and the second largest railway bridge. The Torrejón de Ardoz hangars, with their structural panache, were completed in

Town planning is the preconcerted disposition of urban living-space. Already in the tight society in the years prior to 1800, consideration was given to the building of cities in a manner which could be termed planning. The planned layout of a town, however, was such a self-evident part of government that any special discipline concerned with the technical or economic questions of town layout or planning was simply not referred to.

Even the distinction between towns that have grown and those that have been planned was only invented by art historians of the last century, attempting to demonstrate, for some of the historical towns at least, an ideal conception of their time, 'growth from the free interplay of forces'. Ungeometrical towns were said to have 'grown', in contrast to those with geometrical shapes. Today, however, we know that towns of both basic shapes, regular and irregular, have been planned at some time or other, and that an act of foundation preceded the existence of each town. Most town extensions, too, were planned or comprised in an overall scheme. The common interest of all citizens in effective defence by a system of fortifications made it necessary to conform to a plan.

For a long time the irregularly shaped town was thought to represent an earlier stage of development, the regular shape a later one. No single form, however, has exclusively prevailed at any time. Aristotle, who summarized the whole scientific knowledge of antiquity and remained a supreme authority throughout the Middle Ages, declared that both methods had their advantages and disadvantages, and both might be used according to local conditions. The irregular shape is said to be the more economical one. The necessity for defence and the prevalence of emotional tendencies certainly led to a predominance of ungeometric shapes in the early periods of town development, while the rational and economic tendencies of later epochs displayed a preference for geometric formations. Changes in society have also played their part in the differentiation of town shapes.

After 1800, the last effective possibility of controlling town growth in Central Europe was lost. With the removal of fortifications and quick growth due to increased prosperity as a consequence of industrialization, cities spread rapidly along their main arteries, beyond their former limits. Property speculators provided hastily erected tenement houses, badly lighted and cramped, for the mass of people streaming into the towns from the country. Building by-laws which permitted a shameless exploitation of people and sites left their mark on the appearance of these districts. The grid-type layouts of the surveyors, the unvaried street widths and heights, and the squares dotted here and there without rhyme or reason, were meant to be neutral, so as to avoid obstructing the action of economic forces. The fate of the town was thus left to chance and speculation, and it grew in unconnected single phases.

Around the year 1900, movements for social reform attempted to remedy the poor living conditions of the towns (E. *Howard, H. George, Damaschke, Fritsch, Eberstadt and others). The science of town planning was gradually developed; with the foundation of town planning associations the recognition emerged that town and country must complement each other and be subjected to a common plan (Unwin, Schumacher). Traffic considerations came first, closely followed by economic factors. For a time, living conditions occupied the focus of attention, then politico-sociological aspects of the town and finally the demand for green belts and landscaping. Only a team consisting of every kind of specialist (mining engineers, surveyors, architects, economists, sociologists, doctors, lawyers

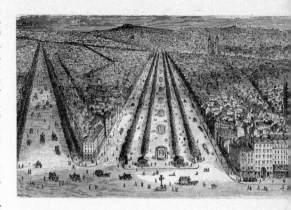

Georges-Eugène Haussmann. Boulevard Richard-Lenoir. Paris, 1861–3. Remedial measures are confined to cutting new streets through

and landscape architects) is in a position to grasp such a complex problem as the town of today, and to work out a plan that does justice to all these aspects of development. Academies and associations such as *CIAM (with its *Athens Charter) drew up minimum requirements and optimum conditions for the renewal or reconstruction of cities. A recognition of the basic needs a town has to provide for (work, living, traffic, leisure) and their correct coordination with each other was a start. Minimum health requirements for sunshine, daylight, dust and noise abatement, green belts and open spaces, were formulated. The subdivision of the town into organic units with service centres featuring schools, churches, cultural buildings and shops, separated from other such units by belts of parkland, became a further instrument of urban design. In this conjunction the problem arose of how to ensure the best use of city sites. City centres needed thinning out, while denser development was called for on the peripheries; hence internationally valid specifications for optimum land use were involved.

The 'floorspace index' represents the ratio of the total floor area of a building to the area of its site, and may vary from 2.0 to approximately 0.2 in areas with main services (highest in business areas; City of London currently 6.3!). These rules have become necessary not only to ensure sufficient ventilation, sunshine, daylight and parkland; they are an essential consequence of the ever-increasing density of traffic. For volume of building and volume of traffic are interrelated: by reducing the volume of building, a reduction of traffic density can be achieved. A floor-space index of 1.0, which may be regarded as the upper limit for purely residential areas, corresponds to a population density of 200 inhabitants per net acre, and a building density of about 60 dwelling units per acre, while the cities of Central Europe have maximum population densities of 400 an acre.

In urban residential districts supplied with main services, FSI 0.2 should not be exceeded (giving a plot area of about 360 square yards) as otherwise the town spreads out uneconomically. No type of development is more expensive than the type of 'suburban sprawl' generally encountered today, with detached private houses on 1,200 square yard plots. While it is essential to thin out the unsanitary and overcrowded tenements that often survive in central zones, a denser development of the outlying suburbs is currently aimed at by planners. By adjusting both extremes, towns with an average FSI of 0.4 would not have to extend beyond the present boundaries of their built-up areas. In Berlin, the most densely populated district of Kreuzberg has 480 dwelling units per acre, while that of Zehlendorf has only 5. If the regulations for distances between buildings and the restrictions on density are adhered to, the problem of correct orientation for blocks of flats or rows of houses is no longer a difficult one. The most favourable disposition in the British Isles is without doubt a south-west aspect, but others are also possible and have advantages for certain occupations or members of the family. One thing must however be avoided, living-rooms facing north!

The type of building presents another problem, whether multi-storey, medium-high or low. Where no specific housing tradition prevails, as it does in countries such as England, the United States and Holland where low structures are the general rule, the type of building to be erected is determined by considerations of profitability to the landlord and ease of running. Sociological and biological factors

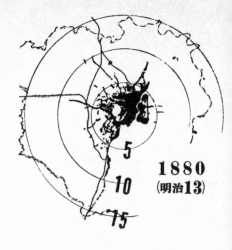

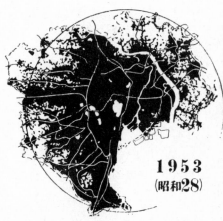

Area of Tokio in 1880 and 1953. An increase in radius from 5 to over 15 km.

should, however, be the criterion. Low buildings are usually better for people with children and dependents who feel united as a family. Multi-storey blocks of flats are more suitable for childless couples, unmarried people and families whose jobs require them to move about. The medium-high building has become almost meaningless, and simply serves to make the supply of accommodation of various types appear the more diverse. In cities and metropolitan areas, the number of people requiring flats in multi-storey blocks may be estimated at 20–30 per cent, naturally higher than in medium-sized towns (5–20 per cent). In small towns the demand goes down virtually to zero, corresponding to the considerably larger number of people living in families. The method previously used of classification according to social strata and equivalent types of accommodation has all the disadvantages of a monolithic social system. Within a neighbourhood unit—preferably in a group of about 100 dwellings—every type of professional and family combination on the social scale should be included.

In the last century, industries were sited in the immediate neighbourhood of residential districts, as had been the custom of the old craft manufactories. It was not due to the resultant inconvenience but to the lack of space for extension that factories were moved to the outskirts and into industrial districts. With the introduction of electrical power, dust-extraction plants, and the sub-division of industry into smaller factory units, partial decentralization of industry becomes possible: either in the shape of small industrial plants attached to the neighbourhood units or by transference to the country. Only heavy industry, complex processes and offensive trades are tied to actual industrial districts. For the rest, industry can become the most flexible unit in the town, as its buildings usually have to be replaced after ten to twenty years.

Town planning measures are most easily realized nowadays in matters of traffic engineering, which everybody can understand. In the last thirty years enormous sums have been spent in the United States on the provision of highway facilities, but without remarkable success. The lesson to be learnt from this by European town planners is the need to avoid excess traffic by advance planning, thinning out congested areas and redirecting traffic sources and their destinations. Journeys to and from work make up 60–70 per cent of all the traffic in a town. Consideration of how living and working zones might be related to each other, and how change of workplace and removal from home could be coupled, is of such significance that it cannot be rejected by references to individual liberty. Shopping, school and leisure

J. H. van den Broek and Jacob B. Bakema. The Lijnbaan pedestrian street. Rotterdam, 1953

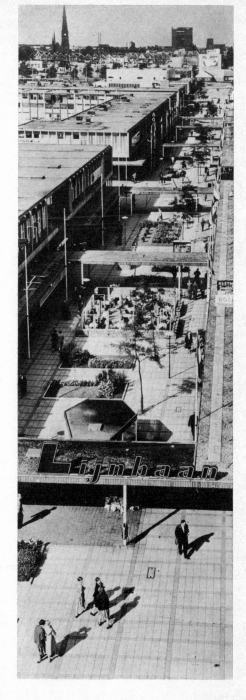

journeys can be reduced by planning (gardens surrounding houses, parks accessible on foot, shopping centres, schools and cultural facilities within the district). What essential traffic remains should be directed via differentiated lanes (motorway to residential street) so that its main stream makes contact with the town according to its nature. The town itself should be divided into traffic-free precincts, in which only pedestrians, cyclists and emergency traffic (doctors, police) are permitted. On the edge of the pedestrian precincts there should be adequate parking facilities.

Parks as recreational areas in the centre of a town have only been called for in our own times. It is the town planner's task today to link up incidental open spaces such as parks, cemeteries, the areas between buildings, allotments, sports grounds, and rivers and lakes with their banks into an interconnected green network. Like the traffic network, the green network should pass through each district so that each part of a town, and the countryside also, may be reached on foot via one of these links. These green belts should contain all secondary schools, sports facilities and baths, and any woodland in the town. Apart from them there are the green areas inside the individual districts, which accommodate playgrounds, primary schools and nursery schools. These constitute the actual centre of the district.

The vast extension in the size of towns means that the city centre forfeits its vitality. Hence the city must be decentralized, i.e., on the one hand it must be afforded increased ground space to accommodate ever-growing public and private services; on the other hand, all functions which have no definite central character can be moved into the suburbs. Satellites or New Towns are built to relieve the city's burden.

In Great Britain the New Town Act of 1946 provided for the development of a series of townships, each with populations of between 30,000 and 50,000. Apart from the usual apparatus of civic amenities, each town was designed to attract its own

Stockholm City Planning Office; Chief Architect: Sven Markelius. Satellite town of Vällingby, near Stockholm, commenced 1953. Site plan

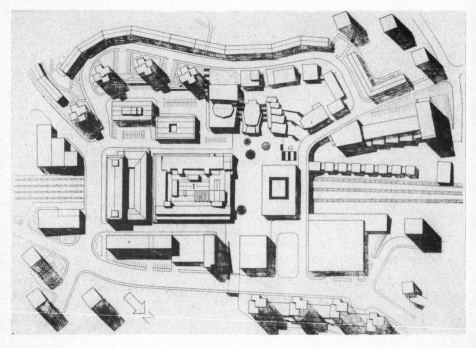

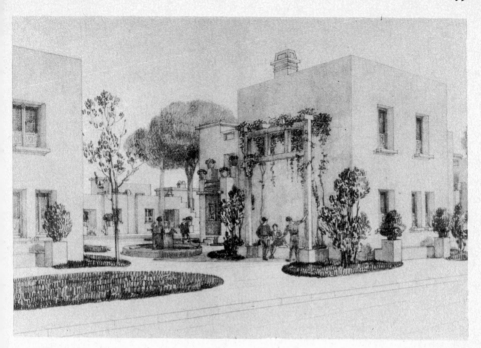

Tony Garnier. Residential district. Cité Industrielle. 1901–4. Project

industries of various types, to prevent it from lapsing into a mere dormitory. Projects include Basildon, Stevenage, Harlow (chief planner: F. Gibberd), Hatfield (L. Brett), Peterlee, Newton Aycliffe and Corby in England; East Kilbride and Glenrothes in Scotland; and Cwmbran in South Wales. The standard of achievement, varies, but the more successful express considerable urban distinction. Their example, and the progressive legislation which underlies them, have inspired other countries, Scandinavia in particular. Germany, too, has recently built a number of satellite towns in the neighbourhood of the larger cities.

A comprehensive advance in planning law is marked by the 1947 Town Planning Act, which lays an obligation on all planning authorities in Great Britain to produce a plan for their areas. This has given a great impetus to town planning practice, since many local authorities have had to set up planning departments for the first time. The development plans they are expected to work out, are based on a simple form of comprehensive survey, showing the future policy of land use in each area, and indicating where development or redevelopment is expected to take place; these plans are reviewed at five-yearly intervals. In addition, the 1947 Act provides for the safeguarding of trees and woodlands and the protection of buildings of historic interest, which it requires to be listed; it also embodies powers for the control of outdoor advertising.

Subsequent legislation includes the 1951 New Streets Act, which ensures that private developers do not leave their highways unadopted, and the 1952 Town Development Act, designed to facilitate the planned expansion of towns chosen to receive overspill populations.

Many schemes for the comprehensive redevelopment of central areas have been drawn up in recent years, frequently in collaboration with property companies.

Bibliography: Lewis Mumford, *The Culture of Cities*, New York 1938; Roland

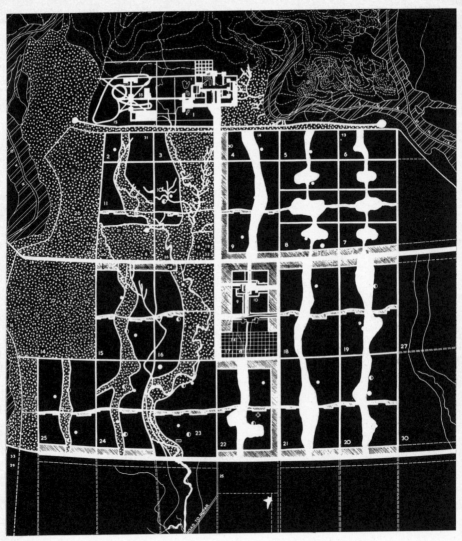

Le Corbusier. Chandigarh, commenced 1950. Site plan

Rainer, *Städtebau und Wohnkultur*, Tübingen 1948; Frederick Gibberd, *Town Design*, London 1953; 4th edition 1962; Hans Bernhard Reichow, *Die autogerechte Stadt*, Ravensburg 1959; Fritz Jaspert, *Vom Städtebau der Welt*, Berlin 1961; Gordon Cullen, *Townscape*, London 1962.

HUBERT HOFFMANN

Townscape. Concept evolved in the late forties by analysing examples of consciously or unconsciously successful town design in terms of the progressive revelation of space and function to the moving spectator; influenced in part by the theories of English 18th-century landscape architects, which are transferred to an urban setting.

Invaluable discipline for the appreciation of historic towns, and the application of the lessons so learnt to the design of new ones.

Bibliography: Gordon Cullen, *Townscape.* London 1961.

HAROLD MEEK

Urbanism. *Town Planning.

USA. American architecture was for a long period an outpost of the European mainstream. During the colonial era (17th and 18th centuries) the styles were scarcely more than echoes of British practice at the same moment. With the coming of the Revolution, the influence of France became momentarily predominant. Then, for the first three-quarters of the 19th century, building developments in the United States followed the pace established both by British and French designers. The classical and Gothic revivals were succeeded by those mid-century Victorian fashions that were championed by Ruskin, Eastlake, *Morris and other writers, while Parisian influences in the guise of the Second Empire style were equally pervasive.

While it would be an exaggeration to maintain that American architecture had attained independence as well as maturity by the time of the Philadelphia Centennial Exposition of 1876, the date can be taken as symbolic of a new turn. At this juncture, American artists became aware of the unique character of their own colonial past, and, while in the process of making this discovery, they came under the influence of the new English taste for vernacular post-medieval styles, a revival movement that is generally if not especially accurately referred to as the Queen Anne. These two phenomena, in effect complementary manifestations of the same late 19th-century eclectic development, were present in varying degrees in the work of the three major American architects of the period, Henry Hobson *Richardson, Louis *Sullivan, and Frank Lloyd *Wright. Wright not only played a major creative rôle in the domestic architecture of the 1890s, but continued in both a creative and patriarchal capacity to mould and influence architecture in America and in Europe well past the middle of the 20th century.

It is conceivable that Richardson was the first architect of the post-Renaissance period to whom the word 'genius' is not inappropriate. In his ponderous, taciturn style were united the moralistic, revivalistic and rational principles of diverse earlier tendencies. However, above and beyond its manifold sources, the personal style of Richardson is remarkably fused, and the inner conflicts latent in its origins are so reconciled and submerged that it is eclectic and revivalistic only in methodology. In actuality these robust masonry or wood shingle forms are among the most disciplined and unified creations of the last century. It was the example of Richardson that helped to clarify the somewhat less certain taste of Louis Sullivan, who had been at first inspired by a Victorian architect of almost grotesque power, Frank *Furness, and only subsequently by the new technology of the steel-framed tall office building, which was invented and popularized in Chicago in the 1880s, a rational type of design that is identified by the sobriquet *'Chicago School'. Sullivan's most striking accomplishments of the 1890s in commercial architecture were echoed in the perceptive if less elegant skyscraper designs of Daniel H. *Burnham and John W. *Root, whether in the dense masonry structure of the Monadnock Building (1891) or in the expressive steel-framed Reliance Building (1890–4), a glazed thirteen-storey shaft. In contrast to these striking manifestations of commercial efficiency in a materialistic era, the early tall office buildings in New York were less boldly simplified in aspect, though their greater attention to variety of detail, as in Richard Morris Hunt's Tribune Building, New York (1873–5), was more original than is generally realized.

Frank Lloyd Wright is the third and most spectacular of this triumvirate in American architecture. An assistant of Louis Sullivan until he established his own practice in 1893, Wright subsequently devoted most of his efforts to domestic architecture, and if his position long went largely unrecognized in the USA—although his work always earned a degree of respect and admiration, if usually qualified in tone— the brilliant spatial inventions of his suburban Chicago houses of the period 1893–1909, culminating in the Robie House of 1909, were of immeasurable influence in Europe. These works were published and exhibited in Germany in 1910–11, and to

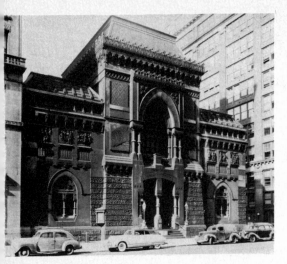

Frank Furness. Pennsylvania Academy of Fine Arts. Philadelphia, 1872–6

Louis H. Sullivan. Auditorium Building. Chicago, 1886–9

judge from the works of the masters of the *International Style, together with their subsequent testimony, they had a tremendous impact. Wright's domestic architecture of 1900 was complemented by the work of others in his immediate circle, and his principles were echoed on the west coast in the domestic work of Charles and Henry *Greene, notably the Gamble House, Pasadena (1908–9), in which seemingly exotic oriental elements are successfully blended with an indigenous offshoot of the Queen Anne known as the 'Shingle Style', a mode originally popularized by Richardson. A similar independence was manifested by Bernard R. *Maybeck in his Christian Science Church, Berkeley (1910), in which a concrete structure is enriched by provocative medievalizing timber details. Equally picturesque effects, but in an academic, indeed, Imperial Roman garb, were produced by Maybeck in his Fine Arts Building for the 1915 San Francisco Exhibition, a temporary structure in pink stucco that still stands, albeit in a ruinous state.

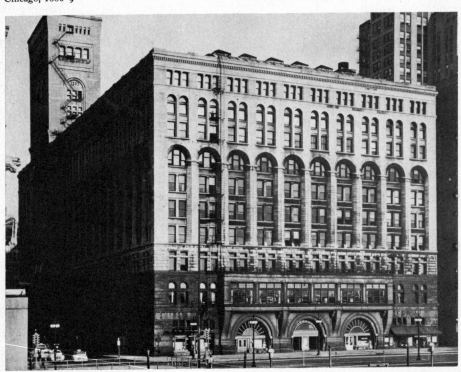

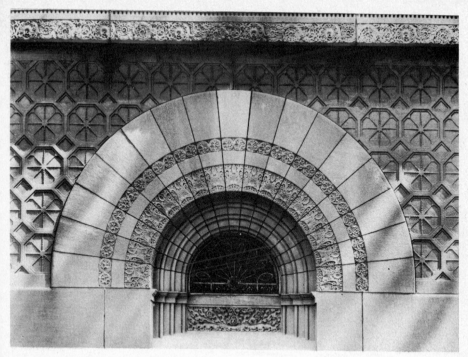

Louis H. Sullivan Getty Tomb. Chicago, 1890

The taste which stands behind the general style if not the personal feeling expressed in Maybeck's Fine Arts Building had earlier been crystallized at the World's Columbian Exposition, Chicago (1893), where a group of architects led by the fashionable academic firm of McKim, Mead and White (who had begun as disciples of Richardson) produced the famous 'White City' of Imperial Classicism in plaster and lath. Largely if not completely divorced from this *beaux-arts* design discipline was Sullivan's Transportation Building, with its intricately detailed round-arched portal which was admired by European if not by American visitors.

With this unmistakable 'revolution' in favour of the classical modes, which in a decade spread across the country, Sullivan and other independent-minded architects gradually lost contact with what seemed at the time to be the main stream of modern architectural design, a main stream which

produced buildings such as the Pennsylvania Station, New York (1906–10), by McKim, Mead and White, which was not only stylistically neoclassical but went so far as to seek identity with a distant past through the imitation of certain portions of a typical Roman bath. Such accomplishments almost totally eclipsed for the moment the works of Sullivan's old age, such as the National Farmers Bank, Owatona, Minnesota (1907–8). Here the block-like design cut with a massive round arch bears analogies not so much to the current academic fashion, as to the earlier idiom of Richardson. Sullivan's work of this period is in effect a vital, organic outgrowth of the late-19th-century traditions, whereas that of McKim, Mead and White is a largely sterile, even if scholarly, product of the same tradition.

If Wright, the Greene brothers, Maybeck and a few others clearly belong to an independent movement in architecture around 1900, along with Sullivan, the same

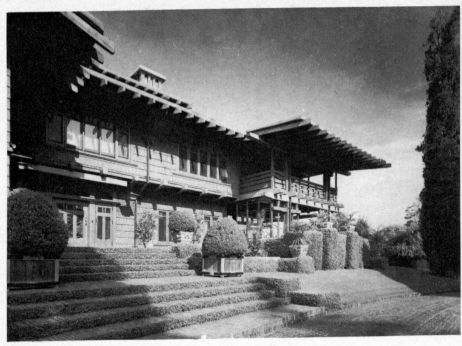

Charles and Henry Greene. Gamble House, Pasadena, 1908–9

cannot be said for a host of other interesting architects active during the first two or three decades of the 20th century in the USA. Among the domestic specialists of the period, few seem in retrospect to have been so able and craftsmanlike as the Philadelphia firm of Mellor, Meigs and Howe. Their abilities to produce a bland if arcane eclecticism are amply illustrated in the house of 1914 at Chesnut Hill, Pennsylvania, built for George *Howe, the junior member of the firm, who was later to reject this tentative style for a more forthright modernism.

Monumental architecture at this epoch is represented by Cass Gilbert's (1859–1934) Gothic skyscraper, the Woolworth Building, New York (1913); Bertram Grosvenor Goodhue's (1869–1924) tentatively 'modernistic' Nebraska State Capitol and Los Angeles Public Library of the 1920s, in which the departing spirit of 19th-century eclecticism makes one last effort to survive in a provocative compromise form; or in James Gamble Rodgers's (1867–1947)

numerous designs for Yale University, beginning in 1917, which depend for their sense of medieval authenticity upon a particularly luxuriant texture and carefully studied detailing. The classical tradition was maintained by Henry Bacon's (1866–1924) Lincoln Memorial, Washington (1914–22), and by John Russell Pope's (1874–1937) National Gallery of Art, Washington (1937), both extraordinarily pure revisions of the academic formula. Most of these able designers were nearly exact contemporaries of Wright, and it is therefore all the more interesting to compare the latter's idiosyncratically monumental Hollyhock House, Los Angeles (1920), with the more customary monumentalism of the others. Another contemporary of Wright, Albert *Kahn, had a rather different contribution to make to the growth of recent American architecture. From the first decade of the century his vast organization specialized in large-scale industrial work, and continued the process of developing the large office which had been inaugurated by the academically inclined firms of the 1880s and 1890s.

However, the work of the 1920s in the USA, curious and interesting as it is, completely lacks the forthright intensity of the new architecture that was then emerging in Europe. Indeed, the work of Wright at this time, even when viewed in the context of the more traditionally oriented buildings of the day, was less acutely creative than at an early or at a later period. But already there were signs that this era of somnolence was not destined to last. In 1923 the Finnish architect, Eliel *Saarinen, settled in America, representing the vanguard of a coming wave of distinguished European émigrés. While his work never quite fulfilled the promise of his earliest endeavours in Finland, and instead appears tentative in style if forthright in its programmatic solutions, a rather different and more unmistakable contemporaneity was to be found in the designs of Rudolph *Schindler and Richard *Neutra, two architects of Viennese origin whose particular dispositions were influenced by such disparate stimuli as Otto *Wagner, Adolf *Loos, and Frank Lloyd Wright. The houses built first by Schindler and, subsequently, by Neutra in and around Los Angeles, were the very earliest manifestations in the USA of the technique and taste that were later identified as the *International Style. The clear, unmistakably pure character of their works demonstrated that the tentative modernism of a Goodhue or an Eliel Saarinen would become outmoded along with the more literal sort of historicism as soon as the new architecture had spread.

The speed with which the new ideas and motifs took hold can be illustrated in the transformation of Raymond *Hood's widely admired skyscraper designs, which changed from a neo-Gothic mode in the Chicago Tribune (1923, with John Mead Howells, b. 1868), to a simplified abstract mode which is, albeit superficially, both functional and futurist, in the New York Daily News Buildings (1930). A much more profound essay in 'Skyscraper International' was the tower of the Philadelphia Savings Fund Society by George Howe and William *Lescaze of 1932, whose expression of vertical structural members on one side is set in contrast to the horizontal expression of cantilevers on

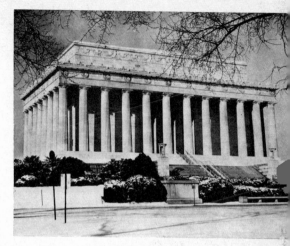

Henry Bacon. Lincoln Memorial. Washington, 1914–22

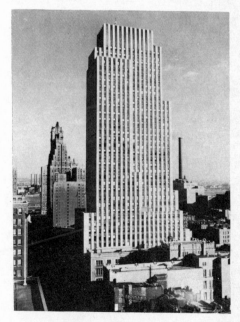

Raymond M. Hood. Daily News Building. New York, 1930

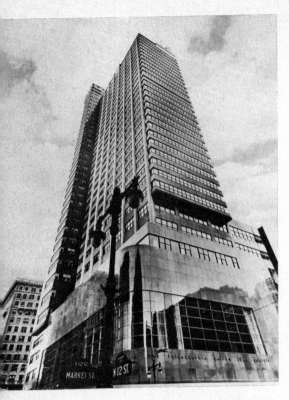

William Lescaze and George Howe. Philadelphia Savings Fund Society Building. Philadelphia, 1932

another. Such integral relationships between the frame of the building and its surface is analogous to the practice of the earlier Chicago School, although the formal vocabulary conforms with the new European fashion. This unusually frank design is in distinct contrast with the tallest of all tall office buildings, the Empire State Building, New York, by Shreve, Lamb and Harmon (1930–2), which manages to be 'traditional' without being recognizably revivalistic in style.

The 1930s were marked by two events which had the dual effect of releasing contemporary American architecture from the predominantly tentative statements of modernism, and of forming the basis from which the post-Second World War leadership of the USA in the development of world architecture would suddenly grow. The first of these was the renaissance of

Frank Lloyd Wright (no other word will suffice), which reached an initial climax in the Kaufmann House, Falling Water (1936), a building in which the organic, naturalistic features inherent in Wright's design philosophy were reconciled with the machine-like clarity characteristic of the European modern movement. Seconding this noteworthy achievement in the re-integration and development of 20th-century American architecture was the arrival in the USA of several of the chief mentors of the International Style itself: Walter *Gropius and *Mies van der Rohe were joined by others of more Expressionist leanings like Erich *Mendelsohn or by their younger disciples such as Marcel *Breuer. Gropius continued his rôle as an educator which he had begun in the *Bauhaus by taking charge of the Architectural School at Harvard, while Mies assumed a similar rôle at the Illinois Institute of Technology, Chicago. Both contributed to the development of American modernism at this juncture with distinctive and influential buildings. Mies's master plan for the new campus of IIT, perfected in 1940, did not exert a great influence for perhaps a decade, and then, suddenly, its cool, pristine, stately geometry became the paragon of new architecture in the 1950s. More immediately influential were a series of houses designed by Gropius in collaboration with Breuer in the neighbourhood of Boston, Mass. in the late 1930s and early 1940s, houses in which the severe geometry of the International Style was tempered and transformed by the native wood-frame traditions of New England domestic architecture.

This transplanted style quickly evolved in the direction of something more organic and romantic in the post-1945 houses of Breuer, and was in fact anticipated in the domestic architecture of the Western States, generally known as the Bay Region Style. The restrained manner of William W. *Wurster and the more personal styles of Hartwell Hamilton Harris and John Yeon represented, throughout the 1940s, one of the most vigorous schools of domestic architecture; it remains far more memorable than the much publicized Scandinavian 'New Empiricism' of the same epoch. However, few works of this group were quite so remarkable as developments of the fluent, interlocking spatial

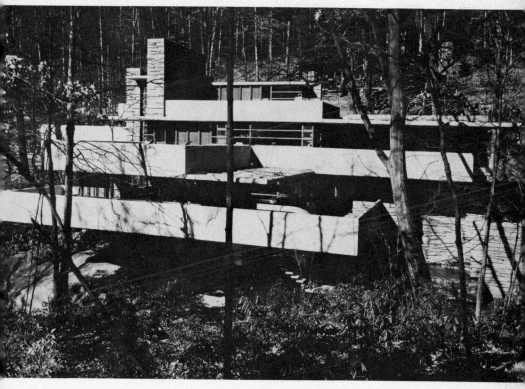

Frank Lloyd Wright. Kaufmann House, 'Falling Water'. Bear Run, Pa., 1936

schemes of the International Style as were the southern California villas of Richard Neutra that date from the late 1940s. At the same period there are other more novel developments in domestic architecture that are due to Frank Lloyd Wright, whose second house for Herbert Jacobs, Middleton, Wis. (1948), is, in its fortress-like, primitive character, an extraordinary reaction against the openness and sophisticated modernism of Neutra's contemporary dwellings. Indeed, in many of his more monumental designs of the 1940s and 1950s Wright seems to be continuing and reinterpreting the massive and closed 19th-century forms of Richardson and Sullivan, giving them a new contemporary relevance rather than merely 'reviving' them.

Other characteristics of this varied and formative period can be seen in two academic buildings in Cambridge, Mass.:

Alvar *Aalto's Dormitory for the Massachusetts Institute of Technology (1948) and Walter Gropius's Harvard Graduate Center of 1950. The former, a tawny brick serpentine slab, represents the continued growth of the romantic, empirical strain (as opposed to the more provocative personal mode of Wright) in American architecture. On the other hand, the layout and elevations of the Harvard Graduate Center are dependent upon the tradition of purged and simplified geometry that was earlier realized in the Bauhaus itself, but with one important difference: the contrasts between the shapes and locations of the various elements are less harsh and bold. Each of these buildings illustrates in its own way an aspect of 20th-century modernism that was on the wane in the late 1940s.

The immediate future was destined to be predicated upon two much more simple and intellectual domestic designs of the period: Mies van der Rohe's Farnsworth House (1946–51) and Philip *Johnson's Glass House, New Canaan, Connecticut (1947–9). In many respects the spatial and planning techniques of these two highly specialized dwellings are dependent upon a half-century of the machine aesthetic, and as such are outgrowths, if not ultimate manifestations, of the International Style. However, the reduction and simplicity of the cubic form, and the crystalline uniformity of the enclosing glass introduces a degree of regularity in both houses that is in contrast to the more diverse and irregular shaping and surfacing of the 'functional' architecture of the 1920s. The new architecture of the 1950s was to learn much from this carefully stated neoclassicization of the machine aesthetic. Equally, the precision with which these and other works by Mies and Johnson were rendered was an external and easy-to-imitate element that was swiftly turned into a popular fashion in the commercial architecture of the period. The firm of *Skidmore, Owings and Merrill—in effect a latter day successor to both the academicism of McKim, Mead and White and the utilitarianism of Albert Kahn—dominated this side of American

architecture, especially through the quality of its commercial designs, and it continued to be acutely sensitive to shifts of taste when, in the late 1950s, its manner edged away from the glass box to more solid-seeming forms.

The early 1950s also witnessed the emergence of Eero *Saarinen, son of the pioneer Finnish architect. His General Motors Technical Center, Warren, Michigan, has a superficial Miesian character, but the varied proportions indicate a certain freedom of stylistic disposition which would lead to a pronounced design eclecticism in the late 1950s. This direction is amply documented in his new residential colleges for Yale University (1962) in which an abstract and empirical design is made to blend subtly with the elegant historicism of James Gamble Rodgers's collegiate Gothic of a generation before. A similar testing of various modernist idioms, together with a tentative eclecticism, is revealed in the designs of Paul *Rudolph, who had achieved considerable success as a designer of houses about 1950, and who, in the subsequent decade, has made interesting contributions to the expansion of the contemporary idiom in larger buildings. In particular, Rudolph has

Alvar Aalto. Students' Hostel, Massachusetts Institute of Technology. Cambridge, Mass., 1948

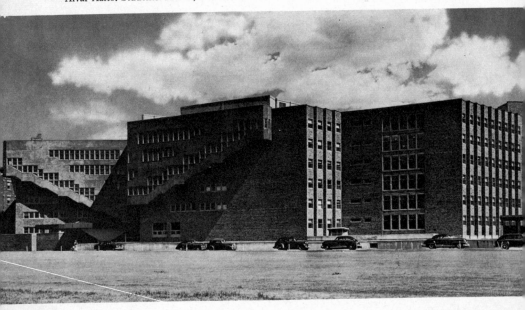

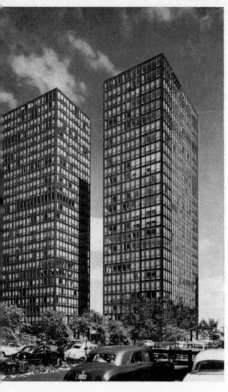

Ludwig Mies van der Rohe. Lake Shore Drive Apartments. Chicago, 1950–1

recently made an effort to transpose the vigorous late style of Le Corbusier in designs for religious, educational and commercial buildings.

The most fashionable of recent architects have tended towards a certain decorative elaboration in the composition of façades. Perhaps the most successful of these designers a few years ago was Edward D. *Stone, whose American Embassy in New Delhi, India (1958), was the first of a series of endeavours to create an officially endorsed modernism. A more recent example is Saarinen's Embassy in London (1960). However, the opulent yet brittle mannerisms of Minoru *Yamasaki, with façades protected by metal grilles and thinly disguised historical motifs, is perhaps an even more potent fashion in the early 1960s. In spite of these somewhat frigid, superficial efforts to create a revisionist movement in contemporary archi-

tecture, the older practitioners have tended to hold fast to the creative basis if not to the external appearances of their previous work. In his ultimate works, Wright created a dazzling array of forms, but they were invariably imagined upon the basis of previous designs. Mies's latest projects have been for buildings abroad, notably in Mexico and Germany, and thus his tenacity in holding to the style he perfected twenty years ago, especially in the face of change reflected both in the ephemeral work of the 1960s, and of normal development in the work of direct followers such as Johnson, and Skidmore, Owings and Merrill, is particularly noteworthy.

As if to compensate for Mies's relative inactivity recently in the USA, *Le Corbusier, the most distinguished of the veteran modernists remaining in Europe, was invited to design a new Art Center at Harvard in 1960. The characterful forms of this new building will thus form a challenging comparison with the other significant contemporary works of the last decade in Cambridge, Mass., those of Gropius, Aalto and Eero Saarinen. However, to the dynamic inflections of a sculptural sort that are now being introduced into American architecture by way of Le Corbusier, there is another, equally rugged, manner that is to be seen almost exclusively in the new work of Louis I. *Kahn. Hardly known a decade ago, except to a loyal band of young students, by the

Paul Rudolph. Cultural Centre, Wellesley College, Mass., 1955–9

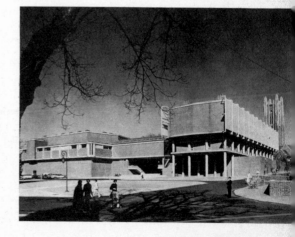

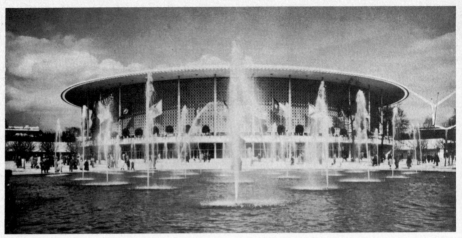

Edward Durell Stone. US Pavilion at the International Exhibition. Brussels, 1958

late 1950s his fame was already assured. Kahn's forthright concrete frame structures possess the semblance of a design philosophy relevant for their period and a final outward appearance which appeals both to a taste for contrasts of form and for certain kinds of justifiably accidental effects. Consequently, Kahn's few executed buildings may well turn out to be the most historically important if least typical designs of the early 1960s. Indeed, the nature of his style is such that it suggests the fulfilment of a century of American architecture, subsuming some of the profoundest lessons of Wright, Sullivan, and Richardson, and reaching so far back as to make relevant once again the century-old Victorian 'realism' of Sullivan's early mentor, Frank Furness.

The other side of the current picture is also traditionalist, but, it would seem, takes its cue from the alternate, academic current of the American development. The handsome, tasteful designs for Lincoln Center, New York, the work of several architects, including Wallace *Harrison, Max *Abramovitz, Philip Johnson, Skidmore, Owings and Merrill, and the late Eero Saarinen, seem to represent a blend of the challenging modernist discipline of a quarter-century ago with the half-century-old security of academicism as earlier represented by McKim, Mead and White. Of all the buildings at Lincoln Center, only Johnson's Theater of the Dance seems to

be the outcome of anything more than the most superficial decorative approach.

Under these confusing and rather inconsistent circumstances it is not easy succinctly to characterize the American scene in the 1960s. However, it is clear that an epoch of assimilation is past and the modern movement, brought to a climax in Europe in the 1920s and 1930s, has been incorporated into the evolving tradition of American architecture. The latter has, thereby, achieved new responsibilities through a generally recognized world-wide leadership which places new demands as well as a new dignity upon its subsequent development.

Bibliography: E. B. Mock, Built in USA 1932–1944, New York 1944; Henry-Russell Hitchcock and Arthur Drexler, Built in USA: Post-war Architecture, New York 1952; Lewis Mumford, Roots of Contemporary American Architecture, New York and London 1952; Ian McCallum, Architecture USA, London 1959; Wayne Andrews, Architecture in America, New York 1960; Esther McCoy, Five California Architects, New York 1960; 'America', Zodiac 8 (special number), Milan 1961; John Burchard and Albert Bush-Brown, The Architecture of America, Boston and Toronto 1961; C. W. Condit, American Building Art, Vol. I, The 19th century; Vol. II, The 20th century, New York and London, 1960 and 1961.

JOHN M. JACOBUS, JR

Utzon, Jørn, b. Copenhagen 1918. Utzon is the most original talent in modern Danish architecture. From the earliest years of his career he was possessed by an organic sense of architecture which was inspired by Frank Lloyd *Wright and Alvar *Aalto and strengthened by a period of study in the USA and six months' work in Aalto's Helsinki drawing office (1946).

For the young Utzon the functionalism of the thirties had ended in formalism, and the traditionalism of the forties, a consequence of the isolation and restrictions caused by the war, was totally lacking in relevance to the technical and scientific developments of the times. He considered that a progressive architecture could be learned from the laws of nature, and that new materials should be used in accordance with their own properties. He was himself able to live up to these very ambitious demands thanks to his originality, imagination and professional skill.

Utzon completed his secondary education in 1937 and entered the architectural school of the Academy of Arts, where he was taught by Kay *Fisker and Steen Ejler Rasmussen. He qualified in 1942 and then worked for three years in Stockholm, where his encounter with Gunnar *Asplund's architecture in particular influenced his development. In the following year he received prizes in a series of competitions for projects worked out in collaboration with Tobias Faber and submitted a design for the Crystal Palace in London together with Faber and Mogens

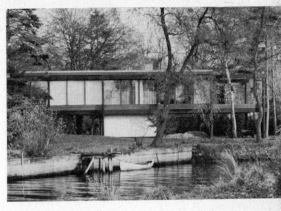

Jorn Utzon. House. Holte, 1952–3

Irming. Also important at this time was his friendship and collaboration with the Norwegian architect, Arne Korsmo.

In 1952 he built his own house in Hellebæk on a southward facing slope at the edge of a wood; the spaciousness and open ground-plan were quite new to Denmark at that time. A little later, 1952–3, he built a house in Holte, whose inspiration was more Japanese. Its concrete frame holds the otherwise timber-clad house a storey above the ground. During the first half of the fifties he received prizes in several Swedish competitions, including a plan for the Elineberg housing estate, which was subsequently realized (in collaboration with E. and H. Andersson).

Jorn Utzon. Opera House. Sydney, 1956. Model

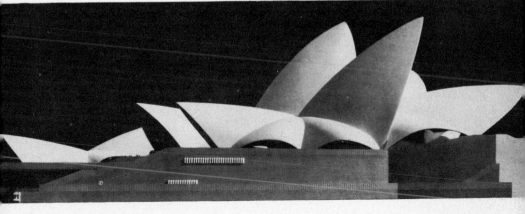

In 1956 Utzon received first prize for a highly original plan in the international competition for a new Sydney Opera House, to be placed on a mole in the middle of the city's harbour. The opera house, concert hall and foyers are to lie under shells 200 feet in height on an extensive stepped platform. This platform will serve as the cover for a lower level with experimental theatre, access for vehicles, extra space, etc. The shells are planned according to a bold and original scheme developed in collaboration with Ove Arup in London. The project was hailed by Harry *Seidler as 'pure poetry', but the detailed planning shows the presence of a logical and realistic architect, able to turn his visions into reality. In a number of projects from 1958 to 1960 Utzon varied the idea of raised platforms or bastions, with vehicular access below and the building proper above (Højstrup Workers' High School, 1958; a row of buildings in Frederiksberg, near the centre of Copenhagen, 1959; International Exhibition in Copenhagen, 1960). Smaller, but no less characteristic, is the plan for the Melli Bank in Teheran (1958).

While Utzon was working on these dynamic and imaginative projects, two housing estates in northern Zealand were erected—Kingohusene near Helsingør (1957–60) and the Danish Co-operative Building in Fredensborg. Both are chains of houses with courtyards or gardens, staggered to fit the topography. Each house and garden is enclosed by yellow brick walls of various heights. The houses are small and inexpensive and remind one of a North African village.

                                        TOBIAS FABER

Vago, Pierre, b. Budapest 1910. Came to Paris at eighteen years of age to study under Auguste *Perret at the École Spéciale d'Architecture. While still a student, in 1932, he became editor-in-chief of the journal L'architecture d'aujourd'hui. In 1934 designed a prefabricated all-metal house. Town planning, schools, housing (in Berlin 1957, with flat-units one and a half storeys high), churches (Basilica of Pius X at Lourdes, commenced 1954, with *Freyssinet as engineer).

Van de Velde, Henry, b. Antwerp 1863, d. Zurich 1957. Henry van de Velde was the apostle in theory and practice of func-

tional aesthetics and 'pure form'; between 1900 and 1925 he exerted a decisive influence on architecture and the applied arts, particularly in Germany. Born of a middle-class Flemish family, van de Velde was attracted to music, literature and painting before turning to architecture. He was a student at the Académie des Beaux-Arts at Antwerp in 1881, where he attended the painting classes; he continued with Carolus Duran in Paris from 1884 to 1885. He made contact with the Impressionist painters and Symbolist poets, and was particularly impressed by Seurat, whose pointilliste technique seemed to embody a spatial concept capable of opening up new prospects in architecture. Returning to Antwerp, van de Velde took part (1886) in founding the cultural circle named Als ik Kan (after Van Eyck's motto), and a year later, L'art indépendant, an association of young neo-Impressionist painters. From 1889 onwards he took part in the international activities of the famous avant-gardist Brussels group known as Les XX, where he discovered the synthetical art and flowing hand of Gauguin, the English *Arts and Crafts Movement, and the socially orientated work of William *Morris. Towards 1890 he became associated with the journal Van Nu en Straks, for which he devised a revolutionary layout, new typography and woodcut ornaments in a style derived from Gauguin. This undertaking, which played an important rôle in the renaissance of Belgian book production, started van de Velde on the road to the craft side of art. Henceforth, following the example of William Morris, he gave up painting (1893) and concentrated on illustration. He designed a mural tapestry, 'The Angels' Vigil' (1891, Zurich, Kunstgewerbemuseum), and went on to three-dimensional work with the creation of his first pieces of furniture (1894), the last stage before entering, shortly after his marriage, on the royal road of architecture proper.

In 1895 (two years after *Horta's Hôtel Tassel) van de Velde built his own home, 'Bloemenwerf' at Uccle near Brussels. It is designed as an organic whole and completely fitted out (joinery, hardware, furniture, carpets, curtains, dinner service, glasses, silver) in a uniform style of English inspiration, thus conforming with the theories which he set out in his own

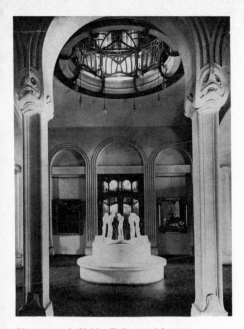

Henry van de Velde. Folkwang Museum.
Hagen, 1900–2

structures imbued with the rhythm of a linear ornament. This failing that characterizes my first works has nothing to do with the rise of Art Nouveau, which certain writers have fathered on me, and which enshrined an amalgam of the type of ornamentation I was using around 1894 and the kind of floral ornament associated with the drawings of long-haired women that Otto Eckmann was turning out in Berlin at the same period, and which he had borrowed from the English Pre-Raphaelites.'

The fact remains that van de Velde's cult of linear ornament, of the undulating line, was strengthened by his enthusiastic adherence to the neo-romantic theory of empathy, formulated by Lipps in 1903. The originality of his designs soon caught the attention of the art historian Julius Meier-Graefe and the art dealer S. Bing, who helped to ensure their international popularity. In 1896 Bing invited van de Velde to fit out four rooms of a shop he was opening in Paris under the name of *L'Art Nouveau*. His robust and curvilinear furniture, in a style very like that introduced by the young Liége-born designer Georges Serrurier-Bovy in 1894, aroused much

publications (*Déblaiement d'art*, *L'art futur*, *Aperçu en vue d'une Synthèse d'art*). Noteworthy features include a return to a rational style that 'frankly and proudly' displays the processes of manufacture in all fields, an uncompromising logic in the use of materials, and a rejection of all ornament inspired by nature and all historic detailing. But van de Velde's renewed awareness of structural function, his desire to cast off dead tradition and his basic rationalism still retained sentimental overtones. His thought was instilled with German romanticism. 'Whether it was a matter of the works of German, Austrian or Dutch artists', he wrote later, 'we were all more attached than we thought to a kind of romanticism which would not allow us to consider form "without ornament", we were too much painters, too much wedded to literature, to glimpse the necessity of abandoning ornament and decoration . . . the temptations and subconscious insinuations of romanticism prompted us to bend and twist our structural schemes and present them as ornaments acting as structural elements, or as

Henry van de Velde. Art School. Weimar, 1906

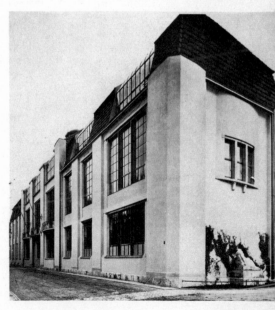

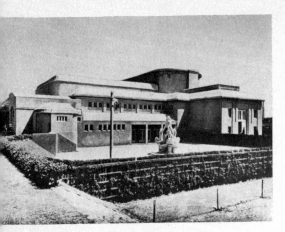

Henry van de Velde. Werkbund Theatre.
Cologne, 1914

enthusiasm at the Dresden Exhibition of
Applied Arts in 1897.

Henceforth, van de Velde's path was clear:
he would make his career in Germany.
Before he left Belgium (1899), Meier-
Graefe commissioned him to do the
interior decoration of the *Maison Moderne*
he had founded in Paris, and introduced
him to the *Pan* group in Berlin, where he
also won many commissions (Hohen-
zollern Craftwork Shop, 1899; Haby's
barber shop, 1901; premises for the
Habana Tobacco Co., 1900; Esche House,
Chemnitz, 1902). During the winter of
1900–1, he undertook a lecture tour in
Germany, during which he explained his
artistic principles (published in 1902 under
the title of *Kunstgewerbliche Laienpredigten*).
At the instance of K. E. Osthaus, he undertook the internal layout and decoration of
the Folkwang Museum at Hagen (1900–2;
exhibition rooms, glass cases, stairs, handrails, decorative glazing, mouldings, furniture, etc). The strong modelling and curved
ornamentation of this building are typically Art Nouveau, and mark the culminating point of the first phase of van de
Velde's career, which closes with the rest
room he designed for the Dresden Exhibition of Applied Arts in 1906.

The second phase, from 1906 to 1914, is
opened by the foundation and building of
the Weimar School of Applied Arts,
thanks to van de Velde's influence with the
Grand Duke of Saxe-Weimar, to whose
court he had been attached since 1901 as

artistic counsellor, charged with raising the
level of design in local industry. Here he
found an ideal field for exercising his
vocation as a teacher. He introduced a new
system of instruction based on the development of spontaneous feeling and a constant
recourse to the student's powers of invention, avoiding the use of models from
the past and the study of historic styles.
These methods gave rise to new forms,
which German industry was not slow to
adopt. 'We shall be obliged to recognize
one day,' van de Velde subsequently
observed, 'that these objects with their
rational shapes prepared the way for the
advance of a rational type of architecture,
and largely contributed to its general
diffusion. Their principles are the same as
those that modern architecture was based
on afterwards.'

The design of the Weimar school buildings
clearly expresses in itself the development
of van de Velde's architectural thought.
Although traditional building methods are
employed, a surer sense of space and
volume is evinced. The straight line returns,
ornament is purified and stress laid on
plastic expression, as in the Werkbund
Theatre. This celebrated building, now
destroyed, was built for the Werkbund
Exhibition of 1914, in Cologne. Laid out
on a symmetrical plan, with a heavy traditional shell, albeit of original appearance,
it embodied numerous innovations that
provided a brilliant answer to the requirements of the dramatic art of its day:
auditorium in the shape of an amphi-
theatre, independent proscenium, circular
horizon, and, in particular, tripartite stage.
Van de Velde, who was friendly with
Gordon Craig and Max Reinhardt, had
already in 1911 drawn up the first plans
for the Théâtre des Champs-Élysées,
Paris.

The outbreak of the First World War marks
the commencement of the third and final
phase of van de Velde's career (1914–57).
He moved to Switzerland in 1917, where
he became intimate with Romain Rolland
and E. L. Kirchner. In 1921 he transferred
to Holland, where he was commissioned by
the Kröller-Müller family to design a
museum, which he ultimately built, to a
modified plan, at Otterlo (1937–54). This
building is a work of great simplicity and
harmony, free of all rhetorical efforts; it is
perfectly adapted to its site and function

(one level throughout, main and secondary circulation, top lighting, etc.).

Van de Velde returned to Belgium in 1925. With the support of the Minister C. Huysmans, he was given the opportunity once more of carrying out the experiments he had conducted at Weimar: in 1926 he founded the Institut des Arts Décoratifs de la Cambre, which later became the École Nationale Supérieure d'Architecture et des Arts Décoratifs. He was the principal of this school until 1935; in addition, he occupied the chair of architecture at the University of Ghent from 1926 to 1936. He settled at Oberägeri in Switzerland in 1947, where he began writing his memoirs.

Van de Velde's work is dominated by his controversial and acute writings. His thought is condensed in the *Formules de la Beauté architectonique moderne* (Weimar 1917), revised and re-issued as *Formules d'une Esthétique moderne* (Brussels 1923), which stands to early-20th-century architecture as do Maurice Denis's *Théories* (1890) to the painting of his time. Among van de Velde's most important collaborators and pupils may be mentioned Victor *Bourgeois, J. J. Eggerick, R. Verwilghen, and L. Stynen.

Bibliography: Henry van de Velde, *Déblaiement d'art*, Brussels 1894; Henry van de Velde, *L'art futur*, Brussels 1895; Henry van de Velde, *Aperçu en vue d'une Synthèse d'art*, Brussels 1895; Henry van de Velde, *Geschichte meines Lebens*, Munich 1962; Karl Ernst Osthaus, *Henry van de Velde. Leben und Schaffen des Künstlers*, Hagen 1920; J. Mesnil, *Henry van de Velde et le Théâtre des Champs-Elysées*, Brussels; O. J. Maurice Casteels, *Henry van de Velde*, Brussels 1932; 'Henry van de Velde', Special Issue of *La Cité*, Brussels 1933, No. 5–6; Herman Teirlinck, *Henry van de Velde*, Brussels 1959.

ROBERT L. DELEVOY

Viganò, Vittoriano, b. Milan 1919; garduated there 1944. Residential and sports buildings. His Istituto Marchiondi (Milan 1957) with its dramatically accentuated structure, heavy massing and untreated, exposed concrete is regarded as the Italian variation of *Brutalism.

Villagran Garcia, José, b. Mexico City 1901. Studied architecture at Mexico University. Teacher of most modern Mexican architects and pioneer of modern architecture in *Mexico. Numerous schools, public and welfare buildings.

Villanueva, Carlos Raúl, b. Croydon, England 1900. More than any other individual architect Villanueva has been responsible for the impressive development of modern architecture in Venezuela. He studied at the *École des Beaux-Arts in Paris. In a way typical of his generation throughout Latin America, his early work was an attempt to renew, with discriminating connoisseurship, the traditions of local colonial architecture. Quite soon, however, he came to a deep understanding of the new ways of thought in architecture and devoted himself with a missionary ardour to the spread of modern architecture in his own land.

To the inspiration received from the great masters of his time Villanueva adds characteristic personal elements: a dynamic and spontaneous quality in structural design, forcefully expressed in exposed concrete; a catholicity of taste reflected in extensive collaboration with many painters and sculptors as well as in a daring use of polychromy; and a feeling for large-scale composition which enables him to cope with the enormous building programme resulting from the rapid development of the country. Villanueva's impact is also felt in the fine architectural tradition established by the housing authority, the *Banco Obrero*, whose gigantic operations on a consistently high level have enabled many younger architects to start promising careers. Among Villanueva's most important work the buildings for the University City in Caracas obviously come first. The Olympic Stadium (1950–1), with its daringly cantilevered marquees, built in shell concrete, with exposed ribs, and the Auditorium and the Covered Plaza (Aula Magna and Plaza Cubierta, 1952–3) are the best known. The Aula Magna, one of the most beautiful assembly rooms in the world, has a clean white curved ceiling against which float a large number of variously coloured and shaped panels, designed by Alexander Calder (with R. Newman as acoustics specialist). The austerity of the exterior, emphatically expressing the structural framework, is compensated by the gaiety and airiness of the Plaza Cubierta, the large semi-enclosed

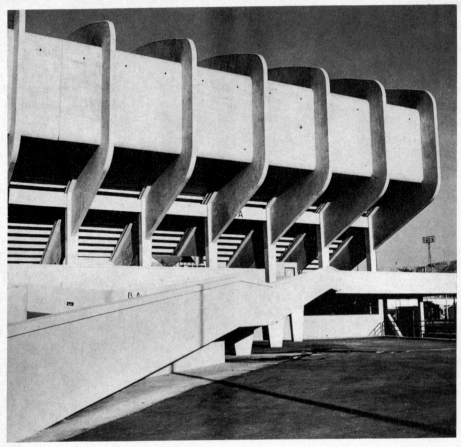

Carlos Raúl Villanueva. Olympic Stadium. Caracas, 1950–1

foyer, displaying works of art by Arp, Léger, Vasarely, and others. In all the other buildings, such as the library, the hospital, the various schools, an individual theme is carried through, the result of special research into each particular programme, boldly expressed in a framework of exposed concrete, often filled in with variously coloured panels covered with mosaic.

Of Villanueva's huge housing projects, called for by the rapid growth of Caracas (163,000 inhabitants in 1936, 359,000 in 1941, 718,000 in 1951, and 1,300,000 today) at least two, located in this city, must be mentioned as examples: the 'Dos de Diciembre' Housing Estate, with 2,366 dwellings for 12,744 people—400 persons per hectare—designed in collaboration with José Manuel Mijares, José Hoffman and Carlos Branco; and the 'El Paraiso', a smaller estate, with duplex units in a four-storey and a sixteen-storey building, (the density only 200 people per hectare), designed in collaboration with Carlos Celis and José Manuel Mijares. In both, the provision of ancillary facilities, social and commercial, is typical of the architect's humanistic approach. The extremely frank expression of the structure distinguishes these buildings, like most of Villanueva's, from the work of other Venezuelan architects such as Bernardez, Vegas and Galia, or Guinand and Benacerraf, which

seems closer to an international idiom. But it is precisely this distinction that lends to Villanueva's work its characteristic pioneering and dynamic spirit.
Bibliography: Henry-Russell Hitchcock, *Latin-American Architecture since 1945*, New York 1955.

HENRIQUE E. MINDLIN

Viollet-le-Duc, Eugène Emmanuèle, b. Paris 1814, d. Lausanne 1879. In 1840 began a series of important restorations of medieval buildings, of doubtful quality, however, by current standards of conservation; these include Vézelay, Carcassonne, Amiens, Pierrefonds, Notre-Dame de Paris. He had controversies with the *École des Beaux-Arts, to which he was appointed in 1863. His influential writings (*Dictionnaire de l'Architecture*, 1854f., *Entretiens sur l'Architecture*, 1863–72), although supporting the tendencies to stylistic copyism of the times, went far beyond Viollet-le-Duc's own work in their demand for rationality of structure.

Vlugt, L. C. van der, b. Rotterdam 1894, d. Rotterdam 1936. Housing and schools. From 1925 onwards in partnership with Johannes Andreas *Brinkman.

Voysey, Charles Annesley, b. Hessle, Yorkshire, 1857, d. Winchester 1941. Architect and designer of great influence on English and Continental *Art Nouveau. His private houses, mostly small, go back to the tradition of the English country house and are examples of building 'from the inside out' in their functional design.

Wachsmann, Konrad, b. Frankfort on the Oder 1901. Wachsmann has been a pioneer of industrialized building in theory, practice and teaching. He has always advocated that the scientific and technical resources of mass production should be applied to the processes of building, and he holds a corresponding structural and aesthetic conception of architecture. He came straight from building in timber to the problems of prefabrication. Trained as joiner and carpenter, Wachsmann was a student at the Arts and Crafts Schools of Berlin and Dresden (under Heinrich Tessenow) and at Berlin Academy of Art, where he was a star pupil of Hans *Poelzig's. From 1926 to 1929 he worked as chief

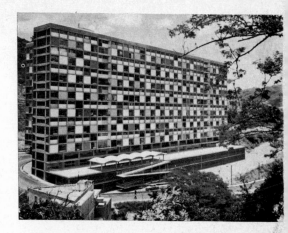

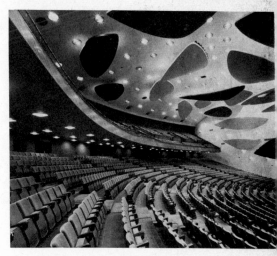

Carlos Raúl Villanueva, Carlos Celis and José Manuel Mijares. El Paraiso Flats. Caracas

Carlos Raúl Villanueva. Building for the Faculty of Architecture and Town Planning of the University. Caracas, 1957. Large Hall.

architect for the firm of Christoph and Unmack who were the largest manufacturers of timber buildings in Europe at the time. In 1932 he was awarded the Rome Prize by the German Academy in Rome. In the years following, which he spent in Rome, he was occupied with building blocks of flats in reinforced concrete. Emigrating to the United States, he founded a partnership with Walter

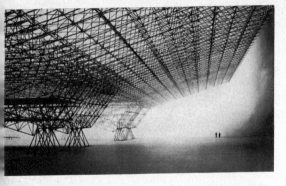

Konrad Wachsmann. Structural system for halls.
1950–3. Model

*Gropius from 1941 to 1948, from which
emerged the General Panel Corporation,
the first fully automated factory for the
production of prefabricated building components. In 1950 Wachsmann, who has
been an American citizen since 1946 and
who lives partly in America and partly in
Europe, was appointed professor at the
Illinois Institute of Technology at Chicago
and director of the Department of Advanced Building Research. Since then,
with the support of the American Government, he has directed architectural semi-

Konrad Wachsmann. Perspective of a structural
unit. 1953

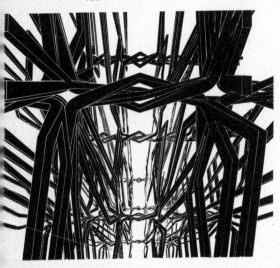

nars at universities and colleges in Japan,
Israel, Austria and Germany. In recent
years he has conducted research on town
and country planning in the United States,
and on multi-storey building in Europe.
Wachsmann's research has concentrated on
the basic character of universal elements in
building construction which can be mass
produced. His starting point is 'modular
coordination', which governs the relationship of the various building components to
each other. These components should be
as simple as possible and capable of as
many different combinations as possible.
A 'universal module', identical with the
'planning module', comprises all the
modular categories (material, performance,
construction, installation, etc.). The resulting abstract data are carried over into the
concrete conception of a standard form.
Wachsmann's research has found a practical
application above all in the General Panel
System, which is made up of prefabricated
timber units. In the forties, he was commissioned by the US Air Force to develop
the 'Mobilar Structure', a system for the
construction of aircraft hangars to any
required size by the addition of steel
struts, whose tubular diameter possesses
extremely favourable static properties. He
made a special study of the nature of the
connections and joints of cellular structures
such as Buckminster *Fuller's geodesic
domes or Le Ricolais's space structures,
built up from similar elements. In 1951,
he worked out a classification system for
modular coordination for the Federal
Housing Agency in Washington as an
example of the rational planning of vast
building programmes.
Wachsmann carried out part of his research
in the form of team-work with his students
in the course of his teaching activities. On
the rôle of the architect within the industrialized building process he says: 'It will
be the task of the universal planner to
combine the requisite technological components by a creative act into a complete
whole. The universal planner becomes part
of the creative team, combining prefabricated parts and planning with them in the
widest sense.' He has anticipated the future
time and again with his apparently utopian
projects, and has stimulated discussion,
beyond the limits of architecture, on the
problem of the spirit in a technical
civilization.

Bibliography: Konrad Wachsmann, *The Turning Point of Building*, New York 1961; Konrad Wachsmann, *Aspekte*, Wiesbaden 1961.

MARGIT STABER

Wagner, Martin, b. Königsberg 1885, d. Cambridge, Mass. 1957; 1926–33 City Architect of Berlin, where he was closely associated with *Gropius, *Häring, *Mies van der Rohe, *Poelzig, *Scharoun. Emigrated to the United States. Lecturer at Harvard University (1936–50).

Wagner, Otto, b. Penzing, near Vienna 1841, d. Vienna 1918. A precursor of 20th-century architecture and town planning, Wagner was the founder of the Vienna School, which rose to fame through its most brilliant disciples: Adolf *Loos, Josef *Hoffmann and Joseph Maria *Olbrich. He was the spiritual heir of *Viollet-le-Duc, and played a part in Austria equivalent to that of *Sullivan in the United States, van de *Velde in Belgium and *Berlage in the Netherlands. His work is based fundamentally on a renewed awareness of the plan, adapted to the requirements of social progress and current advances in technology; it expresses an unerring renewal of architectural thought and symbolizes the great changes in taste that were taking place at the turn of the 19th and 20th centuries.

Wagner began his studies in 1857 at the Vienna Technical College. He spent some time in 1860 at the Berlin Academy of Building, and completed his training at the school of architecture of the Vienna Academy from 1861 to 1863. The first phase of his career is marked by a historical outlook. He adopted a form of classicism derived from the Tuscan and Florentine High Renaissance: closed plans that were lucid, logical and very severely geometrical. His work earned him such a reputation that he was commissioned in 1890 to draw up a scheme for completely remodelling the city of Vienna. Of this, the only item to be carried out was the construction (1894–7) of the Stadtbahn, or metropolitan railway network, intended to provide rapid communication with the suburbs and to thin out city traffic.

In 1894 he was appointed head of a special class in architecture at the Vienna Academy. This year also marked the opening of a

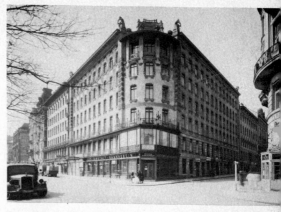

Otto Wagner. Majolika-Haus. Vienna, *c.* 1898

second phase in the development of his work (1894–1901), characterized firstly by his assumption of a definite theoretical standpoint and next by his adherence to the system of aesthetics proclaimed at Brussels, Paris and Munich by the adepts of *Art Nouveau. While van de Velde was

Otto Wagner. Post Office Savings Bank. Vienna, 1904–6

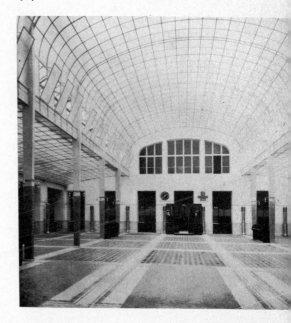

opening his famous campaign in Brussels to purify the language of architecture (*Déblaiement d'art*, 1894), Wagner put forward in his inaugural lecture at Vienna Academy (1894) a doctrine that has become famous under the title of *Moderne Architektur*. In his view, the new architecture must take the requirements of modern life as its point of departure, and find adequate forms to express them. Two years after Sullivan's plea (*Ornament in Architecture*, 1892), and three years before the first statements of Loos, Wagner was extolling horizontal lines, flat roofs, and a stripped-down style that would draw its powers of expression from a striking affirmation of structural principles and the loyal use of materials, with steel in particular affording solutions that were new and bold.

The Stadtbahn station in the Karlsplatz (1899–1901) may serve to illustrate this transitional period. The use of a steel frame, in accordance with current French practice at the time, requires all archaeological reminiscences to be dispensed with; but by combining the straight line and the curve in floral ornamentation, a compromise is struck between doctrinal rigour and the inflections made fashionable by Art Nouveau.

Wagner went on to adopt a more radical attitude in full conformity with the principles he defended. The Post Office Savings Bank in Vienna (1904–6) dominates the third and last phase of his career; the economy of its trapezoidal plan, developing harmoniously around a central hall, the feeling for monumentality, the flexible handling of space, the complete eschewal of ornament and the perfect integration of steel and glass all go to make this building an unmistakable landmark in the history of contemporary architecture.

Bibliography: Otto Wagner, *Moderne Architektur*, Vienna 1896; 4th Edition: *Die Baukunst unserer Zeit*, Vienna 1914; Joseph August Lux, *Otto Wagner*, Munich 1914; Hans Tietze, *Otto Wagner*, Vienna 1922.

ROBERT L. DELEVOY

Warchavchik, Gregori, b. Odessa 1896. Trained in Rome. Warchavchik, who published a 'Manifesto of Functional Architecture' in 1925, built private houses in Brazil in the *International Style in the late twenties.

Webb, Philip, b. Oxford 1831, d. Worth, Sussex 1915. Assistant of G. E. Street, in whose office he met William *Morris. Associate in the Morris Company. Webb built town and country houses, in which he employs late-medieval building methods to create unconventional designs without resorting to historical copyism. The Red House near Bexley Heath, Kent (1859).

Weese, Harry, b. Chicago 1915. Trained at Massachusetts Institute of Technology and at Harvard University, Cambridge, Mass. Collaborated with Gordon *Bunshaft (*Skidmore, Owings and Merrill). Houses, schools, project for US Embassy at Accra (Ghana).

Wendingen. Dutch architectural journal (until 1936) which served as the focus for a group of architects in Amsterdam.

Werkbund. *Deutscher Werkbund.

Williams, Sir E. Owen, b. Tottenham, London 1890. Reinforced concrete structures important in the development of modern English architecture. Boots' factory at Beeston near Nottingham (1932), Empire Swimming Pool, Wembley (1934), Peckham Health Centre (1936), aircraft hangars in London (1955).

Wright, Frank Lloyd, b. Richland Center, Wis. 1867 or 1869, d. Taliesin West, Ariz. 1959.
After Frank Lloyd Wright's death at the end of an architectural career that had continued for more than seventy years, he was very generally considered the greatest American architect and one of the three or four greatest architects of the 20th century. Yet recurrently, and to the end, his work had been the subject of controversies and it is unlikely that in the future all those controversies will be resolved in his favour —nor perhaps would he have wished it to be so. Even the date of his birth is disputed —he believed he was born in 1869, but evidence in the family records indicates 1867. Of English origin on his father's side and Welsh on his mother's, it was the Celtic strain in his temperament that dominated; at the same time he considered himself the most American of Americans, or as he was inclined to put it, Usonians. His remarkably long career not unnaturally

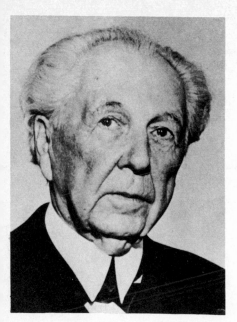

Frank Lloyd Wright

which naturally increased in volume after his break with Sullivan in 1893, many influences other than Sullivan's are evident, notably from such architects of the eastern seaboard as *Richardson, Bruce Price, and McKim, Mead and White. Following on the apprentice work of the nineties, in which his own studio in Oak Park (1895), the windmill for his aunts at Spring Green (1896), and the River Forest Golf Club (1898) may be cited as especially significant, he came to maturity almost precisely in 1900.

In that year the Bradley and Hickox Houses in Kankakee, Ill. and the design for 'A Home in a Prairie Town' (published in the *Ladies Home Journal* in February 1901) initiated the series of his Prairie Houses, his earliest major contribution to modern architecture. In the Prairie Houses, of which the most notable were perhaps the Willitts House in Highland Park, Ill. and the Heurtley House in Oak Park (1902), the Martin House in Buffalo, New York (1904), the Glasner House in Glencoe, Ill. (1905), the Coonley House in Riverside, Ill. and the Isobel Roberts House in River Forest, Ill. (1908), and above all the Robie House in Chicago and Mrs Thomas Gale's House in Oak Park (1909), the American house was revolutionized with results that later affected house-design internationally. Characteristically the plans of these houses were articulated in X, L, and T shapes, with free spatial flow between the principal living areas. Externally they were low and horizontal, with windows arranged in continuous bands under the wide-spreading eaves of low hipped or gabled roofs which also subsumed porches within the carefully ordered compositions. Except for leaded-glass windows with delicate geometrical patterns, there was usually no ornament whatsoever and, except for occasional bold cantilevering of the roofs, no real modification of standard American building methods.

Already in 1901, however, he had published in *The Brickbuilder* a project for a cast-concrete bank and in non-domestic work was soon exploiting *reinforced concrete structure. When his work was brought to the attention of European architects by the Wasmuth publications of 1910 and 1911, the Larkin office building in Buffalo, New York (1904), the Unity Church in Oak Park (1906) and even the

divides into a succession of phases, from his education in the 1870s and 1880s in which his exposure to the Froebel kindergarten system and his reading of such architectural writers as *Ruskin and *Viollet-le-Duc seem to have played as great a part as the two years he spent studying engineering at the University of Wisconsin, to the final florescence of the 1950s. Nor, on the testimony of his remarkable autobiography can the ambience of his grandfather's farm near Spring Green, Wisconsin, be ignored in the early formation of his agrarian preferences and his special attitude towards nature and the nature of materials.

After a very brief initial period of work in the office of the minor 'Shingle Style' architect J. L. Silsbee in Chicago, he entered in 1888 the employ of Louis *Sullivan, the greatest American architect of the day, always to Wright the *Lieber Meister*. In that office he was early entrusted with the domestic commissions, notably the Charnley House in Chicago of 1892. But in his personal work, which began with the construction of his own house in Oak Park, Illinois, in 1889 and

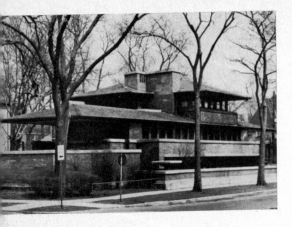

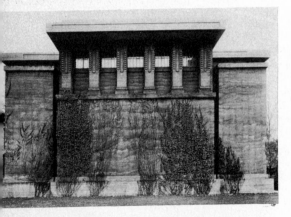

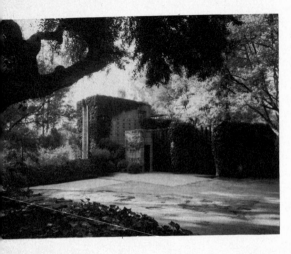

small hotel in Mason City, Iowa (1909) were perhaps more influential than the domestic work. Their complex cubic forms, spatial development in three dimensions, and expressive exploitation of new building materials and methods appealed strongly to younger architects abroad, and this influence played some part in the adumbration of the *International Style in Europe in the following fifteen years.

For various reasons personal and general the next decade was less productive for Wright. But to these years, often considered his 'Baroque' period, belong the destroyed Midway Gardens in Chicago (1913), in which the sculptured and painted decoration paralleled and even prefigured aspects of post-Cubist art in Europe, and the big Imperial Hotel (1916–22) in Tokyo.

With his return to America in the early 1920s came a group of concrete-block houses in California, the most notable the Millard House in Pasadena (1923). Here a new setting and a new material induced a total revolution in his house design, with crisper forms, all-over patterned surfaces and invisible flat roofs. His own house, Taliesin, near Spring Green, Wisconsin, first built in 1911 and rebuilt after fires in 1914 and 1925, was more in the line of the earlier Prairie Houses, but characteristically adapted to a hillside and making expressive use of the local limestone.

In the mid and late 1920s Wright's career seemed for some years to have come to an end and he was already considered an 'old master', left behind by the new developments in architecture of that decade. Projects, however, notably that for the Noble apartment house in Los Angeles of 1929, indicated his will to rival, if not to imitate, the new architecture that he scorned as mere 'boxes on stilts'; and when the curve of his production turned up once more in the mid 1930s two extraordinary works, Falling Water, the Kaufmann House in the Pennsylvania woods (1936) and the S. C. Johnson & Son administration building in Racine, Wis. (1936–9) indicated in

Frank Lloyd Wright. Robie House. Chicago, 1909

Frank Lloyd Wright. Unity Church. Oak Park, 1906

Frank Lloyd Wright. Millard House. Pasadena, 1923

their totally different ways—extravagant exploitation of cantilevering; utilization of free-standing mushroom columns—the assurance with which he was now ready to handle reinforced concrete. In their almost total avoidance of ornament, in the subtle handling of a wide gamut of materials—from the Taliesin-like stonework of the core of Falling Waters to the metallic slickness of the glass-tube fenestration of the Johnson Building—these works displayed the ever-increasing range of his sensitivity to materials both old and new.

Also to the late 1930s belong his 'Usonian' houses with walls of wooden-sandwiches and flat roofs of crossed wooden scantlings, modest dwellings built at surprisingly low cost in which his planning reached its extreme of openness with the substitution of clerestory-lighted 'work-spaces' attached to the main living areas for conventional kitchens. The range and size of his commissions was already widening. But more significant perhaps for the final florescence of his last twenty years than the large project of 1938 for a new campus for Florida Southern College in Lakeland, Fla., where construction started in 1940 and continued into the 1950s, was the variety of response evoked by the opportunity to work in sharply contrasted natural settings: the desert of Arizona, where he began his own winter establishment 'Taliesin West' at Scottsville in 1938 and the exemplary Pauson House of 1940 at Phoenix, making use of 'desert concrete' in which large rough blocks of local stone were laid up loosely in forms with a minimum of cement binding; the hills of Los Angeles, where the Sturgis House (1939), a 'box without stilts', although visibly of brick and redwood, was cantilevered by hidden stall beams even more boldly than the terraces of 'Falling Water'; not to speak of Florida, where the warm climate and the lush foliage encouraged a return to the patterned block-work of the earlier California years.

Parallel to this was an extraordinary increase in the range of geometrical and structural themes which he was to continue to develop to the end of his life. In addition to the rectangular forms characteristic of his work in the first quarter of the century, he now became fascinated with plan-patterns based on 60°–30° angles, on circles, and even on spirals. Early instances

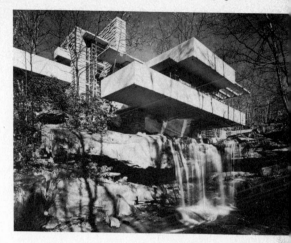

Frank Lloyd Wright. Kaufmann House, 'Falling Water'. Bear Run, Pa., 1936

of these new approaches can be found in the projects of his fallow 1920s, but their full exploitation came only with the years after the Second World War. The 60°–30° angles appeared first in the San Marcos, project for a resort in Chandler, Ariz. in 1927 and were first carried to execution in the Hanna House in Palo Alto, Calif., in 1937. The circle and the helix were the theme of the Strong Automobile project for Maryland (1925), but came to ultimate realization in the Guggenheim Museum, designed 1943–6 and built 1956–9.

Frank Lloyd Wright. Taliesin West. Scottsville near Phoenix, Ariz., 1938

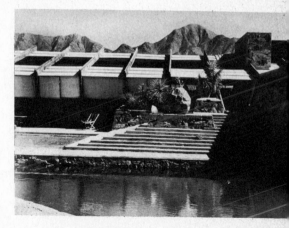

The remarkably prolific and varied production of Wright's last decade of activity, including several major works such as the County Buildings for Marin County, California, which are still in construction, has not yet been sorted out and published in dated sequence.

In the vast variety of his plans, which included fantastic urban projects for Bagdad as well as for Pittsburgh and Madison, Wis., not to speak of a Mile High Skyscraper, it is difficult to see what were the main lines along which he was moving. Responsive, perhaps, to the new international architectural climate of the 1950s, as he had once before been to the climate of the late 1920s and early 1930s, he seemed ready to initiate a new style with each major project. Yet more careful study of the drawings of his earlier periods of activity often reveal that what seemed to be wholly new developments of his later decades were in fact the realizations of ideas long nurtured; thus the design of the Price Tower at Bartlesville, Okla. (1955) can be traced back through several intervening versions to the St Mark's Tower project for New York (1929).

In conclusion it should be noted that Wright was not a silent creator. Difficult as it may be sometimes to see precisely how, in detail, his ambitions for a universal

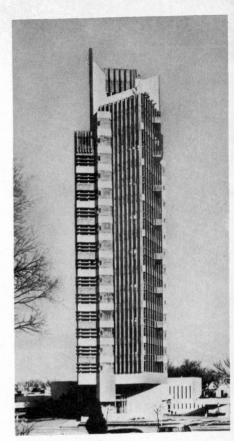

Frank Lloyd Wright. Price Tower. Bartlesville Okla., 1955

Frank Lloyd Wright. Beth Sholom Synagogue. Elkins Park, Pa., 1959

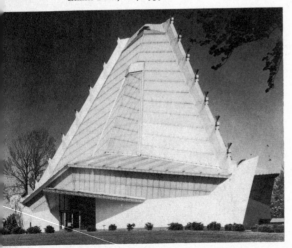

'organic architecture' of the 20th century reached the particular expression that they did in his own works, his career owed much to what he said and wrote. Posterity will have more material concerning Wright than can be readily digested for a long time in a tremendous *œuvre*, a vast volume of intrinsically fascinating drawings, and a written gospel, on which to base a later judgement on this great architect, who was also perhaps the greatest American of his generation.

Bibliography: *Frank Lloyd Wright on Architecture*, ed. Frederick Gutheim, New York 1941; Henry-Russell Hitchcock, *In the Nature of Materials, 1887–1941, The Buildings of Frank Lloyd Wright*, New York 1942; Frank Lloyd Wright, *Auto-*

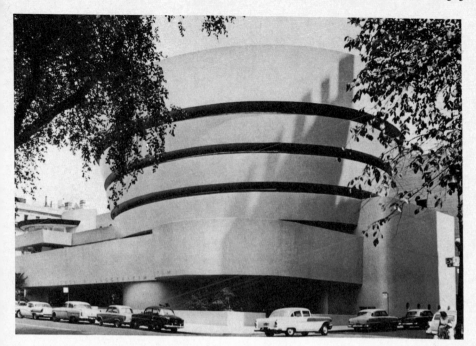

Frank Lloyd Wright. Guggenheim Museum. New York. Designed 1943–6, built 1956–9

biography, New York 1943; Frank Lloyd Wright, *Testament*, New York 1957; *Drawings, Frank Lloyd Wright*, New York 1959; *The Drawings of Frank Lloyd Wright*, ed. Arthur Drexler, New York 1962; Vincent J. Scully, Jr, *Frank Lloyd Wright*, New York 1960, Ravensburg 1961.

HENRY-RUSSELL HITCHCOCK

Wurster, William Wilson, b. Stockton, Calif. 1895. Studied at the University of California. Independent practice from 1926; since 1945 in partnership with Bernardi and Emmons. Wurster, who was influenced by *Maybeck, is an exponent of the 'Bay Region Style', the Californian variant of modern American architecture. He became known through his town and country houses which are distinguished by their modesty, adaptation to environment and consideration of locally prevailing social, economic and climatic conditions. Wurster, who thinks of *Aalto as a like-minded person, talks of an 'every-day-architecture' which is more concerned with function than form.

Yamasaki, Minoru, b. Seattle 1912. Studied at the Universities of Washington and New York. Worked in the offices of the Empire State Building architects Shreve, Lamb and Harmon; with *Harrison, Fouil-houx and *Abramovitz; and with Raymond Loewy Associates. He achieved inter-national notice together with Hellmuth and Leinweber, his partners at the time, for the airport at St Louis (1953–5) whose recep-tion halls consist of a series of intersecting barrel vaults.

Yamasaki is an admirer of *Mies van der Rohe, although he aims increasingly at a 'richness' which 'would make Mies frown' (Yamasaki). A characteristic feature of his style is the dissolution of the wall into an apparently textile-like fabric, which veils the structural members: umbrella walls made of profilated blocks at the Society of Arts and Crafts and at the American Concrete Institute (1958) at Detroit; metal grilles in the Reynolds Metals Office in Detroit (1959). Axial plans, silhouettes enlivened by turrets or top lighting visible from the exterior, and exuberant layouts

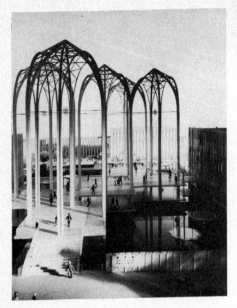

Minoru Yamasaki. Century 21 Exposition.
Seattle, 1962. Model

Yorke, Rosenberg and Mardall. London
(Gatwick) Airport, Stage 1. 1958. Terminal
Building and Central Pier

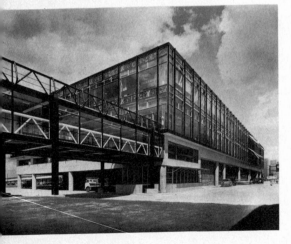

with gardens and pools contribute to the
impression of contrived elegance which is
typical of Yamasaki's later designs. Cano-
pied structures for the American pavilion
at the New Delhi Fair (1960) and the
Century 21 Exposition at Seattle (1962).

Yorke, Francis Reginald Stevens, b. 1906,
d. 1962. Studied at Birmingham University
School of Architecture. Founder member
of MARS (British section of *CIAM) and
pioneer of modern architecture in *Great
Britain, with his reinforced concrete
houses at Gidea Park, Essex (1933, with
W. *Holford, G. Stephenson and A. Adam)
and house at Nast Hyde, Hatfield (1935).
In partnership with Marcel *Breuer, 1935–
37, and from 1944 with Eugene Rosenberg
and Cyril Mardall, in the firm of Yorke,
Rosenberg and Mardall, which has been
responsible for many important projects,
including schools at Stevenage (1947–9),
Oldbury, and Pool Hill, Salop. (1955–7,
with extensive use of timber cladding),
academic buildings in London, Merthyr
Tydfil and Leeds; housing at Stevenage,
Harlow and the Hansa district of Berlin;
hospitals at Londonderry, Crawley and
Hull; a department store at Sheffield, and
Gatwick Airport, Sussex. The firm's own
office in London, a restrained but finely
proportioned and detailed building, was
awarded the RIBA Bronze Medal for 1962.
Yorke was the editor of the annual volume
Specification from 1935 to the time of his
death, and was the author of standard
works on modern houses and (with
Frederick *Gibberd) modern flats.

HAROLD MEEK

Zanuso, Marco, b. Milan 1916; graduated
there 1939. Olivetti factory at São Paulo
(1956–8), a scheme consisting of honey-
comb cells, roofed with thin shell vaults.
Also worked as a journalist.

Zehrfuss, Bernard, b. Angers 1911.
Studied at the École des Beaux-Arts,
Paris. Awarded the Rome prize of the
French Academy in 1939. Unesco build-
ing, Paris (1953–7, in collaboration with
*Breuer and *Nervi). Exhibition building
of the Centre National des Industries et
Techniques, Paris (1958, in collaboration
with Camelot and De Mailly). Industrial
buildings (Renault Works at Flins, 1953;
Mame Printing Works at Tours).

Selected bibliography on the history of modern architecture

See also the bibliographies at the end of individual articles

Banham, Reyner, *Theory and Design in the First Machine Age*, London 1959.

Banham, Reyner, *Guide to Modern Architecture*, London 1962.

Behrendt, Walter Curt, *Modern Building. Its nature, problems and forms*, New York 1937.

Benevolo, Leonardo, *Storia dell'architettura moderna*, 2 volumes, Bari 1960.

Blake, Peter, *The Master Builders*, New York 1961.

Conrads, Ulrich and Hans G. Sperlich, *Phantastische Architektur*, Stuttgart 1960.

Darmstaedter, Robert, *Künstlerlexikon. Maler-Bildhauer-Architekten*, Berne and Munich 1961.

Dorgelo, A., *Modern European Architecture*, Amsterdam 1959.

Enciclopedia Universale dell'Arte. Encyclopaedia of World Art. Venice, Rome, New York, Toronto, London 1959 ff.

Francastel, Pierre (editor), *Les Architectes Célèbres*, 2 volumes, Paris 1959.

Giedion, S., *A Decade of New Architecture —Dix Ans d'Architecture Contemporaine*, Zurich 1954, 1st edition 1951.

Giedion, S., *Space, Time and Architecture*, Cambridge, Mass. 1956, 1st edition 1941.

Gropius, Walter, *Internationale Architektur*, Munich 1925.

Handbuch moderner Architektur, Berlin 1957.

Hilberseimer, Ludwig, *Internationale Neue Baukunst*, Stuttgart 1926.

Hilberseimer, Ludwig, *Grosstadt-Architektur*, Stuttgart 1927.

Hitchcock, Henry-Russell, *Modern Architecture, Romanticism and Reintegration*, New York 1929.

Hitchcock, Henry-Russell, *Architecture: Nineteenth and Twentieth Centuries*, Harmondsworth 1958.

Hitchcock, Henry-Russell and Philip Johnson, *The International Style. Architecture Since 1922*, New York 1932.

Joedicke, Jürgen, *A History of Modern Architecture*, London 1959.

Jones, Cranston, *Architecture Today and Tomorrow*, New York 1961.

Kultermann, Udo, *Baukunst der Gegenwart*, Tübingen 1958.

Pevsner, Nikolaus, *Pioneers of Modern Design. From William Morris to Walter Gropius*, London 1936.

Platz, Gustaf Adolf, *Die Baukunst der neuesten Zeit*, Berlin 1927.

Richards, J. M., *An Introduction to Modern Architecture*, London, Baltimore 1953.

Roth, Alfred, *La Nouvelle Architecture— Die neue Architektur—The New Architecture*, 4th edition, Zurich 1948.

Sartoris, Alberto, *Gli elementi dell'architettura funzionale*, 3rd edition, Milan 1941.

Sartoris, Alberto, *Encyclopédie de l'architecture nouvelle*, 3 volumes, Milan 1954–57.

Sartoris, Alberto, *Introduzione alla architettura moderna*, 3rd edition, Milan 1948.

Scully, Vincent, *Modern Architecture*, New York 1961.

Siegel, Curt, *Strukturformen der modernen Architektur*, Munich 1960.

Smith, G. E. Kidder, *The New Architecture of Europe*, London 1961.

Taut, Bruno, *Die neue Baukunst in Europa und Amerika*, Stuttgart 1929.

Thieme, Ulrich and Felix Becker (editors), *Allgemeines Lexikon der Bildenden Künstler von der Antike bis zur Gegenwart*, 37 volumes, Leipzig 1907–50.

Wasmuths Lexikon der Baukunst, 5 volumes, Berlin 1929–37.

Whittick, Arnold, *European Architecture in the Twentieth Century*, First Vol.: *1800–1924*. Second Vol.: *1924–1933*, London 1950–53.

Zevi, Bruno, *Architecture as Space*, New York 1957.

Zevi, Bruno, *Storia dell'architettura moderna*, 3rd edition, Turin 1955.

Photograph sources

The publishers are indebted to all individuals and institutions listed below who have kindly supplied photographs for publication in this book and especially to the Rijksvoorlichtingsdienst, The Hague; the Suomen Rakennustaiteen Museo, Helsinki; and to Mr Edgar Kaufmann jr., New York.

A.C.L., Brussels; Agtmaal, van, Hilversum; Aistrup, Wedboek; Annan, Glasgow; Apollo, Helsinki; Architectural Photographing Company, Chicago; Architectural Review, London; Beider, Basel; Bentham-Moxon Trustees, London; Beratungsstelle für Stahlverwendung, Düsseldorf; Bildarchiv Foto, Marburg; Bladh, Bromma; Borremans, Cachan; British Features, Bonn; Bulloz, Paris; Casali, Milan; Cellard, Bron; Cetto, Mexico City; Checkman, Jersey City; Chevojon, Paris; Deutsche Presse-Agentur, Frankfurt; Diederichs, Berlin-Lankwitz; Dino, Milan; Doeser, Laren; Dotreville, Brussels; Dumont, Royan; Dupain, Sydney; Dyckerhoff und Widmann, Munich; Faigle, Stuttgart; Farbwerke, Hoechst; Finsler, Zurich; Fortunati, Milan; Fotogramma, Milan; Friedrich, Berlin-Lichterfelde; Futagawa, Tokyo; García Moya, Madrid; Gasparini, Caracas; Gautherot, Rio de Janeiro; Georges, New York; Gerlach, Vienna; Giraudon, Paris; Gmelin, Dornach; Grünert, Zurich; Guerrero, New York; Hanley; Havas, Helsinki; Hedrich-Blessing, Chicago; Heidersberger, Braunschweig; Held, Weimar; Helmer-Petersen, Copenhagen; Hervé, Paris; Høm, Copenhagen; Hubmann, Vienna; Ingervo, Helsinki; Jacobs, Berlin-Lichterfelde; Joedicke, Stuttgart; Jonals, Copenhagen; Josuweck, Cologne; Kersting, London; Kidder Smith, New York; KLM Aerocarto, Amsterdam; Köster, Berlin-Lichterfelde; Korab, Birmingham, Alabama; Kunstgewerbemuseum, Zurich; Laboratorio Fotografico, Rome; Landesbildstelle, Hamburg; Larson, Stockholm; Lazi, Stuttgart; Lens Craft, New York; Library of Congress, Washington; Luckhaus, New York; Madenskey,

Vienna; Mäkinen, Helsinki; Maltby, London; Manchete, Rio de Janeiro; Mango, Neapel; Maré, London; Mari, Rome; Martin, Paris; MAS, Barcelona; Michel, Rio de Janeiro; Møller, Århus; Moisio, Turin; Molitor, Ossining; Moosbrugger, Basel; Moncalvo, Turin; Moscardi, São Paulo; M.R.L., Strassburg; Müller, Alfred, Rio de Janeiro; Murasawa, Tokyo; Museum of Modern Art, New York; National Buildings Record, London; New York Daily News; Nilsson, Stockholm; Ojen, van, The Hague; Österr. Nationalbibliothek, Vienna; Pfau, Mannheim; Pietinen, Helsinki; Pfriem, Paris; Publicam, Hilversum; Reens, New York; Renes, Amsterdam; Roos, Helsinki; Roubier, Paris; Ryan, Minneapolis; Schiller, Mill Valley; Schwab, Stuttgart; Science Museum, London; Shokokusha, Tokyo; Shulman, Los Angeles; Sibbelee, Amsterdam; Smith, Wilton; Sörvik, Göteborg; Souza, Rio de Janeiro; Spaziani, Rome; Spreng, Basel; Steiger, Stuttgart; Steuer, Chicago; Stillman, Litchfield, Connecticut; Stoedtner, Düsseldorf; Stoller, Rye; Strüwing, Copenhagen; Sturtevant, San Francisco; Sundahl, Stockholm; Syndicat d'Initiative, Évian; Szarkowski, Ashland, Wisc.; Urbschat-Fischer, Berlin-Charlottenburg; USIS, Bad Godesberg; Vasari, Rome; Velin, Helsinki; Versnel, Amsterdam; Victoria and Albert Museum, London; Villani, Bologne; Viollet, Paris; Volkart, Stuttgart; Vriend, Amsterdam; Vrijhof, Rotterdam; Wåhlén, Stockholm; Wahlström, Helsinki; Wasastjerna, Helsinki; Whittick, Crawley; Wickberg, Helsinki; Winkler, Stuttgart; Wölfl, Vienna; Wrubel, Düsseldorf; Zerkowitz, Barcelona; Zumstein, Berne.

Index of names

Architects whose names appear in italic have individual entries. Figures in roman type indicate text references; those in bold type refer to the illustrations.

Aalto, Aino 64
Aalto, Alvar 19–20, 28–32, 64, 100–1, 103, 147, 240, 307, 309, 311, 325, **18, 28–31, 103, 154, 220, 308**
Abel 126
Aberdeen 32
Abildgård 160
Abramovitz 32, 81, 147, 310, 325, **81**
Adam, A. 326
Adam, H. G. 108
Adler 32, 69, 128, 275–6
Åhrén 283
Aillaud 107
Albers 46
Albert, Edouard 107
Albini 32–3, 155, 158, **33**
Albuquerque 54
Alexander 215
Allison, J. T. 88
Almqvist 33, 282–3
Alvarez 188
Amis 151
Andersson, E. 311
Andersson, H. 311
Angeli 208
Antonelli 33
Apel 127
Arbeitsgruppe 4, 42, **42**
Arcon 98
Arnodin 105
Aronco, d' 34, 155, 262, **156**
Arp 87, 316
Arsène-Henry 108
Artaria 286, **286**
Artigas 55, 188
Arup 312
Ashbee 12, 36–7, **37**
Ashihara 164
Aslin 38, 73, 136, **136**
Asplund 17, 21, 33, 38–40, 133, 160, 282–5, 311, **38, 39, 281**
Astengo 158
Atelier 5, 287
Attolini Lack 188

Aubert **20**
Auböck 42, 232

Backström 285, **283–4**
Bacon 304, **305**
Badovici 105–6
Baines 98
Bakema 42–3, 60, 73, 212–13, **42, 61, 212, 297**
Balat 149
Baldessari 43, 156, 158
Balla 114
Baltard 130
Banfi 47, 158
Bardi 156
Barillet 133
Barnes 58
Baroni 257
Barragán 188
Bartning 43, 97, 126, 133, 244, **271**
Bartoli 208
Baruel 31
Basile 34, 43, 155, 262
Bassi 158
Baudot, de 43, 208, 234, **235**
Bauersfeld 257, **256**
Baumgart 216
Baumgarten 126
Baur, Hermann 287, **286**
Baur, H. P. 287
Bauschinger 234
Bayer 46, 87
BBPR 47, 158, 240, 244, **25, 159**
Beaudouin 47, 106–7, 177, 231, 240, **106, 108**
Bega 132, 240
Behrens 14, 20, 34, 36, 47–8, 50, 79, 85–6, 93, 97, 123–4, 132–3, 139, 145, 152, 170, 189–91, 202, 238, 244, 271, **48–50**
Bélanger 267
Belgioioso 47, 158
Belluschi 50, 80, **81**
Belmont **232**

Benacerraf 316
Bentsen 82
Berg 50, 93, 123, 236, **124, 237**
Berghoef 212
Bergsten 33, 280, 282, **280**
Berlage 14, 33, 50–1, 104, 130, 169, 191, 209–10, 222, 242, 271, 280, 319, **51, 209**
Bernardes 55
Bernardez 316
Bernardi 325
Bernasconi 80, 158, 219, **80, 157**
Bernoulli 285
Beuté 107, 177
Beyaert 145
Bieber 40
Bijvoet 88, 210
Bill 51, 286–7, **287**
Bindesbøll 82–3, **82**
Bing 313
Black **99**
Blomstedt, Aulis 103, **104**
Blomstedt, P. E. 100
Bo 84, **84**
Boberg 279–80
Boccioni 114
Bodiansky 67, 107, **108**
Bogardus 51, 132, 268, **267**
Böhm 51–2, 126
Boileau 130, 268, **268**
Bolonha 55
Bon 68, 137
Bonatz 52, 93, 248, **96**
Bordenave 235
Borromini 166
Bottoni 158
Boullée 9
Boulton 266, **266**
Bourdon 267
Bourgeois 52, 71, 315
Bradshaw 258
Bragaglia 115
Bramante 204
Branco 316
Bratke 55

Bräuning 287
Brechbühler 287
Brenner 40
Brett 299
Breuer 46, 57–60, 76, 87–8, 125, 133, 135, 142, 164–5, 205, 208, 212, 219, 240, 255, 258, 306, 326, **57–9**, **77**
Brinkman 60, 133, 317, **211**
Broek, van den 43, 60, 212–13, **42, 61, 212, 297**
Brown 98
Brugger 286
Brunel 130, 267
Brunet 267
Bryggman 28, 64–6, 100–1, **65**
Bunshaft 66, 168, 261, 320
Burckhardt 286
Burle Marx 56
Burnham 6, 66, 69–70, 79, 132, 177, 245, 270, 278, 301, **68–9**
Burton 129, **129**
Bürck 48

Caccia Dominioni 158
Calder 315
Calini 157, **157**
Camelot 109, 231, 326
Camenzind 286
Camus 32
Cancellotti 157
Candela, Antonio 66
Candela, Félix 66–7, 188, 240, 258, **66–7**
Candilis 67, 73, 107, **108**
Capon 34
Cardoso 215
Caretta 288, **288**
Carloni 286
Carminati 292
Casson 67, 98, 134
Castañedo 188
Castellazzi **157**
Castiglioni 67, 158
Castrén 241
Castro Mello 55
Celis 316, **317**
Celsing 285
Cessart, de 267
Cetto 188
Cézanne 30, 35, 74
Chamberlin 68, 137
Chance 223

Chareau 106
Chemineau 107
Chermayeff 185
Chiattone 68, 114, 116, 250, **114**
Chitty 291
Choisy 105, 165
Christiansen 48
Cocchia 158
Cocke 34
Coignet 234, 235
Colbert 89
Conder 67, 134
Connell 135
Contamin 7, 35, 79, 130, 234–5, **235, 269**
Cook 258
Cooke-Yarborough 34
Correia Lima 54, **52**
Costa 20, 54–6, 77–8, 172, 215–16, 219, 232, 238, **53, 78**
Coulon 108
Coyne 107
Crabtree 136, 138, **136**
Cragg 266
Craig 314
Crane 37
Cret 167
Cuijpers 78, 208, **208**

Damaschke 295
Daniel 138
Dark 98, 138, 204
Dastugue **20**
David 254
Davies 204
Davis 138
Debat-Ponsan 118
Deilmann 82
Deitrick 82, 219, 240, 278, **279**
Delaunay 91
Denis 315
Depero 114–15
Dichinger 66, 257–8
Dickens 36
Dillon 267
Diulgheroff 114
Dixon 138
Döcker 86, 125, 244
Dodd 266
Doesburg, van 75, 87–9, 177, 210, 222, 242, 272–3, **88, 272**
Dondel **20**

Dony 67
Drake 111, 291
Drew 88, 98, 111
Drexler 198
Dubuffet 62
Dubuisson 107
Dudok 79, 88, 211, **210**
Dugdale 291
Duiker 88, 133, 210, 238
Duran 312
Durand 9, 202
Duret 286
Dürig 287
Dutert 7, 35, 79, 130, **269**
Duthilleul 108
Düttmann 127

Eames, Charles 89
Eames, Ray 89
Eastlake 301
Easton 134
Eastwick-Field 274
Eberstadt 295
Ebert **144**
Eckmann 92, 313
Ecochard 107
Eesteren, van 43, 71, 73, 75, 87, 89, 210, 242, **272**
Egender 286, 287
Egger 107
Eggerick 315
Ehmcke 85
Eiermann 89–90, 127, **89–90**
Eiffel 6, 35, 90–2, 105, 130, 268, **90–1, 268**
Eijck, van 73, 92, 213, **212**
Einstein 201, 221
Ekelund 101
Ellis 179
Ellwood 92
Emberton 135
Emmons 325
Endell 34, 92, 123, **35, 123**
Enfantin 5
Eriksson 284
Ervi 92, 101
Esquillan 258
Estellita 218
Estrella 54
Eyck, van 312

Faber 311
Fadigati **157**
Fahrenkamp 96
Fairbairn 234, 266
Farmer 98, 138, 204

Feininger 15, 45, **15**
Fellerer 42
Ferreira 54
Fietz 287
Figini 99, 104, 145, 157–8, 226, 291, **159**
Fillía 114–15
Finsterwalder 66
Fiocchi 80, 104, 158, 219, **80, 157**
Fischer, Florian 286
Fischer, Theodor 51–2, 85, 93, 104, 146, 183, 221, 290
Fischli 286
Fisker 82, 104, 282, 312, **83**
Fletcher 288
Fontaine 129
Fontseré 119
Förster 10, **10**
Fouilhoux 147, 325
Fox and Henderson 223
Frank 40, 86, 253
Frette 145, 291
Freyler 42
Freyre 52
Freyssinet 107, 109–11, 206, 225, 236, 257, 294, 312, **110**
Friedhoff 211
Fritsch 295
Frosterus 28, 100
Fry 88, 98, 111, 135, 142
Fuller 64, 111–12, 229, 264, 272, 318, **111–12, 229, 264**
Furness 113–14, 275, 301, 310, **302**

Gabo 74, 76
Gabriel 225
Galia 154, 316
Gallé 34
Gallén-Kallela 99
Garcia Roza 55
Gardella 20, 116–17, 133, 158, **116**
Garden 70, 237
Garnier 7, 105, 117–19, 170–1, 202, 235, **9, 117–18, 236, 299**
Gärtner 8
Gaudí 14–15, 35, 67, 119–23, 151, 262, **13, 36, 119–21**
Gauguin 35, 312
Gellner 158
George 295
Gerson, Hans 96–7
Gerson, Oskar 96–7
Gesellius 99, 248

Gibberd 128, 138, 299, 326, **128**
Gibson 73, 128, **99, 128**
Giedion 61, 70–3, 203
Gieselmann 127
Gilbert 304
Gill 128
Gillet 107, 231, **108**
Gilly 9, 122, 254, **9**
Ginsberg 107
Godwin 12
Goeritz 188
Goff 134
Gollins 134, 138
Gomis 107
Goodden 98
Goodhue 304–5
Goodwin 274
Gores 58
Gottwald 40, 42
Gowan 274
Granpré Molière 211
Gravereaux 80, 107
Greene, Charles Sumner 139, 302–3, **304**
Greene, Henry Mather 139, 302–3, **304**
Greenham 188
Grice 34
Groenewegan 210
Gropius, Martin 139
Gropius, Walter 14, 16–17, 20–2, 24, 35, 43–6, 50, 57–8, 73, 79–80, 86–7, 95–6, 111, 116, 124–6, 132, 134–5, 139–46, 148, 152, 155, 162, 164, 189–90, 194–5, 205, 212, 219, 229, 237–8, 244–5, 258, 274, 282, 288, 306–7, 309, 317–19, **15, 45–6, 80, 139–41, 144, 152, 229**
Gruen 145
Guadet 202, 225
Guevrekian 106
Guimard 12, 34, 105, 123, 145, **35, 105**
Guinand 316
Gunnløgsson 84
Gutbrod 126
Gutmann 73

Hack 82
Haefeli 286–8, **286, 288**
Haertl 40
Haesler 125, 244
Hahr 282
Haller von Hallerstein 9

Hankar 34, 145–6, **145**
Hansen 83
Harding 291
Häring 97, 124, 146–7, 244, 319, **146**
Harkness 288
Hartley 266
Harmon 306, 325
Harris 306
Harrison 32, 80–1, 132, 147, 310, 325, **81**
Hausen, von 82
Haussmann 10, 147, **295**
Havlicek 147
Hawksmoor 61
Helg 33
Hellmuth 258, 325, **259**
Henderson, W. A., 136
Hennebique 234–6, **235**
Henrion 98
Hentrich 80, 126, **126**
Hepworth 122
Herbé 107, 231
Herholdt 82
Hermant 108
Hilberseimer 86, 125, 147, 244, 253
Hitchcock 17, 165
Hittorff 8
Hoch 42
Hoff 83, **83**
Hoff, van't 210, 242, 272, **273**
Hoffmann, Josef 34, 40, 85–6, 147–9, 155, 170, 178, 248, 319, **148**
Hoffmann, Ludwig 93, 146
Hofmann 286
Höger 96–7, **95**
Holabird 69–70, 149, 214, 270
Holford 149, 326
Holzbauer 42
Holzmeister 41, 149
Honegger 107, 177, 288
Honeyman 179
Hood 147, 149, 305, **305**
Horeau 5
Horiguchi 162–3
Horta 12, 34, 79, 104, 123, 132, 145, 149–51, 270, 312, **36, 129, 149–51, 270**
Hottinger 287
Howard 100, 151, 295
Howe 151, 167, 177, 271, 304–5, **306**
Howell 73, 151
Howells 305
Hruban 258

Hubacher 286, **286**
Huber 48
Hubsch 122
Hunt 69, 301
Huszar 272
Hutchinson 179
Huttunen 100
Huysmans 315
Hyatt 234

Imai 162
Irming 311
Ishimoto 162
Israel 179
Israels 47
Ito 162
Itten 44–6

Jacobsen 83–4, 154, 159–61, **160–1**
Jäntti **102**
Järvi **101**
Jeanneret, C. E. *Le Corbusier
Jeanneret, P. 106, 170, 256
Jefferson 167
Jenney 6, 69, 79, 132, 149, 164, 177, 270, **6**
Johansen 58, 164, 204
Johnson 17, 58, 165–8, 195, 205, 245, 308–10, **165–7, 204**
Johnson-Marshall 183
Josephson 280
Josic 67
Jourdain 79, 105
Jung **99**

Kahn, Albert 167, 304, 308
Kahn, Louis 62, 147, 167–9, 205, 309–10, **168–9, 205**
Kampmann 82
Kandinsky 45, 97
Karsten 210
Kaspé 188
Kaufmann 9
Kazis 108
Keppie 179
Ketterer 42
Khnopff 34
Kikutake 164, **164**
Killick 151
Kirchner 95, 97, 314
Kishida 163
Klaarhamer 242
Klaudy 42
Klee 45

Klenze 8
Klerke, de 33, 169, 209–10, **14, 96, 210**
Klimt 34, 147, 178, 180
Klint, Jensen 82, 169, **83**
Klint, Kåre 82
Kneese de Mello 218, **55, 216**
Koch 180
Koechlin 91
Koike 163
Kok 272
Kokko 240
Kokoschka 95
Kolbe 194
Korsmo 311
Kosaka 162, **162**
Kraemer 126, 169, **127**
Krahn 126
Kramer 33, 209
Kreis 96
Kröller 191
Kromhout 34
Küpper *Doesburg, van
Kurrent 42

Labrouste 6, 43, 105, 133, 169, 242, 268, **105**
Lafaille 107, 257
Lagneau 107
Lamb 306, 325
Lambot 234
Larco 145, 291
Larsson 279
Lasdun 111, 137, 291, **138**
Lassen, Flemming 160
Lassen, Mogens 83
Latis 158
Laugier 205
Laurence 133
Lauritzen 83, **83**
Leão 54
Leck, van der 272
Le Corbusier 9, 11, 15–20, 22, 24, 26, 47, 50, 54, 58, 61, 67, 70–1, 73, 75–80, 83, 86–8, 104–7, 111–13, 119, 126, 130, 132–3, 137, 139, 146–8, 150, 152, 155, 160, 162–3, 168–76, 181, 183, 187, 190, 200–3, 206–7, 215, 217, 225, 236–8, 240, 246, 256, 258, 271, 282–4, 286, 288, 309, **16, 19, 27, 53, 62, 106, 132, 152, 169–76, 201, 203, 238, 300**
Le Couteur 107
Ledoux 9, 166–7

Leemann 288
Léger 133, 316
Legorreta 187
Lehmbrock 126
Leibl 47
Leinweber 258, 325, **259**
Lemmen 34
Lemos 218
Leonhardt 127
Leonidow 17
Lepère 8
Le Play 7
Lequeu 9
Le Ricolais 92, 264, 279, 318
Lescaze 151, 167, 177, 271, 305, **306**
Lethaby 37
Leuzinger 182
Levi 54, **52**
Lewerentz 33, 38, 177, 282, 284–5, **284**
Libera 145, 291
Lichtblau 40
Lindegren 30, 100, 103, **102**
Lindgren 99, 248
Lindquist 99
Lindström 285
Lingeri 156, 158, 292
Lipps 313
Lipschitz 165
Lissitzky 17, 74–6, 177, **76**
Llorens y Barba 119
Lodoli 63
Lods 47, 106–7, 177, 231, 240, **106**
Loewy 325
Loghem, van 210
Loos 14, 40, 42, 105, 118, 128, 147–8, 150, 152, 155, 177–8, 180, 202, 213, 250, 305, 319–20, **14, 40, 177–8**
Lopez 80, 107, 231
Lorenz 42
Lotufo 218, **55, 216**
Louis 267
Lozeron 288
Lubetkin 291
Luccichenti 157
Luckhardt, Hans 96, 124, 178, 244
Luckhardt, Wassili 96, 124, 178, 244
Lund 83
Lundsten 241
Lundy 179
Lurçat 106, 148, 179, **107**
Lutyens 37, 264

Lynn 62, **62**
Lyons, Edward D. L. 179
Lyons, Eric Alfred 179

Maaskant 43
Macdonald, Frances 180
Macdonald, Margaret 180
Machado Moreira 54, 55, **53, 54**
Mächler 124, 252
Mackintosh 12, 14, 35–7, 48, 123, 179–81, 248, **180–1**
Mackmurdo 34
Maekawa 163–4, 181, 288, **163**
Magistretti 158
Magnant 107
Maillart 181–3, 206, 225, 236, 240, 258, 285, **182**
Mailly, de 109, 231, 258, 326
Makkinheimo 31
Makowski 264
Malevich 17, 74, 183, 278, **76**
Mallet-Stevens 106, 183
Mandrot, de 70
Mangiarotti 158
Marc 97
Marchi 114–15
Marcks 45–6
˜Marcos 188
Mardall 326, **326**
Marinetti 114, 116, 202, 251
Marinho 54–5
Markelius 183, **282, 298**
Marot 108
Marsio *Aalto, Aino 28
Martin 70, 237
Martinez de Velasco **188**
Matisse 133
Matthew 137, 183, **137**
Maus 34
May 71, 125, 183, 244
Maybeck 183, 226, 302–3, 325
Mayer 219
McKim 303, 308, 310, 321
McMillan 288
McMillen 288
McNair 179
Mead 303, 308, 310, 321
Meier-Graefe 313–14
Meigs 151, 304
Mellor 151, 304
Melvin 134, 138
Mendelsohn 15, 17–19, 48, 95, 97, 124–5, 133, 135, 140, 183–6, 214, 220–1, 237, 244, 271, 306, **97, 184–6, 220**

Merkelback 210
Merrill (SOM) 23, **23**
Mesquita dos Santos 54
Messel 93, 186
Meuli 288
Mey, van der 33, 209
Meyer, Adolf 80, 86, 139–41, 152, 189, **15, 140, 152**
Meyer, Hannes 46, 71, 125, 189, 286, **189**
Michelangelo 220
Michelucci 158, 189
Mies van der Rohe 15–17, 20–4, 46, 50, 61–2, 78, 80, 84, 86–7, 89, 92, 95, 107, 122, 124–6, 132–3, 139, 146, 152, 155, 160, 162, 165–8, 177, 189–99, 202, 204–5, 212, 214, 224–5, 231, 237, 240, 244–6, 250, 252, 255, 261, 271, 282, 306, 308–9, 319, 325, **21–2, 95, 125, 130, 133, 153, 190–9, 203–4, 272, 309**
Mijares, José, 316, **317**
Mijares, Rafael **187**
Milà y Fontanals 119
Miljutin 252
Mills, Edward David 98, 200
Mills, Mark 262, **263**
Mindlin 55, **55**
Mirabaud 107, 231
Mizutani 163
Moberley 136, **136**
Moholy-Nagy 45–7, 87
Moll 252
Møller, C. F. 82, 84, 104, **83**
Møller, Erik 84, 160
Mollino 158
Moltke, von 58
Monaco 157
Mondrian 75, 206, 243, 272–3
Monier 234
Montuori 157, **157**
Moore 122
Mora, de la 187, **67**
Moral, del 187–8, **187**
Morancé 105
Morandi 158
Moretti 157
Morgenthaler 287
Morisseau 258
Morris 11, 34–7, 84–5, 202, 280, 301, 312, 320
Moser, Karl 177, 202, 238, 285, **285**
Moser, Koloman 147

Moser, Werner 286–8, **286, 288**
Moya 137, 228
Muche 45, **44**
Munch 35
Murata 164
Muthesius 37, 48, 84–7, 123, 202, 211
Muzio 157

Nairn 274
Nash 8, 202, 267, **8**
Nelson 202
Nervi 20, 58, 77, 111, 155, 158–9, 181, 206–9, 225, 227, 240, 258, 272, 326, **158, 206–8, 229, 239, 258**
Neutra 17, 40, 133, 148, 213–15, 271, 305, 307, **213–14**
Newman 73, 315
Nicholson 67
Nielsen 84
Niemeyer 20, 54–6, 77–8, 128, 172, 215–19, 238, 255, **53, 55–6, 216–18**
Nilsson 280
Nizzoli 80, 104, 158, 219, **80, 157**
Nolde 97
Nouguier 91
Novarina 133, **231**
Nowicki 82, 219, 240, 278, **279**
Noyes 219
Nunes 54
Nyrop 82
Nyström 99

Obrist 11, 92
Oddie 61
Oesterlen 126
O'Gorman 63, 187–9, 219, **188**
Olbrich 34–5, 40, 48, 92, 147, 178, 219–20, 319, **12, 219**
Oliveri 104, 219
Olivio D' 158
O'Rorke 98
Östberg 282
Osthaus 314
Otaka 164
Otto 127, 221, 279
Oud 18–19, 86–7, 133, 152, 155, 210–12, 221–2, 272–3, **14, 221–2, 273**
Overbeck 119
Owings (SOM) 23, **23**
Ozenfant 105, 170

Pagani 158
Pagano 156–7, 227, 292
Paillard 288
Paine 267
Palanti 55
Palladio 61
Pani 188
Pankok 92
Pannaggi 114
Partridge 151
Pasmore 138
Paul 190
Paxton 5–6, 79, 111, 129, 207,
    223–4, 267, **5, 223, 228**
Pei 224
Peressutti 47, 158
Perkins 70
Perrault 234
Perret 79, 83, 104–6, 118, 133,
    152, 170, 202, 224–5, 235,
    238, 240, 312, **224–5, 237**
Perriand 108
Perrin-Fayolle 231
Persico 156–7, 227
Petäjä 241, **241**
Petersen 82
Petschnigg 40, 80, 126, **126**
Pevsner, Antoine 74, 91
Pevsner, Nikolaus 203
Pfeffer 42
Phidias 202
Piacentini 156–7, 203, 258
Piccinato 157
Pickett 6
Pingusson 106
Pintonello **157**
Piot 67, **108**
Piscator 141
Pison 106
Poelzig 48, 85–7, 93, 97, 124,
    226, 244, 255, 271, 317, 319,
    93, 226, 270
Polk 79, 132, 226
Pollini 99, 104, 145, 157–8,
    226, 291, **159**
Pollock 62
Ponti 156, 158, 208, 226–7,
    240, **226–7**
Pope 304
Popp 133
Portinari 56
Powell, Geoffrey 68, 137
Powell, Philip P. 137, 228
Powers, M. A. R. 34
Prampolini 114–15
Price 321
Prieto 188

Prouvé, Henri **231**
Prouvé, Jean 106–7, 230–2,
    231–2
Prouvé, Victor 231

Quaroni 157

Rabut 109
Rading 86, 252
Rafn 82
Rainer 41–2, 232, **41**
Ramirez Vázquez 189, **187**
Rasmussen 311
Rava 145, 291
Rave 82
Redig de Campos 55
Redslob 45
Reichow 126
Reidy 54–5, 232–4, 238, **53,**
    55, 233
Reifenberg 98
Reilly 136, **136**
Reinhardt 226, 314
Reinius 285, **283–4**
Repton 267
Revell 101, 240–2, **104, 241–2**
Ribeiro 55
Ricci 63
Richardson 6, 50, 69, 104, 242,
    248, 276, 279, 301–3, 307,
    310, 321, **68**
Rickman 267
Ridolfi 157
Riemerschmid 85, 92, 123, 242
Rietveld 75, 148, 152, 155,
    210, 213, 242–4, 272–4,
    243–4
Riihimäki 240
Rivera 188
Roberto, Marcelo 54
Roberto, Milton 54
Roberts 258
Robertson 134
Robson 258
Roche 69, 70, 149, 214, 270
Rocher 133
Rodgers 304, 308
Rogers 47, 72, 158, 244
Rolland 314
Root 6, 66, 69–70, 79, 132,
    177, 245, 270, 301, **68–9**
Rosen 83, 188
Rosenberg, Eugene 326, **326**
Rosenberg, Léonce 105
Roth, Alfred 286, **57**
Roth, Emil 286–7, **57, 286**
Rouhault 129

Roux-Spitz 106
Rowe 204
Rudolph 26, 58, 245, 308, **309**
Ruf 90
Ruhnau 82
Ruskin 5, 35–7, 301, 321
Russell 98

Saarinen, Eero 26, 155, 167–8,
    225, 245–8, 258, 272, 308–
    10, **24, 154, 245–7, 250**
Saarinen, Eliel 99–100, 245,
    248–50, 305, **249–50**
Saarnio 30
Saavedra **188**
Sakakura 164
Saldanha 55
Salvisberg 286
Samonà 158
Samuel, Godfrey 291
Sánchez 188
Sant' Elia 15–16, 68, 114, 116,
    152, 155, 171, 202, 250–2,
    115, 251
Sarger 258
Sartoris 114–15, 158
Saskelin 64
Sato 163
Saturnino de Brito 54
Saugey 286, 288
Saulnier 79, 268, **79**
Sauvage 106
Scalpelli 157
Scarpa 133, 158, 252
Schader 287
Schaefer 258
Scharoun 86, 89, 96, 124,
    126–7, 147, 244, 252–4,
    319, **94, 125, 253–4**
Schein 107
Scheper 46
Schimka 42
Schindler 17, 40, 214, 254,
    305
Schinkel 7–9, 21, 122, 165,
    191, 193, 202, 225, 254–6,
    123
Schleget 83
Schlemmer 45, **43**
Schmidt, Friedrich 8
Schmidt, Hans 286, **286**
Schmidt, Joost 46
Schmidt, Karl 85
Schmidt, Richard E. 70, 237
Schneck 86
Schneider 96
Schneider-Esleben 132
Scholer 52, 93

Schröder-Schräder 242
Schumacher 93, 97, 125, 295
Schuster 40–1
Schütz 287
Schwanzer 42, **41**
Schwarz 126–7, 255, **127**
Schwippert 255
Séguin 267
Seidler 40, 255, 312, **255**
Sekino 162
Sekler 42
Semper 256, **9**
Senn, Otto 286
Senn, Rainer 108
Serrurier-Bovy 34, 313
Sert 72–3, 205, 256
Seurat 312
Severud 82, 219, 240, **279**
Shaw 12, 84, 134–5, 248, 256, **256**
Sheppard 258, 260
Shreve 306, 325
Silsbee 321
Silvy **232**
Simberg 30
Simon 258
Sipari 241
Siren, Heikki 101, 260, **103, 230**
Siren, J. S. 100
Siren, Kaija 101, 260, **103, 230**
Sirvin 107
Sitte 118
Sive 107, **231**
Sjöstrom 65
Skidmore, Owings and Merrill (SOM) 23, 66, 80, 126, 132, 164, 245, 260–2, 308–10, 320, **23, 81, 260–2, 271**
Skinner, Francis 291
Slater 136, **136**
Sluyterman 34
Smith 62, **62**
Smithson, Alison 61, 64, 73, 137, 204, 262, **63, 205**
Smithson, Peter 61, 63–4, 73, 137, 204, 262, **63, 205**
Soane 8, 9, 12, 166, 205, 262
Sobre 9
Soeiro 54
Soleri 63, 262, **263**
Sommaruga 34, 155, 262
Sonck 99, **99**
Sonrel 108
Soraja y Matyas 252
Sordo Madaleno 188
Soufflot 234

Spalt 42
Spence 98, 133, 138, 264, 266, **265**
Stam 60, 75–6, 86, 177, 210, 286, **76**
Stegmann 82, 104, **83**
Steiger, Peter 288, **287**
Steiger, Rudolf 286–8, **286–8**
Steinbüschel 40
Steiner 14, 96, 237, **97**
Stenhammar 280
Stephenson G. 326
Stephenson, Robert 267
Stillman 274
Stirling 274
Stone 24, 26, 90, 274, 309, **23, 310**
Stonorov 167
Street 202, 320
Strengell 100
Strnad 40
Stubbins 26, 274, **274**
Stucky 288
Studer 288, **288**
Stuijt 221
Stynen 315
Sullivan 6, 32, 69–70, 113–14, 128, 132, 151, 177–8, 220, 248, 270, 275–9, 301, 303, 307, 310, 319–21, **275–8, 302–3**
Summerson 63
Sundahl 283
Syllas, de 34

TAC 23, 144, 288, **143–4**
Takizawa 162
Tange 164, 181, 288–90, **163, 289–90**
Taniguchi 163–4
Tarjanne 99
Tassel 34
Tatlin 74, 76, 177, 290, **75**
Taucher 100, **101**
Taut, Bruno 15–16, 19, 22, 86, 124, 163, 244, 252, 290, **130**
Taut, Max 86, 124, 244, 290
Tavio 30
Tecton 135, 137, 291, **135–6**
Tedesco, de 235
Telford 266–7, 291, **6**
Tengbom 282
Terragni 64, 145, 155–6, 158, 203, 291–2, **291–2**
Tessenow 85, 211, 317
Thiersch 183

Thompson 288
Thomson **8**
Tijen, van 43, 60
Torroja 20, 66, 240, 258, 292–4, **257, 293–4**
Trucco 156, 236, **156**
Tschernykhov 76
Tsuchiura 164
Tubbs 98
Turner 129, **129**
Turnock 133
Tyrwhitt 72

Uchôa 218, **55, 216**
Ungers 127
Unwin 295
Ursault 107
Utzon 84, 311–12, **311**

Vago 107, 312
Välikangas 100–1
Valjus 241
Vanbrugh 61
Van Gogh 35
Vantongerloo 75, 272
Vasarely 316
Vasari 220
Vasconcellos 54, 238, **53**
Vegas 154, 316
Vegter 212
Velde, van de 11, 34–5, 37, 43, 47–8, 85–6, 92–3, 100, 123–4, 145, 220–1, 312–15, 319, **313–14**
Verwilghen 315
Vesnin, Alexander 76, **75**
Vesnin, Vladimir 76, **75**
Viard **20**
Viénot 108
Viganò 63, 158, 315, **24, 63**
Villagrán Garcia 187–8, 219, 315
Villanueva 315–17, **26, 316, 317**
Villar 119–20
Viollet-le-Duc 43, 78, 104, 112, 119, 149, 183, 209, 225, 317, 319, 321, **266**
Vital Brasil 54
Vitellozzi 258, **157–8, 258**
Vitruvius 220
Vlugt, J. A. van der 210
Vlugt, L. C. van der 60, 133, 210, 317, **211**
Voelcker 73,
Voysey 12, 35, 37, 84, 134–5, 151, 202, 248, 317, **11**

Wachsmann 92, 144, 229, 264, 272, 317–19, **263, 318**
Wagner, Martin 125, 252, 319
Wagner, Otto 34, 40, 130, 147, 155, 178, 213, 219, 250, 254, 271, 305, 319–20, **40, 319**
Wahlman 282
Wallot 104, 202
Walton 37
Warchavchik 54, 77, 232, 320
Ward, Basil 135
Ward, Edmund Fisher 134, 138
Ward, Ronald 138–9
Wasmuth 321
Watt 266, **266**
Wayss 234
Webb 84, 134–5, 202, 248, 320, **37**
Weber 127
Weese 320
Weideli 287
Weinbrenner 9

Westman 280
White 303, 308, 310, 321
Wickman 279, 282
Wiebinga 210
Wiener 54
Wilde 35
Williams 134–5, 238, 320, **134**
Wils 87, 210
Wimberley 258
Windbrechtinger 42
Windinge 83, **83**
Wittkower 204
Wittwer 189, **189**
Wogenscky 107
Wohlert 84, **84**
Wolf 34
Wolske 127, **127**
Woods 67, **108**
Wörle 42
Wren 34
Wright 12, 14, 18, 20, 22, 68, 70, 84, 104, 112, 133–4, 146, 152, 163, 168, 176, 214,

220–1, 238, 248–9, 252, 254, 262, 274, 280, 288, 293, 301–7, 309–11, 320–5, **12, 19–20, 131, 220, 307, 321–5**
Wurster 306, 325
Wyatt 130

Yamada 162, 164
Yamasaki 25–6, 258, 309, 325–6, **25, 259, 326**
Yamawaki 163
Yáñez 187
Yeon 306
Yorke 58, 326, **326**
Yoshida 162, 164, **162**
Yoshimura 164

Zanuso 158, 326
Zavanella 158
Zehrfuss 58, 109, 208, 231, 240, 258, 326
Zevi 157, 159, 203
Zweifel 286